Community Health Nursing Practice

Second Edition

RUTH B. FREEMAN, R.N., Ed.D.

Professor Emeritus
The Johns Hopkins University
School of Hygiene and Public Health

JANET HEINRICH, R.N., Dr. P.H.

Consulting Nurse
Division of Nursing, United States Public Health Service
Department of Health and Human Services

1981   W. B. SAUNDERS COMPANY
PHILADELPHIA/LONDON/TORONTO/SYDNEY

W. B. Saunders Company: West Washington Square
                            Philadelphia, Pa. 19105

                            1 St. Anne's Road
                            Eastbourne, East Sussex BN21, 3 UN England

                            1 Goldthorne Avenue
                            Toronto, Ontario M8Z 5T9, Canada

                            9 Waltham Street
                            Artarmon, N.S.W. 2064, Australia

Library of Congress Cataloging in Publication Data

Freeman, Ruth B

Community health nursing practice.

1. Community health nursing.   I. Heinrich, Janet, joint
   author.   II. Title. [DNLM: 1. Community health nursing.
   WY 106 F855c]

RT98.F73 1981   610.73'43'0973   80-52769

ISBN 0-7216-3877-5

The opinions expressed in this book are those of the authors and do not necessarily represent the official policies of the Division of Nursing of the United States Public Health Service.

Listed here are the latest translated editions of this book together with the language of the translation and the publisher.

Spanish (*1st edition*) — Neisa, Mexico City, Mexico

French (*1st edition*) — Lu Ediciones, Holt, Rinehart et
                         Winston, Limitee, Anjou, Montreal,
                         Canada.

Community Health Nursing Practice   ISBN   0-7216-3877-5

Last digit is the print number: 9   8   7   6   5   4   3   2   1

PREFACE

The traditional function of community health nursing is to help others help themselves. To achieve any degree of self-reliance, people need to cultivate their own resources, both human and material, at all stages and phases of development. The purpose of this book is to describe the unique blend of nursing and public health practice aimed at developing and enhancing the health capabilities of people, either singly as individuals or collectively as families, special populations, or communities.

The community health nurse as practitioner, teacher, interpreter, stimulator, listener, and organizer is a significant factor in determining the success or failure of the health effort. The nature of this effort will be constantly challenged and changed by the goals, resources, and constraints of the socioeconomic, ideological, and political situation. The practice of community health nursing will need to remain fluid and flexible if it is to be consistent with community needs, available resources, new scientific knowledge, and the capabilities of the people being served.

As in the previous edition, the intent of this text is not to tell "how to do it!" but rather to assist readers in thinking about the process and some of the strategies for working with others in solving community health problems. These approaches, many proved successful over time, are applied to our current health problems, delivery systems, and special populations. Frequently encountered environments of community health nursing are described as they pertain to providing care to a variety of groups — those in a specific developmental period, in a particular locale, or with a particular kind of health or illness problem.

A systematic approach to assessing the community health status, identifying families and population groups at risk, planning programs and services, and constantly monitoring the relationship between needs and services, between resources and consumer demands, and between goals and results is stressed throughout. Emphasis is placed on the full use of informal resources, the family, and the neighborhood as well as on shared professional action to meet the needs of people.

The revision for this edition has been sweeping, yet there are always concerns of omissions and inadequacies when we review the extraordinary development of community health nursing over the past decade. The text is only a point of departure for further independent study and professional growth. We hope that this is a book students and practitioners can refer to as they encounter problems and search for solutions in the care of families and communities. If we convey the excitement of the challenge inherent in community health nursing, and if we stimulate readers to listen, to question, to see the multiple dimensions of nursing practice, and to assume responsibility for assessing the total environment and for seeking ways to effect change for better health for all people, this book will serve its purpose.

We wish to express our gratitude to all the community health nurses who are "doing it," who try new ideas and discover old ones, who seek the unusual, who are concerned about the development of others, and who have so richly shared their experiences, thoughts, and probing questions with us.

We are particularly grateful to Anna Scholl, who has been our "rock" to touch base with, always encouraging us when we needed it most. Special thanks are due to Velena Boyd, Margaret Kauffman, Mabel Morris, Patricia Deiman, Tom Phillips, and Gretchen Osgood for their belief in nursing and preventive care and their thoughtful reading of parts of the manuscript. Many people in the Division of Nursing, HRA, DHHS, helped in many ways, providing information and support. We would like to thank Charlotte Eliopoulos, Consultant in Gerontological Nursing, State of Maryland Department of Health and Mental Hygiene, and Rosemary Wood, Chief, Nursing Services Branch, Indian Health Service, for sharing with us their special expertise. We also thank Marie Lowe and Amelia Maglacus, who have made many contributions over many years as colleagues and friends and have a sustained interest in the potential of community health nursing.

We are indebted to the staff of W. B. Saunders Company, especially to Robert E. Wright for his sustained encouragement and to Kathy Pitcoff and Ilze Rader for their enduring patience in seeing this revision to completion.

Working together has been an exciting and profitable collaborative effort, for us as individuals as well as for our families. The experiences and talents of one have helped and supported those of the other, confirming our belief in the meshing of problems and resources of a multitude of developmental ages and stages. We would like to thank our families and good neighbors for their indulgence, if not always patience, in seeing us through this effort. Nancy Smith, editor as well as daughter, and Laura Heinrich, friend as well as sister, deserve our special thanks for their thoughtful assistance. But most of all, we are indebted to those amiable tyrants, Anselm Fisher and James C. Cobey, who have judiciously badgered, bolstered, and consoled us in our efforts.

RUTH B. FREEMAN
JANET HEINRICH COBEY

CONTENTS

CHAPTER 1

PERSPECTIVES

Intelligent participation in any human enterprise requires that it be seen from the perspective of its time, setting, and probable future. The pattern of community health nursing will grow from its own historical antecedents, from the broad socioeconomic-ethical trends that affect all human services, from the biological and environmental threats that determine the focus of health efforts, and from the organizational systems through which health resources are applied to human problems.

Today, virtually every country of the world sponsors a group of nursing personnel engaged in some form of work that can be called *community health nursing*. They are distinguished from other nursing groups by the locus of their work (outside the hospital for the most part), by the scope of their concern (the total health spectrum from crisis care to the promotion of wholesome healthiness), and by their commitment to the entire population as distinguished from a designated case load.

However, within this broad definition of community health nursing, there is wide variation in programs, personnel, and organization. Programs may range from massive efforts directed toward control of a specific disease or threat to survive, to large-scale preventive measures geared to comprehensive care for the community as a whole, to work with a limited group of people or a family on a purely local problem. The nursing personnel can range from a largely short-trained or "middle level" staff (such as aides or indigenous midwives), with a sprinkling of professional nurses, to what is essentially a professional service, with a small supporting staff who have lower levels of preparation.

Community health nursing may be organized as a country-wide, government-sponsored operation or as a conglomeration of voluntary and government agencies that function independently. This variation exists because change comes in local as well as global sizes; and the opportunities and constraints imposed by these changes will be interpreted and implemented in very different ways, depending upon the

1

values, the economic-technical-political capability, and the nursing leadership of a particular population at a given time.

A TROUBLED WORLD FACES A PROTRACTED PERIOD OF CRISIS AND MASSIVE CHANGE

There is a strong indication that for some years ahead many, if not most, of the countries of the world will be faced with problems of runaway inflation, recession, shortages of essential goods or foods, and unstable or poorly supported governments. These changes are being brought about by a combination of developments, none of which appear to be short-range in their consequences.

A Galloping Technology Must Be Tamed as Well as Tended

The incredibly rapid progress of technology is expected to continue well into the future, and may even be acclerated. The day is not so far off into the future when we can expect to hear about such possibilities as the following: a computer technology that permits computers to help teach the young, diagnose the sick, or plan family menus; the discovery of a safe, lasting, and fool-proof contraceptive; or the development of new food-producing techniques that will make it possible to feed many more people with available arable land. We envision, almost greedily, the potential benefits to society of such developments. Increasingly, however, it is recognized that exploitation of technologic advances may prove a mixed blessing. While scientific discovery and improved production methods have brought conveniences and a longer life expectancy, it is not clear that the effect on the *quality* of life has indeed been a positive one.

Technologic assistance to other countries has created more consumer goods but, often, has not narrowed the gap between the affluent and the poverty-stricken. Improved transportation and roads have moved people more quickly — and more dangerously. Human labor has been greatly reduced by the use of machines and new management techniques — and unemployment soars. The gross national product goes up, while the drain on nonrenewable natural resources proceeds at what is almost certainly an intolerable rate. Disposable packaging, high obsolescence, and continually shifting work patterns reduce the effort required to produce or use goods, but also increase pollution and create anxieties. As Barry Commoner has said, "There is no such thing as a free lunch."[1] We have to impose some sense of balance between technology for its own sake and technology for true progress.

The "good" health care made possible by medical advances may also prove to have hollow benefits. The ability to prolong the life of a greatly impaired aged person or of a grossly malformed and defective child may absorb limited resources that are badly needed elsewhere, without providing any meaningful life for the recipient of the care. Reduction of infant mortality may produce population levels incompatible with food resources — and, thus, result in disaster rather than human gain. It is frustrating and disappointing when technologic advances in health care outrun the available material or human resources required to put discoveries to work; this problem is increased if, at the same time, improved and highly available communication media are informing the public of great gains, thus stimulating interest and raising expectations. The result of this process can be public dissatisfaction, which in turn may create pressure to allocate scarce resources unwisely to meet the demand for "instant solutions."

The development of national policies and priorities in technologic development, as well as careful planning for the introduction of technologic change, will be a vital problem in the decades to come.

There is increasing concern for the *lagging social technology*. While scientific and production technology has developed rapidly, there has been no corresponding achievement in social technology. For example, in the area of automobile accidents, the techniques for counting, classifying, predicting, and caring for accident victims have advanced dramatically, but no comparable methodology has evolved for altering health-threatening driving habits. The procedure for diagnosis and treatment of disease is described and documented, often by computerized data and analyses. However, professionals still rely largely on intuition to establish understanding and productive decision making between consumers and personnel in a health center. There is little precise and reliable knowledge about the prevention of crime or child and drug abuse. Hospitals provide elaborate and definitive care for acute complex diseases, but neither health nor educational systems can teach people how to *live*. Indeed, modern patterns of education at grade school, high school, and college militate *against* the development of learning habits so necessary for the decisions that must be made over a lifetime in an increasingly complex world.

War is perhaps the most awesome and incongruous of all human efforts. The creation and elaboration of weaponry move inexorably forward at a terrifying pace, but little or nothing is done to develop some rational base on which to build the skills of peace — dialogue, negotiation, and open and mutually supportive relationships. These are the talents that are needed to create a more just and equitable society; they are also the skills that can be put to use in dealing with problems of community development and of intergroup relations within cities and in persuading people to relinquish some immediate convenience for the benefit of the community, the city, or the environment as a whole.

Looking ahead, it seems inevitable that there will be — there *must* be — fundamental changes in the areas of education, international relations, and human services.

Rapidly Expanding Populations and Industrialization Strain the World Supply of Natural Resources and Set Limits to Growth

The Club of Rome is an informal multi-interest, multinational group of scientists, educators, humanists, industrialists, and civil servants who are deeply concerned with "the predicament of mankind." A 1972 report generated by this association warns that the world's nonrenewable natural resources (oil, arable land, air, water, and essential minerals) are being depleted rapidly. They estimate that if present trends in population growth and industrialization continue, the limits of growth on this planet will be reached within the next hundred years.[2] While there is much disagreement about the immediacy and the exact extent of the danger, there is little argument that a crucial problem does exist requiring immediate action.

This realization has had some important repercussions. Resource-rich developing countries are in a much better bargaining position than in the past; and, for some, this has meant moving from relative poverty to noticeable affluence in a very short time. Conversely, high consumer countries are encountering the reality of finite supplies and escalating demands for resources; they face the probability of a considerable reduction in their standard of living as measured by the acquisition of material goods. The United States is a high consumer of many raw materials, especially oil, and is dependent upon other countries for resources. Most economists believe that this consumption of material goods must be cut down substantially. This is regarded by some as the end of the great "joy ride" of the sixties, and a healthy return to simpler ways of life. By others, it is seen as a giant step backward.

New Problems Create a Global Imperative

Many of the pressing issues facing civilization today will require remedies that are globally oriented and massive in scale. World hunger is an example, with food production and poverty in every country impacting on the problem. International economies and energy resources are issues for all of mankind and can only be dealt with by countries acting in concert.

The development of new resources involving the use of the sea bed or outer space cannot be the prerogative of a single country. There is a growing belief that such resources should be considered as "the common heritage of mankind" rather than as a property to be parceled out to individual nations.[3] The exploration of new sources of energy will often require a multinational effort. In addition, there are moral and humanistic considerations with these problems. A country that is poor in resources must be protected from sudden or drastic withholding of essential food or energy supplies for political purposes. Nations with high levels of industrialization and abundant resources must learn to share with countries less well endowed, even if this entails some sacrifice.

This global imperative is not solely the problem of international diplomats or planning groups; its effects can be felt in very specific ways in the daily life of the average man. For example, if large quantities of grain are exported to combat starvation in another country, citizens at home may have to make do with less or be willing to pay more for what they buy. As world oil resources drop and more international sharing is required, two-car families may become one-car families or may use bikes. People accustomed to affluence may have to accept restriction in their right to acquire certain goods, which they can afford, that cannot be spared if the more urgent needs of others are considered, or that would contribute to pollution or inflation.

HUMAN RIGHTS AND HUMAN NEEDS ARE BASIC CONCERNS

There is no movement more significant for the future of health services than the current worldwide appraisal of the dimensions of human rights. This movement is revolutionary in force and pervasive in scope. The rights of poor countries in the family of nations, of specially disadvantaged groups within the population, of those suffering deprivation from causes beyond their control, of every individual for human dignity and self-determination — all of these are factors in establishing goals and programs. More recently, these concerns have broadened to include the rights of women to equal treatment; the rights of children, born and unborn; the rights of the physically and mentally handicapped; the rights of political dissidents, welfare recipients, and prison inmates. This surge of interest has occasioned new programs to correct inequities and avoid or repair the damage of dehumanizing policies of the past.

Advanced communication technology has given these problems greater visibility. Television has brought into the American living room the meaning of war, starvation, brutality, and joblessness as well as the agonizing decisions regarding abortion or commitment to mental institutions. Willingly or not, a large proportion of the population becomes at least tangentially involved.

Traditional Goals and Values Are Being Challenged

Young people are weighing the relative virtues of patriotism and personal responsibility to act in opposition to the horrors of war; religious leaders and novices are seeking a more meaningful relationship between the world of the spirit and doctrine and that of personal conscience and social action; medical personnel as well as families are confronting the moral issue of the right to die as well as the right to live and questioning whether limitation of family size is a matter of personal choice or of social policy.

Belief in the *work ethic* (a conviction that work is intrinsically good) has long been ingrained in the collective thinking of many countries, including the United States; however, this concept is being seriously challenged. The concern of many workers for early retirement and freedom from overtime, a refusal to accept "demeaning" work, and the high rates of absenteeism attest to a lowering of esteem for work. Indeed, the work ethic has been supplanted in many areas by the "welfare ethic" — a conviction that steady work is to be avoided.[4] Welfare is a necessary support for honest workers caught between jobs or stranded in periods of unemployment; when it develops into a way of life, however, it becomes a character-destroying force.

Another element affecting the old "work ethic" is the fact that free time may constitute the greater part of the individual's schedule. Futurists believe that continuing technologic advances will further reduce the human energy required to perform a job, and, even with population stabilization, a considerably smaller proportion of time will be needed for productive work. Already some employers are studying the implications of a three-day work week.

There Is Growing Disillusionment With Future Prospects and With Institutions

The glowing optimism of the sixties is being replaced by a more sober view of the future, sometimes accompanied by disillusionment. Yost speaks of "a rise of falling expectations" that is affecting both the highly industrialized and the developing nations.[5] The likelihood of continuing inflation and world shortages of food and energy appears to be accompanied by a lack of confidence in the ability of governments to deal with these problems. Politicians are held in low esteem. Correspondingly, there is little public confidence in the educational system, and less and less faith in the value of advanced degrees.

Neither the public nor the private sector is able to resolve the issues of relatively slow growth and persistent high rates of inflation. Distrust of government and the perceived self-interest of big business seem to be producing a growing feeling that the only long-term hope for improving the state of affairs is to rely on oneself. Amara predicts a shift toward tradition, conservatism, self-reliance and greater individual participation in decision making, particularly in the work place.[6]

A "sense of community" seems to be diminishing, particularly in urban areas. This is the experience of being a part of the community, an expectation of giving and receiving support from community members, a feeling of involvement and pride in and concern for one's own immediate environment. Some sociologists correlate this absence of a community affiliation with a rise in antisocial behavior and crime. Homey, neighborly tasks — such as tending the sick, visiting the lonely, participating in activities to improve the neighborhood, or providing child care — have been relinquished to professionally staffed agencies. This not only increases the burden on the agencies, but leaves the individual with a sense of rootlessness and an impaired perception of identity. A "dont't-give-a-damn" attitude toward the quality of work, the welfare of others, and the existence of starvation abroad and injustice at home is costly to production, dangerous to public safety and health, and fatal to a free society. If health is considered to encompass social health, then the lack of a sense of community might well be the number one health problem.

THE CHANGING NATURE OF DECISION MAKING AFFECTS ACTION PLANNING

It is fair to say that, in the past, decisions regarding community action and the major areas of family life were made by adult men, and (in the case of the community) persons of influence and prestige. Patterns of accepted practice did not vary greatly from place to place. Recently, leadership appears to be distributed much more widely. One feature is the tremendous worldwide improvement in the status of women, a long-time concern of the United Nations and the International Labour Organization as well as of national governments. Substantial corrective legislation has been stimulated in recent years by public agitation on the part of women's organizations; International Women's Year; and, in the United States, the ferment created by activities surrounding the proposed Equal Rights Amendment to the Constitution.[7]

During 1979, which was the International Year of the Child, the U.N. Commission on Human Rights considered a proposed draft convention on children's rights, highlighting issues of poverty, disease and malnutrition, education, and child labor.[8] The young are certain to play a larger role in leadership in all fields. Mead points out that children live in a world their parents never knew as children, and thus parents may not necessarily be the best judges of what is appropriate in this untested atmosphere.[9]

Perhaps the strongest new voice in decision making is that of the consumer. Consumer organizations are increasing in size and power; the neighborhood health center board, the League of Women Voters, Common Cause, and Public Citizen are examples of such organizations.

This changing nature of decision making will have a tremendous effect upon the direction and management of health services. The role of the professional in health management will become more and more one of shared leadership.

In considering these broad trends as they affect community health nursing, it is important to keep in mind Rene Dubos' dictum, "Trend is not destiny."[10] Man can invent rather than submit to his future. Trends may be changed or even reversed by science, political movements, or new approaches to social action. Accommodation to reduced natural resources may lead to happier rather than diminished living styles — for example, more walking is definitely beneficial to health; fewer gadgets can simplify the work of the homemaker; and new urban planning influenced by energy shortages may provide more humanizing environments. What is certain is that the changes in the coming decades will be fundamental and massive; there can be no returning to the good old days.

A GROWING POPULATION APPEARS TO BE MOVING SLOWLY TOWARD STABILIZATION

Population growth has become a primary international policy issue. World population increased from approximately one billion in 1830 to two billion in 1969, reaching 4.4 billion in 1979. The projected median population of the world by the year 2000 is estimated by the Population Division of the U.S. Census Bureau to be 6.4 billion. Table 1–1 shows birth rate, death rate, and infant mortality for selected countries. Natural increase (the excess of births over deaths) added an estimated 1,405,000 persons to the United States population in 1978. The United States rate of increase was 6.5 persons per 1,000 population in 1978. The average world rate of natural increase was 19 per 1,000 population between 1970 and 1977.[11] Population growth in the United States has been dramatic — rising from 3.9 million in 1790, to 76 million in 1900, and then to approximately 218 million in 1978.

Future trends in population are hard to predict because of uncertainty about the *fertility rate* (the number of births that 1000 women would have in their lifetime if, at each year of age, they experienced the birth rate occurring in the specified year), which is largely determined by individual choice. The Bureau of the Census projects a slight rise in the rate of natural increase from 6.6 per 1,000 population in 1977 to 7.8 by 1983, largely the result of higher birth rates as large numbers of women enter their childbearing years.[12] Economic trends of inflation and

Table 1-1   BIRTH RATES AND DEATH RATES PER 1,000 POPULATION AND INFANT MORTALITY PER 1,000 LIVE BIRTHS IN SELECTED COUNTRIES, 1978[1]

Country	Birth Rate	Death Rate	Infant Mortality	Country	Birth Rate	Death Rate	Infant Mortality
Africa				Norway	12.7	9.9	9.2
Egypt	37.6	10.5	101.3[2]	Poland	19.0	9.3	22.5
Mauritius[2]	26.8	7.9	45.6	Portugal	16.8	9.8	38.9[4]
Nigeria[2]	49.2	20.7	–	Romania[2]	19.7	9.7	31.2
South Africa[3]	43.1	13.9	–	Spain	17.2	7.9	15.0
Tunisia[2]	36.4	7.9	54.9[4]	Sweden	11.3	10.8	8.0[2]
Asia				Switzerland	11.2	9.0	9.8[2]
Cyprus	19.3	8.4	17.5	United Kingdom	12.3	11.7	14.2
Hong Kong	17.5	5.2	11.6	Yugoslovia	17.4	8.7	35.2[2]
Israel	24.8	6.8	16.5	North America			
Japan	15.0	6.0	8.9[2]	Antigua[2]	19.7	6.8	24.5
Kuwait[2]	41.5	4.8	39.1	Bahamas, The[2]	22.1	4.9	28.3
Philippines[4]	26.7	6.3	58.9[5]	Barbados[2]	16.0	8.0	25.0
Singapore	16.9	5.2	12.6	Canada	15.2	7.3	12.4[2]
Syria[4]	50.4[2]	14.8	112.5	Costa Rica[6]	29.3	4.6	33.6
Taiwan	19.2	4.7	12.9[6]	Cuba[6]	19.8	5.6	22.9
Thailand[6]	24.1	5.5	25.5	El Salvador[2]	41.7	7.8	59.5
Europe				Guatemala[6]	42.6	13.1	76.5
Austria	11.3	12.5	16.9[2]	Jamaica[6]	29.8	7.1	20.4
Belgium	12.4	11.7	11.6	Mexico[6]	34.6	6.5	54.7
Bulgaria	15.5	10.5	23.7[2]	Panama[2]	28.8	4.8	28.5
Czechoslovakia	18.4	11.5	18.7	Puerto Rico[2]	22.6	6.0	20.1
Denmark	12.2	10.4	8.9	United States	15.3	8.8	13.6
Finland	13.5	9.2	12.0[2]	Oceania			
France[2]	14.0	10.1	11.4	American Samoa[2]	36.5	4.4	18.8
Germany, East	13.9	13.9	13.1[2]	Australia	15.7	7.6	12.5[2]
Germany, West	9.3	11.8	15.5[2]	Fiji[2]	27.0	3.9	14.5
Greece	15.6	8.7	19.3	Guam[6]	32.8	5.0	18.0
Hungary	15.7	13.1	24.3	New Zealand[2]	17.4	8.4	14.2
Iceland	18.6	6.5	10.8	Pacific Islands,			
Ireland[2]	21.4	10.5	15.7	Trust Terr. of[2]	29.2	4.3	31.2
Italy	12.5	9.4	17.6[2]	Western Samoa	14.0	2.6	16.3
Netherlands, The	12.6	8.2	9.5	U.S.S.R.	18.3	9.8	27.7[5]

[1] Registered births and deaths only.
[2] 1977.
[3] 1975–1980 UN estimate.
[4] 1975.
[5] 1974.
[6] 1976.
Sources: United Nations, *Population and Vital Statistics Report;* various national publications.

recession could reduce this projected increase. It is clear, however, that for the immediate future, the population will probably continue to grow.

The Composition of the Population is Changing

America is "graying." Improved social conditions and medical advances have pushed life expectancy from 54.1 years (as of 1920) to 69.7 years in 1960 and to 73.2 in 1977.[13] Average life expectancy at birth for selected countries is presented in Table 1–2. A lower birth rate has led to some decrease in the younger age group. About 7 per cent of the

Table 1-2   LIFE EXPECTANCY AT BIRTH, IN YEARS, FOR
SELECTED COUNTRIES[1]

Country	Period	Male	Female
Africa			
Burundi	1975–80	41.4	44.6
Egypt	1975–80	53.7	56.1
Liberia	1975–80	44.4	47.6
Madagascar	1975–80	44.4	47.6
Nigeria	1975–80	41.9	45.1
Upper Volta	1975–80	37.5	40.6
Asia			
Hong Kong	1976	68.0	75.5
India	1976–81	53.8	52.6
Indonesia	1975–80	48.7	51.3
Israel[2]	1977[3]	71.9	75.4
Japan	1977[3]	73.1	78.2
Korea, South	1975	66.0	70.0
Pakistan	1975–80	52.4	52.1
Taiwan	1976[3]	68.8	73.7
Thailand	1975–80	57.6	63.2
Europe			
Albania	1975–80	68.0	70.7
Austria	1975–80	68.7	75.5
Belgium	1968–72	67.8	75.5
Bulgaria	1974–76	68.9	73.9
Czechoslovakia	1977[3]	66.7	73.6
Denmark	1967–77[3]	71.2	77.1
Finland	1976[3]	67.5	76.1
France	1976[3]	69.2	77.2
Germany, East	1976	68.8	74.4
Germany, West	1975–77	68.6	75.2
Greece	1970	70.1	73.6
Hungary	1974	66.5	72.4
Iceland	1975–76[3]	73.0	79.2
Ireland	1974–76[3]	66.8	70.7
Italy	1970–72	69.0	74.9
Netherlands, The	1976[3]	71.5	78.0
Norway	1975–76	71.8	78.1
Poland	1977[3]	69.2	74.6
Portugal	1975–80	66.1	72.7
Romania	1975–77	67.5	72.1
Spain	1970[3]	69.6	75.1
Sweden	1976[3]	72.1	77.9
Switzerland	1968–73	70.3	76.2
United Kingdom	1974–76	69.4	75.6
Yugoslavia	1970–72	65.4	70.2
North America			
Barbados	1975–80	68.0	73.0
Canada	1975–80	69.6	75.6
Costa Rica	1975–80	68.5	72.1
Cuba	1970[3]	68.5	71.8
Guatemala	1975–80	54.9	56.6
Mexico	1975–80	63.6	67.4
Panama	1975–80	66.3	69.5
Puerto Rico	1975–80	70.6	75.3
United States	1977[3]	69.7	77.1

Table continued on next page

Table 1-2 LIFE EXPECTANCY AT BIRTH, IN YEARS, FOR
SELECTED COUNTRIES[4]—*Continued*

Country	Period	Male	Female
Oceania			
Australia	1975–80	69.7	76.0
New Zealand	1975–80	69.4	75.6
South America			
Argentina	1975–80	66.1	72.9
Brazil	1975–80	60.7	66.7
Chile	1975–80	61.3	67.6
Peru	1975–80	56.3	60.0
Suriname	1975–80	64.8	69.8
Uruguay	1975–80	67.3	73.3
Venezuela	1975–80	64.6	68.3
U.S.S.R.	1971–72[3]	64.0	74.0

[1] Projection.
[2] Jewish population only.
[3] Actual.
Sources: United Nations, *Selected World Demographic Indicators by Countries, 1950–2000;* official country sources.

population in 1976 were under 5 years of age, 24 per cent were under 15 years of age, and 11 per cent were 65 years of age and over. This age distribution is expected to change, with a considerable increase in the portion of the population 25 years and over. In the year 2000, there will be a 56 per cent increase in the number of people 25 to 44 years of age, a 41 per cent increase in those 45 to 60 years of age, and a 58 per cent increase in those 65 years of age and over, compared with 1970 statistics.[14] This shift has great importance for health planning, since those 65 or over generally require more and different service from that of the other age groups.

Women outnumber men, especially in the older age group. In 1910 there were 106 males for each 100 females. In 1976, the number of males residing in the U.S. was about 5 per cent less than the number of females. The sex ratio decreases as age increases — i.e., there were about 105 males per 100 females at birth, about 100 at 20 to 24 years, about 79 at 65 to 69 years, and about 47 at 85 years and over.[15]

Families have become very mobile. Many families migrate to other states or regions. Movement seems to be related to available work, but a variety of factors affect family plans. International migration has been escalating, particularly in Indochina as well as in the South American countries. According to the United Nations High Commission for Refugees, more than 13 million people left their homes because of political or religious beliefs in 1979. The physical and mental health of these displaced persons, as well as many children left unprotected in refugee camps, is a serious international problem.[16]

Although total enrollments have decreased, education continues to be an important component of American life. There were 58.4 million students in U.S. classrooms at the beginning of the 1979 to 1980 school year. Thirty per cent of the population were involved in education as students, teachers, or administrators.[17] This is an important population for planning health services and health education.

CHANGING LIFE STYLES AFFECT GOALS AND PROGRAMS

A changing environment is producing marked changes in styles of living. Four areas of change appear to have relevance for human health services: (1) patterns of consumption, (2) marriage and the family, (3) work and play, and (4) community relationships.

An Affluent Society Faces Shortages and Inequities

Among the world nations, the United States is one of the more affluent. Despite the shifting locus of the world's wealth, it is likely to remain one of the richer countries. The personal income per capita in the United States was $3,893 in 1970 and $7,836 in 1978.[18] There are indications that the real income of families has declined during a period of high inflation with particular implications for the poor and those on fixed incomes (such as the elderly).

Imbalances between the white population and minority groups continue to exist. Historically, the largest minority group has been and continues to be the black population. An estimated 23 million blacks represent 11 per cent of the population. About one-half of the black population now lives in the South. Blacks and other minority groups are much more urbanized than whites. Approximately half of the black, Hispanic, and Asian populations live in center cities as opposed to 24 per cent of the white population.[19]

Table 1–3 presents selected socioeconomic characteristics of the principal minority groups. The socioeconomic status of minorities is generally low, except for relatively high incomes and education levels of the Asian population. The proportion of black families with incomes less than $5,000 is about three times the proportion of white families; for Hispanics, the proportion is about two times that of the white population. Blacks and Hispanics are underrepresented at the higher income and educational levels.[20]

Americans are accustomed to high consumption. Over 95 per cent of all households have television sets, telephones, and one or more cars. High levels of consumption are also reflected in the purchase of household equipment (dishwashers, clothes washers, dryers), and in the number of swimming pools, recreational vehicles, and second homes.

Table 1-3 PER CENT OF POPULATION WITH SELECTED SOCIAL AND
ECONOMIC CHARACTERISTICS, ACCORDING TO RACE OR ETHNICITY:
UNITED STATES, AVERAGE ANNUAL 1976–1977

Social and Economic Characteristic	Race or Ethnicity			
	Black	Hispanic	Asian or Pacific Islander	White
Family Income	*Per Cent of Population*			
Less than $5,000	30	19	12	11
$5,000–$9,999	29	33	18	19
$10,000–$14,999	19	24	20	23
$15,000 or more	22	24	51	47
Educational Attainment[1]				
High school graduate or more	50	42	78	70
College graduate	7	5	30	15
Employment Status[2]				
Unemployed	12	9	8	6
Marital Status[1]				
Married, spouse present	47	63	65	67

[1] Persons 17 years and over.
[2] Persons 17 years and over in the labor force.
NOTE: Racial and ethnic categories are mutually exclusive.
Source: Division of Health Interview Statistics, National Center for Health Statistics:
Data from the Health Interview Survey.

There are some indications that the "addiction to the abundant life" is
decreasing slightly. It is becoming increasingly clear that production
must be adjusted to correspond to available natural resources, and
account must be taken of the costs in terms of pollution.

Marriage and Family Style Offer New Options

The majority of Americans live in nuclear families and maintain
traditional family roles — the father as primary breadwinner and the
mother as socializer and home manager. This pattern persists, in many
instances, even when both parents are employed. In 1976, about 63 per
cent of the population aged 15 or older were married. Table 1–4 shows
these changes in the proportion of people, adults and children, living in
households with husband-wife families, other types of families or
households headed by primary individuals.[21] In 1975, there were
1,036,000 divorces — a rate of 20.3 per 1,000 married women 15 years of
age and older.[22]

While it is likely that the traditional family will prevail for some
time to come, there are pressures for change. Labor-saving equipment,

Table 1-4 PER CENT OF POPULATION LIVING IN HOUSEHOLDS, BY TYPE OF HOUSEHOLD AND RACE: 1960 and 1976

	Whites			Blacks		
Type of Household	1960	1976	Change	1960	1976	Change
Total	100	100	—	100	100	—
Husband-wife family	87	80	−7	72	55	−17
Female-headed family	6	9	+3	19	32	+13
Male-headed family	2	2	—	3	3	—
Female primary individual	3	5	+2	3	5	+2
Male primary individual	2	4	+2	3	5	+2

—Entry represents zero.
Source: Bureau of the Census, *1960 Census of Population*, Public Use Sample Tape; *Annual Demographic File*, March 1976.

early school admissions, and public recreational facilities have reduced the time required for homemaking (and also much of its challenge as a vocation). The reproductive research now underway offers the hope of greater alternatives in childbearing — more precise methods of fertility control, expanded use of artificial insemination, and even surrogate childbearing and "test tube" babies modified by cloning techniques. Cultural change has also brought sanction for greater experimentation, and the sexual revolution encourages it. "Spinsterhood" is no longer a disgrace (the term itself has an archaic sound; it is more usual today to call both unmarried women and men "singles"), and the dangers of overpopulation make family limitation and childless marriage more acceptable than in the past.

The growing involvement of women in the labor force made possible by these developments is producing more and more two-career families. Projections of the size of the labor force by sex indicate that by 1990, there will be 43.7 million women in the labor force, a 22 per cent increase from 1974. In 1975, 37 per cent of the women with children under 6 years of age were in the labor force, and 52 per cent of women whose children were of school age. The rate of working mothers has tripled since 1950.[23] In the past, it was common for the working wife to continue to assume the traditional homemaking responsibilities in addition to her job. More recently, there has been a trend toward the sharing of parental roles. Children are also encouraged to adopt a more self-reliant stance and assume chores that might otherwise be undertaken by their parents.

Traditionally, the parents establish social and moral values. Today, as family roles are shifting, children are becoming partners in guiding their own development.

There are many exploratory marriage patterns reflecting attempts of individuals or groups to bring greater meaning into marriage and family life. News media are peppered with references to contract marriages, which substitute an expressed time limit for "Til death us do part" and practical operating agreements for the usual vows; to unisex marriage; to "open marriage," which affords sexual freedom within a continuing relationship; to group marriage and the resulting extended family; and to the nonkinship commune which may serve the social functions of the more typical family unit.[24] These developments and their ramifications are of particular concern to community health nursing, since the family is still the primary unit of service.

Less Work and More Play?

Work is an important part of the life experience for most people. The great majority of workers are in organized industries rather than in individual enterprise. While workers have made great advances in controlling the conditions of work, there is still much that remains out of their control, and indeed outside the control of the industry itself. General economic conditions, changing public tastes, availability of raw materials, and strikes in related industries are some of the factors affecting the work situation.

Unemployment is another threat. The unemployment rate between 1947 and 1972 varied from 6.8 per cent in 1958 to a low of 2.9 per cent in 1953. The rate in 1972 was 5.6 per cent; it topped 8 per cent in 1975 and continues today near that level. Since unemployment is not distributed evenly, in some localities there will be much higher rates than in others, with consequent stress and uncertainty. Relocation of industry is relatively frequent; and this, added to rapid obsolescence in methods of production, places more strain on the workers involved.

Work hours have decreased significantly from an average of 48.5 hours per week in 1943 to 39.4 hours in 1980. Most futurists feel that work hours may be shortened drastically in the future as less manpower will be required for standard jobs.

In summary, work will most likely require far less time in the future; however, stress may be high due to uncertainties, mobility, and constant technologic change. The *intrinsic* satisfaction in work has been falling, but it is hoped that managerial measures may counteract this trend. What is certain is that much of the time formerly allocated to work will now be released for leisure uses.

The use of leisure time has real significance for health. It may contribute to health through providing opportunities for self-development, or it may exert a negative force through encouraging the harmful habits of inactivity or of dangerous activities. The public has a large investment in recreation, both in tax dollars and participation — in state and national parks, playgrounds, symphony orchestras, theaters, museums, and a vast array of related educational facilities.

Information about the response of people to leisure opportunities is fragmentary, but there are some indicators that seem important. Passive rather than active recreational pursuits seem to predominate, even though we see a number of people out "running." Estimates for the number of hours spent watching television run very high, especially for children (5 to 6 hours a day). A balance between active and passive "play" is needed at all age levels.

The Individual-Community Relationship Is Changing

The traditional community that provided dependable support to its members, unambiguous definition of "acceptable" behavior, and a forum for decisions has been a casualty of the industrial era and its associated depersonalization. Neighborly closeness is hard to achieve when people live in one place and work in another, when no adult is at home during the day to respond to requests for help, and when relatives and friends are scattered or frequently on the move. Professional services have moved into many areas that were formerly the province of neighborly helpers, so that the pattern of helping has a different focus. The nursing home has replaced the family as caretaker for the elderly; the homemaker service is more likely to be called upon in an emergency than is an aunt, a grandmother, or the lady next door.

Recently there have been attempts to revive the neighborhood as a functioning community. Great impetus was given this movement under the provisions of the Economic Opportunity Act of 1964, which required "consumer" representation in planning and action. The impact of this Act has been diluted since it was administratively transferred to the Department of Health, Education, and Welfare in 1972.

Neighborhood health centers, operating under the auspices of the Economic Security Act or the provisions of other bills, have consistently included consumer involvement and fostered a neighborhood approach.

Much thought is being given to what communities should do vis-à-vis their members and the larger units of social organization, to the purposes that should be served and the structure required to realize that purpose. There is a renaissance of interest in planning for communities that provide for small, interacting clusters of population, offering opportunities for individuals to live and work together on a human scale. There is a strong feeling that decisions made directly and personally by the people involved tend to be more workable, and that the opportunity for citizens to have access to information about conditions that may mandate or constrain certain actions will create a better understanding between the population and its institutions. The objective is to promote participation in seeking solutions to problems geared to specific communities. The great American dream of a little house in the suburbs is no

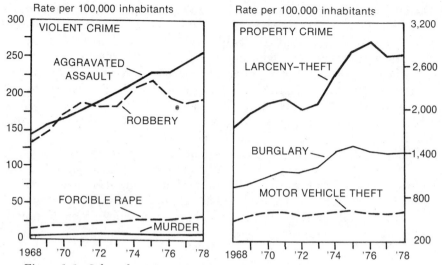

Figure 1-1 Selected crime rates: 1968 to 1978. (Based on chart prepared by U.S. Bureau of the Census; data from U.S. Federal Bureau of Investigation.)

longer feasible for many young couples. New approaches to multiple-dwelling systems, combining central facilities for recreation and social action, may be a solution to housing needs and may contribute to a new community identity.

Violent crime against people and property continues to rise despite the strong efforts at controlling it. Statistics on four types of violent crime (murder and negligent manslaughter, forcible rape, robbery, and aggravated assault) show that the rate per 100,000 of the population rose from 49 in 1940, to 160 in 1960, and then to 459 in 1974. The rate continues to rise despite increases in the size of police forces and efforts aimed at prevention. Crime was most prevalent in cities with populations over 250,000. (The incidence of motor vehicle thefts and burglary also continues to rise; see Figure 1-1.)

Unfortunately, little is known about the prevention of crime, except for certain tactics of "defensive living." Arguments rage among the advocates of different curative measures (ranging from those demanding tougher cops and public whippings to those emphasizing rehabilitation and abolition of prisons), but in the meantime the public has come to accept crime as a fact of life which they must cope with by putting bars across their windows and installing burglar alarms.

This, then, is the "people" parameter of community health nursing in the United States. There is an increasing, aging, mostly urban population, slowly moving toward a stable birth rate. By world standards, the people have a high standard of living and an elevated real income, with unmatched access to material goods. Educational opportunities are abundant, and the level of completed education is high.

Despite this, there is a persistent and substantial portion of the population who do not enjoy their fair share of the available resources, and who live in poverty. There is also a likelihood — indeed, almost a certainty — that greater austerity will continue to be part of the future.

There is constant testing of and experimentation with basic institutions in an effort to make them more responsive to the needs of different groups. There is unprecedented leisure, and little comprehension of how to use it. Living with crime is accepted, but methods for crime control are undeveloped. Communities, for the most part, do not establish a sense of affiliation or affinity among their members.

The speed of change; the uncertainties of the social order; the helplessness and lack of control the individual confronts in many aspects of his life; the pervading sense of disillusionment, disappointment, and distrust of institutions — all these combine to produce an environment riddled with stress.

DEATH, DISABILITY, AND DANGEROUS BEHAVIOR: THE CHALLENGERS

As populations move to more favorable levels of economic stability aided by advanced technology, the scope and direction of health management must also change. In this regard, the problems of "developed" countries may be very similar.

The Killers

The four major causes of death continue to be diseases of the heart, cancer, cerebrovascular diseases, and accidents. Table 1–5 describes major causes of death, according to life stages, for 1977. From adolescence through early adulthood, accidents and violent death take the largest toll. Infants under one year die because of prematurity, birth-associated problems, and congenital birth defects. There is much that can be done to prevent these deaths. Among those 65 years of age and older, influenza and pneumonia were the fourth leading cause of death.

The major causes of death may not reflect those of *preventable* death, which must be the principal public health concern. The Surgeon General's Report, published in 1979, set the major public health goals to be reached by 1990. Specific areas suggested for disease prevention were: hypertension, family planning, pregnancy and infant health, immunization, sexually transmitted disease, toxic agent control, occupational safety, accident prevention, smoking, alcohol and drug abuse, nutrition and physical fitness, stress, fluoridation, and control of infec-

Table 1-5 CAUSES OF DEATH BY LIFE STAGES, 1977

Age Groups → Problem	Infants (Under 1) Rank	Rate[1]	Children (1-14) Rank	Rate[2]	Adolescents/ Young Adults (15-24) Rank	Rate[2]	Adults (25-44) Rank	Rate[2]	Adults (45-64) Rank	Rate[2]	Adults (Over 65) Rank	Rate[2]	Total Population (All Ages) Rank	Rate[2]
Chronic Diseases														
Heart Disease			7	1.1	6	2.5	2	25.5	1	351.0	1	2334.1	1	332.3
Stroke			8	.6	9	1.2	8	6.1	3	52.4	3	658.2	3	84.1
Arteriosclerosis											5	116.5	9	13.3
Bronchitis, Emphysema, & Asthma									10	12.2	8	69.3		
Cancer			3	4.9	5	6.5	1	29.7	2	302.7	2	988.5	2	178.7
Diabetes Mellitus					10	.4	10	2.4	8	17.8	6	100.5	7	15.2
Cirrhosis of the Liver							7	8.6	4	39.2	9	36.7	8	14.3
Infectious Diseases														
Influenza and Pneumonia	5	50.6	6	1.5	8	1.3	9	3.0	9	15.3	4	169.7	5	23.7
Meningitis			8	.6										
Septicemia	6	32.7												
Trauma														
Accidents														
Motor vehicle accidents			2	9.0	1	44.1	3	23.1	7	18.3	10	24.5	6	22.9
All other accidents	7	27.7	1	10.8	2	18.4	4	18.5	5	25.5	7	78.1	4	24.8
Suicide			10	.4	3	13.6	5	17.3	6	19.1				
Homicide			5	1.6	4	12.7	6	15.6					9	13.3
Developmental Problems														
Immaturity-associated	1	407.7												
Birth-associated	2	294.4												
Congenital Birth Defects	3	253.1	4	3.6	7	1.6								
Sudden Infant Deaths	4	142.8												
All Causes		1412.1		43.1		117.1		182.5		1,000.0		5288.1		878.1

[1]Rate per 100,000 live births.
[2]Rate per 100,000 population in specified group.
Source: Based on data from The National Center for Health Statistics, Division of Vital Statistics.

tious disease.[25] Certainly, many deaths from accidents might be considered preventable; and a large proportion of deaths from breast cancer and, to some degree, lung cancer may be considered preventable in the light of present available knowledge. The rate of death from diabetes is increasing despite the present advanced level of medical expertise, indicating that a higher rate of control should be possible. Although the rate of infant deaths in the United States (deaths among children under one year of age per 1,000 live births) has fallen from 47 in 1940 to 14.0 in 1977, there are indications that many deaths are still preventable. For example, a persistent gap exists between white and nonwhite infant deaths that could be reduced with the application of preventive care strategies. In 1977 the infant death rate for black infants was 23.6 per 1,000 live births and that for white infants was 12.4 deaths per 1,000 live births.[26]

The Disablers: Thieves of Time

In 1976, there were 18.2 restricted-activity days per person per year, with 7.1 of these days indicating time spent confined to bed. Limitation of activity was largely accounted for by chronic conditions, 14.3 days per person per year. Respiratory problems accounted for the most frequent acute condition.[27]

Of the chronic conditions encountered, those most likely to cause physical limitation were heart conditions (17.3 per cent), arthritis and rheumatism (9.9 per cent), old age (5.9 per cent) and mental and nervous conditions (5.3 per cent); next in frequency were cerebrovascular disease and emphysema.[28]

While there is no measure of the proportion of those affected with some disabling condition who require assistance, it seems likely that the need for supportive and preventive care is well above the level provided.

The Risk Makers: Health-Threatening Environment or Behavior

The community health nurse must be involved not only with health problems that are already apparent, but also with potential dangers and risks. This is the essence of preventive care. The threat of death, illness, injury, developmental aberration, or substandard health can be heightened by: a nonsupportive environment, health-threatening personal behavior, public or personal negligence, and low value placed on health in respect to other personal or social goals.

The *environment* may threaten health in many ways: pollution of the water, soil, or air; unsafe buildings or roads; uncontrolled population; and extreme poverty with its attendant prevailing mood of discontent and despair. Noise pollution has also been recognized as a serious problem: planes, traffic, machinery, radios, even vacuum cleaners contribute to the continual din. Water pollution may result from effluents discharged into lakes and rivers by factories or public sewerage systems, from chemical substances that become dangerous only when other chemicals are present, from oil spillage from tankers, and from agricultural pesticides that contaminate streams. An estimated 3½ billion tons of nonreturnable bottles, cans, and cartons create further disposal and aesthetic problems.

The slum or ghetto may in itself create a complex environmental threat. Substandard housing, peeling lead paint, overcrowding, fire hazards, and an uncontrolled rat population are obvious dangers. Equally hazardous may be poor housekeeping habits, drug addiction or alcoholism, a sense of hopelessness, a lack of community identity as a result of transient living, the immediate reward of crime. All of these can be more catching than measles — and more deadly.

The rural community also has problems, arising from careless use of pesticides, dilapidated equipment, and poor water supplies. Equally harmful in their own way are elements such as inadequate educational facilities, stereotyped behavior, and frozen or rigid social patterns that create an inflexible class society.

Lawton points out that unfavorable environments may hasten symptoms of aging. He notes that an environment tolerable to the nimble and energetic young may prove hazardous to the elderly, who feel unable to contend with high-speed transportation, crowds, smog, and thunderous music. He suggests that environments should be deliberately planned to elicit "behavior elevating" responses. Although he was referring particularly to the elderly, the principle could be applied to all ages.[29]

The environment must be seen as a whole — the land, the air, and the water; the people who occupy the space; and the relationship between the two. As Train says, "Our air, and water, and soil, and cities are sick, and the sickness is people."[30]

Health-threatening personal or community behavior is a matter of worldwide concern. Documentation of the effects of certain kinds of behavior is gradually growing. There is no doubt that cigarette smoking, drug abuse, recklessness in driving or in sports, negligence and nonadaptive life styles can and do result in premature death, disability, and decreased vitality.

Cigarette smoking has shown a satisfying decline. Among adults in the United States it was estimated that in 1966, 42.2 per cent were cigarette smokers; by 1978 the proportion had dropped to approximately 31 per cent. A decrease in smoking among teenagers since a peak in 1974 has resulted in 11 per cent males and 13 per cent females using cigarettes today.[31] The problem, however, remains a critical one. Despite the demonstrated linkage between cigarettes and diseases, intensive educational programs, and warning statements in advertising and on cigarette packages, more cigarettes are being sold in the United States than ever before.

Drug abuse has emerged as a global problem and a major threat affecting all groups of the population. Alcohol is by far the most popular of the addictive drugs and is of enormous economic importance because of its relationship to driving accidents, impaired work performance, and the devastating effect of alcoholism on family stability. It is estimated that improper use of alcohol costs the nation 43 billion dollars annually — in lost production, medical services, accidents, crime, and other problems.

Abuse of drugs other than alcohol is a growing problem and one for which control measures still appear to be inadequate. Over the past 20 years, there has been a tendency for drug use to start at earlier and earlier ages, and it has spread to contaminate virtually every social and cultural group. Estimation of the size of the drug problem is hampered by the illicit nature of much (but not all) drug use, the enormous differences in the effects of various drugs, the tendency of patients and families to deny that a problem exists, and the unclear terminology — a "user" may be a person who experimented once with a drug, or someone who resorts frequently to drugs, or a habitual and hopeless addict. Reported incidence of drug addiction seems to underestimate the problem; however, some concept of its magnitude may be gleaned from the following statistics: between May 1976 and April 1977, there were an estimated 7000 to 8000 deaths and approximately 300,000 medical emergencies related to drug abuse. An estimated 2,500,000 persons (2 per cent of the population 18 and over) are having serious drug problems; of these, 450,000 are heroin-dependent.[32] There is no question that drug dependence is a prevalent, complex, and largely unsolved public health problem.

Recklessness in driving, in sports, and in handling machinery is a big factor in accidental deaths. Driving at excessive speeds, failure to use seat belts or to carry or wear life belts in boats, attempting new or dangerous sports without proper preparation or training, swimming in unknown waters, daredevilling with a tractor, or playing "chicken" in city traffic — all are escapades which invite injury or death.

Negligence is an all too frequent cause of illness, injury, or premature death. Common examples of negligence are: failure to carry out regular self-examination of the breast among women, delay in seeking medical care in pregnancy, or failure to respond to a recommendation for further examination following a positive cervical smear for cancer diagnosis. Similarly, failure to follow advice to increase exercise and decrease weight may invite hypertension, heart disease, or unmanageable stress. Such negligence is rarely limited to a single episode of ignoring medical advice; it usually represents customary behavior on the part of the individual. Normally, negligence is not the result of a lack of knowledge, but rather an unwillingness to face the possibility of a specific illness, or a feeling of invincibility ("it can't happen to me"), or a lazy habit of just not getting around to things. Sometimes it is based on the belief that medicine cannot help — so why bother?

Overwork or poor pacing of life activities is another pitfall. The harried administrator who needs six hours of sleep and only gets three, the hard-working mother who "lives for her children" and never has time for leisure or self-development, the politician who ignores the physiologic realities of jet lag, and the adolescent who laps up every possible new experience at the expense of sleep or introspection are all vulnerable candidates for illness.

Lowered expectations regarding health are usually realized. If the individual or community does not expect to be healthy in the sense of Halbert Dunn's "high level wellness,"[33] either will be content with inadequate health care. The individual will accept as inevitable constant low back pain, headaches, or fatigue; the community will not protest about unimmunized children, or wide disparity between the poor and the well-to-do in the medical care available, or callous and negligent treatment of the elderly.

The public needs to have its health consciousness raised. Fortunately, many health professionals are succeeding at this by expressing concern for the problems of people who are technically healthy but who, nevertheless, suffer from low energy, anxiety, or debilitating minor stress.

In planning community health nursing strategies, it is imperative to include consideration of the various threats to health, as well as the actual disruptions of health. Only in this way will it be possible to move toward positive health goals.

THE HEALTH CARE SYSTEM: THE MEANS

The health care system is the means by which the community acts to realize its program for health action. This includes the great, interacting complex of health facilities; private, voluntary, and public agencies and services; health manpower; the consumers of health care; and the formulation of comprehensive policies for health management. To the degree that this system is adequate, viable, and integrated, the health program is able to realize the goals of the people.

At present, the United States has no clearly defined national health policy, although there has been congressional effort to create a national council for health policy and health development.[34] Public statements by health and government leaders and declarations of purpose in the many and scattered laws relating to health management indicate a concern for a planned health care system, comprehensive in both content and coverage; but we are still waiting. President Franklin Roosevelt called upon Congress in 1944 to establish "the right to adequate medical care and the opportunity to achieve and enjoy good health." In 1971, four basic elements of a national health strategy were presented: assuring adequate access for all, balancing supply and demand, organizing for efficiency, and building on strengths by a pluralistic rather than a monolithic system.[35]

The basic assumption is that health care is a right and that the government has an obligation to remove barriers to needed health care. This concept is reiterated in the original Social Security Act of 1935 and its many subsequent health amendments, including Medicare and Medicaid; the Economic Opportunity Act of 1966, the specific laws providing care for special groups such as migrants or Indians, and many more. This vague definition of policy, however, may in part be responsible for the piecemeal and erratic way in which health programs have developed.

Public desire for health care is reflected in the degree to which medical care is funded, both publicly and privately. In 1978, health expenditures totaled 192.4 billion dollars, an increase from 74.7 billion in 1970. The proportion of the gross national product (total monetary value of all final goods and services produced in a country during one year) related to health care rose from 7.6 per cent in 1970 to 9.1 per cent in 1978.[36] Senator Abraham Ribicoff commented, "If cost were any indication of quality, then America would be the healthiest nation in history."[37] Unfortunately, this is not the case, and citizens and professionals alike are dissatisfied.

People are dissatisfied with the high costs and care which they consider minimal. We also know that access to services is not equally distributed to all groups in society.

Third-party payments for medical care continue to account for an increasing proportion of personal health care expenditures (67.1 per cent in 1978). Public sources paid 38.7 per cent of the total expenditures, with the federal government share continuing to increase, especially since the advent of Medicare and Medicaid programs.[38] All institutional care — i.e., hospital and nursing homes, — has shown tremendous cost increases. For example, in 1977, it cost $173.25 per in-patient day in short-stay hospitals, an increase of 13.8 per cent from 1976.[39]

Pressure from the general public and legislators is heavy for some rationalization of this sprawling and spotty system. The Comprehensive Health Planning and Public Health Service Amendments of 1966 (PL 89–749) were viewed as an effort to bring some order into the chaotic health services picture. This law provided grants to states for planning comprehensive health programs. Recent health planning law has expanded the responsibilities of the Health Service Agencies created for planning and organizing services at the local level. To date, results have been less than spectacular. This may be the result of meager funding, the strength of entrenched institutions, lack of authority in the provisions of the planning agencies, or poor planning skills.

It seems highly likely that some form of national health insurance program will develop in the relatively near future that will serve to weld together the many bits and pieces of the present system. The presence of common themes that link most consumer and legislative proposals indicates a strong movement toward a health policy that would insure basic health care for all. This care would be built on insurance mechanisms; it would provide for participation at all levels of government and would mandate a strong consumer voice in policy and administrative decision making. Bills continue to be introduced, some more comprehensive and expensive than others. Until more is known about how to effectively contain costs while maintaining quality and accessibility, there is a reluctance to commit ourselves to what promises to be a very expensive program.

Health Facilities Are Assuming New Configurations

Compared to other countries of the world, the United States is well supplied with facilities for preventive and curative services. However, problems involving distribution, lack of coordination, and sometimes lack of vision (with respect to care of the healthy population) create shortages in some localities and for some types of service.

Basic to the health facility system is a countrywide network of national, state, and local official *public health agencies*, which are legally responsible for protecting the public health. These agencies study the health problems of the nation, promulgate laws and regulations to protect health, support and coordinate services afforded by other agencies, and represent the interests of the population as a whole. About 92 per cent of the population is covered by such organized health services. These agencies should be of great strategic importance in health planning and evaluation and in the stimulation of action among other health facilities. There is presently much concern about defining the role of these agencies and developing a clearer mandate for them in order to utilize their leadership potential.

A large and dispersed *hospital* system is also reviewing its role. In 1977 there were 1,088,348 hospital beds in the United States available in 3,781 hospitals for short-stay. This represents a slight increase from 1972, when there were 1,004,854 beds. There are currently approximately 4.6 short-stay beds per 1,000 population. In 1977, there were 597 hospitals classified as "long-stay," with 277,278 beds. There are approximately 1,402,400 nursing homes in the country — 21 per cent are certified as a skilled nursing facility; 39.2 per cent are classified as skilled and intermediate care; 27.9 per cent are certified as an intermediate care facility; and 11.9 per cent are not certified.[40]

Almost every acute hospital includes an out-patient facility. For many people, especially urban dwellers, the out-patient facility has become a substitute for the physician's office.

The *health maintenance organization* (HMO) has had strong governmental support as a mechanism for providing comprehensive care. The Health Maintenance Organization Act of 1973 (PL 93–222) provided 375 million dollars to be spent over a five-year period for grants and loans designed to stimulate the expansion and development of HMO's.

The HMO is a prepaid medical service capable of providing or arranging for all health services that may be required by a specific enrolled group. The HMO serves individuals or families who have voluntarily entered into a contract with the organization to pay (or have paid on their behalf) a fixed sum for an agreed upon set of services. Many kinds of health delivery systems qualify as HMO's: hospitals, group health associations, private medical group practices, or networks of community facilities organized into cohesive service structures. However, all are required to meet defined prerequisites. They must:

1. Assure services as needed 24 hours a day, 7 days a week.
2. Provide comprehensive service coverage, including preventive care. (As a minimum, provision must be made for physicians' services, in-patient care, emergency care, and out-patient services. Many include much more than the minimum.)
3. Demonstrate proper management and fiscal viability.

Proponents of the HMO system believe that it provides more efficient use of available health resources and manpower and more comprehensive care; that it affords easy access to health care for the consumer; that it reduces the general demand for hospital care; and, because of prepayment, that it relieves the enrolled subscriber of worry about costs. Opponents of the system are critical because it does not cover the entire population; because care can be depersonalized, since the doctor is employed by the organization; and because services vary from one organization to another, leaving many gaps and deficiencies.

"Free clinics" are a modern phenomenon, unusual not only because they are, for the most part, free of cost to the patient, but also because they have developed a distinctive character. These facilities serve a group which would not otherwise be reached. Originally they evolved to meet the needs of hippies and other exponents of youthful underground subcultures who felt alienated from or distrustful of conventional medical sources. They continue to attract a clientele that is largely young and critical of orthodox living standards. Their patients are usually seeking help for drug abuse or venereal diseases, or counseling during pregnancy, though they also require the whole range of medical care. Outreach and advocacy are usually part of the care provided. Easy access and lack of pressure to pay are characteristic. Much of the care

provided is given during evening hours. There is no red tape and no eligibility requirement for service.

Conditions in free clinics are far from ideal. Facilities are often makeshift, and provision of supplies can be erratic. The staffs are largely volunteer, with patients themselves often helping out. Nevertheless, they provide essential services to a group that is particularly vulnerable. It has been estimated that there are approximately 200 such clinics in the country, treating over two million people a year.[41]

The *neighborhood health center* is an old idea rediscovered and updated. In the early 1900's, neighborhood health centers, supported largely by philanthropy, were established as a means of reaching the poor who were plagued by disease and malnutrition among infants. In the sixties, the idea was revived as a means of aiding the poor or otherwise disadvantaged groups who were not utilizing available health care resources. As part of its work in the war against poverty, the Office of Economic Opportunity encouraged the use of such neighborhood-based activities, providing a model widely copied by other health centers not sponsored by OEO funds.

Sponsorship is diverse: schools, citizen's groups, community corporations, hospitals — as well as Economic Opportunity agencies — are among the initiators and supporters. The range of services varies widely, as do operating policies. However, there is general acceptance of the following criteria:

1. Provision of comprehensive care, either directly or through referral.
2. Maximum accessibility in hours of service and availability of personnel.
3. Involvement of the community in policy and administrative and allocative decisions.
4. Use of residents of the community as paid and/or volunteer workers.
5. Flexibility and modification concerning the application of traditional programs or methods.
6. Decentralization of control.

To date, the neighborhood health center has been used largely as a means of reaching low-income groups, but health professionals believe that the concept would be acceptable to other groups as well.

The development of *community mental health centers* has been promoted by provisions of the Retardation Facilities and Community Health Centers Act of 1963 (PL 88–164) as a means of increasing the impact and relevance of mental health services. These centers share much of the philosophy of the neighborhood health center except that, because of the specialized nature of their concern, the catchment area is larger; hence, direct community involvement is more difficult. The community mental health center is considered by many to provide a valuable bridge between the hospital and the community and a means of early recognition of need for hospital or adjunct care.

Home health agencies are another form of care being revitalized from the past. Spiraling hospital costs, the particular nature of health care needs of the elderly, and a growing appreciation of the importance of other in-home services have led to pressure for alternatives to hospital care. Senate Committee Reports and special studies have emphasized the importance of in-home care as an integral part of a comprehensive care plan and have urged the creation of a national advisory committee to develop standards and policies for such service.

The Council of Home Health Agencies and Community Health Services of the National League for Nursing has developed a model for the delivery of home health services.[42] The home health agency, as currently conceived, may vary greatly in sponsorship, program, and coverage; however, each offers skilled nursing care. To qualify for reimbursement from Medicare, the agency must provide at least one additional service, such as home health aides or physical or occupational therapy, and must meet certain requirements regarding policies, clinical records, and local licensure regulations. The League model suggests that much is required from a truly comprehensive agency.

There are, of course, many types of agencies involved in certain aspects of home care. The American Red Cross provides instruction in home care of the sick; Alcoholics Anonymous provides crisis intervention services to alcoholics; and churches or civic assocations may provide visiting and supportive services. A thorough investigation of all local volunteer and professional health services will normally reveal a substantial number that can be utilized for home care.

Voluntary health organizations play an important role in health care. They can provide health education and promotional programs in their field of interest; specific help, such as supplies or counseling services; and interpretation of local problems for legislative and funding organizations. The National Health Council is an organization for national agencies in the health field; and it provides coordination, exchange of information, and advice to voluntary groups. A recent compendium describes many voluntary associations, professional societies, and other groups concerned with health, medical, hospital, pharmaceutical and related fields throughout the country.

The American people have a substantial investment in health facilities. However, for the most part, these services are poorly supported, unevenly distributed, and devoid of any common framework of policy. The potential of these agencies and services to meet the needs of the population will be severely hampered unless some kind of rationale becomes possible.

HEALTH WORKERS: THE ACTIVATORS

Three kinds of participants are involved with health care: the client or user of service and his representatives, the professional and related personnel who provide care, and the planners and legislators who integrate health concerns with other political action.

The Consumer

Health care groups and institutions have traditionally involved community representatives in their work, as Board members, volunteers, or advisory and consultant committee members. For the most part, those involved were deeply committed to the cause of health improvement, but they were also usually prestigious and economically favored individuals. Beginning in the 1960's, the concept of consumer participation shifted, and more emphasis was placed on involvement of users of the services and residents of the areas served. Consumer involvement was mandated and prescribed in detail in considerable health legislation. The Community Mental Health Centers Act (PL 94–63), for example, states that community action agencies must provide for the "maximum feasible participation of residents of the area and of the group served." This involvement was eagerly sought by many consumers who had not previously been consulted about either the needs or the administration of programs, or, if consulted, did not participate in the decisions that were ultimately made. This emphasis on involvement has introduced large numbers of consumers into the health system.

The individual rights of patients or groups have also been clarified. A publication of the National League for Nursing, "What People Can Expect of Modern Nursing," and a more recent statement by the American Hospital Association, the "Patient's Bill of Rights," spell out the right of the consumer to be treated with dignity and to make decisions about his own health care.[44]

A relatively new phenomenon is the *consumer organization* (such as Common Cause and Public Citizen) that provides a strong and powerful voice in health decisions at the community or national level. Whatever channel or role the consumer selects, it is clear that he no longer believes that the doctor always knows best!

Health Professionals Are Becoming More Numerous and Diversified

The number of people employed in the health care industry is 6.7 million as of 1978; more than half of the total were working in hospitals.[45]

The special needs of a changing society, a sophisticated level of care, and extended research involvement require contributions from many different service levels; and high costs have led to additional employment of short-trained workers of all types. By comparison with other countries, the United States is well supplied in all major man-power groups, although there is a continuing disparity between the work force available and the demands for care.

The number of *physicians* in the United States has increased in both absolute numbers and in the ratio of physicians to population. In 1950 there were 232,697 physicians (including Doctors of Medicine and Doctors of Osteopathy), or 14.2 physicians to each 10,000 of the population. By 1977 the number had risen to an estimated 424,000, or 17.9 for each 10,000 of the population; and it is projected that by 1990 this number will reach 594,000, or 24.4 physicians for each 10,000 of the population.[46] Among the approximately 359,515 active *Doctors of Medicine* in 1977, the majority of these were in individual practice. However, group medical practice among active physicians is increasing, from 18 per cent in 1969 to 25 per cent in 1975. Some policy makers suggest that creation or expansion of group practice would alleviate shortages in rural and inner city areas.[47]

The trends in physician specialty from 1970 to 1977 remain fairly constant for the proportion in primary care (approximately 40 per cent). Primary care specialty includes internal medicine, pediatrics, and general practice. About one third of active physicians are in surgical specialties with general surgery showing the largest increase (18 per cent) since 1970. Another one third of active physicians are in "other" specialties — i.e., anesthesiology, psychiatry, radiology, and so forth.[48] (The "family doctor," however, is still a scarce commodity.)

Despite this plentiful supply of physicians, surveys have found that distribution is very uneven. Geographic variations in the ratios of physicians and specialists to population changed the most in the southern United States and the least in the Northeast, which has the highest ratio of physicians to population. In fact, there has been very little progress made toward a more even distribution of physicians.[49]

The work of the physician is supplemented by *physician's assistants*, who perform delegated duties under the physician's supervision; *medical assistants*, who have a more limited role; and the aid of expanded nursing care. A survey in 1978–1979 reported 8,000 physician's assistants and medical assistants (MEDEX), and an unknown number of assistants and aides working in special medical services. Physician's assistants are trained solely to assist or substitute for the physician in the performance of certain medical tasks.[50]

The Supply of Registered Nurses Has Also Grown Rapidly

In 1974 there were an estimated 857,000 active registered nurses in the United States. This number has more than doubled since 1954, increasing the nurse to 10,000 population ratio from 25.1 to 40.7 in 1974.

About 66 per cent of all registered nurses are employed by hospitals, 8 per cent by nursing homes, 7 per cent by public health agencies and doctor's offices, and much smaller percentages (approximately 4 per cent) in nursing education, occupational health, and private duty.[51]

Projections of the future supply of registered nurses have provoked much debate over numbers of inactive registered nurses, distribution, educational preparation, and entry level into practice. Despite an encouraging picture based on preliminary figures for 1979, the concerns remain about the supply of nurses.[52] One fear is that the supply does not allow for an adequate pool for the leadership that will be required to give direction to nursing effort in the future. As of 1974, 3.3 per cent of registered nurses had a master's or doctoral degree; 15 per cent had a baccalaureate degree; 75 per cent had diplomas; and 6 per cent had associate degrees.[53] A baccalaureate degree is considered basic to the development of a leadership career. Another concern for policy makers has been high turnover rates and decreased job satisfaction for nurses working in hospital and community settings.

Geographic distribution is also a concern, especially in underserved areas. Wide acceptance of nurse practitioners who provide nursing care as well as perform certain medical functions in rural areas and other underserved areas has been seen by policy makers as a way of reducing the physician maldistribution. In 1979, there were 16,240 nurse practitioners — 89 per cent with certificates and 64 per cent with master's degrees.[54]

The work of registered nurses is augmented by *licensed practical nurses* and other short-trained personnel. The pool of auxiliary workers has been increasing rapidly: the number of licensed practical nurses in practice was 427,000 in 1972;[55] projections for 1979 to 1980 show only slight increases.

There Has Been a Modest Increase in the Number of Nurses in Community Health

Figures from 1972 surveys reported 7 per cent to 9 per cent of registered nurses as working in community health.[56] Preliminary data from 1979 surveys of community health nursing support this rate, although actual numbers of nurses have increased slightly.[57] The ratio of community health nurses to population has almost doubled since 1947, from 1.3 per 10,000 population, to 2.1 in 1972.[58] The numbers of nurses working in community health do not provide for equitable access or flexible utilization. As in all areas of health manpower, geographic distribution is ragged.

Efforts are being developed to plan and project the future requirements for nursing on a more rational basis. The term "requirements," as developed by a WICHE (Western Interstate Commission for Higher

Education) project, refers to the numbers of nursing personnel needed to meet stated goals. The Requirements Projection Process consists of five major steps: (1) differentiating the client population, (2) examining health status indications, (3) choosing realizable health goals, (4) developing a health strategy, and (5) planning appropriate staffing patterns.[59]

Table 1–6 presents projections of needs for community health nursing according to four basic functional areas: home visiting, clinic services, school health, and occupational health. In some areas, such as home care for the population over 64 years or care for the at-risk maternity population, the projected need is far beyond current resources.

In essence, nursing practice and programs must be molded by all of the following conditions — the times, the people, the threats to health, and the resources for health care.

An uneasy world is creaking under the burden of swift and drastic change, and we are faced with an unprecedented adaptation of fundamental assumptions and life styles, requiring new and complex networks of interdependent action for individuals, groups, and nations. In the United States (as in most industrially developed countries) people are, for the most part, well fed and enjoy a high standard of living. But the *quality* of life has not shown comparable improvement. Inequities persist, so that many are still denied the benefit others enjoy. Apparently, a well-financed, heavily staffed health system is neither meeting the needs for care as seen by professional health workers nor satisfying the public. This is the result of poor distribution, imprecise goals, scattered

Table 1–6 COMMUNITY HEALTH NURSE REQUIREMENTS FOR 1982 ACCORDING TO FOUR BASIC FUNCTIONS

Function	Population Base	Population	RN/10,000 Pop.	Total FTE° RN
1. Home visiting				
A. Home health care	Total population	224,785,000	0.65	14,611
	Over 64 years	25,295,000	2.29	5,792
B. General public health	Live births	3,985,800	4.52	1,801
	Infant deaths	66,000	23.90	157
	Under 17 years	59,351,000	1.29	7,656
	17 years and over	165,434,000	1.29	21,340
2. Clinic	Total population	224,785,000	0.95	21,354
3. School health	Under 17 years	59,351,000	5.14	30,506
4. Occupational health	Age 17–64 years	140,139,000	2.48	34,754

°FTE = full-time equivalent.

Information taken from Elliott, J. E., and Kearns, J. M.: *Analysis and Planning for Improved Distribution of Nursing Personnel and Services—Final Report.* Public Health Service, U.S. Department of Health, Education, and Welfare. Washington, D.C., U.S. Government Printing Office, Pub. No. (HRA) 79-16, December 1978, p. 112.

efforts, and a paucity of proven treatment and preventive measures for behaviorally induced health problems. It is within this framework that community health nursing must look toward the future in order to establish the same degree of accommodation that it has brought to bear in earlier periods of crisis.

REFERENCES

1. Commoner, B.: *The Closing Circle: Nature, Man and Ecology.* New York, Alfred A. Knopf, Inc., 1971, Chapter 1.
2. Meadows, D., Meadows, D. L., Randers, J., and Behrens, W.: *The Limits to Growth: A Report for the Club of Rome's Project on the Predicament of Mankind.* New York, Universe Books, 1972, pp. 23–24.
3. Borghese, E. M.: Who owns the earth's resources? Vista, 9:13, 1945.
4. Lasch, C.: *The Culture of Narcissism: American Life in an Age of Diminishing Expectations.* New York, W. W. Norton & Co., Inc., 1979.
5. Yost, C. W.: The rise of falling expectations. The Interdependent (published by the U.S. United Nations Association), 1:2, 1974.
6. Amara, R. C.: 1985, in *Britannica Book of the Year.* Chicago, Encyclopedia Britannica, Inc., 1980, pp. 142–143.
7. U.S. Commission on Civil Rights: *A Guide to Federal Laws Prohibiting Sex Discrimination.* Washington, D.C., U.S. Government Printing Office, 1974.
8. Harrison, P.: The International Year of the Child, *in Britannica Book of the Year.* Chicago, Encyclopedia Britannica, Inc., 1980, pp. 15–19.
9. Mead, M.: *Culture and Commitment: A Study of the Generation Gaps.* Garden City, N.Y., Doubleday and Co., 1970.
10. Dubos, R.: Man and environment: Scenarios for the future. NYU Educ. Quarterly, 11:2, 1971.
11. United Nations: *Population and Vital Statistics Reports.* New York, United Nations.
12. *Health in the United States: Chartbook.* Washington, D.C., U.S. Government Printing Office, DHEW Pub. No. (PHS) 80-1233, 1980.
13. *Monthly Vital Statistics Report – Advance Report: Final Mortality Statistics, 1977.* National Center for Health Statistics, DHEW Pub. No. (PHS) 79-1120, 28:2, 1979.
14. Public Health Service, U.S. Department of Health, Education, and Welfare: *Health – U.S. 1978.* Washington, D.C., U.S. Government Printing Office, DHEW Pub. No. (PHS) 78-1232, 1978, p. 138.
15. Ibid., p. 138.
16. United Nations High Commission for Refugees, New York, United Nations, 1979.
17. *Britannica Book of the Year,* 1980, p. 333.
18. *Bureau of Economic Analysis Survey of Current Business.* Washington, D.C., U.S. Department of Commerce.
19. Public Health Service, U.S. Department of Health, Education, and Welfare: *Health – U. S. 1979.* Washington, D.C., U.S. Government Printing Office, Pub. No. (PHS) 80-1232, p. 4.
20. Ibid., p. 5.
21. Bureau of the Census: *Conference on Issues in Federal Statistical Needs Relating to Women.* Washington, D.C., U.S. Department of Commerce, Current Population Reports Special Studies, Series P-23, No. 83, December 1979.
22. Public Health Service, U.S. Department of Health, Education, and Welfare: *Vital Statistics of the United States, 1975, Vol. III – Marriage and Divorce.* Washington, D.C., U.S. Government Printing Office, Publ. No. (PHS) 79-1103, 1979.
23. Bureau of the Census: *A Statistical Portrait of Women in the U.S.* Washington D.C., U.S. Department of Commerce, Current Population Reports Special Studies, Series P-23, No. 58, April 1976, p. 26.
24. Francoeur, R. T.: *Eve's New Ribs – Twenty Faces of Sex, Marriage, and Family.* New York, Harcourt Brace Jovanovich, Inc., 1972.
25. U.S. Department of Health, Education, and Welfare: *Preventing Disease/Promoting Health, Objectives for the Nation* (draft). August 1979.

26. Public Health Service, U.S. Department of Health, Education, and Welfare: *Health in the U.S.: Chartbook*. Washington, D.C., U.S. Government Printing Office, DHEW Publ. No. (PHS) 80-1233, 1980.
27. Public Health Service, U.S. Department of Health, Education, and Welfare: *Current Estimates from the Health Interview Survey*. Washington, D.C., U.S. Government Printing Office, Pub. No. (PHS) 78-1547, 1976.
28. Ibid. (current estimates).
29. Lawton, M. P.: Social ecology and the health of older people. Am. J. Pub. Health, 64:259, 1974.
30. Train, R.: Prescription for a planet. Am. J. Pub. Health, 60:433, 1970.
31. *Health in the U.S.: Chartbook*, p. 23.
32. *Promoting Health/Preventing Disease*, p. 84.
33. Dunn, H.: *High Level Wellness*. Arlington, Va., R.W. Beatty Co., 1961, Chapter 1.
34. The National Health Policy and Health Development Act of 1974, HR 12053, 93rd Congress.
35. Message from the President of the United States: Building a national health strategy, HR Document 9294, 92nd Congress.
36. Public Health Service, U.S. Department of Health, Education, and Welfare: *Health – U.S. 1980*. Washington, D.C., U.S. Government Printing Office, p. 244.
37. Ribicoff, A.: The healthiest nation myth. Sat. Rev. 53:18, 1970.
38. *Health – U.S. 1980*, p. 237.
39. Ibid., p. 238.
40. Ibid., pp. 221 and 231.
41. Amenta, M. M.: Free clinics change the scene. Am. J. Nurs., 74:284, 1974.
42. *A Prospectus for a National Home Care Policy*. National League for Nursing, New York, Pub. No. 21 — Pros, 1978.
43. U.S. Department of Health, Education, and Welfare: *Consumer Heaalth Education. A Directory*. Washington, D.C., U.S. Government Printing Office, Pub. No. (HRA) 77-607, 1976.
44. Quinn, N. and Somers, A., The patient's bill of rights. Nurs. Outlook, 22:240, 1974.
45. *Health – U.S. 1980*, p. 205.
46. Ibid., p. 213.
47. Ibid., p. 207.
48. Ibid., p. 215.
49. Bureau of Health Manpower: *A Report to the President and Congress on the Status of Health Professions Personnel in the U.S.* Hyattsville, Md., Health Resources Administration, DHEW Pub. No. (HRA) 79-93, 1979.
50. *Health – U.S. 1980*, p. 71.
51. Public Health Service, Department of Health, Education, and Welfare: *Source Book: Nursing Personnel*. Washington, D.C., U.S. Government Printing Office, Pub. No. (HRA) 75-43, 1974, pp. 61–67.
52. Divison of Nursing, Bureau of Health Professions: *Preliminary Data*. Health Resources Administration, Department of Health, Education, and Welfare, 1979.
53. *Source Book: Nursing Personnel*, p. 69.
54. *Health – U.S. 1980*, p. 74.
55. *Source Book*, p. 61.
56. Ibid., p. 187.
57. Division of Nursing, Bureau of Health Professions, 1979.
58. Source Book, p. 197.
59. Elliott, J. E., and Kearns, J. M.: *Analysis and Planning for Improved Distribution of Nursing Personnel and Services — Final Report*. Public Health Services, U.S. Department of Health, Education, and Welfare. Washington, D.C., U.S. Government Printing Office, Pub. No. (HRA) 79-16, December 1978, p. 9.

SUGGESTED READINGS

Davis, K.: *National Health Insurance: Benefits, Costs and Consequences*. Washington, D.C., The Brookings Institution, 1975.
Davis, K., and Schone, C.: *Health and the War on Poverty*. Washington, D.C., The Brookings Institution, 1978.

Fitzpatrick, M. L.: *The National Organization for Public Health Nursing, 1912–1952: Development of a Practice Field.* New York, National League for Nursing, 1975.

Fuchs, V. R.: Economics, health and post-industrial society, Milbank Memorial Fund Quarterly/Health and Society, 57:153, 1979.

Kalisch, P. A., and Kalisch, B. J.: *The Advance of American Nursing.* Boston, Little, Brown and Co., 1978.

Lasch, C.: *The Culture of Narcissism: American Life in an Age of Diminishing Expectations.* New York, W. W. Norton & Co.. Inc., 1979.

Milio, N.: A framework for prevention: Changing health — damaging to health — generating life patterns. Am. J. Pub. Health, 66:435, 1976.

Rice, D. P., Feldman, J. J. and White, K. L.: *The Current Burden of Illness in the United States.* Washington, D.C., Institute of Medicine, National Academy of Sciences, 1976.

Rosen, G.: *From Medical Police to Social Medicine: Essays on the History of Health Care.* New York, Neale Watson Academic Publ., Inc., 1974.

Spitz, B.: When a solution is not a solution: Medicaid and health maintenance organizations. J. Health Pol., Policy and Law 3:497, 1979.

Wald, B., and Dubos, R.: *Only One Earth: the Care and Maintenance of a Small Planet.* New York, W.W. Norton & Co., 1972.

Wortman, S., and Cummings, R. W.: *To Feed This World.* Baltimore, The Johns Hopkins University Press, 1978.

CHAPTER 2

THE NATURE OF COMMUNITY HEALTH NURSING: DEFINITION AND ROLE

Community health nursing is more than simply nursing outside a hospital. It is more than the implementation of measures for the protection of public health. It is a unique blend of nursing and public health practice woven into a service that, properly developed and applied, can have a tremendous impact on human well-being.

The *basic purpose* of community health nursing is to further community health through the selective application of nursing and public health measures within the framework of the total health effort.

The nature of any human service will, of course, be constantly challenged and changed by the goals and constraints of the social milieu in which it functions and by the varying capabilities and commitments of those who provide the service. However, it is essential to consider the phenomenon of community health nursing as it operates (or purports to operate) today in order to understand the dynamics of practice in this field. The discussion that follows is based upon a number of assumptions:

1. Community health nursing is a recognizable, though not sharply defined, area of health practice.
2. Community health nursing operates as a subsystem of the health and human services systems.
3. Community health nursing is responsive to the expectations of society and the professions and shapes its roles accordingly.
4. Community health nursing accomplishes its purpose through the application of a defined process.

Definition Is Difficult

As the health services move strongly into a systems organization, the blurring of professional lines is inescapable, and a clear definition of practice for any group of workers becomes difficult. For example, community health nurses may provide primary health care — but so do many physicians, short-trained primary health workers, indigenous healers, or hospital-based nurses. Preventive nursing may be hard to distinguish from preventive medicine, and nursing consultation from health education or social work. Responsibilities and roles can change so rapidly that any definition is obsolete even before it is generally accepted. Certainly, *definition,* in the sense of "to fix the boundaries of" or "to fix or lay down definitely," is impossible. Nevertheless as Helvie and coworkers point out, there are some differences between community health nursing and nursing in another setting: in patterns of practice, in the relative emphasis, and in the nature of the caseload.[1]

Fortunately, the dictionary provides another meaning for *to define* — "to explain the nature and the essential qualities of."[2] In this sense, it is possible to provide a descriptive definition for community health nursing as a service and as a field of professional practice, considered within the context of today's industrialized country.

COMMUNITY HEALTH NURSING: A DESCRIPTIVE DEFINITION

Community health nursing is an area of human *services* directed toward developing and enhancing the health capabilities of people — either singly, as individuals, or collectively, as groups and communities. The goal of community health nursing is to enable people to cope with the discontinuities in and threats to health in such a way as to maximize their potential for high-level wellness as well as to promote reciprocally supportive relationships between people and their physical and social environment.

Community health nursing has a responsibility for the total population within a defined area or environment as well as to the individuals and families whose well-being is essential for community health. It is concerned primarily with conditions that are continuing rather than episodic and with situations in which the results of care depend predominantly upon the decisions and responses of the people involved rather than upon the highly specialized personnel and "hardware" characteristic of the large hospital or medical center.

Community health nursing represents a subsystem to the larger health and human services system of the community, and consequently, is committed to share responsibility for the health program as a whole, and to interdependent as well as independent action in the accomplishment of its own purposes.

Community health nursing is also an area of professional nursing and public health *practice* characterized by the systematic application of selected nurturing, medicotechnical, educational, or social-action skills for the analysis and amelioration of personal or community situations inimical to preserving health. Community health nursing action may be directed toward inciting or managing change in the health status or health behavior of a designated population, or in the physicial or social environment in which the population functions. In addition, community health nursing may be directed toward changing the relationship between the population and the health or health-related care systems developed to serve it.

The definition just outlined suggests certain characteristics that might be expected of community health nursing.

Community Health Nursing Focuses On the Community

Implicit in this definition is the precept that the focus of community health nursing is the community: the direction of the nursing program is shaped by the needs of the community as a whole and by the nature of the total community health effort.

The health of the community is as much the product of its physical and social environment, institutions, and interactions as it is that of the condition of health of its population. The interchange between the individual and his environment— whether the microcosm of family and immediate neighbors or the macrocosm of the city, county, or country— is a determining factor in family and community health. Improving that relationship is one of the major channels for improving health.

A Family Service Unit

The problems encountered in community health nursing are such that their origin, impact, and solution are familial rather than individual. The obese person needs help from other family members on the problems of dietary control. The family must be willing to remove the temptations to overeating, to provide approved foods, and to encourage restraint. This concept is not synonymous with a family *focus* — in which one looks at the family to see how it relates to the care of an individual member; rather, it concerns the care of the family as a whole, including all of its individual members, and the dynamics of interacting and decision making through which the family operates.

A Wide Range of Problems

Whether in Taiwan or New York City, the community health nurse cannot limit her attention to the individuals or families in her caseload.

She must be equally concerned with those who may need care but have not sought it or have been unable to find it. It is not enough to give the very best and most complete care possible to a small segment of the population, while others are left without any care at all; nor is it possible to limit community health nursing to "patient" care. The community health nurse must be as concerned with the safety implications of a new swimming pool and the alienating effects of ghetto psychology as she is with the individual who has a diagnosed illness. She must also be concerned with health-related factors such as the ways in which welfare money is administered — since this affects family budgeting and buying habits and, consequently, the family's ability to remedy nutritional deficiencies — or the degree to which the school is involved with the community — since this affects the recreational and social behavior of the adolescent population and may therefore have a part to play in the control of venereal disease or pregnancy among unmarried teenage girls.

Special Skills Required

Just as surgical nursing involves some procedures that are common to both the surgeon and the nurse, and just as psychiatric nursing requires some procedures that are common to the psychiatrist and the nurse, so community health nursing involves some procedures, skills, and knowledge that are common to all public health practitioners. The diagnosis of community health problems — the institution of measures designed to evaluate, protect, and advance the health of the population as a whole — requires special competence in epidemiologic methods, in the interpretation of biostatistical reports, and in community organization and planning. None of these special skills can replace the basic nursing skills, which are equally important in the provision of community nursing service; rather, they are necessary supplements, which are especially useful when the community health nurse is working in a small agency with minimal immediate nursing and public health supervision.

Nursing skills required in community health nursing may also differ from those in other fields. Care of minor diseases rarely seen in the hospital, management in delegating care to others and coordinating services from many other sources, estimation of vulnerability (either general or specific), and investigation of precursor symptoms — all are areas of nursing practice prominent in community health nursing.

A Generalized Approach

Although community health agencies may include specialists on their staff, community health nursing, on the whole, is a generalized practice. As will be discussed further on, community health nursing may be provided through many different services and under many sponsorships within a given locality. However, the community health nursing effort for the community as a whole must be involved in the entire spectrum of health services, since the object of the service — the community — is made up of people of all ages who are afflicted with a variety of diseases; faced with a multitude of genetic, psychological, social, and environmental threats to health; and hampered or helped by many different sorts of health practice.

Many of those served by the community health nurse will not be sick at all, but may need preventive supervision during periods of stress. Vulnerable groups (as, for instance, children coming from broken homes or suffering from physical or emotional deprivation) may require special protection. Anticipatory guidance, such as preparing a geriatric patient for problems associated with the aging process or readying the family of a hospitalized psychiatric patient for his return, takes an important place in health care. The community health nurse must be concerned with pre-disease manifestations or indications for preventive or supportive medical care that, in other settings, would be recognized by the physician or noted in routine medical or laboratory examinations.

At the same time, the community health nurse will be increasingly concerned with a variety of illnesses and injuries being cared for outside the hospital. In one day, she may serve families who are coping with a variety of situations — tuberculosis, pregnancy, mental illness, or the supervision of a healthy school child. Thus, it can be seen that, above all, the community health nurse is a generalist.

A Long-Term Commitment to Care

Several factors combine to produce a long-term commitment in community health nursing service. The high level of chronic illness and disability due to aging requires care over a long period of time. The advantages of health care outside the hospital place many of those needing help within the jurisdiction of the community health nurse. The importance of developmental guidance throughout the life cycle and recognition of the basic obligation of each family and group to take responsibility for its own health offer new opportunities for community health nursing in terms of extended monitoring and counseling. It is also important to know that the future of preventive care depends, in large measure, upon behavioral changes in the population — the wise use of alcohol or drugs, the avoidance of creating risks to others, and the habit of mutual help for common problems — behavior that must be developed over long periods of time.

Independent and Interdependent Action

Much of the work of community health nursing is performed in the home or in small groups. Thus, it is not always possible to anticipate the problems that will arise. In these situations, the community health nurse will not have immediate access to the advice of a physician or a senior nurse. As a result, she is likely to be called upon to make decisions or to take action on her own initiative to a greater degree than might occur in another setting. She may be expected to make a decision on referring a child to a physician after a school mishap or on advising a family to stop medication pending investigation of symptoms by the physician.

The community nurse, like all nurses, is accountable to her client. However, lines of authority in the community setting may be different from those in the hospital or other work settings. There may be a framework of legislative requirements within which the work must be carried out; for example, health laws and regulations may require periodic vision and hearing tests for school children, or they may specify the procedures to be followed in the care of patients with communicable diseases.

In some instances, the community nurse will be accountable to more than one person. Certain aspects of her work may involve the school authorities, the family physician, or the medical director of the health unit. Although the nurse supervisor or administrator may be the mediator in the large agencies, in many instances the nurse will work within a general policy developed by her agency, and her responsibility in regard to another person or agency will be immediate and personal. Care of the individuals and families she serves may be shared by several other agencies or departments with whom she must find ways of working and coordinating.

Whatever the setting, the community health nurse must relate not only to the family as a unit of service but also to many individuals and special groups within the community and to the community as a whole. For example, the nurse in a rural county will work with individual families to provide preventive and curative nursing measures; she will also collaborate with teachers and other groups within the school to develop the nursing program, and with agricultural extension programs and community action groups to plan health education activities. Even though the distribution of effort and time among these various arenas will vary with different settings, community health nursing, by its nature, requires such collaboration.

In maternal care, for instance, the nurse may work with indigenous midwives. She may help plan for the development of better facilities for intrapartum care or, as a part of an effort to improve the statistical base for program planning, gather information about health problems related to pregnancy. She may also work with community resources for employment, housing, and welfare.

Activities Are Based in the Community Rather than in the Hospital

While some community health nurses function in hospitals, the great majority operate from a facility in the community that is close to those being served. Hospitals or professional schools that offer community health services as part of their general or educational program sometimes provide a separate community facility for this work. Many planners and practitioners believe that the community locus has many advantages over the more complex hospital center. Where "outreach" is important, this community locus places the workers close to their clients — where they identify with the community — and enables them to work in a setting that is conducive to informal relationships.

Community health nursing is a diffuse and highly diversified activity. Its commitments are broad, general in scope, and inclusive. The network of action through which its objectives are achieved involves many individuals, organizations, and institutions. In all areas of the work, collaboration with others is of primary importance.

COMMUNITY HEALTH NURSING: SYSTEMS, NOT SOLO PRACTICE

Community health nursing is not an individual and isolated action involving only the nurse and the client. It is a care *system*, operating within a galaxy of related care systems. The term "system," as used here, is defined as a collection of people, resources, and policies or processes united by a common purpose and organized to do a specific job.

The community health nursing system is a subsystem of the larger health system; it interacts with other systems operating in the community that are concerned with health or health-related problems. The family system, the larger community system, the hospital and medical care systems, the welfare system, and the political action system are all examples of related systems.

The personnel in a local community health system will vary in degree and length of experience. Staff may include administrators, clinical specialists, community health nurses and family health practitioners, registered nurses, practical nurses, aides, physical therapists, consumer advisers, and many more. These people may actually be employed by the agency, or they may be available to the agency through reciprocal agreements. In other instances, the local system may consist of a single community health nurse, supported by the supervisory and consulting personnel of a state agency, a part-time clerical worker, and volunteer workers recruited locally.

The physical plant and resources may be equally diverse; office space, records, supplies, equipment, and transportation may range from elaborate to minimal. The interrelating mechanisms — including such things as policy statements, procedural guides, interagency agreements or contracts, methods of communication and referral, collective bargaining structures, and fee arrangements — may also vary widely.

However simple or complex the system, each member must be able to function knowledgeably within it, recognizing the opportunities as well as the constraints such a systems orientation provides. An established relationship between the community health group and a welfare group that has been working with low-income families may provide an opportunity to consider innovative community health nursing measures in conjunction with the welfare program. However, an individual nurse should not take action independently. She should not, for instance, rush into offering evening services not previously afforded by the agency without realizing the effect such action might have on the insurance or maintenance costs of the agency, the demands that might arise within other groups, or her own availability for the regular work of the agency. These considerations are not necessarily restricting — it might be possible to set up an exploratory service, which later could be continued or possibly extended. The system should function so as to avoid premature or conflicting action, without discouraging initiative.

Families and communities also operate within their own systems. An understanding and appreciation of these systems and of the methods of moving within them are an integral part of community health nursing practice. The availability of resources will differ widely from one family to another. For purposes of planning, it is important that the nurse learn the different ways in which families go about the business of family life.

Community health nursing is part of the larger health and community system, the hospital and medical system, and the school and industrial health system. For instance, a plan to extend or exchange community health services for maternity patients and their families would be related to the programs being developed in the hospital, or perhaps to existing patterns of medical practice.

Interactions between the community health nursing system and the nursing and public health systems are particularly important. The basic nursing educational programs, the development of specialist roles for nurses, the standards set by professional nursing associations, the scope of services afforded in nursing as a whole and the health/manpower goals and programs — all affect what can be done in community health practice and service. Similarly, areas of intersection between the community health nursing system and the public health system include the expansion or contraction of the public health component, the admission polices of schools of public health, and the introduction of new categories of public health personnel.

The community health nurse should be prepared for intersystems action, so that she can work with existing systems and help to shape them. Simple communication and exchange of information facilitate intersystem action. In the service sector, intelligent referral practices, case conferences, and collaboration with an industrial personnel office are simple examples of intersystems effort. In the administrative sector, *ad hoc* committees representing several systems may be created to deliberate and suggest joint action on specific problems; participation may be sought in developing an overall policy for dealing with such things as methods of financing, services, exchange of documents, and documentation linkage with other agencies.

THE COMMUNITY HEALTH NURSE'S ROLE IS VARIED, DYNAMIC

The community health nurse plays an important role in the health system, and she herself is the heart of the community health nursing system. Her role will be influenced by several factors:
1. The nature of the health needs of the population.
2. The specific goals of the health care system in general and those of the system in which the nurse is working. The commitment to care may range from a total coverage program to one limited to emergency situations and major preventive measures for a selected high-risk population. Within the large system, the specific goals of the agency will affect the role of community health nurses.
3. The number and preparation of community health nurses, and of personnel in other categories that have overlapping or supplementary responsibilities (such as patient representatives or physician's assistants).
4. The customary patterns of practice and attitudes of other health care providers such as physicians, health educators, and indigenous health practitioners.
5. Public understanding and acceptance of or confidence in the community health nurse.

Clarification of the role of the community health nurse today is conditioned by an expansion of the nursing role in general, and by roles that the public has come to associate with community health nursing in the past.

An "Expanded Role" Creates New Boundaries, New Depth for Traditional Roles

Throughout its history, community health nursing has consistently enlarged its role in health care. However, during the last decade there has been a massive movement to enlarge and extend the role of nurses that is unprecedented both in scope and in potential impact. The stimulus for change came from many sources — physicians, nurses, administrators, and institutions. The causes were also mixed — to reduce the cost of medical care, to extend the scope of existing agencies, to reach populations currently unserved, to improve those aspects of health care not related to disease, and to provide a rewarding career for nurses whose primary interest lay in practice rather than in administration.

There was prompt and widespread endorsement of the idea. A committee convened by the Secretary of the U.S. Department of Health, Education, and Welfare in 1971 urged action to further expand the nurse's role.[3]

A host of programs under many types of sponsorship bloomed overnight — everything from short-term, on-the-job training in specific techniques such as physical examination or dialysis to lengthy, academic-based, degree-granting programs. A new (but far from descriptive!) title was devised — "nurse practitioner." The term "nurse practitioner" generally describes the nurse who has received education beyond the basic requirements for licensure as a registered nurse to prepare for expanded functions in diagnostic and treatment needs of patients — i.e., history taking, physical examination, ordering laboratory tests, and assuming responsibility for medical management of selected cases with emphasis on primary care. Many subspecialties have developed within this expanded role. These include pediatric, midwifery, maternity, family, adult, psychiatric, and emergency nurse practitioners.[4]

As of 1977, there were approximately 200 nurse practitioner programs in existence. A survey of these programs in 1977 projected that by the end of 1979, 16,000 nurses would have graduated from these programs with approximately 10.8 per cent employed in health departments and home health agencies and another 25.6 per cent employed in community-based clinics.[5]

New approaches to preparation were introduced.[6] Currently, certificate programs in various specialties are available that award continuing education credit, ranging in length from 9 to 12 months. These programs require licensure and malpractice insurance carried by the individual nurse. There are also a number of master's degree programs that offer an opportunity for more in-depth physiologic and behavioral science study as well as for longer periods of supervised clinical practice. Funds were made available at the federal level to stimulate development of nurse practitioner programs under the Nurse Training Act of 1975.

Certification of nurse practitioners to practice has not been uniform across the United States. A voluntary national certification program was begun by the American Nurses Association in 1973. The basic requirement is current licensure as a registered nurse and provision of direct patient care in the field in which certification is sought, as well as documentation of completed course work in an approved program. Alternative opportunities for certification are available to maternal-gynecologic-neonatal nurse practitioners through the Nurses Association of the American College of Obstetricians and Gynecologists, and to pediatric nurse practitioners through the National Board of Pediatric Nurse Practitioner/Associates. Some states also issue a certificate in addition to the registered nurse license. Nearly all states have made some attempt to consider and deal with the expanded role of nurse practitioners. Current revisions of Nurse Practice Acts are broadly worded and lessen restriction on nurses' activities, thus moving the legal definitions more in line with the scope of nursing projected for the future.

Nurse-midwifery also has experienced significant changes. The nurse-midwife is a registered nurse who has had formal theoretical and clinical preparation in the comprehensive care of mothers and infants throughout the maternity cycle. Her training includes management of delivery, procedures for the relief of pain and provision of assistance with family planning. She works with the obstetrician in sharing the responsibilities for the family under care. Nurse-midwifery has been shown to be a useful facet of care, and some reports indicate that it could be a factor in reducing the present infant death rate.[7]

Professional certification is mandatory rather than voluntary for nurse-midwives. All but two states, Kansas and Wisconsin, permit the full practice of certified nurse-midwives. These states require certification by the American College of Nurse-Midwives, in addition to current state nurse licensure.[8]

Unlike most countries, the United States has been slow to develop nurse-midwifery, and the use of lay midwives appears to be approaching the vanishing point. However, within this new climate of change and expansion, it seems inevitable that the approximately 1200 nurse-midwives practicing in the United States will be increased substantially.

There has been some concern about the development of these expanded roles for nurses, centering largely upon the unpredictability of the product of the educational programs, and the fear that the added responsibilities might actually reduce rather than enhance the nursing aspects of care.[9] But, on the whole, the record of experience with nurse practitioners has proven them to be attractive and productive members of the health care team; and they are generally accepted by other health care providers, by consumers, and by nurses themselves.

It is apparent that there is no such thing as the "typical" nurse practitioner; however, the following elements seem to recur consistently:

1. Inclusion of elements of practice (e.g., judgments, activities) traditionally considered as part of medical rather than nursing practice.
2. Increased independence of the nurse practitioner in the management of health care, with consequently increased accountability.
3. A collaborating rather than implementing relationship between the nurse and the physician.
4. Increased scope of concern in health care, especially in relation to the non-medical aspects of care.
5. In most instances, a commitment to the traditional nursing aspects of care.
6. An overflow effect from programs designed to prepare community health nurses at the specialist level into the area of more general

practice, so that the phenomenon of role enlargement affects all community health nurses to some degree.

The Community/Family Health Nurse Practitioner: Common Characteristics

An increasing number of service and educational agencies are engaging in the preparation of family and/or community health nursing practitioners. The variation in sponsorship, goals, curricula, and results is very great. There seems to be, however, some consistency in the conception of the role. In general, the practitioner is expected to perform essentially the same roles as the community health nurse, only more so. Primary care, for example, has long been a function of community health nursing — the nurse was often the first person on the scene in times of illness and the first to discover problems as she engaged in outreach activities. She was expected to use clinical judgment in deciding whether a patient needed a referral for medical care or in determining whether the school playground constituted a threat to health. Care of the unhospitalized sick has been a traditional area of community health nursing practice. The practitioner has enlarged this role by assuming management responsibility for the total health situation, by engaging in interventions formerly performed by physicians, and by enlarging the areas of personal decision in the total care process. Also, in the community phases of care, all community health nurses may engage in epidemiologic investigation, community organization and action, and management. The practitioner often brings greater knowledge and skills to the task and, thus, is able to operate at a more independent level.

The relationship between the skills and capabilities of the community health nurse and those of the community/family health nurse practitioner is such that it is fruitless to try to define two different sets of roles. Rather, it can be assumed that the roles will differ in scope and depth, depending on the preparation of the particular nurse.

CURRENT ROLES OF THE COMMUNITY HEALTH NURSE

Provider of Primary Health Care

Primary health care is the initial service provided when a client (either an individual or a family) enters the health care system seeking help with a particular episode of illness or a general health problem or disability. Primary health care is also the provision of continuing surveillance and management of problems in health maintenance.[10] In the past, these aspects of care have been managed rather haphazardly, with several different health care practitioners assuming some portion of the responsibility. All too often, the result was partial, fragmented, uncoordinated, and impersonal care. Later, it was recognized that designating one primary care referent (or source) would be a far more effective means of conserving professional effort and of motivating the client to use the health system wisely. This establishment of a "primary health care provider" assigns one person (who is both part of and accountable to the health care system) to perform this initial service. That individual (whether community health nurse, physician's assistant, physician, short-trained health worker, or other type of health personnel) becomes the person whom the client will first turn to for help in whatever health problem may arise. The client should expect the problem to be dealt with either by prompt provision of care or consultation or by referral to other sources of care.

When the community health nurse is the primary provider of health care, she is expected to ascertain from the client just what the problem is and what action seems indicated; she is expected to provide immediate assessment or care, which may be sufficient to deal with the problem or may lead to more intensive or different care. She is expected to serve as a triage agent in determining the relevance of available resources for the problems encountered; to effect referrals as necessary, with supporting data secured in the primary encounter; and, in general, to serve as a bridge between the client and the health care system.

In some settings, the level of knowledge and skills required for primary health care may go beyond that expected of the community health nurse. The skills required may be those traditionally found in medicine, social work, or public health practice, and the nursing skills required may go beyond those included in the basic community health nursing preparation. In such cases, additional preparation will be needed to fulfill this role.

Provider of Personal Care to the Unhospitalized Sick or Disabled

To many people, the words "nurse" and "care of the sick" are inseparable. Care of the sick, the disabled, and the dying has been a historical concern of community health nurses and remains a basic commitment. The current trend toward less indiscriminate use of hospitalization places new emphasis on this role. There are more sick and disabled people choosing to remain at home or in some informal community facility than has been true for several decades. Also an increasing number of people are choosing to have their babies at home or to die at home. The increased life span has resulted in a larger number of disabled elderly who need additional care.

In the early days of the visiting nurse, nursing was primarily seen as a service to the poor. However, it is recognized today that the need for nursing care at home or in a community facility exists at all economic levels. Diversification of the nursing staff has resulted in the delegation of some of the responsibility to other personnel — whether a registered nurse, a clinical nurse specialist, or a nursing aide. But caring for the unhospitalized sick remains an important obligation of every community health nurse.

A Willing, Knowledgeable, and Aggressive Advocate

With the advent of specialization in medical practice and the consequent fragmentation of health and other human services, the community health nurse is often seen as an advocate of and mediator for those being served. She is a kind of ombudsman in the home, solving a variety of problems — for example, she will try to explain to the doctor the difficulties of following a prescribed treatment regimen, expedite welfare action for the Medicaid patient, prod the housing authority to correct violations of the code, arrange for the sanitarian to visit the rural school, or talk to the school authorities when a student is repeatedly kept out of school to care for the home when someone is ill. The community health nurse is seen as someone who can stand between the family and the frustration, delay, and confusion caused by fragmented and depersonalized health services. She can speak for the client or, more importantly, help the client to speak for himself, when his needs are not being met, or for others, when community action (such as installation of a traffic light at a busy intersection) is needed.

An Approachable and Concerned Adviser

From the viewpoint of the recipient of community health nursing care, perhaps the most significant role attributed to the nurse is that of, as Gerald Caplan has called it, a "wise older sister." This implies a commitment to the individuals being served that goes beyond a casual interest or an impersonal provision of services. It involves identification with the problems that concern the patient and his family. The relationship is not one of equal exchange, however, because of the nurse's professional preparation; there is, in fact, a kind of claim on the part of the family for the nurse's concern, interest, and intervention on their behalf. The role of the nurse lies somewhere between that of teacher and collaborator, or between that of counselor and friend. This relationship can best be illustrated by the different ways in which patients approach the physician and the nurse. They generally regard the doctor as distant, formidable — someone not to be bothered with trivia. Patients are not afraid, however, to reveal themselves and their concerns to the nurse or to discuss problems with her which they might consider "too silly" to take to the physician.

Coworkers also use the nurse as an adviser. For instance, the health director may use her as a source of information about planning aspects of an immunization program; the school principal may consider her to be someone knowledgeable about the detection of disease among school children; the industrial physician may see her as a mediator who can anticipate problems in securing employee compliance with a cancer-screening program among workers; and the health council member may regard her as an alert observer who knows both the needs of the community and the reactions of the local population to health programs.

A Sensitized Observer

For other members of the health team, particularly the medical care team, the community health nurse's role as a sensitized observer is very important. The physician assumes that the nurse will be alert to any deviation from expected behavior in regard to illness, growth and development, response to drugs, and general well-being. He is also dependent upon the nurse to be sensitive to behavioral patterns and environmental conditions and to report those which are of importance in managing the case or in locating possible precursors of disease. In other words, he expects that she will be able to sort out and transmit to him those observations which are relevant to the situation.

Since the physician's contacts with the patient and his family may be brief and infrequent, the nurse's observations are especially needed concerning the home. For example, the pediatrician may rely on the nurse to evaluate the degree to which the father of a family is supporting the preventive care recommended for the children, the capacity of the family to carry through medical recommendations, and the degree of confidence the family has in the treatment he has recommended. Families, too, share this expectation of the nurse as an alert observer — frequently they will say of her, "I'm glad she came; she'd know if anything was wrong."

This role of sensitized observer extends to the community as well. It is assumed that the community health nurse will be aware of and will report any unusual occurrence of disease symptoms, environmental threats, or family and community stresses that may indicate a need for further epidemiologic, social, or environmental study or for political or neighborhood action.

One Who Influences Decisions and Produces Change

The community health nurse, by virtue of her expertise in public health practice as well as in nursing, is expected to influence decisions at the individual, family, and community levels and to effect change for more beneficial health care.

At the time that rural health services were being developed, the public health nurse was frequently the only representative of community health services. The employment of a public health nurse usually increased the likelihood of a more comprehensive health organization, and led to more medical supervision and prenatal care and a higher incidence of immunization.

Currently, as health care becomes more and more dependent upon the willing and informed action of the public, the community nurse has a more central role in enabling the individual, family, or group to make wise decisions about health, to take appropriate and prompt action, and to deal constructively with inescapable illness and death. Lundberg calls this role the "potentiator" — someone who serves as a catalyst and who is able to make others more effective.[11]

The community health nurse is expected to do the following: to increase the capacity of both the family and the community to cope with their health problems, as well as to provide them with care herself; to help school children utilize the educational facilities of the school more effectively; to bring accident control programs into the homes, schools, and industries of the community; and to encourage support and participation in the total health program. She faces a variety of problems: some are questions of logistics, such as poor scheduling in a crippled children's clinic; some are questions of attitude, such as distrust of any authoritative figure on the part of a low-income family. Still, the nurse is generally expected to "do something about it." She is relied upon to try to overcome whatever stands in the way of progress.

It is also expected that the nurse's efforts on behalf of change will extend to promoting action on more general fronts as she sees, interprets, and urges action with respect to unmet human needs or incongruous community responses to health-care requirements.

An Organizer and Manager

Whether in caring for a family or carrying out agency responsibilities in homes, schools, and places of employment, the community health nurse often performs as an organizer who welds the many aspects of service into some kind of suitable pattern.

She may be the person who keeps the clinic running smoothly, or the one who gathers together all of the many strands of care provided to a particular family, or the one who organizes and supervises auxiliary workers. She may identify, interpret, and maintain the linkages between hospital and community nursing services or between developments in professional nursing practice and the health agency program. In general, the nurse is the one who keeps things "under control."

Most importantly, the community health nurse is the natural partner of the family in establishing and maintaining a family health care program that brings to the family the health system. As a result, health status is monitored; appropriate preventive measures are taken; health deviations are promptly detected and treated; and, as much as possible, "habilitation" is substituted for "rehabilitation."

An Informed Participant in Community Planning and Action

Within deliberative groups in the agency and in the community, there is almost always provision for "a representative of nursing" or for someone who can provide the "nursing point of view."

The contribution provided by the community health nurse is important in molding decisions about not only nursing but also community health, and both the health and health-related facets of education and welfare programs. The community nursing representative can provide essential information for others to act upon, or she can be an active member of a deliberative group; in either capacity, the community health nurse is rarely absent from the decision-making arena.

Nursing knowledge and experience are important. Decisions concerning the timing of a particular program, the methods of approach that might be used in securing community participation and support, or the people who might be appropriately involved in carrying through community action programs all require both general professional skills and specific local knowledge. However, it must be added that the nurse's role as a decision-maker is sometimes clearer to the nursing profession than it is to others involved in the decision making!

Political intervention, as well as professional or technical, may be necessary. Public health is a political phenomenon, and advances in community health services often depend upon political action. Without engaging in partisan politics, the community health nurse can refer problems for consideration to appropriate political and bureaucratic groups. Feelings of alienation from the community, indifference to health care, or distrust of health service representatives are legitimate political concerns. Because of her close and continuing relationship with families, the community health nurse is apt to be aware of the need for political action before the point of confrontation has been reached. By providing information, suggesting positive action alternatives, or helping community groups to exercise their rights and obligations as citizens, the community health nurse may help relate humanistic goals to political reality and, thus, play a part in securing desirable health action.

A Contributor to Knowledge

The community health nurse is also expected to contribute to new knowledge — by conducting direct research or field studies, by contributing pertinent data to the research of others, by working on epidemiologic investigations, or by participating in multidiscipline or evaluative studies. The research most needed in public health today is in areas where community health nurses function primarily — areas involving the effects of behavior on health, the causative conditions or agents of disease, and the establishment of more useful indices of health.

Provider of personal care, advocate, teacher, counselor, observer, potentiator, organizer, and decision maker — in different ways and in varying degrees, the community nurse is expected to fill all of these roles. The nature and the scope of these expectations have a strong effect on what the community health nurse is able to do. The degree to which the expectations of others are congruent with those of the nurse herself will have much to do with the satisfaction she derives from her work.

REFERENCES

1. Helvie, C. O., Hill, A., and Bambino, C.: The setting and nursing practice, Parts I and II. Nurs. Outlook, *16*:27, 1968 and Part II *16*:35, 1968.
2. *Random House Dictionary of the English Language,* unabridged edition. New York, Random House, 1967, p. 379.
3. U.S. Department of Health, Education and Welfare: *Extending the Scope of Nursing Practice: A Report of the Secretary's Committee to Study Extended Roles for Nurses.* Washington, D.C., U.S. Government Printing Office, 1971.
4. Sultz, H. A., et al.: *Longitudinal Study of Nurse Practitioners, Phase III.* Washington, D.C., U.S. Government Printing Office, DHEW Pub. No. HRA 80–2, 1980, p. 44.
5. Ibid, p. 104.
6. See Chow, R. K.: Research + primex = improved health service. Int. Nurs. Rev., *19*:314, 1972; Coulehan, J. L., and Sheedy, S.: The role, training, and one year's experience with a medical nurse practitioner. Health Services Rep., *88*:827, 1973; State laws recognize expanded role of nurses, Am. J. Nurs., *73*:1169, 1973; and Kelly, L.Y.: Nurse practice acts. Am. J. Nurs., *74*:13, 1974.
7. See Record, J. C., and Cohen, H. R.: Introduction of midwifery in a prepaid group practice. Am. J. Pub. Health, *62*:354, 1972; Meglen, M. C., and Burst, H. V.: Nurse midwives make a difference. Nurs. Outlook, *20*:386, 1974; and Levey, B. S., Wilkenson, F. S., and Marine, W. A.: Reducing neonatal mortality rate with nurse midwives. Am. J. Obstet. Gynecol., *109*:50, 1971.
8. *Supplemental Information on Nurse Practice Acts.* Washington, D.C. American College of Nurse-Midwives, 1980.
9. See Rogers, M.: Nursing — to be or not to be? Nurs. Outlook, *1*:42, 1972 and Weston, J.: Whither the "nurse" in nurse practitioner? Nurs. Outlook, *23*:148, 1975.
10. Extending the Scope of Nursing Practice, op.cit., p. 8.
11. Lundberg, H. G.: A community health potentiator. Nurs. Outlook *14*:43, 1966.

SUGGESTED READINGS

Anspach, E., Casbeer, M. E., Halfman, J., and Landholm, J.: Johnny and the school nurse practitioner. Am. J. Nurs. *74*:1099, 1974.

Archer, S., and Fleshman, R.: *Community Health Nursing.* North Scituate, Mass., Duxbury Press, 1979.

Berger, M., Rennert, E., George, H., and Schwartz, B.: A case study in professional collaboration. Nurs. Outlook, *20*:714, 1972.

Bernstein, L., and Dana, R. H.: *Interviewing and the Health Professions.* New York, Appleton-Century-Crofts, 1970.

Birckhead, L. M.: Automation of the health care system: Implications for nursing, Part 1. Int. Nurs. Rev. *22*:28, 1975.

Blair, K. K.: It's the patient's problem — and decision. Nurs. Outlook. *19*:587, 1971.

Bullough, B.: Is the nurse practitioner role a source of increased job satisfaction? Nurs. Res., *23*:14, 1974.

Burnett, R. D., and Bell, L. S.: Projecting pediatric practice patterns. Pediatrics, *62*(Supplement):625, 1978.

Cady, L.: Extending the role of public health nurses. Nurs. Outlook. *22*:636, 1974.

Cleland, V.: Implementation of change in health care systems. J. Nurs. Admin., *2*:64, 1972.

Congressional Budget Office, Congress of the United States: *Physician Extenders: Their Current and Future Role in Medical Care Delivery.* Washington, D.C., U.S. Government Printing Office, 1979.

Davidson, N.: Definition of an expanded role: The nurse midwife. Nurse Pract., *1*:26, 1975.

Diers, D., and Molder, S.: Some conceptual and methodological issues in nurse practitioner research. Res. Nurs. Health, *2*:73, 1979.

Farrand, L. L., and Cobb, M.: Perceptions of activities performed in ambulatory care settings. Nurs. Pract., *1*:69, 1975.

Freeman, R. B.: *Some Observations on the Use of Nurse Practitioners in Community Health Nursing.* New York, National League for Nursing Pub. (21–1570) 57–64, 1975.

Ford, L. C.: A nurse for all settings: The nurse practitioner. Nurs. Outlook, *27*:516, 1979.

Hall, V. C.: *Statutory Regulation of the Scope of Nursing Practice: A Critical Survey.* Chicago, National Joint Practice Comm., John Hancock Center, 1975, p. 51.

Hall, V. E., and Weaver, B. R.: *Distributive Nursing Practice: A Systems Approach to Community Health.* Philadelphia, J. B. Lippincott Co., 1977, Chapter 11.

Health Care in the 80's, Who Provides? Who Plans? Who Pays? New York, National League for Nursing, Inc., NLN Pub. No. 52–1755, 1979.

Henry, D. M.: Progress of the nurse practitioner movement. Nurse Pract., *3*:4, 1978.

Lewis, C. E., et al.: Activities, events and outcomes in ambulatory patient care. New Engl. J. Med., *280*:645, 1969.

Nuckolls, K. B.: Who decides what the nurse can do? Nurs. Outlook, *22*:626, 1974.

Strovan, C., Anderson, E. T., and Gottscholk, V.: Community nurse practitioner: An emerging role. Am. J. Publ. Health, *64*:847, 1974.

Slone, C., et al.: Effectiveness of certified nurse-midwives: A prospective evaluation study. Am. J. Obset. Gynecol. *124*:177, 1976.

Spitzer, W. O., et al.: Burlington randomized trial of the nurse practitioner. New Engl. J. Med. *290*:251, 1974.

Health — United States, 1979. Chapters on Manpower. DHEW, PHS. National Center for Health Statistics. Washington, D.C., U.S. Government Printing Office, 1979.

CHAPTER 3

COMMUNITY HEALTH NURSING: THE PROCESS

Community health purposes and goals are realized through engagement in a process: an orderly series of steps that, if taken, are expected to lead to a desired result. The process is generic to problem solving, and predictably the steps will have much in common with the processes found in other helping professions such as medicine and social work. The uniqueness of the process as used in community health nursing will depend on the nature of both the end, which is the best possible application of nursing to the community's health problems, and the means, which is a synthesis of nursing and public health skills.

Six major steps may be identified in this process:

1. Establishing, reinforcing, or maintaining working relationships with clients, coworkers, and the public.
2. Assessing the situation as it relates to health and nursing care as well as to the balance between health conditions and the reinforcing or countervailing forces that mediate them.
3. Developing and negotiating action goals with clients and coworkers.
4. With collaboration of client and others involved in the process, deciding among possible courses of action.
5. Developing a step-by-step course of action, including check points.
6. Validating or evaluating the action taken.

Even though the problems confronting the nurse will vary considerably, the process by which she moves to deal with them should remain constant. Whether she is working with an individual being treated in a venereal disease clinic or with a community organizing to prevent accidents on the highway, the same steps will be utilized in moving toward a solution.

The process by which an effective community health nursing program is established involves the integration of the decisions and actions of many workers, both professional and nonprofessional. The decisions of the client — whether a family, a fellow health professional, or a community committee — must be developed and reconciled with those of the nurse in a way that makes the final action satisfactory to both parties.

The family, as well as the nurse, decides the kind of relationship or interchange that will be acceptable as a "working" relationship; the community planning committee, as well as the nurse, will define the goals that should govern the action to be taken; the medical director, as well as the nurse, will be involved in determining the effectiveness of the nursing services provided.

A WORKING RELATIONSHIP IS ONE THAT WORKS

A "working relationship" is one that permits both provider and user of care to clarify and accept their perceptions and feelings, and to mobilize and fuse their efforts to improve the situation. It rests upon four basic assumptions:

1. The sovereignty of the client in making health care decisions (so long as these decisions do not endanger other people).
2. The obligation of the professional to resist "overselling" the client on a particular plan or course of action — health is a factor that may affect the quality of life, not an inevitable good.
3. The economy of coordinating and conserving the efforts of multiple sources or providers of service.
4. The uniqueness of every situation, mandating a wide variation in possible interaction.

A good working relationship is the base on which to develop the ability and willingness of individuals, families, and community groups to make careful decisions, to persist in a long course of action, or to change fundamental patterns of living. To achieve this base, the nurse must draw out and clarify the attitudes and feelings that influence the client's evaluation of the problem. A good relationship helps accomplish the goals of the community health nursing service and becomes the foundation for all subsequent nursing action.

Characteristics of a Working Relationship

Productivity

The primary criterion for a working relationship is that, in the long run, it produces the intended results. Thus, when an emergency makes immediate hospitalizaton imperative but both patient and family are too distraught to think clearly, an authoritarian or "hard sell" approach may be entirely appropriate. However, if the situation involves the need to find a nursing home for a geriatric patient whose presence in the home is threatening the well-being of other family members, an authoritarian relationship may be totally inappropriate. A commanding manner may produce immediate results in terms of initiating nursing-home care, but the *decision* will not have been made by the family; moreover, all of the possible factors will not have been discussed and evaluated in advance. Consequently, the long-term result may be the return of the patient to the home, or the development of emotional problems among guilt-ridden family members as a result of a lack of confidence in the decision that has been made. The situation may thus be aggravated, not improved.

Mutual Trust. Trust is the *sine qua non* of any truly joint endeavor. If the family members see the nurse as a representative of the authorities who have the power to cut off welfare aid or if they see her as someone too well-off, too young, or too protected to accept them as they are and to appreciate real-life problems, they are unlikely to trust her sufficiently to reveal their true feelings. If the nurse expects her clients to be lazy, unwilling, or unable to do what is expected of them, she too will find it hard to deal openly and objectively with the problems at hand. Both the nurse and the client must be confident of the other's basic integrity. Even though differences in cultural or educational background may create differences in value concepts or in behavioral patterns, mutual respect is imperative before a working relationship can be established.

If they are to work together effectively, the recipient of care must feel that the nurse's main concern is the good of the family (or the good of the agency or the community) and that her primary objective is to help. The nurse, in turn, must feel that those with whom she is working sincerely desire to improve the situation and that each individual with whom she deals is a person of worth and consequence.

These concerns are important in other relationships as well. The physician-administrator must trust the nurse to share a commitment to the program as a whole, and the nurse must trust the administrator's good faith in decisions affecting nursing; agencies must trust in the good intentions and integrity of other community institutions.

Trust must be earned — it isn't provided free, although the traditions of nursing may give the community health nurse a head start. Simple courtesy, rigorous fulfillment of commitments, explicit explanation of the reasons underlying a particular attitude or decision, patience, respect, and tolerance — all are required to earn the trust that must exist.

Empathy. Empathy is an essential ingredient in any helping relationship. As a basis for planning specific health care, it is necessary to see another person's problem through his eyes and to try to understand his attitudes. The professional health worker who is trying to make joint decisions with care recipients must have an undistorted picture of how his clients feel about their health problems and about the health-care system. This kind of understanding rests for the most part on the ability to sense the feelings of others — to accept, rather than to judge, the ways in which people relate to their world. The health professional must have the capacity not only to emphathize with another person but also, when the occasion demands, to become an objective observer and planner.

"Getting involved," once considered a hazard to sound decision making, has become respectable. The advocacy and political action roles of nurses have become clearer, and they have gained greater experience in nursing estranged groups.

Outreach

Outreach — i.e., taking the initiative, as in introducing discussion of a problem or in offering assistance — has assumed greater importance. Recent studies of the failure of community services to reach certain segments of the population suggest that many families and groups, especially those living in poverty, take a passive role with respect to the community services offered to them. There may be many causes for this: a failure to recognize that a problem exists; a feeling that clients are expected to be grateful and undemanding; or an inability to articulate needs. In such cases, the service personnel must take the initiative rather than wait for requests for care or for information to be volunteered. The nurse must undertake the responsibility to visit families not currently under care, or to introduce the topic of birth control, or to propose greater involvement in specific health matters.

Open Communication. Open communication is basic to all nursing practice. It is characterized by a willingness to reveal one's self to others — to take the risk of exposing feelings, attitudes, and anxieties through verbal or nonverbal means. It occurs between groups or among members within a group, as well as on a one-to-one level.

When one of the communicators is a professional, communication can present particular problems. The community health nurse, through education and experience, has accumulated a store of information and skill that can "help" others, and she will be anxious to share this knowledge. The client may see the nurse as an expert, someone who can give advice or provide answers. Often, unwittingly, the nurse becomes a teacher or rescuer; ideally, she should play the role of supporter, helping the client to understand his situation and thus gain mastery over his problems.

All too often, open communication is not achieved. Constant vigilance is required to avoid premature professional intervention: impatience, hastiness, cutting short the exploration and verbalization of feelings by premature "reassurance" or summarization and interpretation. What is desired is a comfortable relationship through which the client gains confidence in his own capacity to deal with the problems facing him.

Confidence. A working relationship must be based on the assumption that the relationship is worthwhile, that something will come of it. Both the nurse and those with whom she works must be convinced that the nursing input (that is, what the nurse does) has relevance and is likely to help. The family must feel that the nurse's advice regarding prenatal supervision is truly germane to their well-being; the public health physician consulting with the nurse must feel that the suggestions she offers are practically related to the problems of the program as a whole.

On the other hand, the nurse, too, must have confidence in those she serves. She must accept the validity of a parent's estimate of the probable behavior of his offspring. She must accept behavior different from that which the nurse herself would find natural — for example, the overstriving of the suburban middle class parent or the all-or-nothing orientation of an adolescent — without letting this difference undermine or distort her belief in the basic competence of most people to make wise decisions and to consider the alternatives in a rational way.

Fostering Development

A working relationship is one in which those involved build upon one another's abilities so that each grows through encounter with the other. The ego-damaged parent living in a low-income area may gain strength and self-confidence through the way in which the community health nurse provides help. If the nurse is willing to expose her own thoughts and feelings, she may promote a similar response on the part of the client. This, in turn, will increase the nurse's ability to help both family and community.

Moreover, a building relationship is concerned with general as well as specific development. The abilities to solve problems, to deal with daily tasks more effectively, and to gain a little insight into problems in wider spheres of action are as important in building health competence as they are in providing satisfactory measures of personal development.

A Working Relationship Is Developed, Not Discovered

Few practitioners develop their capacity for using interpersonal relationships to the fullest. Certainly, the ability to use one's relationship with others as a means of achieving service goals should continue to grow with professional maturity and experience. However, it cannot be assumed that experience alone will assure this growth. There is need for a firm conviction that such relationships are an integral part of successful practice and that a persistent effort toward improvement of interpersonal skills is both necessary and rewarding.

Stop, Look, Listen — and Wait

Health problems that, at first glance, seem glaringly apparent and amenable to a quick solution may prove much more involved when the situation is carefully reviewed. Stereotyped views of thinking can produce quick responses — e.g., babies born out of wedlock are unwanted; black families are matriarchal; politicians care only for votes; nurses are highly motivated to do good — but these attitudes are likely to lead to irrelevant care for the client, and to careless observation in general. Each person, each situation, and each community must be seen as unique. For example, it is helpful to know that many unemployed men who are heads of families may feel inadequate and that this feeling could be reflected in their relationships with professional personnel and neighbors; however, what is basic to establishing a working relationship is how *this* particular breadwinner feels about his inability to provide for *his* family, and how these feelings are likely to affect his dealings with the providers of health care.

Observation. Learning about diseases is relatively easy; learning about people, considerably less so. Much will be learned by observation — the way a mother holds her infant; the pride or exasperation in the voice of a patient telling about the members of her family during the taking of a family history; or the presence or absence of hobby equipment, play facilities, and religious artifacts in a home. But observation alone is not enough; the nurse must be willing to relax, to absorb atmospheres, to "sop up" the moods and manners of her clients. She must temporarily put aside all of the pressures of her own work in order to tune in the family or group to understand what they are trying to communicate — though this communication may involve no words, or words that express something quite different from their literal meaning.

In any interpersonal exchange there are clues to meaning that are essential guides. Hodgins explains this well when describing the silent patient who may be saying by his silence that he thinks no one wants to help, that no one can help, or that no one can be trusted to deal with him honestly. The family member who agrees too quickly to suggestions that are bound to be hard to carry out, the family physician who talks about the "wonderful girls in the VNA" but who seldom refers a patient, the adolescent who shows no concern over the possibility that he has contracted gonorrhea: each is saying something of importance; and, by the way they select what they say or do not say, they are expressing the quality of the relationship that has been developed.[1] The virtue of quiet repose — listening without talking — cannot be overestimated as an investigative method.

In community health nursing, getting to know the patient also involves becoming acquainted with the environment in which he lives. A patient divorced from his environment cannot be accurately evaluated. Nor, for that matter, should a particular social climate be condemned at first impression. An environment that, to the nurse, seems grossly inadequate for the needs of the community may in fact be the lesser among the available evils. Peripheral benefits such as reliable neighbors or a strong sense of community may be more important to some groups than physical amenities. How the environment affects the nurse is not germane; what is important is how it affects her patients.

Service records and conferences with other workers who have known the family are excellent sources of information. Reading about cultural patterns that prevail in subgroups of the population will also help in understanding the families with which the nurse works, thereby making it easier to build bridges between her own experiences and values and those of her clients.

Declare in Explicit Ways the Intention to Help

There are many ways of declaring oneself as committed to helping. Some of these are verbal, such as invitations to communicate ("Would you like to talk about it?" or "I would like to try to understand") or offers to initiate action ("Perhaps it would help if I talked to the school physician" or, to a committee, "I will try to get the reports we need from the Health Department").

However, there is also great force in nonverbal expression. Johnson points out the significance of touch in nursing practice.[2] Similarly, the nurse's facial expression (such as one showing shock or disapproval), her manner of wearing a uniform, her style of dress when not in uniform, or her bodily posture (such as a pose that suggests she is ready for flight) may all serve to alienate the family.

When there are obvious differences in the backgrounds of the nurse and her client, the identification of shared interests (such as raising children, cooking, or growing plants) may diminish barriers and indicate the nurse's intention to establish some common bonds.

Doing something tangible to help is one of the most effective means of developing a successful working relationship. Whenever possible, nursing service should provide immediate and responsive action. For example, it may be possible to provide help with a problem immediately instead of putting it off until another visit, or to provide treatment in the home rather than in a clinic (particularly if getting to the clinic involves a long tedious trip across town). Agency policies may not foster this kind of action (especially in the latter case), but if it appears to be a helpful approach, the field nurse may urge that policies be revised.

On extremely rare occasions, mandatory actions required for the protection of the public may be resisted by an individual or group, and the nurse may be regarded as an enforcer rather than as a helper. For example, certain immunizations may be required as a prerequisite for admission to school, and some parents may believe that the requirement is unnecessary or goes against their religious principles. In these instances, mediation and explanation of the rights of others in the community may do much toward securing voluntary compliance and preserving the threatened relationship. Should all efforts at voluntary compliance fail, a full explanation of the nurse's obligation to report the incident and her acknowledgment of the right of the individual to hold an opposite view (even if it could not prevail) may leave a foothold for more productive relationships at a later time.

Go the Second Mile

> Whosoever shall compel thee to go a mile,
> Go with him twain.
>
> (ST. MATTHEW, 5 V. 41)

For the professional health worker, the development of a relationship with others may require that she go more than halfway. This second mile may be the willingness to take the initiative in offering help or to wait for another individual to reach the point of being able to engage fully in an interchange or to offer help over and over again in different forms if there is evidence of need for such help and if there is the possibility of making it acceptable to the recipient.

The desired goal is to make the client able to manage his own health problems through use of the services available to him. In order to achieve this, the relationship must be one that fortifies rather than diminishes the patient. Hodgins illustrates this with the example of a professional who refuses to share what he knows with a stroke patient while engaging in an exclusive medical discussion about the patient at his bedside; this diminishes the sufferer and makes him less able to deal with his already severe problems of adjustment.[3] The failure to listen to the family's plan for treatment before proposing action or to view family health care as a concern of the father as well as of the mother may be equally diminishing and, hence, may move one away from the goal rather than toward it.

The Nurse Must Teach Others How to Establish and Maintain Working Relationships

A relationship is something that cannot be created by one person. Parents must develop a working relationship with their children; they must earn trust, learn to communicate, and remember the importance of interpersonal relationships in the development of children. The nurse's aide or home nurse must learn to use her relationship with the patient in a knowledgeable way and balance her own need to be appreciated and liked with the patient's need to develop self-reliance.

Thus, the community health nurse must teach as well as practice the development and maintenance of working relationships. Such teaching should serve to deepen her own understanding and skills as well as to increase the interpersonal capabilities of her clients.

ASSESSMENT IS MORE THAN A LAUNDRY LIST OF PROBLEMS

Assessment — defining the nature and the essential aspects of the problem to be dealt with — determines the conditions for nursing intervention. Precision in selecting the amount and type of nursing intervention to be employed, efficient definition of the nurse's case load and priorities, and valid evaluation of the results of service are all dependent on this first critical step. In future chapters, we will consider the application of assessment to family and community health; the purpose here is to discuss the nature of the assessment process.

A Tool for Action

The purposes of nursing assessment are, first, to provide an estimate of the degree to which a family, group, or community is achieving the level of health possible for them; second, to identify specific health deficiencies or guidance needs; third, to identify reinforcing or mitigating forces within this situation; and fourth, to estimate the probable effect of nursing intervention. In other words, the overall purpose is to evaluate the extent to which a community health nursing effort may be expected to close the gap between present and potential levels of health or between health behavior and health understanding.

The process of assessment is based upon the following assumptions:

1. The health conditions and problems in any situation are inextricably interwoven with social, cultural, economic, and environmental conditions.
2. Health problems and health needs are not synonymous:
   a. A health *deficit* occurs when there is a gap between actual and achievable health status.
   b. A health *need* exists when there is a health deficit that can be alleviated with present or probable levels of medical or social technology.
   c. A health *problem* is a situation in which there is a demonstrated health need combined with actual (or potential) resources to apply remedial measures and a commitment to act on the part of provider and/or user of care.

3. A variety of remedial measures exist for most health problems, as well as a variety of methods for applying these measures.
4. Perceptions of health problems vary widely among individuals, institutions, special populations, and societies.

Nursing assessment in community health situations differs somewhat in content, though not essentially in process, from that of acute care situations. Problems in community health lie more frequently within the areas of non-acute or minor illness and health maintenance and, therefore, tend to be less urgent. Many problems are amenable to care of the patient by his family, with support from the professional health worker. Many problems are anticipated rather than immediate. Clients contribute a major proportion of the care, with the professional standing by to reinforce and support.

Participation in the management of disease and disability is one important aspect of the work of the community health nurse. The nature and extent of illness and disability in a family, group, or community are vital determinants of nursing need and, therefore, represent data essential to the nursing assessment. But the nursing diagnosis focuses as much on the relationship between demands imposed by the disease, and the willingness and the capability of the family to deal with those needs, as it does on medical management. In fact, many of the situations with which the community health nurse will be concerned are not characterized by the presence of any illness or disability. Reducing smoking among school children, offering health guidance to expectant parents, promoting a screening program in a presumably healthy population, and improving relationships between generations in families are all examples of situations in which the emphasis is on *prevention of problems* rather than on the care of illness or disability.

Assessment is more than a "laundry list" of medical diagnoses or problems. Rather, it is a reasoned analysis of the health status of a particular client (whether an individual, family, or community) at a particular point in time as perceived by those responsible for dealing with the problems, and as related to the ability of providers and consumers of health care to deal with the situation.

The assessment process involves five steps; each step is taken with the active participation of the client (individual, family, community) in the decisions made and the conclusions reached.

1. Collection of subjective and objective data relating to health and illness, including social, environmental, or personal conditions that may be favorable or prejudicial toward health maintenance.
2. Identification of health deficits, health threats, and foreseeable crises or stress points. Health deficits have been defined above. Health threats are conditions that promote disease or injury and prevent people from thriving or realizing their potential. Health threats exist when the population is inadequately immunized against preventable disease, or when an individual (or group) smokes cigarettes, or when a new high-speed highway is installed. Other examples are: obesity

in an individual with a family history of diabetes and highly competitive social behavior in an upwardly mobile family. Foreseeable crises include stressful occurrences such as the death of a family member, relocation in a distant community, retirement, or abortion.

3. Exploration and evaluation of possible precursors of the health deficits noted, such as frequent headaches or gastric upset after starting a new job, a history of repeated infections or miscarriages, and inadequate parenting.

4. Estimation of the capability of the family or community with respect to the conditions identified. The health-care problems facing a community or family may range from a critical and urgent need for medical care to a lack of appreciation of the importance of social or intellectual development. In nursing assessment, it is important to focus on the nursing *problem* of the family or community rather than on the underlying *condition* that may have precipitated it. For example, pregnancy among young unmarried women is not a problem in the nursing or medical sense, if "problem" is defined in operational terms. It is a condition that may or may not produce problems of alienation, increased social dependency, or additional need for health and medical supervision. Thus, in this instance, the nursing problem is one of enabling the family to deal with its problems and properly utilizing health services rather than one of illegitimacy *per se*.

A typology developed by the nursing staff of the Richmond, Virginia Community Nursing Service suggests that family problems in nursing care management may be considered generically within a nine category system that is independent of any medical or developmental diagnosis. These problem categories are shown in the Appendix, The Family Coping Estimate. In practice, this model has proven to be useful in delineating the specific difficulties families face in managing their health problems and as a guide for nursing intervention.

The capacity of the family or community to cope with its problems and the description of the specific areas in which difficulty occurs are the next concern. In many instances, families or communities with rather substantial health problems may manage exceedingly well without assistance. The diabetic patient or his family may be perfectly able to provide the required care at home; they may know how to use the family or clinic physician wisely and may have adapted to the condition intelligently and serenely.

5. Estimate the impact of the health deficits identified, and the likelihood of reducing the impact through community health nursing action. Impact will vary not only with the nature and severity of the health deficit or threat but also with the strength or vulnerability of those affected by it. For example, a death in the family may have less impact if each member has a positive attitude toward death and the physical and spiritual strength to make the transition a reasonably comfortable one. Heavy cigarette smoking or failure to seek medical care for an undiagnosed lump in the breast has a high impact, both to

the individual who stands to lose his or her life and to the community in terms of economic loss. The relationship between deficit and coping may produce a situation that is threatening, disruptive of customary work or family life, stressful, costly, and diminishing to self-esteem.

The likelihood that community health nursing might reduce the impact of these conditions depends upon the ability of the family to cope with the situation, the availability of skilled nursing personnel, and the adequacy of community resources to deal with the immediate problem and with relevant causative factors.

With nursing assistance, the management of health care could be improved for the great majority of families and communities. However, there will be situations or aspects of care which, because of the nature of the problem or because of a dearth of health resources, no amount of professional health service could change. For example, the senile and slightly disoriented woman living alone, even with plentiful help from warm and responsible neighbors, may have unclean living quarters, a poor diet, and inadequate general supervision. However, if the patient values her independence above all else, if habits of hoarding and erratic eating are deeply rooted, and if the community cannot provide adequate care facilities, there is little likelihood that the nurse will be able to improve the situation.

It is important to determine the barriers and the strengths, internal or external, that block or invite achievement of satisfactory health action. Such barriers may be physical, social, economic, or perceptual; and they may exist in either the recipient or the provider of the care. It is at this point that the nurse should look realistically at what she can offer and the probable effect of such nursing intervention. The question is not what kinds of nursing action are *possible* in this situation but, rather, what kinds of nursing intervention are *likely to be effective* in this situation.

Based on the preceding considerations, the nurse should develop a problem list. This is a list of conditions prejudicial to health, with which the family or community cannot cope without help, which are likely to improve with help, and have or are likely to receive a commitment to action.

The diagnosis of many of these problems — such as the existence of pregnancy, the child already known to the courts as unruly, or a specific illness — involves data that are essentially objective or previously defined. However, diagnosis may also involve data that are more subjective, more subtle, and hazy. There is no statistical measure of how deeply the family feels about a particular problem, how far they are willing to go toward self-help, or whether the recommendation made by the "health establishment" is really relevant to them when all factors in the situation are considered.

In general, the problem list will be developed jointly by nurse and client. However, the nurse may recognize "incomplete" problems — situations where, although help is needed, there is no commitment to act because the community or family is already overwhelmed or resources are not yet available. In such instances, the nurse may put these problems aside until a more favorable time.

Thus, the process of assessment in community health nursing includes not only intensive fact finding, but also the application of professional judgment in the estimation of (1) the meaning and importance of these facts to the family and community, (2) the possible avenues of nursing service, and (3) the degree of change which nursing intervention can be expected to effect.

STATED GOALS GUIDE ACTION DECISIONS

A goal is, in effect, a declaration of purpose or intent that gives direction to action. Whether the service unit is an individual family, a community, or a nation, the development of clear-cut, feasible, and acceptable goals is basic to planning. Goals set the criteria for selecting an appropriate choice among possible courses of action, and also provide a yardstick for measuring progress. The joint development of goals by nurse and client may also provide a valuable experience in problem solving and decision making — general skills much needed by health care consumers.

Goals exist at all levels — ranging from the broad statement of the purposes of a program to the most explicit statement of desired results for an immediate and specific action. Frequently, there is an unfortunate tendency to concentrate on defining immediate and measurable results in order to get on with the job without clarifying the more general goals, which are sometimes described as "academic." However, it is usually true that specific goals have meaning only in the context of the general goals.

For example, placing an individual under care for gonorrhea may be an immediate goal, i.e., a response to the immediate task that has been assigned. However, broader goals — i.e., those concerned with preserving the family and enhancing individual potential — impose new responsibilities and constraints upon the nurse. Nursing care must, of course, be directed toward assuring necessary treatment for the individual and preventing the spread of infection by identifying and treating any of the patient's contacts who may also need care. However, in terms of the more comprehensive goal, the nurse's concern extends to more general problems related to the illness — such as its effect on the patient's self-image, its effect on his family relationships, and the need of his family and contacts for support and understanding. It involves trying to understand the situation more deeply: whether the infection is incidental or symptomatic of more fundamental emotional problems — for example, promiscuity growing out of a sense of frustration and isolation that, in turn, may have been engendered by unemployment.

Thus, the task of the nurse might involve supporting the family, helping the patient to express his concerns, or referring the patient to a community agency for job training, counseling, or psychiatric help.

Goals for health care will represent only one area of aspiration. The nurse will have goals relating to her personal or family life that may occasionally compete with the goals of her profession. A family may be committed to unusual responsibility for older dependent family members and yet want a college education for their children. The agency wants a broad spectrum of health services in which nursing constitutes only one part. The community wants roads and schools and welfare as well as health programs. Thus, the problem of formulating goals involves an understanding of the broader scene into which the nursing-care goals must fit.

Goals Should Be Set by Those Responsible for Their Implementation

In community health, the achievement of health is primarily the responsibility of the family or community and secondarily that of the health professional. Thus, families under care or community residents and groups eligible for care should have a major role in developing action goals. When professional goals are being set (e.g., for improvement of the quality of care or reorganization of the methods by which care is provided), the professional may have the major responsibility; nevertheless, the user or potential user of care also has an important part to play.

In collaboration with the nurse and/or other health professional, the family can decide what they most want to achieve in health care and the goals that must be reached to meet that end. The nurse provides necessary information, interprets the community health program, and guides the family by making sure they have considered all possible courses of action. The resulting goals are not the exclusive property of the nurse or the family but represent a fusion of judgment and commitment that provides a solid base for future action.

While "consumer inputs" are increasingly mandated in sponsored programs, not all families or community representatives are ready to participate fully. They may need to revise their concept of the nurse's role, or they may not be prepared to engage in joint decision making.

When Possible, Goals Should Be Stated in Behavioral Terms and with Specific Time Limits

Vague goals (such as "To improve the maternity experience") are not very useful in measuring the results of care — which is one of the functions a goal should fill. More explicit goals, such as "Encourage relaxed relationship with the baby" or "Dispel fear of leaving the baby with a qualified sitter" are more measurable. Setting a time limit is also useful; a goal such as "Enroll in mothers' class *next week*" may really bring results.

Health Goals Should Mesh with Other Goal Systems

Family nursing goals must be consistent with overall program goals, standards of care, and broad community goals. For example, goals for prenatal monitoring should be compatible with goals of the nursing profession regarding standards of care; goals for maternity care should be compatible with the medical goals for care and also with community goals concerned with protection of mothers and children as well as population control.

Statement of Goals Does Not Assure Acceptance

The community health nurse has special knowledge and, often, a kind of status that may cause families or community representatives to defer rather than contribute to her definition of goals or agree with her verbally without any true commitment to action. It is important, therefore, that the community health nurse learn as much as possible about the general goals of the family or community, so that she can judge whether the plans proposed are reasonably consistent with these goals. If there appears to be a discrepancy, this should serve as a signal to take another look.

It may be desirable to compromise on goals, even when no compromise is requested. For example, the nurse may see the need for an elderly disabled woman to become more independent, even though this independence will cost much effort and pain. The family may concur verbally, while actually holding the view that they should do everything possible for a beloved parent, relieving her of effort or pain whenever possible. The perceptive nurse may sense this, and in the interests of harmony put aside her plans for the time being. With experience, the family may come to realize the larger goal of the patient's needs.

To proceed on the basis of goals that are not understood and accepted by the recipient of care is likely to be a wasteful tactic. It must be recognized that the professional worker, despite his or her training, *can* be wrong.

A distinction must also be made between setting goals and then securing the compliance of others, and truly mutual goal setting. One of the goals in the process is to clarify and make explicit the commitment to action that is implied in the goal. In a successful coalition, the abilities and commitment of both nurse and recipient are merged to produce a viable objective.

Goals As Well As Performance Must Be Evaluated

Unrealistic goals exert a negative effect because they lead to disappointment, frustration, and a loss of confidence. In nursing care today, it is important that what is "reasonable" or "possible" is not confused with what can be done *under the present level and type of nursing intervention*. There is a danger of underestimating, as well as overestimating, the capacity of a family or group for self-help or for decision making, particularly if the family has fallen out of the habit of self-reliance or if the nurse has adopted an overly helpful stance that inhibits family initiative. Constant testing is required to see whether the goals really *can* be achieved and if the goals are challenging enough to stretch the capabilities of those involved.

The objective of goal setting in health care is to secure commitment to a clearly defined, desired outcome that is compatible with the life goals of the recipients of care and with the reality of the situation.

CONSTRUCTING A PLAN FOR ACTION

Planning for nursing care should be based on certain "watch words" that help to direct choices in the planning process:

1. **Self-help.** Promoting the capability of families and communities to deal with their own health problems is essential to assure coverage of the total population, to effect cost controls, and to help individuals achieve their potential more fully.

2. **Conservation.** Even in an affluent country, the need for care exceeds the available resources. The greatest possible conservation of human and material resources is essential to bring to the public the greatest possible return on its health care investment.

3. **Restraint.** It is important to be frugal when choosing between possible courses of action, so as to use the least costly approach that is most likely to produce the desired result.

4. **Accommodation.** To be effective, a program must be palatable to many diverse groups — the providers and consumers of health care, the poor and the well-to-do, the agency and the community, urban and rural dwellers. It must accommodate a variety of needs and a complexity of motives.

5. **Innovation.** The exploration of new strategies as well as the continuous refinement and modification of existing strategies is essential if programs are to remain relevant.

The planning phase of the community nursing process is concerned with:

1. Choosing among possible courses of action.
2. Selecting appropriate types of nursing intervention.
3. Identifying appropriate resources for care.
4. Developing an operational plan.

CHOOSING AMONG COURSES OF ACTION

In most instances, there will be more than one course of action that appears suitable to the problem. For example, five possible plans for providing personal care to the incapacitated arthritic patient could be considered: care could be furnished by the nurse herself, by a home health aide supervised by the community nurse, by a registered nurse who would provide care without the supervision of the community nurse, by a member of the family, or by some combination of the four. The selection of one course of action over another in this case would depend upon many factors — such as the acceptability of a specific plan to the family, the amount of expertise required in care and the seriousness of possible error, the expectation of the community, the availability of community nursing services, the sources of payment for nursing care, and the stamina and commitment of the family nurse. A limited range of possible choices in nursing action may result in stereotyped or ritualistic practice, which tends to diminish the relevance and impact of the action taken.

For most actions, there are negative as well as positive consequences: the elderly patient who is being encouraged to do more for himself may feel deserted or rejected; the decision to keep a patient at home may place additional strain on an already overburdened wage-earner or homemaker; a permissive approach to child rearing may create problems with grandparents; home psychiatric care may lessen the stress for the patient but increase stress for his family.

The positive consequences anticipated must be seen against these possible negative aspects. Selecting one of several choices involves weighing the positive and negative values of each and attempting to identify the "best buy." For example, if a severely handicapped mother is cared for by her daughter, this may be the most economical use of scarce nursing time, but it may have a negative effect on the daughter's emotional health. The provision of care by the nurse herself might be most satisfying to the family, especially if they have known her in other situations, but this responsibility may take the nurse away from concerns of higher priority. The use of a home health aide may not be acceptable to the family, particularly at first, but this plan would be most economical of nursing time if the aide is capable of meeting the needs of the patient satisfactorily. Within the community, a "comprehensive nursing-care" approach may meet the needs of a particular family, but it might reach only a fraction of those who need help. The essential relationship to be considered is that between the *cost* of a given course of action, in terms of effort or money, and its *benefits*, in terms of the improvement that action is expected to produce.

"Benefits" cannot always be neatly categorized. For instance, when a family is encouraged to take the responsibility for selecting a given course of action, the action selected could in fact be less productive than one the nurse would have chosen; however, the value of improving the ability of the family to solve its own problems and make decisions in health matters may outweigh the "efficiency" of the nurse's method.

Selecting Appropriate Types of Nursing Intervention

Nursing intervention may be of three types: supplemental, facilitative, or developmental.

Supplemental intervention means doing things that the family, group, or community cannot do for itself. It may take the form of providing personal or therapeutic care for the sick, planning a community program when the community is not organized to participate through its own representatives, or making decisions when the head of a household is immobilized in the face of a crisis.

Facilitative intervention is concerned with removing barriers to care — whether these barriers are economic (lack of carfare to get to the source of medical care), social (culture-linked resistance to necessary change), or behavioral (a lack of information or motivation on the part of those who are expected to take the necessary action).

Developmental intervention is based on improving the capacity of the recipient to act on his own behalf. Teaching families and groups to make responsible health decisions, supporting them in developing a sense of identity and worth, and guiding them in dealing with predictable crises or points of stress are examples of developmental intervention.

Most nursing service will, of course, involve elements of all three types of intervention. It is important, however, to be sure the intervention used is indeed suitable to the situation. A prolonged use of supplemental intervention, for example, may prevent progress toward independence; whereas trying to encourage self-help by withdrawing supplemental assistance too early may create negative responses, which will interfere with future utilization of needed nursing services.

Identifying Appropriate Resources for Care

In addition to the nurse and other members of the nursing team, there will be many other individuals, agencies, or groups involved in accomplishing health objectives. First and most central are the recipients of care — the patient, his family, the neighborhood, the school, the industrial population — who are called upon to make relatively sophisticated judgments and to take responsible action on their own behalf.

Second, the whole medical care system — the hospitals, health departments, clinics, private and group practitioners of medicine, and the health units of welfare departments, voluntary health agencies, and health-related agencies — serves as a resource that must be selectively used and activated.

The third group of resources are the nonhealth facilities — such as the social case work, educational, and counseling services — that are essential to the well-being of the population.

Developing an Operational Plan

The components of the plan for implementing nursing care need to be drawn together into an organized schedule for action. This procedure will involve the establishing of priorities and the phasing and coordinating of activities.

Establishing *priorities* is achieved by ranking the various aspects of care in terms of urgency or impact in order to determine those which warrant the earliest and most inclusive attention. The relative importance of a particular problem depends upon the degree to which it actually threatens health or the danger it raises. Thus, for a family in which a member has active tuberculosis, the highest priority would certainly go to establishing and maintaining an adequate drug regimen. In an area with a very low level of productivity, the first priority might be assigned to improving the health of those in the producing age groups — the young and middle-aged adults who are most involved in the production of food and goods — in order to provide an adequate base for maintaining life and health in the rest of the population. In a neighborhood where sanitation is very poor, the control of rats may assume such importance that all other measures must take a second place.

The *phasing* of nursing action is a threefold process. First, multifaceted problems must be broken down into manageable units. Second, these units must be organized into a reasonable sequence in which each step depends upon that which precedes it. Finally, phasing involves the establishment of checkpoints that permit periodic evaluation and replanning.

Some phases of care may be postponed in order to keep the problem manageable from the family's point of view. If the family is facing multiple problems, it is often wise to take one problem at a time, deferring consideration of others until the family is feeling less demoralized.

Coordinating is important in planning for community health nursing. In many localities, the extreme fragmentation of health care creates a multitude of incursions on the family and community, each demanding some sort of response. All too often, there is no place where the patient or family can go to be put together again. The community may have no way of preventing or regulating the wasteful proliferation of basically worthwhile, but scattered and incomplete, health-care services. The community nurse is in a position to keep the many, varied forces in some sort of ordered relationship. Through observation, consultation, and various reporting systems the nurse can detect inconsistencies or inadequacies in the health care provided; and she can report these failings to appropriate sources.

IMPLEMENTATION, THE ACTIVE PHASE OF THE PROCESS

In community health nursing, implementation may be directed toward the following objectives:
1. Doing what is required (supplementary intervention).
2. Getting others to do what is required (facilitative or developmental intervention).
3. Documenting needs and care and the relation between them (facilitative intervention and assessment).
4. Monitoring the action taken (facilitative intervention, prelude to evaluation).
5. Modifying the pattern of care as necessary (evaluation and the planning phase).

The pattern of intervention is determined by the goals that have been set and is guided by the "watch words" that govern planning. As in all nursing, the process should be subject to constant review; it should adapt to changes in the situation or to evidence that the methods chosen are not effective.

Doing what is required — providing personal or therapeutic care, securing needed information, organizing direct community action — may take many forms. It may consist of providing physical care that cannot be found elsewhere, or communicating the concern of the agency and the commitment of the nurse to help, or reassuring an anxious patient or family. In some instances, this action may provide a favorable environment for the development of trust or the improvement of communication.

Getting others to do what needs to be done is a major concern in community health nursing. Since the nursing action is usually of short duration — and the problems presented are often amenable to care by non-nursing personnel — the great bulk of care is provided by the family or other nonprofessionals, with assistance from the nurse. Because the needs of clients are so diverse and because the causative or influencing conditions are so widespread, other health or health-related sources of care are often required.

The community health nurse is obligated to assure that, as far as possible, the care from all sources is relevant and adequate in both quantity and quality. Three approaches to utilizing the work of others may be identified:
1. Motivation — incitement to action
2. Mobilization
3. Delegation

Measures for Inciting Action Are Essential

The identification of appropriate resources for care must be accompanied by measures to enlist their aid — *to incide (or motivate)* them to act with respect to the problems identified. Decision to act will depend upon whether (1) the care agent feels the action is worth taking; (2) whether he is *able* to take the action required, or whether the action is *possible;* and (3) whether taking the action will be *rewarding.* Unless all three conditions are met, the action may be incomplete or fragmented.

Thus, a discouraged mother must be persuaded that it is worth the exceptional effort it may require to talk and play with her baby; that she *can* find a way to do it; that it is related to her goals for the family; and that, if she does indeed set aside time for this action, it should be a pleasurable experience for her and an important factor in the social development of her child. A neighborhood group must be sure that they can deal with the rat population in their neighborhood through a concerted and intensive attack; that it will be worth doing for health and aesthetic reasons; and that the very process of taking action will be a satisfying experience. Sometimes the required action may mean a substantial change in attitudes, life style, or environment.

Mobilization is the involvement and organization of varied resources to deal with health and health-related problems in a concerted way. As mentioned earlier, these resources may include many types of care-givers. The various members of a family may be mobilized to care for a mentally retarded child; efforts may be pooled by the community health nurse and the community to seek better day-care facilities for children; or the nurse might join with hospital staff, residents of a particular community, and school personnel to provide needed support to unwed adolescent mothers.

The community health nurse can do much to weld these many sources of care into an operating team. She may do this by alerting agencies, groups, or families to the anticipated or actual needs for service. She may keep various participants informed about the whole care picture or about certain aspects of the problem of special interest to one or another of the resources; she may coordinate efforts through developing case conferences, or opening lines of communication to help synchronize efforts at care.

Delegation is one of the most potent and frequently used community health nursing tools. By far, the majority of nursing required for family health care is carried out by someone other than the professional nurse — by the mother or other family member, or by another member of the nursing team such as a licensed practical nurse or aide. In very few instances, is it possible for the nurse to provide constant surveillance or hour-by-hour supervision. An adequate delegation process will assure that the individual can carry out the delegated functions safely and without undue burden on the family. A simple definition of delegation is not easy; *who* does *what*, and just what is done, will vary from family to family. "Standing orders" or "standard operating procedures" are seldom applicable.

What is delegated will depend upon the complexity of the functions to be delegated, the capability and willingness of the given family, the availability of services from non-family members, and the costs of a particular delegation pattern. The community health nurse may be providing personal care to an arthritic patient who has considerable pain and requires constant encouragement to maintain as much motion as possible. The only other family member in the home may be a distraught daughter who is attempting to provide care while holding a job. If the nurse is there only for a short period of time on most days, the main burden of feeding, positioning, and assisting with patient's toilet use will fall to the daughter. In this instance, the community health nurse may continue to provide personal care, or she may have a nursing aide or a member of the staff take over, supported as necessary by the nurse. If such services are available in the community, she may delegate care to a homemaker; this would have the additional value of relieving the daughter. Another arthritic patient with different family circumstances may require establishment of a totally different arrangement.

Costs, too, may differ widely. For example, analysis of services required by a particular family may indicate that a good part of the nursing care could be safely handled by a short-trained worker rather than by a professional nurse. The costs of care, however, might rise if additional training, supervision, and travel were required.

Among those to whom some part of care may be allocated are:

(1) Family members (sometimes including extended family members, one of whom might relieve the principal home nurse one day a week).

(2) Another member of the nursing staff: licensed practical nurse, aide, nurse specialist (who may assume responsibilities in an area where the main family nurse feels she herself is not competent), or nursing student.

(3) A homemaker: homemakers usually spend several hours in the home caring for the patient and helping with meal preparation or light housework. A homemaker may be a part of the health agency, another community agency, or attached to an employment registry. The organization, duties, and method of payment vary from community to community.

(4) Volunteers, individually or as members of an organized service or group, offer myriad services — friendly visiting, personal care, support (such as members of "like experience" Ostomy groups or visiting grandmothers), or direct nursing care. There is great disparity in the preparation and commitment of volunteers, and in the screening and supervision they receive from their sponsoring agencies.

(5) Other health professionals may also be co-opted to provide nursing attention on an occasional or continuing basis. In a rural area, for example, the community health nurse may ask the environmentalist or sanitarian to check progress of designated students with the local teacher, or a social worker in frequent contact with a particular family may take on certain surveillance tasks on behalf of the nurse. Interchanges such as these are reciprocal, and at times the nurse will in turn fill in for the sanitarian, social worker, or public health physician. These interchanges may be called lateral rather than hierarchical delegation.

This relationship also characterizes delegation to nurse specialists. The person accepting the assignment is not directly or generally responsible to the person seeking help. The same steps, however, are taken in the actual delegation process with both groups.

The *delegation process* is designed to safeguard the client and to use personnel wisely.

The first step is to *analyze the job* to be delegated. Is the job a technical one, with defined procedures and little judgment required? Is judgment needed to differentiate between significant and insignificant symptoms? Will it be necessary to persist with certain procedures even if the patient objects? Is precision required in giving medication? On the basis of answers to such questions, the nurse can decide whom to delegate to and what level of delegation is indicated. If the job requires considerable judgment and if the consequences of misjudgment are great, delegation should be limited to professional level personnel or to a family member or agency worker who has previously shown that he or she is capable of sound judgment.

The *level of delegation* may vary. The community health nurse may delegate *full responsibility* for the activity, retaining only minimal supervision so as to remain accountable for the case. In other cases, delegation may be made on a more *partial* basis, with the delegate performing only specified tasks related to the case, or working under the continuing supervision of a nurse. This might be called "task assignment." There has been, in the past, an unfortunate tendency to regard the job of the professional nurse as dealing with *cases*, and the job of the auxiliary staff or of the family as dealing with the *case*. Categorization of this sort may lead to poor use of the abilities of both professional and non-professional personnel.

Based on this analysis, and taking into account the options available in the scope of delegation, a suitable person should be identified and recruited. It may be that there is no suitable delegate within the family, and the most qualified person would be a licensed practical nurse — someone who could be given maximum freedom in the case. However, if a licensed practical nurse is unavailable, an aide could be used; this would require an adjustment of the professional input to include intensive supervision. In some communities, there may be a choice between the services of a homemaker or a practical nurse. The best choice might be the homemaker if the patient were living alone, requiring some care but also likely to benefit from the longer working day of the homemaker, and the nursing tasks were not beyond those that the homemaker could develop with some training and supervision.

The next step is to analyze the present capabilities and *training needs* of the delegate. This is usually best done in conference with the assigned person. In delegation, it is important to judge not only what the individual was *taught* to do but also what she *can* do. For example, the nursing care may require administering medication by hypodermic, a procedure included in the training of nursing aides. If the aide has had no experience (or no recent experience), re-education is definitely indicated. Attitudinal as well as technical status may be important. One aide may react positively to the idea of working with children, while another may find satisfaction in care of the elderly; it is not always possible to choose, but when options are open, "matching" makes for good family/agency relations.

Once the needs have been determined, an *educational plan* can be developed. This plan should assure that the home nurse, aide, or other person has the knowledge, skills, and attitudes that the job requires. For example, a volunteer friendly visitor who falsely believes that the elderly should be coddled and not "made" to do uncomfortable things, such as exercise, could do more harm than good in a situation involving an aged patient.

At this point, it is well to *review* the level of delegation and re-examine the capability of the assignee after the training period. The delegate may prove to be entirely capable, or it may be necessary to reduce her freedom or limit the boundaries of her responsibility and increase the amount of supervision.

When some or most of the care is provided by the family, family members should be told exactly when the nurse will be available to them, and whether or not she plans to continue visiting. If another worker (practical nurse or aide) provides care, the family should know the extent to which the community health nurse will be involved — as a frequent visitor, a regular consultant, or available only when called upon. It is important that the family be able to identify the *primary source of care* — the person they should turn to if problems develop. Even with maximum delegation, a regular interchange of information is desirable for as long as the case is open, in order to make sure that the situation has not changed.

Delegation has a strong impact on the quality and quantity of care provided. It is a vital tool in preparing families for self-help and neighbor-help in times of crisis or illness. It can also lead to a release of scarce nursing time, which can then be applied to other efforts. In short, it allows the community health nurse to do more.

Referral Procedures Clarify Expectations and Facilitate Use of Resources

Referral systems are the bridge between families or groups and the organizations serving them. The referral process includes not only an exchange of forms documenting requests and responses for service but also ongoing counseling that prepares families to analyze their health problems and take responsibility for health action. Its success depends upon open communication and information exchange between the community health nurse and other health or health-related care providers.

The object of referral is to introduce the client and the resource, clarify their respective expectations, and facilitate coordination of the care to be provided. To ensure these results, referral procedures should meet the following criteria:

1. The referral should provide *specific* information; time, place, person to see, (if indicated) travel instructions, needed documents (e.g., medicaid card, clinic identification card), or any other information that may be requested.
2. The referral should *interpret* the needs, constraints, and coping level of the family; it should explain the reasons for and expectations of the referral. It should interpret to the family the agency's expectations, procedures, and constraints.
3. The referral procedure should *inform* the agency regarding other care being provided, so that the referral for care can be seen in the context of the total care process.
4. The referral procedure should provide for return of information through reports or record exchange, as a basis for evaluating the results of care.

EVALUATION IS A CONTINUING PROCESS

Evaluation is interwoven with every nursing activity and every step of the community health process. Each nurse-client encounter, each new method or program introduced, and each new aide's progress during her introduction to the service deserve evaluation to test the usefulness of what has gone before and to serve as a basis for improvement in the future. In addition, at stated times (as when a family is moving from active to inactive service classification), at stated checkpoints in the care of long-term patients, and at significant points in the nurse's career, a more intensive evaluation is again imperative.

Evaluation involves:

1. Devising objective, observable indicators of achievement that document progress toward the established goals for care.
2. Continuing observation and documentation of changes in health

condition or health behavior, and of developments or care experiences that may have affected these changes.

3. Continuing analysis of the nursing methods or processes as related to service and to the costs of care.

4. Periodic audit of overall performance, including case or work load, family progress, effectiveness and cost of care strategies used as compared to possible alternatives, unmet or projected needs of the population under care.

There are two major approaches to the evaluation of community nursing services: the first is based on evidence of effectiveness of the service provided, and the second is based on evidence of excellence of professional practice.

Effectiveness of Service

Changes in those aspects of health that can be controlled by the client or the nurse are without doubt the most relevant measures of the effectiveness of nursing care. At the same time, these are the most frustrating of measures to apply: first, because it is difficult to establish objective indicators of results; and second, because many factors other than nursing may affect the changes that occur.

Changes that occur in the course of nursing service may also be a valuable source of evaluation data. Many efforts are being made to develop more sensitive indicators of health and general welfare.[4] These efforts have great relevance for nursing. Roberts and Hudson have developed a method of measuring patient progress based on the reduction of nursing needs in the course of care.[5] By estimating the reduction of needs, as reflected in changed conditions or behavior, it is possible to estimate the impact of nursing service. Mager suggests that evaluation may be predicated on simple indicators, not inclusive in themselves, based on answering the question, "What will the learner be doing when he is demonstrating that he has attained the objective?"[6] Thus one might say, "The mother who has learned to communicate with her infant will cuddle and talk to the baby." Such limited indicators, if accumulated and classified, may make good measures of broader attainments.

Sometimes it is useful to look at secondary indicators of change. One such measure that is widely used is compliance with medical recommendations.[7] Satisfaction with the care received — another frequently used measure — is of more doubtful value.

Much research has focused on the evaluation of nursing intervention, and more is needed. Even though the literature is peppered with studies that failed to show the anticipated results, many things have been learned from them. And those studies with positive findings are encouragement to continue the search for more refined measures of achievement.

However, certain guidelines should be observed if evaluation is based on change in a patient, family, or community:

1. The change to be measured should be one that is largely dependent on nursing intervention. For example, the nurse might be very influential in changing patient and family behavior with respect to following a prescribed medical regimen for tuberculosis. Moreover, changes involving the regularity of taking drugs or reporting to a clinic might constitute a legitimate measure of nursing effectiveness. However, nursing care would not be expected to influence directly the actual progress of the disease; this is much more a factor of the drug prescribed and the basic condition of the patient. Thus, to evaluate nursing care by the degree to which the patient's physical condition improves may not be appropriate. The measurement of changes affected by nursing may include changes in behavior that are related to health.

2. When changes are observed over a period of time, it is important to establish data collection at the point when nursing service is initiated. Only by knowing what the situation is at the start of service is it possible to document and interpret the extent and direction of the changes that occur.

3. In relating changes in the family or community to nursing, it is also important to take account of other conditions that may be influencing the situation. For example, the patient-physician relationship may produce strongly positive or strongly negative reactions to the care prescribed. The support or non-support of the family may facilitate or impede conformity to recommended health practice. Economic constraints may interfere with proper nutritional practices. Sometimes these other forces are so strong, they outweigh any effect that community health nursing might be expected to produce.

4. The reliability of information relating to change should also be scrutinized. The two most frequent sources of data about the change are the nurse herself and the family or the representatives of the community being served. Both sources are obviously subject to bias in reporting: the nurse — since she is involved, and may see what she hopes to see rather than what is actually there — and the family — since they may not be able to recall the information accurately or to make the observations required with sufficient judgment or skill.

"Quality" of Care Is an Elusive But Critical Component of Service

What we define as "good quality" is determined by value judgments that can vary widely with time and among different groups. In the 1930's, for example, there was much talk of "forceful" teaching, "persuasive" approaches, and "pre-set" objectives for care — all of which would be highly questionable today. Community health nurses would greatly benefit from defining for themselves the meaning and the indicators of high quality nursing practice. The definition should incorporate, but not be limited to, mandated performance standards such as departmental regulations or the reviewing requirements of federally funded programs or projects.

The indicators of "quality" are elusive. Evaluation of the quality of nursing practice rests on the assumption that "quality" has a positive relationship to effectiveness; that is, that improving the quality of practice actually improves the service given. Unfortunately, scientific support for this relationship is still rather weak. It is not clear that the family care provided by "qualified" community health nurses is indeed better than that provided by nurses who lack such training or that sophisticated approaches to a particular situation are more satisfying to the recipient or more productive than relatively simple interventions. The effects of good quality nursing may appear as purely serendipitous benefits of care — in an improved sense of community, a new level of self-respect and self-confidence, and an increased ability to manage stressful situations.

Despite the complications, it is possible to identify some criteria that are useful in evaluating the quality of care.

1. *Conformity to accepted nursing and public health standards of practice.*

Adoption of a truly *comprehensive approach* in the care of families and communities is basic. This requires recognition of both family and community as interlocking systems with interdependent functions. Community action for environmental control can succeed only if each family's concern for the environment is consistent with the overall community program; conversely, only community action via city planning can eliminate the dangerous environment of the ghetto. Indicators of a comprehensive approach might include services provided to family members other than the index case (the primary person referred for care), enlistment of formal and informal resources in the community to deal with conditions in which nursing is not required or needs to be supplemented, and imaginative development of new resources — high school students who volunteer to visit or shop for the elderly, for example. High among the indicators of comprehensive care is evidence of intervention addressed to increasing the general capability of families to deal with their own health problems.

Sensitivity in providing care — demonstrating respect for individuals and confidence in their ability to deal with their problems — is an important quality. Care that goes beyond what is usually offered can be seen in the extra visit, for example, or the phone call to make sure that all is well.

Consideration of the needs of the *population as a whole* and for the *environment* reflects a basic obligation of public health workers. The needs of the total population provide the backdrop for case planning. As one nurse-midwife commented, "In the hospital, I was concerned with the patients who were admitted to care and in some degree with their immediate families; here [*in a community health agency*] I have to worry about all those people out there — the expectant mothers, the may-be mothers, and the infants!"

Outreach activities — taking the initiative in providing care for groups who need but have not sought care (and, indeed, might distrust the providers of care) — are essential if the community needs for community health nursing are to be met. Outreach also implies adaptation to the particular attitudes, conditions, culture, and demands of the recipients of care.

A well-defined *priority system* in planning care is vital in community health nursing, since it is highly unlikely that there will ever be resources adequate to care for everyone in an equally comprehensive way.

2. *Responsible stewardship.*

Good stewardship involves conservation of the community's material and human resources for health care. This is much more than saving paper clips or turning out lights. The primary responsibility is to conserve one's own time and effort. *Reduction of non-effective time* offers great potential for conservation. Time spent in travel or visits wasted — because of insufficient planning or because materials or information were not available — all represent time lost to productive nursing. Much time may be lost, too, if care is prolonged beyond the point when it is needed or useful. Uselessly expensive methods of care (such as making a home visit when a telephone call would have been equally effective) also steal time from productive work.

Acceptability of nursing care by clients is also evidence of capable stewardship, since families and community groups will not be accepting of care if the care does not meet their needs.

3. *Continued refinement and enlargement of practical skills.*

It is expected that members of professions will continually enhance and extend their skills and knowledge through continued field experience and a program of continuing education. It is assumed that these efforts will constantly improve the quality of care provided.

Basic to any evaluation of professional growth is the periodic, *systematic review of performance* — undertaken with or without the assistance of a supervisor, consultant, administrator, or peer group. Norms for comparison may include published regulations or criteria and standards provided by professional associations, service and funding agencies, or legislative provisions. Seeking new information through reading; attending meetings, seminars, and workshops; and using consultants are also indicators of increasing performance skills.

Developing *innovative or investigative possibilities* on the job is also an indication of professional growth. Volunteering to try out new methods of health care or record keeping, taking on a new population group, or critically analyzing one's own case load are indicators of innovative effort.

Gortner proposes that the evaluation of practice in a systematic and cumulative way (or "scientific accountability") is important to the tradition of nursing and is an imperative for the improvement of nursing.[8] Such accountability may be exercised by individuals or groups through responsible and rigorous research or through the development and use of individual capabilities for self-study and constant reappraisal of practice. While not all nurses will necessarily engage in research *per se*, the application of a scientific approach to the evaluation of practice should be an essential component of the nursing process.

THE PROCESS — A NEED FOR GREATER PRECISION

This, then, is the process involved in community health nursing practice: relating, assessing, goal setting, planning, implementing, and evaluating. Each step is essential for the accomplishment of the others; each step is related to all of the others.

Although the explanation may seem lengthy and involved, with experience the sensitive nurse comes to apply some parts of the process more and more intuitively and to recognize and respond to complex situations in a synoptic fashion.

Intuitive response, however, is reliable only if it is firmly rooted in mastery of the scientific and the behavioral content basic to nursing and to public health practice. It is important to know the nature of the process by which this content is transformed into the professional practice of community health nursing.

Undeniably, there is need for much more precision in evaluating the many aspects of community health nursing. Achieving greater exactness will, however, rest on the acquisition of much more detailed knowledge of the nature of the community health nursing contribution, a more precise definition of the changes that may be classified as measures of nursing achievement, and the application of comparative "cost" and "benefit" estimates as they apply to the realization of stated goals for community nursing care. Whether in the field or in the research laboratory, community health nurses must continue to address this vexing and complex problem.

REFERENCES

1. Hodgins, E.: Listen: The patient. New Eng. J. Med., 274:657, 1966.
2. Johnson, B. S.: The meaning of touch in nursing. *In* Stewart, D., and Vincent, P. (eds.): *Public Health Nursing.* Dubuque, Iowa, William C. Brown Co., Publishers, 1968, p. 59.

3. Hodgins: *op. cit.*
4. See, for example, Office of Management and Budget: *Social Indicators.* Washington, D.C., U.S. Government Printing Office, 1973; and Goldsmith, Seth A., A re-evaluation of health status indicators. Health Services Reports, 88:937, 1973.
5. Roberts, D. and Hudson, H.: *How to Study Patient Progress.* Washington, D.C., U.S. Government Printing Office, Public Health Service Publication No. 1169, 1964, p. 1.
6. Mager, R.: *Preparing Instructional Objectives.* Palo Alto, Calif., Fearon Publishers, 1962, p. 14.
7. See, for example, Lowe, M. L.: Effectiveness of teaching as measured by compliance with medical recommendations. Nurs. Res., 19:59, 1970.
8. Gortner, S. R.: Scientific accountability in nursing. Nurs. Outlook., 22: 796, 1974.

SUGGESTED READINGS

American Nursing Association: *Standards of Nursing Practice.* Kansas City, Mo., 1973.
Aradine, C. R., and Pridham, K. F.: Model for collaboration. Nurs. Outlook, 21:655, 1973.
Archer, S. E.; and Fleshman, R. P.: *Community Health Nursing Patterns and Practice,* 2nd ed. North Scituate, Mass., Duxbury Press, 1979, Chapter 13.
Bailit, H., Lewis, J., Hochheiser, L., and Bush, N.: Assessing the quality of care. Nurs. Outlook, 23:153, 1975.
Baumann, B.: Diversities in conceptions of health and physical fitness. *In* Skipper, J. K., and Leonard, R. D. (eds.): *Social Interaction and Patient Care.* Philadelphia, J. B. Lippincott Co., 1965.
Bernstein, L., Bernstein, R. S., and Dana, H.: *Interviewing: A Guide for Health Professionals.* 2nd ed. New York, Appleton-Century-Crofts, 1974.
Bloch, D.: Some crucial terms in nursing; What do they mean? Nurs. Outlook, 22:689, 1974.
Blum, K. L.: *Planning for Health: Development and Application of Social Change Theory.* New York, Human Sciences Press, 1974.
Brill, N. I.: *Working With People: The Helping Process.* Philadelphia, J. B. Lippincott Co., 1973.
Brunclik, H., Thurston, J. R., and Feldhauser, J.: The empathy inventory. Nurs. Outlook, 15:42, 1967.
Buker, F., and Northman, J. E.: Input-throughput-output evaluation of a school mental health clinic. *In* Schulberg, N. C., and Buker, F.: *Program Evaluation in the Health Field.* New York, Human Science Press, 1979, pp. 319–334.
Cordes, S. M.: Assessing health care needs: Elements and processes. Fam. Com. Health, 1:1, 1978.
Donabedian, A.: *The Quality of Medical Care: Methods for Assessing and Monitoring the Quality of Care for Research and for Quality Assurance Programs in Health.* Washington, D.C., U.S. Government Printing Office, 1978.
Duvall, E. M.: *Family Development,* 4th ed. Philadelphia, J. B. Lippincott Co., 1971.
Flynn, B. C., and Ray, D. W.: Quality assurance in community nursing. Nurs. Outlook, 27:650, 1979.
Foote, N. and Cottrell, L.: Interpersonal competence. *In* Faber, B. (ed.): *Kinship and Family Organization.* New York, John May and Sons, 1966.
Fuller, D. and Rosenaur, J. A.: A patient assessment guide. Nurs. Outlook, 22:460, 1974.
Gebbie, K., and Lavin, M. A.: Classifying nursing diagnoses. Am. J. Nurs. 74:250, 1974.
Geismar, L. L., and LaSorte, M.: "Understanding the Multi-Problem Family," New York, Associated Press, 1964.
Gilman, S., and Nader, P.: Measuring the effectiveness of a school health program— Methods and preliminary analysis. J. School Health, 49:10, 1979.
Hanchett, E.: *Community Health Assessment.* New York, John Wiley & Sons, Inc., 1979.
Hecht, A. B.: Improving medication compliance by teaching outpatients. Nurs. Forum, 13:112, 1974.
Hott, J. R.: Mobilizing family strengths in health maintenance and coping with illness. *In*

Reinhardt, A., and Quinn, M.: *Current Practice in Family Centered Community Health Nursing.* St. Louis, C. V. Mosby, 1977, pp. 101–116.

Januska, C.: *Status of Quality Assurance in Public Health Nursing.* Washington, D.C., Public Health Nursing Section, American Public Health Association, 1976.

Kalisch, B. J.: What is empathy? 73:1548, 1973.

King, S. H.: *Perceptions of Illness and Medical Practice.* New York, Russell Sage Foundation, 1962.

Knight, J. H.: Applying nursing process in the community. Nurs. Outlook, 22:708, 1974.

Kron, T.: *Communication in Nursing,* 2nd ed. Philadelphia, W. B. Saunders Co., 1972.

Kron, T.: *Management of Patient Care,* 5th ed. Philadelphia, W. B. Saunders Co., 1981.

Loomis, M.: *Group Process for Nurses.* New York, McGraw-Hill Book Co., 1979.

Marram, G.: *The Group Approach to Nursing Practice.* St. Louis, Mo., C. V. Mosby Co., 1978.

Parson, T., and Fox, R.: Illness, therapy, and the modern urban family. *In* Gartly, J. E. (ed.): *Patients, Physicians, and Illness.* Glenco, Ill., The Free Press, 1958.

Phaneuf, M. C.: *The Nursing Audit: Profile for Excellence.* New York, Appleton-Century-Crofts, 1972.

Phaneuf, M. C.: Quality Assurance — A Nursing View, *Quality Assurance of Medical Care.* February, 1973.

Pridham, K. F., Hausen, M. F., and Conrad, H. H.: Anticipatory care as problem solving in family medicine and nursing. J. Family Pract., 24:1077, 1977.

Reinhardt, A. A., and Quinn, M. D. (ed.): *Current Practice in Family-Centered Community Nursing.* St. Louis, Mo., C. V. Mosby Co., 1977, Parts III and IV.

Rogers, M. E.: *An Introduction to the Theoretical Basis of Nursing.* Philadelphia, F. A. Davis Co., 1970.

Ruybal, S. E.: Community health planning. Fam. Comm. Health, 1:9, 1978.

Schaefer, J.: The interrelatedness of decision making and the nursing process. Am. J. Nurs., 74:1852, 1974.

Schwartz, D. R.: Toward more precise evaluation of patients' needs. Nurs. Outlook, 13:42, 1965.

Siegel, H.: To your health — whatever that may mean. Nurs. Forum, 12:280, 1973.

Sills, G. M., Cohen, M. W., and Schwebel, A.: A two-stage process for surveying community needs. J. Comm. Dev. Soc., 8:1, 54, 1977.

Simmons, D. A.: *A Classification Scheme for Client Problems in Community Health Nursing.* Springfield, Va., National Technical Information Services, Nurse Planning Information Series No. 14, DHEW 80–16, HRP 0501501, 1980.

Suchman, E. A.: *Sociology and the Field of Public Health.* New York, Russell Sage Foundation, 1967.

Suchman, E. A.: *Evaluative Research: Principles and Practice in Public Service and Social Action Programs.* New York, Russell Sage Foundation, 1967.

Watts, W.: Social class, ethnic background and patient care. Nurs. Forum, 6:155, 1967.

Webb, S. R., Jr.: Objective criteria for evaluating occupational health programs. Am. J. Pub. Health, 65:31, 1965.

Yura, H. and Walsh, M. B.: *The Nursing Process: Assessing, Planning, Implementing, Evaluating,* 2nd ed. New York, Appleton-Century-Crofts, 1973.

CHAPTER 4

THE FAMILY AS THE UNIT OF CARE

As early as 1932, an official publication of the National Organization for Public Health Nursing stated: *"The cardinal principle* of public health nursing which must permeate all consideration of visit content is that *family* health work is the basis upon which all factors rest."[1] The concept of the family as the unit of service was accepted well before the publication of that document and has been reiterated frequently since that time. The importance of the family in community health nursing was again emphasized in a recent World Health Organization expert committee report.[2] Yet despite such widespread acceptance, there are many indications that practice does not always follow precept.

In community health or home care services, those providing care usually think in terms of the family as the basic unit, and records are aggregated in family groups. However, the concept of the family as an interacting system with its own particular problems of maintenance and action is changing, or becoming elusive. One must, therefore, determine whether the idea of the family as a unit of service is as valid today as it has been in the past.

THE FAMILY REMAINS A NATURAL UNIT OF SERVICE

There are cogent arguments for considering the family as the unit of service in community health nursing:

1. *The majority of people continue to live in, and believe in the importance of, a family or a family-like structure.* As suggested in Chapter 1, the *concept* of the family is undergoing great change. The ideal of marriage as a permanent institution and the validity of rigid roles for family members are being challenged. The father is no longer seen as the sole breadwinner in the family, although in many countries he is

most often the principal wage earner. Marital fidelity is no longer assumed to be compulsory —or even, for many, desirable.

At the same time, new configurations appear attesting to the vitality of the family as a basic human organization. Whether we speak of traditional families, extended families, tribal families, open marriages, single sex marriages, or communes, these structures all provide the familial characteristics of intimacy, affectional interchange, mutual responsibility, and reasonable stability. For example, Laucks writes: "The idea of family extension in purely blood tie terms has exhausted itself," and goes on to describe a type of extended family based on "homogenous ideals and purposes."[3] Mead points out that while children must go beyond their parents' orbit in order to develop and grow, without adult care they will die, without affection and stability they will never learn to trust.[4]

There is new interest in the extended family, whether in a natural or contrived form. Konrad Lorenz, the great student of animal behavior, is convinced that in the human family the traditional framework of father, mother, and siblings is not enough to provide for adequate human development. He stresses the need for larger, stable family groups for the survival of human society.[5]

Perhaps the most eloquent defense of the family comes from Pauline Paolucci:

"From the home and family radiate the warmth and concern that keep people human. Home represents the safe harbor from the stress of every day living. It is the harbor where each person can feel he is of value to himself and others. The society of the future will have need for richer, more supportive ties."[6]

Above all, the family provides an opportunity for expression of deeply human attributes — of love, commitment, compassion, and understanding — that are, in the long run, basic to human survival.

The general level of family functioning — the degree to which the family can work as a unit in dealing with its problems and can maximize the potential of each of its members — will profoundly influence its capability in handling health matters. The quality of family functioning is, therefore, a central concern of the community health nurse.

2. *The family as a group generates, prevents, tolerates, or corrects health problems within its membership.* Health problems may be caused by many factors: genetic fault (such as Tay-Sachs disease), alcoholism, behavioral irregularities, or catastrophic illness. Families can cause adverse health conditions: disease may be transmitted from parent to child; or prolonged stress in a family may produce emotional illness in one or more of its members. Conversely, the skill and confidence of a family operating in unison not only may facilitate treatment and provide physical support but also may lend emotional strength to an afflicted member and contribute to the social and psychologic development of the total group. It is usually the family, rather than

the individual, that must exert the energy necessary to achieve health goals.

3. *The health problems of families are interlocking.* It is very likely that the health of any one member of the family will affect the well-being of others. The child with a developmental disability may affect the health of his siblings because he requires an inordinate amount of parental time and energy, or the terminal illness of a parent cared for at home may impair the health of the daughter who is home nurse as well as wife and mother. Whatever happens to one member of the family has some effect upon the family collectively and requires a whole series of accommodations on the part of the other family members. Emotional problems, in particular, appear to be reinforced by family interaction.

4. *The family provides a crucial environmental force.* Each individual member constantly interacts with the physical, social, and interpersonal milieu created by his family. The individual responds in his own way to the particular ambiance of his own family: to slovenly housekeeping or to compulsive conformity to rigid norms, to positive family attitudes of social responsibility or to a sense of social alienation. In turn, each individual affects the family environment by his own behavior. That is, each person serves either to reinforce or to contest the values or attitudes held by the others, to preserve or to modify the existing physical environment, and to strengthen or weaken the cohesiveness of the family as an operating unit. This continual interaction, which exists for the most part within a closed system, influences and molds the individual in myriad ways.

5. *The family is most frequently the source of decisions about health and personal care.* In the long run, it is most often the family unit, not the individual or the health professional, that decides whether or not to seek or use health care. Children, of course, must rely on parental action for their health needs. Often there is one strong character within the family who, through force of personality or traditional position, exerts more influence. A husband's desires may have much to do with his wife's decision to seek care early in pregnancy or to see that the children receive proper immunization; a grandmother may influence child rearing practices; a mother may advocate home remedies or homeopathic medicines.

The family is the most usual source of health care. Care for minor ills, long-term illnesses, or disability and prehospital and posthospital care during acute illness are generally provided for at home by family members. In many instances, no care other than family care is required or sought. Alpert asked 78 low-income families (selected at random from a case pool of 500 families) to record on a calendar the day-by-day health of their members: they were to note *any* indisposition and the manner in which it was remedied. This study revealed that these low-income families sought professional medical help in only 4.7 percent of the episodes of illness; the remaining 95.3 percent of illnesses (most often described as respiratory or gastrointestinal ailments, fever, headache, or accidental injury) were presumably treated by the families themselves. Hence the ability of the family to provide nursing care for its members is an important factor in health care.[7]

6. *The family is an effective and available channel for much of community health nursing.* The community health nurse has the opportunity to develop sustained and close relationships with the families she serves. This relationship in turn enables her to establish communication quickly when it is needed; she can elicit appropriate self-reporting on the part of the family, and she can bring them rapidly into the larger health care system; she can help them in times of crisis, and prepare them for possible future stress. Furthermore, the number of individuals who are reached by care is greater when the family is the unit of service. The family itself becomes the means of extending a nurse's influence to those members she cannot personally see. By working with the family as a whole, she is more likely to fulfill her obligation to reach the entire community.

7. *The family, through its interaction with the larger social system, validates and influences health efforts.* By merely refusing to use an available health service, the family can precipitate a re-evaluation of the usefulness and acceptability of that service. The rural family, faced with erosion of the rural way of life, may evolve new perspectives — or, alternatively, may fail to adjust and create or contribute to new tensions. New industry, factories, strip mining, power plants — all will alter the environment and have a profound effect upon the economic and emotional stability of local families.

The effects of change in the larger system upon the individual family are enormous. A population control policy and program, opportunities for employment of women, and increased educational facilities may lead to smaller families, more working mothers, and changes in family roles — all of which can be either rewarding or threatening. The successful family system must interact internally in a constructive way, but must interact as well with the larger social system with wisdom and foresight.

There will, of course, be instances when the individual, rather than the family, is the logical unit of service. The increasing complexity of care may require the use of clinical specialists in nursing who are not trained to treat the broad spectrum of problems found in family care. Whereas the community health nurse may consider the *family* as her patient, the clinical specialist may consider the *individual* as her patient, thinking of the family only as a tangential influence. The specialist, however, can and should work within the context of the family; that is, she should take into account family concerns that affect the treatment of her patient and try to modify them when they are inimical to the patient's care.

Also, there are crash programs directed at limited phases of health care which tend to focus on the individual, not the family. To be consistent, the community health nurse must, in this setting, focus primarily on the individual. This method of delivering health care sets some constraints on the relationship between nurse and family; however, on the other hand, it may possibly lead to a greater depth in the nurse-patient relationship.

THE FAMILY AS CLIENT

The family consists of a group of individuals in close and continuing association, constantly interacting with one another as individuals and, individually and collectively, with others in their orbit and the community as a whole. Its functioning affects and is affected by the physical, social, and psychological milieu in which it exists.

Through this interaction the family clarifies its goals, values, and purposes, creates its interpersonal style, accommodates to the needs of its members, and determines and implements action on its own behalf.

Changes in any single part of the system affect the total. The health professional must be aware that such changes may greatly affect the health decisions and capability of the family. Thus, if a couple decides that the father of the family shall become the homemaker while the wife works outside the home, the capability within that family for continuing health observation may be reduced. A sharp change in economic status or environment (sudden unemployment, a move from suburb to high rise apartment) will require many adaptations by the family as a whole to accommodate to the new circumstances.

Family Values and Orientations Influence Choice

Each family acts in accordance with its own set of values and orientations to life. The concept of family obligation will differ — ranging from a central demanding concern to an almost casual interest. One family will feel personally responsible for looking after a second cousin living in a distant state and needing help in illness or economic adversity; another family will feel that care of their elderly ailing parents should be the responsibility of the community. "Family" may be seen as the parents and children still at home, or as the entire network of relations.

Different families will assign different values to traits such as honesty, industriousness, independence, and self-reliance; conformity to religious tenets, community norms; or tangible evidence of economic "success."

The Family Develops Its Own Life Style

Each family develops its own patterns of behavior and its own style of life. In some families, there is little or no communication between husband and wife and between parents and children. Each member lives locked up in a private world of thought and feeling, even though the physical aspects of group life go on. In other families, there may be much voluble interchange — where shouts, tears, and recriminations are balanced by overt tenderness, respect, and sharing. In still other families, undemonstrative outward behavior may conceal a depth of understanding and affection not quickly apparent to the observer.

Families also develop their own power systems, which may either be balanced (wherein the father, mother, and children have their own areas of decision and control) or strongly biased (wherein one member gains dominance over the others).

In some instances, power distribution is related to role: the mother may make all decisions regarding management of the home and care of the children, while the father makes decisions regarding the economic aspects of family life. Power struggles within the family are not uncommon, and the ripples from such conflicts may reach every member of the family.

Orientation regarding time may also vary. For some, the focus is only on the present, and problems that might arise in the future have little meaning. If the family has been living precariously, future considerations may have little significance in comparison to the immediate problems of securing food or paying the rent.

In times of crisis or confusion, some families cope well, dealing as a matter of course with problems as they arise. The poor mountain family may manage to survive despite a year of poor crops and little outside work, to find a way to get to the health center when no transportation is readily available, or to improvise a bed for a sick child who ordinarily shares a bed with other children. Other families simply give up when trouble strikes, and wait helplessly for something or someone to come and help.

The Family Accommodates to the Needs of the Individual

Within each family, the individual functions not only as a member of the group but also as a unique human being with his own destiny to fulfill. Each member must assert himself in a way that allows him to grow and develop. Sometimes individual needs and group needs seem to find a natural balance; the need for self-expression does not overshadow consideration for others, power is equitably distributed, and independence is permitted to flourish.

At other times, individual and family needs are not so easily reconciled, and conflict or withdrawal may ensue. The adolescent's need for self-determination may run counter to his parents' need for social acceptance, and the result could be a continuing battle.

The Family Relates to the Community

The family develops a characteristic stance with respect to the community. For some this relationship is wholesome and reciprocal; the family utilizes the community and its institutions and, in turn, contributes whatever it can to improve the community. In some cases there is a firmly rooted sense of family responsibility, often stemming from a tradition of charitable endeavor.

Other families feel a sense of isolation from the community. They may maintain a proud "we keep to ourselves" attitude; or they may be entirely passive, taking the benefits that are offered by the community without either contributing to it or demanding changes in it.

The Family Growth Cycle

Families, like individuals, have their own growth cycles. In the foreseeable future the dominant pattern of the family is expected to be fairly traditional, with most couples married and remaining married, electing to have two or three children. The husband will continue to be the principal breadwinner, although many wives will be employed as well. In this general pattern, a typical cycle may be identified. For about two years, the average couple will be childless; for the next twenty years or so, child bearing and child rearing will be central concerns, followed by about six years when children are leaving home for college, marriage, or careers. For approximately 13 years the old couple will be living alone once more, and for the final 16+ years, the family will be reduced to a widow or a widower.

This pattern is by no means characteristic of all families. Atypical families will face quite different cycles. For example, the childless couple will miss the child rearing and separation phases; the contract of marriage of limited duration may never reach the widow or widower stage because of early termination of the relationship. "Open" marriages create altogether new patterns. There are also many single-member families, or households containing only one person who may be part of a larger family unit living elsewhere — e.g., the career girl, college student, bachelor, and widow. The commune "family" may have a group/children rather than a couple/children pattern, and several phases (child rearing, separation, widowhood, couple alone) may co-exist within the group at any given time. The concept of cycles is useful since each step in the "typical" cycle makes its own demands on care.

The sharp transitions between phases that used to exist have been greatly modified. The smaller average number of children has reduced the dependent period, providing more time for the individual to use at his or her own discretion. Increased technology, improved domestic appliances, and day-care centers permit homemakers to take part-time jobs or engage in civic activities.

In sum, the family is the unit to which the community health nurse is most often addressed. It is a functioning group composed of individuals held together by bonds of kinship or strong emotional ties; a unit in which the action of any member may set off a whole series of reactions within the group; an entity whose inner strength may be its greatest single supportive factor when one of its members is stricken with illness or death.

HEALTH TASKS OF THE FAMILY

The health tasks of the family are a primary concern of the nurse. Each family cares for its health in a manner consistent with its own unique set of values, capabilities, resources, and life styles. These tasks include the following:

1. *Recognizing interruptions of health or development*, such as illness or a child's failure to thrive. Families differ in their concepts of illness and health: for example, backache may constitute an illness in one family but is an expected normal occurrence in another; preventive care may be considered important by some, unimportant by others.

2. *Seeking health care.* The family must decide whether to see a physician, to ask a druggist's advice, to institute home remedies, or to "just wait and see" each time a family member is indisposed. Usually the family is the first to recognize any deviation from normal health; and when necessary, it must take the first step toward getting into the health care system. No amount of professional "outreach" can compensate for family lethargy or resistance to care.

3. *Managing health and nonhealth crises.* Sooner or later, every family will face a crisis. Severe or incapacitating illness, death, childbirth, and hospitalization affect all families at some time. Non-health crises (unexpected unemployment, military service, moving into an unfamiliar community) also have an effect on health since, if poorly met, these episodes place great emotional strain on the family as a group as well as on its individual members.

4. *Providing nursing care to sick, disabled, or dependent members of the family.* Only a small fraction of illnesses are cared for in hospitals or other institutions. Treating minor ills and personal care of the very young or the very old, tending the sick before and after hospitalization, or caring for ambulatory patients who require special treatment — all represent health care demands commonly placed upon the family. Home

care may range in complexity from providing dialysis to caring for a child with a head cold.

5. *Maintaining a home environment conducive to good health and personal development.* The home should be physically safe; a place in which elderly members are protected from falls by sturdy railings and in which young children are not exposed to rat bites or tempted by accessible switches on the gas stove. It should also provide a stable emotional and social environment, an atmosphere of confidence and mutual concern, a modicum of beauty and comfort, and room in which to relax and grow.

6. *Maintaining a reciprocal relationship with the community and its health institutions.* Health care of the family requires intervention from a variety of individuals and groups ranging from the neighbor who baby sits to the sophisticated teaching hospital.

In relating to the community and its institutions, the family must arrive at some realistic basis of expectations. They must learn to appreciate their rights as individuals and at the same time to understand the limits inherent in the community or institutional situation. The family has a right, for example, to expect that those who provide care should be qualified, and that health services be run efficiently. On the other hand, the family should expect to assume responsibility for sending children to school on time, for putting garbage in a covered container, for securing immunization at the proper time, for keeping clinic appointments as scheduled, and for not making unreasonable demands on services that may be understaffed and overworked.

Community involvement is one step toward social health. Unfortunately, opportunities for everyone to contribute to decisions about community programs are not always made available to all segments of the population.

These family health tasks are obviously of great importance, and the community health nurse must be deeply concerned with increasing the capability of each family to perform them. It is not enough to improve the family's ability to care for an elderly and incapacitated patient at home while ignoring the need for changing a home environment that is upsetting the physical or emotional health of its other members. Nor is it enough to deal only with that often chance-selected portion of the population that receives nursing care. This problem calls for special multi-agency planning and action, calculated to reach a substantial portion of the families in the community.

THE COMMUNITY HEALTH NURSE'S ROLE IN FAMILY FUNCTIONING

The extraordinary impact of family organization and functioning upon individual, family, and community health makes it a mandatory concern of community health nursing.

The nurse's responsibility is not limited to using the family as a resource for health care; it also includes the provision of general support for family development. As she builds nursing care on the family's own abilities and supplements their action when the problem is too much for them to manage alone, the nurse is constantly aware of the opportunity for strengthening the family, better equipping it to deal with future problems of health care and family management.

Moral and technical limits restrict action to change family behavior. First, the family's right to freedom of choice must not be abrogated; every family has the right to establish its own values, life style, and patterns of health care, provided they do not harm others. For example, refusal by parents of certain medical treatments for a child may be tolerated so long as the child is not endangered: refusal of routine health examinations may be well within parental rights, whereas, on the other hand, refusal to permit surgery that would prevent blindness in a child may require legal action on the child's behalf to ensure that the required care is provided. An adult deciding for *himself* to refuse such care would be within his rights. Efforts to convert families to the nurse's own concept of desirable family behavior should be suppressed in favor of providing the family with the information they need in order to decide for themselves.

In some instances, problems of severe family pathology may be beyond the nurse's competence, requiring intervention by a social worker or psychiatrist.

Within these caveats, however, the community health nurse can do much to encourage and support general family development as a basis for family health care. By supplying prompt and responsive help or careful referral, she can strengthen the family's confidence in, and its ability to use, community institutions.

In planning her service to families, the community health nurse must work within the framework of the whole structure of family health tasks. She must also understand that the resolution of many health problems will depend upon a family's skills in areas other than health. The family that utilizes health-care services too late or too infrequently may be reflecting a general failure to relate to the community. Through her efforts to solve a particular health problem, the community health nurse can help ameliorate other negative factors.

The family may be helped to discover alternatives to some present patterns and to apply problem-solving approaches in making decisions. They may be helped to see the relationship between health behavior or action of their goals and values. For example, a family that sees material possessions as an index of success may feel that the child entering school must have a new outfit for each day of the first week of classes. In the case of a low-income family, the nurse may be tempted to argue that education, not a competitive fashion show, is the object of going to school. It would be wiser to encourage an early start on savings for this foreseeable financial crisis, or to urge investigation of thrift shops or of sewing classes.

The shift from the concept of care for the individual to the concept of the family as patient is not an easy one. Much of the clinical education of health professionals is carried out in large medical centers that are primarily concerned with serious and acute illness or disability and with the individual as the natural service unit. Thus, the habit of basing treatment on the individual is apt to be well established.

Furthermore, the community health nurse is likely to come from a middle class background and to have values and ways of dealing with family problems that differ from those of the families for whom she cares. She may expect others to hold values similar to her own; for example, in a prosperous population, she may not realize the social pressures placed upon the wife of an executive and may feel that too much of the mother's child-rearing responsibility is being assigned to employees.

At times, the nurse may not be able to separate herself from her own family experiences. If she herself has been caring for a disabled mother while working full-time, she may project her own resentments or frustrations into the observations she makes in the course of her work. She may have stereotyped ideas of what makes a "good" mother or a "cooperative" family, which will hamper her effectiveness.

Also, in many cases, the nurse will be younger and less experienced in handling family situations than is the group she serves. If the nurse has just graduated from student status, she may feel inadequate to the demands made upon her for understanding or for decision-making. A sense of inadequacy can also arise from the feeling that she herself could not muster as much strength and wisdom as the family has done. She may be overwhelmed by their problems and by a lack of confidence in her capacity to help. At times, she may feel helpless in the face of seemingly hopeless situations, even to the degree that her judgment is clouded.

Furthermore, in many cases she will not see any tangible results of her labors. She will observe that in the hospital the patient looks more comfortable, that his treatment is producing the desired result, and that all that has been prescribed has been dispatched with efficiency. Helping a family in the home, however, is often much less visibly rewarding. One is confronted with problems that seem to have no solution: how can one help reduce the anxiety of a mother whose husband is out of work and who has never before experienced the "indignity" of making a welfare application? How can one help the overworked young mother who also has the responsibility of caring for a senile parent who wanders around and needs constant surveillance? When the nurse feels she cannot possibly provide help, she can feel bitterly frustrated — which will make it difficult for her to work productively with the family.

At moments like these, the nurse should remember that very few families are truly helpless or hopeless, and that adversity is part of the learning experience. There will inevitably be setbacks and bleak patches, but the community health nurse never functions entirely alone. She has colleagues within the agency and a host of other professionals to turn to for assistance and advice, plus a broad range of health and welfare resources at her disposal. With time, her own experiences will accumulate and provide a solid base for future assurance and confidence. Nursing has always been a challenging profession, and challenges do not grow from simple conquests and easy solutions.

REFERENCES

1. National Organization of Public Health Nursing: Principles and Practice in Public Health Nursing. New York, Macmillan Pub. Co., Inc., 1932, p. 5.
2. Community Health Nursing: Report of a WHO Expert Committee. Geneva, Switzerland, World Health Organization, World Health Organization Technical Reports, Series 558, 1974, pp. 10–12.
3. Laucks, E.: as cited in Center Rep., 3:14, 1970.
4. Mead, M.: as cited in Toffler, A.: *The Futurists*. New York, Random House, 1972, p. 44.
5. Lorenz, K.: as quoted by Walter Sullivan in Goode, W. J. (ed.): *The Contemporary American Family*. Chicago, Quadrangle Books, 1971, p. 272.
6. Paolucci, P., *In* U.S. Department of Agriculture: *Handbook for the Home*. Washington, D. C., U.S. Government Printing Office, 1973, p. 7.
7. Alpert, J. J., Kosa, J., and Haggerty, R.: A month of illness and health care among low income families. Pub. Health Rep. 82:705, 1967.

SUGGESTED READINGS

Broderick, C. B.: Beyond the five conceptual frameworks: A decade of development in family theory. J. Marriage Family, 33:139, 1971.
Crawford, C. O. (ed.): *Health and the Family: A Medical/Social Analysis*. New York, Macmillan Pub. Co., Inc., 1971.
Duvall, E. W.: *Family Development*, 4th ed. Philadelphia, J. B. Lippincott Co., 1971.
Ferriss, A. L.: *Indicators of Change in the American Family*. New York, Russell Sage Foundation, 1970.
Jackson, J. K.: The role of the patient's family in illness. Nurs. Forum, 1:118, 1962.
Litman, T.: The family as a basic unit in health and medical care: A social-medical overview. Soc. Sci. Med., 8: 495, 1974.
Middleton, R., and Snell, P.: Dominance in decisions in the family, race and class differences. *In* Willie, C. V. (ed.): *The Family Life of Black People*. Columbus, Ohio, Charles & Merrill Co., 1970, pp. 16–22.
Nye, J., and Bernado, F.: *Conceptual Frameworks for the Study of the Family*. New York, Macmillan Pub. Co., Inc., 1966.
Otto, H. A.: A framework for assessing family strengths. *In* Reinhardt, A. M., and Quinn, M. D.: *Family Centered Community Nursing*. St. Louis, Mo., C. V. Mosby Co., 1973, pp. 87–94.
Robischon, P., and Scott, D.: Role Theory and its application in family nursing. *In* Reinhardt, A. M., and Quinn, M. D.: *Family Centered Community Nursing*. St. Louis, Mo., C. V. Mosby Co., 1973, pp. 107–118.
Sussman, M. B.: Family systems in the 70's: Analysis, policies and programs. *In* Hymovich, D. P. and Barnard, M. U.: *Family Health Care*. New York, McGraw-Hill Book Co., 1973.
U.S. Department of Agriculture: *Handbook for the Home*. Washington, D.C., U. S. Government Printing Office, 1973.
Willie, C. V.: The structure and composition of "problem" and "stable" families in a low income population. Marriage Family Liv., 25:440, 1963.

CHAPTER 5

FAMILY HEALTH NURSING CARE: GOALS AND STRATEGIES

The potential of community health nursing for improving the general level of family health care is all too often diluted or squandered because of a lack of *specificity* and precision in use. Essential to the effective use of nursing is a clear understanding of the desired outcomes and the available strategies that can be employed for ensuring these outcomes.

GOALS

The *general goals* of family health nursing care are:

1. To enable families to manage their own health problems, both existing and anticipated, while at the same time preserving family functioning.

2. To conserve and strengthen community services for health care.

This summary indicates the two major claimants on nursing: family and community — the *dyad* with which community health nurses are well acquainted. Sometimes these two claimants are in conflict, and the community health nurse must try to effect a compromise. For example, the community's interests may best be served if a chronically ill person is cared for in his or her home. Though the family may be competent and physically able to provide care, the added burden may deflect attention from other important internal problems — such as an unruly adolescent or a shaky marriage.

Whatever the extent of goals for family health, the needs of both claimants must be satisfied as far as possible. It is poor planning to return elderly sick people to their homes to relieve institutional facilities at the expense of the family. It is equally futile to pour the major portion of nursing support into hospital-based care while neglecting the practice of home care.

Within the framework of these broad goals, each nurse must consider, family by family, what specific goals should be set. For example, the family coping goal may be translated as: "To enable Mrs. A. to provide daily care to the patient with confidence, as demonstrated by the ability to give baths, change dressings, change position, and prevent bedsores." Further goals may be: "To develop supplemental sources of care that will relieve Mrs. A. for at least one day a week," or "To provide such assistance or support as is needed by Mrs. A. to develop a schedule that allows her to conserve her own energies and provides time for special activities with her husband."

STRATEGIES

A strategy is a plan, method, or series of actions designed to lead to a desired outcome. In nursing, strategies represent the general plans or methods by which nursing action may be brought to bear so as to improve the health of families. The community health nurse uses a variety of strategies in the conduct of her work. For example, in a situation where the family is providing inadequate health care to an ill member who appears to be coping at a low level, a nurse may elect to *educate* the family in methods of care and arrange for home health aid assistance for a period of time; or she may elect to *provide direct personal care* herself to reduce the pressure on the family and let them move forward within their capabilities. In a family at odds with itself and manifesting emotional problems, the plan may be to set up a referral for intensive *counseling* to improve communication and understanding or to facilitate other support systems through the aid of extended family members. In a family struggling with a child who has a known developmental disability, the nurse may *provide information* on community resources or act as *coordinator* of a variety of needed services.

Obviously, no one strategy will be used to the exclusion of others, and several will be used in most situations. But an understanding of the different possibilities can help the nurse make deliberate and precise plans with the family.

Among those strategies frequently used are: surveillance or ongoing health supervision of families over time; health education and support of groups to develop self-help and decision-making skills; coordination and referral to best meet family needs and wisely use community resources; direct care to the sick or those in need of habilitation; screening for early detection of disease; research to further refine problems; evaluation of nursing process and development of community health nursing theory;

and modification of the environment, both at the family and community levels. The list is not all-inclusive, but these are the strategies common to nurses working with families. Four strategies are described here, others are discussed elsewhere.

1. Surveillance or ongoing monitoring of family coping with stressors throughout the family life cycle and with illness and threats to health.

2. Assistance to families in developing and maintaining ongoing primary care systems to optimize self-help and community health resources.

3. Health education to increase family capability.

4. Modification of the environment to reduce family health problems to tolerable levels.

HEALTH SURVEILLANCE

The word "surveillance" has different connotations. It is used here in the sense of "to watch over." In this context, *health* surveillance may be defined as a systematic, *continuing* watch for illness, for health-threatening or *diminishing* conditions affecting individuals, families, or population groups.

Surveillance measures are well known among community health nurses; for example, periodic physical examination, hearing and vision tests, observation of mothers and infants, self-examination of the breast, and periodic assessment of family nutritional intake.

For most nurses, however, the many fragments of a surveillance program do not add up to a "continuing watch" of the family's health. Infant health supervision may be well developed, while care for the pre-school or adolescent child is minimal. Cervical smears may be secured once or twice, then forgotten. A mother may report that she "never noticed" that one of her several children had become the scapegoat for his siblings. Surveillance can be a powerful tool in many ways, and the community health nurse can do much to make it more inclusive and persistent.

In some instances — generally, in comprehensive health care centers or H.M.O.'s, or in well-organized private group medical practices — reasonably inclusive and synthesized surveillance has been developed. But all too often, in schools, industries, health departments, and hospital out-patient services, parents and medical advisors go their own way, creating great confusion to the users of the services and wasting scarce health care funds.

Family health surveillance is in no way inconsistent with the concept of the ultimate responsibility and freedom of choice of the family with respect to its own health. Indeed, well-conducted health surveillance should provide incentives and helpful support for the family as it makes health care decisions and plans for its own care.

As with virtually every community health nursing function, the responsibility for health service is a shared one. Family members themselves must be the primary health screening agents. Beyond the family, teachers screen their students for evidence of ill health; special-care clinics, physicians, nurses, and social workers are engaged in multifaceted screening; community screening programs may supply additional family health data. The nurse should concern herself with developing — from whatever resources are available — as comprehensive a data base on the family as is possible.

The *overall purpose* of health surveillance is to help avert, delay, modify, or accommodate to sickness, impairment, decreased vitality, and premature death by providing and analyzing subjective and objective health data over time. "Health data" may include data on disease or malfunction, on health-threatening practices such as alcohol abuse or cigarette smoking; on attitudes, values, and patterns of response to illness with respect to health and health care; and on situational threats to health such as unsafe housing, active illicit drug traffic, and neighborhood decay. Systematically collected, such data provide a sound basis for health planning.

Specifically, health surveillance has the following uses:

1. Surveillance efforts may contribute in many ways to early discovery and treatment of disease. Delayed motor or speech development in a child coupled with a home environment providing little stimulation may alert the nurse to potential problems. A periodic health review may reveal a drinking problem, or incipient psychiatric impairment, or evidence of inadequate parenting. Frequent absence from work and complaints of headache may be symptoms of high blood pressure.

2. Health surveillance efforts may help *identify and correct health-threatening behavior* such as smoking, overeating, or poor managing of aggressive feelings and stress.

3. Family health surveillance may *support the family* in its health tasks — strengthening their observational skills and reinforcing their commitment to health maintenance. Parental concerns that something is wrong with their child may be an alert to real problems. Sharing observations can help the family to make sense of the often chaotic and incomplete health system and enable the members to develop a tenable course of action.

4. Family surveillance activities also *enrich the data base* upon which community and family or personal health care decisions can be made.

For the nurse or other professional worker, such data have great value. Family health surveillance findings over time may reveal behavior patterns within families that supply the clue for remedial approaches or that indicate certain subpopulations in the case load with community-specific problems. Such data may provide information about the direction and rate of change in physical condition. For example, with elderly people — where the effort may be to slow the pace of inevitable functional decline — the pattern over time may have significance. Surveillance efforts may also provide data to identify and characterize the problems of the vulnerable family.

The family health surveillance program as a whole should contain the following ingredients:

1. A cohesive, overall family health surveillance plan.

2. Defined working relationships between community surveillance providers.

3. Training in and interpretation of observations, tests, or processes for participants in the surveillance.

4. A schedule or reminder system for infrequently used measures.

5. A program review system to evaluate usefulness, application, and implication of specific and related outcomes of the program.

In order to develop a *family plan* for surveillance, it is essential that there be some working relationship among the various providers of surveillance. For example, results of a chest x-ray examination should be transmitted to the individual's medical advisor and relayed to the community health nurse as well. Referral and "report back" agreements should be developed. The family should have some idea of how these various parts of the health appraisal system relate to one another, and channels or procedures by which the family is apprised of the results.

For many elements of surveillance, it is necessary to *train* observers or technicians. Volunteer workers can conduct vision-testing programs if they have special preparation in the use of testing equipment. Periodic physical examinations can be provided by community health nurses who have skills beyond that expected of all community health nurses. Teachers may be trained in techniques of observation to detect health problems among students.

There is currently much interest in training family members to provide surveillance formerly left to the professionals, and some health centers have established specific training programs for patients to enable them to check family members' blood pressure or evaluate certain types of symptoms.[1]

Ideally, the *family or individual should take major responsibility;* however, at present, many families are in the habit of depending upon professional health providers to remind them of needed health appointments. They wait to be coaxed into getting care.

For the provider, *periodic review* and evaluation of the surveillance provided are essential. Such a review, often with a responsible member of the family, can reveal the source of problems and misunderstandings on both sides and help the family evaluate the usefulness of surveillance measures.

The Community Health Nurse May Take an
Important Part in the Family Surveillance Program

The community health nurse, working with the family, may *establish the surveillance needs* of the particular family. These needs arise from age-related factors (such as high blood pressure, menopausal stress, and prematurity); individual needs growing out of special problems (e.g., epilepsy, hyperactivity, and pregnancy); and general health threats or environmental hazards (inadequate or unsafe housing, widespread use of illegal drugs, or poor sanitary practices typical of a neighborhood or special group). The availability and accessibility of resources for tests or special observation must also be taken into account; the nurse cannot utilize a non-existent periodic medical check-up, or one that is too costly for the family.

The nurse should point out to the family the *necessity for continuing surveillance measures.* For example, the child with delayed development or speech problems may need semiannual or annual evaluation for assessment of physical development or school placement. Close surveillance can facilitate the proper use of resources to enhance the child's growth potential.

Similarly, the family should understand the necessity of continued observation between scheduled physical examinations. The nurse can increase the awareness of family members to evidence that "something is wrong" or to positive behaviors that should be supported. Training in some techniques of observation may be needed, but mothers particularly must appreciate their own contribution to the discovery and evaluation of illness, developmental disorders, or malfunction. Family members are often the first to note such things as withdrawal from social activities, irritability or moodiness that may signal emotional problems, or the slow progress of an infant. Checking children before they start out for school or observing their eating behavior at mealtimes may do much to promote early recognition of health problems.

Although there will be a health record for those under some form of comprehensive health care, there is much to be said for a family maintained *health record* for all. Such a record should include dates of immunizations, physical examinations, and significant illnesses or hospitalization. This information provides not only a quick source of information but also a stimulus for continuing and inclusive health appraisal. Urging the maintenance of such a reference provides one more way in which the nurse can emphasize the ultimate responsibility of the family for its own health care.

Follow through is an essential part of surveillance — helping families to understand the results of the tests or examinations and planning for subsequent adjustments or action. Some families may require only the knowledge that the nurse is standing by with answers, explanations, and available resources. Others will require that much of the initiative come from the nurse, and the follow-through process may be more intensive.

The community health nurse should be concerned also with the evidence of adequacy, relevance, and quality of measures for continued care, and of the resources available.

A review of surveillance results in groups of families may also be helpful. Problems characteristic of certain groups or localities, or trends in patterns of family action while seeking health appraisal, may be identified. Health surveillance is an exceedingly helpful strategy in the protection and promotion of health — by observing and interpreting health behaviors and caring patterns and life styles of individuals and families. This forms the basis for determining community health needs and program requirements.

Assistance to Families in Developing and Maintaining a Primary Care Network

As mentioned earlier, primary care is subject to various interpretation.

> Primary care is what most people use most of the time for most of their health problems. Primary care is majority care. It describes a range of services adequate for meeting the great majority of daily personal needs. This majority care includes the need for preventive health maintenance and for evaluation and management, on a continuing basis, of general discomfort, early complaints, symptoms, problems, and chronic intractable aspects of disease.[2]

In operational terms, this might mean development of a telephone advisory service to help families evaluate the need for immediate or initial care; the provision of periodic health examinations and special observation clinics for detection of cancer, emphysema, or high blood pressure; the care of non-hospitalized patients by visiting nurses and private physicians; health classes and discussion groups; community Red Cross courses on home care of the sick; and so on. The *totality* of these efforts is not always easy to determine.

Good primary care should be accessible to and affordable by all groups. It should include preventive and health promotion activities adequate to the needs of a particular community; illness care; full use of self-help measures; and economical, selective use of the facilities available.

The primary system or *network* is the complex of the *people* involved as users and as providers of care; the *agencies* or *institutions* through which services are provided, with their special policies and commitments; and the *patterns of interaction* through which people and agencies plan and conduct their respective programs. Thus the *people* are (1) the population served, and (2) the doctors, nurses, health educators, social workers, aides, and engineers — each of whom brings to the equation their particular susceptibilities, capabilities, and skills.

The *agencies* and institutions include the hospitals, clinics, health departments, specialized governmental, voluntary, and professional organizations as well as citizens' health committees, activist groups, and "watch dog" consumer agencies. Each of these agencies will have its own policies, commitments, and style.

Coordinating mechanisms may develop in a helter-skelter fashion or through formal planning sessions.

A small but growing proportion of the population is currently enrolled in some form of comprehensive health care — a health maintenance organization or prepaid high-coverage group medical plan. Most of these plans are designed to provide "one door" services in health. Generally, these services cover only a specified insured population. In some instances, welfare or industrial organizations may enroll their clients or workers in such programs. Most of these health care organizations are committed to comprehensive care, although the health promotional and preventive services vary widely. Another type of total care may be provided for certain "closed" groups — populations in prison, nursing homes, or resident facilities for the mentally retarded. Some industries provide or contract for various forms of health service for their employees (and their employees' families).

Most of the population, however, must at present rely on a patchwork of services from many sources. A father may receive complete care from his employer, while a mother and her children must seek multiagency care from private physicians, clinics, or hospitals. A mother may have excellent health monitoring during the time she is pregnant but not during non-pregnant periods. Middle class families may go to the family doctor for "simple" things, directly to the hospital or a surgeon for any serious problem, or to a specialty clinic for gastrointestinal checkups. Children may be given preventive and health promotional care at school and medical care by a general practitioner, clinic, or specialist (depending on the situation and family income). Often, the only coordinator of these many care providers is the family itself.

When a large proportion of the population is covered by comprehensive care services, coordination may be simply a matter of using "extra" health care opportunities — such as group discussions on child rearing, special clinics for abusive or potentially abusive parents, courses in home nursing or first aid and cardiac resuscitation techniques.

For those families floundering among the unorganized multiple sources of care, much can be done to make the system — or non-system — work for them. The community health nurse may be the key to rationalizing potential resources for the family. Take, for example, the family whose primary source of care is the family physician, with other facilities used at the physician's recommendation. Sometimes the physician is apt to be too burdened to provide in-depth health education for his patients. Through special community clases, school health services, and community health nursing, the physician's contribution can be extended and enriched. Nurses may conduct periodic physical examinations within industries or for groups that do not have access to medical examination services. The school health unit or the school nurse alone may be enlisted to help with health examinations of pre-school-aged children. Examinations conducted by nurses may provide more teaching and preventive content.

Two crucial factors may be identified in putting together the bits and pieces of health care. First, the family must comprehend the entire system. The family needs to know what it can expect in terms of possibilities and limits of available resources and also what is expected of the family. The family's obligation to be alert, supportive, and responsible cannot be overemphasized. No comprehensive care facility can provide good care unless the family itself reports needs for care early, or adheres to treatment plans in a reasonable manner.

A knowledge of the way the system works — who does what and how — is essential to effective use of available resources. The nurse (or other continuing advisor) needs a knowledge of the capabilities and organization of the total system in order to estimate how well the various parts approximate a comprehensive and responsive whole. She must be in touch with all the components of the system and with any coordinating bodies such as councils or planning committees. Only then can she help families to take full advantage of what is available.

The Nursing Response

1. Get a "fix" on the present system: Who are the participants? Who (or what) triggers action or change? What is the family's self-help level? Who does what among the providers? What are the structures and what are their commitments? How complete is available coverage? How is coverage distributed among claimants (viz., those eligible for Medicaid may be getting good coverage, but there is much less for non-subsidized populations)? How well does this compare with respect to the family's needs?
2. Help the family to understand what they can expect from the community system and what they themselves might be expected to do. For example, the provider has a right to expect that the family will be *informative* and *responsible* in seeking early care or keeping appointments.
3. Check — and, if necessary, supplement or encourage — development of services to meet family needs. This would include
   a. *A specific place to call for advice* if a family member is worried or perhaps ill, or when definitive care may be needed.
   b. Routine preventive services — such as developmental assessment of small children, immunization, screening services for glaucoma, diabetes, tuberculosis, cancer, and preconceptional and prenatal supervision.

ACCIDENTS, SURGERY, HOSPITALIZATIONS RECORD
(or other important medical occurrences)

Family Member's Name	Date	Age	What Happened	Severity	Complications

Figure 5-1 Home health history. (From *How to be Your Own Doctor—Sometimes* by Keith W. Sehnert, M.D., and Howard Eisenberg. Copyright © 1975 by Keith W. Sehnert, M.D., and Howard Eisenberg. Used by permission of Grosset & Dunlap, Inc. Reprinted by permission of the author and the author's agents, Scott Meredith Literary Agency, Inc., 845 Third Avenue, New York, New York 10022.

RECORD OF DOCTORS

Keep a record of all doctors you go to. Note when you change doctors. This can help in assuring that medical records can be quickly located and sent for when needed.

Doctor's name and address	Type of doctor	Hours	Office and after hours phone	Date started with doctor, date ended
1. _____				
2. _____				
3. _____				
4. _____				
5. _____				
6. _____				
7. _____				
8. _____				
9. _____				
10. _____				

Figure 5-1 *Continued,* From *How to be Your Own Doctor—Sometimes* by Keith W. Sehnert, M.D., and Howard Eisenberg. Copyright © 1975 by Keith W. Sehnert, M.D., and Howard Eisenberg. Used by permission of Grosset & Dunlap, Inc. Reprinted by permission of the author and the author's agents, Scott Meredith Literary Agency, Inc., 845 Third Avenue, New York, New York 10022.

   c. Programs or advisory services for safeguarding or improving the environment — such as rat control programs, citizens' groups to improve neighborhood sanitation, housing regulatory agencies, traffic safety programs to protect school children, and industrial health services.
   d. Emergency and continuing medical care — such as family physician, clinic, group care agency, rescue squad or other transport, and Medicaid panel.
   e. Sources for nursing and related care of ill or disabled persons at home, visiting nurse service, volunteer services either formally organized or available within an extended family or neighborhood.
4. Coach the family or family surrogate in self-care skills. This might include such things as referral to a community class in home care of the sick, home visits to demonstrate and supervise care, use of hospital or other medical care facility patient-education programs, and maintaining telephone contact with families with marginal health levels (such as the very elderly).
5. Support of families in keeping a family health record (see Fig. 5–1, pp. 108 and 109).
6. Assist the family to develop a calendar of health actions; so, for instance, at the time of one dental checkup the family may record the need to make another appointment.
7. Inform agencies or planning groups of problems that arise in families seeking care: for example, the lack of preventive care for the unemployed individual, or the need to arrange a combined medical visit for the school-age children of one family (to spare the mother from making multiple trips).

   The methods of securing family health care are bound to change, and the strategies for relating family and community programs will also change. However "comprehensive" care is, there is going to be a need for clarification of responsibilities and roles in the health care process.

Changing Family Health Behavior Through Health Education

   The commitment to health education is deeply embedded in current community health nursing practice. New knowledge makes it possible to achieve more in this field.

   A simple definition makes the purpose of health education efforts clear: "Health education is a process that bridges the gap between health information and health practice."[3] Thus, any nursing activity could be considered "health education." For purposes of clarity, the discussion here focuses on three of the major approaches to health education of the family: *health teaching* of skills, knowledge, and values conducive to health; health *counseling* to develop and strengthen family decisions; and *operant conditioning* as a measure for motivation toward desirable health behavior. These and other approaches will be called upon in the total process of changing health behavior through education — sometimes concurrently, sometimes sequentially, depending on the nature of the problem. These measures may be applied to individuals within a family or other group, to the family as an operating system, or to ready-made or specially constructed groups.

The professional health educator has graduate-level preparation in education and usually in public health, and serves as an invaluable resource to the community health nurse. He or she serves in a variety of ways, working directly with families, organizing community programs and action groups, and preparing educational campaigns. The educator is a resource for other staff members, helping with specific health teaching problems, locating references in specific areas where the community health nurse needs further information, and serving as a catalyst to develop the capabilities of others and stimulate new ideas. The short-trained health educator is not widely used in industrially developed countries but, when available, is a good source of information about local needs and values.

Health Teaching

Health teaching is based on the assumption that the nurse possesses special knowledge or expertise, which is different from or more extensive than that of the client. The relationship is that of teacher and learner. Both teacher and learner make equal contributions to the process. The family as learner may want to be shown how to care for a sick person at home, to be reassured that its present information is accurate and adequate for the situation. But the family's knowledge of the costs (in terms of both money and discomfort) for a particular course of action or the tolerance of family members for responsibility and disciplined action will far exceed that of the nurse.

Health teaching requires a set of active *goals,* an *assessment* of knowledge deficits, an *orderly plan* for action, and a concurrent and periodic *evaluation.*

Action goals define the outcomes expected and include quality and time indicators. They are most useful if expressed in terms of the expected *behavior* rather than merely *knowledge* and *skills,* which are the means of acquiring desired behavior. For example, the patient with diabetes should be expected to control and monitor his medication program or to establish food-intake patterns required for control of the disease. Knowing the symptoms of over- and underdosage, and understanding and using a practical exchange diet, are part of the control of his own care.

The goals system will include *contributory* as well as central goals. Such contributory goals may be narrower in scope and may be expressed in terms of *learning* rather than action. For example, the ability to "eat out" wisely, and to apply exchange values to food in this setting.

In most instances, goals will be developed jointly by client and nurse. Some groups have developed contracts between client and nurse for this purpose. Reviewed and modified periodically, they will provide a basis for the action program, referred to in the process of care and again in evaluation.

There will be occasions when the nurse will have goals that are not shared by the client. The nurse's goal may include enabling the individual to self-administer his own insulin safely, comfortably, and on time. If the newly diagnosed diabetic child and his parents are not yet ready to accept this goal, the nurse may shelve the idea temporarily until the family is ready.

Sometimes goals are external to the family. The nurse may want the family to substitute home care for hospital or nursing home-care for a relative, as a measure to reduce pressure on local institutions. Such a suggestion may make the family uneasy, and left with the feeling that their best interests are being subordinated to the interests of the community.

Basic to the establishment of a teaching plan is an estimate of the family's *knowledge, skill,* and *attitude;* and an assessment of what the family *needs* to know and what the family already does know. The amount and extent of knowledge required by the situation must also be part of the equation. In this media-dominated age, nobody starts at square one! An adult woman may *need* to know how to recognize the warning signals of cancer, she may *not* need extensive information on the epidemiology of cancer and ongoing experimental research.

Frequently, knowledge is suppressed. A young girl who really knows the symptoms of gonorrhea may suppress that knowledge to enable her to conceal a suspected infection.

An orderly plan for action helps conserve energy and assure appropriate care. The plan should include *what* should be taught, *who* will do the teaching, and *when* and *how* it will be done.

The "what" in teaching is largely a factor of the learning deficit, as well as of action that is required to protect the community. Sometimes there is a tendency on the nurse's part to introduce too much information into home and family interaction. For example, most expectant mothers do not need to know or want to know much about rare complications of pregnancy, or about maternal and infant mortality statistics. They must know, however, how to secure necessary medical or midwifery surveillance.

The "by whom" involves dividing the teaching tasks among the nurse, a family member, a nurse-surrogate, or a community education facility. For example, in teaching the home care of a sick elderly person, the nurse may set the pattern of care by modeling (providing care without obviously teaching and so setting a model); she may delegate such teaching to a nursing aide, practical nurse, specially trained volunteer, or to an experienced family member. Often there are community agencies that provide teaching support, such as the American Cancer Society or the American Red Cross. Clinics may also offer teaching services, such as classes for diabetics or for recovered cardiac patients.

The "when" depends on the readiness of the learners and the urgency of the need for information or skills. In the case of a child who has not been immunized against polio or measles, the nurse must initiate a prompt program to provide the family with necessary information and assistance. If the case is one of a slightly overprotective mother, the nurse can wait for a favorable time to introduce the subject of a child's need for independence.

The "how" of teaching offers rich variety. Telling, showing, and discussing help define the problem and promote skill and understanding. Television health programs and health classes or group discussion sessions are helpful. "Follow-up" visits afford an opportunity to observe the learner's skills and progress and clarify or expand on the knowledge gained. Just being available in the office at stated times to receive visits or phone calls may be part of the teaching strategy.

Continuing and periodic *evaluation* of the learner's progress is essential. Such evaluation should center on behavior rather than words, and on understanding rather than disparate facts. The evaluative process should involve both teacher and learner and be clearly based on the goals to which both had previously agreed.

People need knowledge to protect their own health, and there is much new information that is not common knowledge. A poll involving 1609 people showed that, despite extremely active educational efforts to teach individuals to recognize and report symptoms of cancer, only 13 per cent knew four or more of the danger signals.[4]

Health Counseling

Health counseling is a helping process through which an individual with special knowledge or skills interacts with a client who has health needs in such a way as to enhance the client's ability to assess and to cope effectively with his health problems.

In counseling, the initiative rests clearly with the client. It is he who must define the meaning and impact of a particular condition, who must decide whether or not to take action, and where and how he will act. The development of independence and skill in matters of health decisions and actions is particularly important when the outcome is dependent upon the decision of the individual — not mandated by legislation or dictated by necessity, such as the treatment of an acutely ill person, or a physical examination in an industrial health service.

Many important health decisions require such initiative and

choice — to smoke or not to smoke, to terminate or not to terminate a pregnancy (when amniocentesis reveals a severely damaged fetus), to seek or reject measles immunization for children. Indeed, mundane decisions may be the most difficult to make. In such instances no one can decide a "right answer" for the individual. Thus it is important that individuals, especially if there are pressing problems already, be prepared to make these decisions wisely, and to take necessary action expeditiously.

Characteristics and content of counseling as they might be undertaken in community health practice can be discussed only briefly.

The essential ingredient in counseling is the relationship between counselor and client. To be effective, the counselor must be seen by the client as a friend with whom it is possible to speak freely and honestly, whose support and respect is unequivocal, and who is informed in health matters and willing to help *on the client's terms.*

The client must be seen by the counselor as someone worthy of respect — as someone who, given the proper support, is able and willing to act on his health problems and whose knowledge of particular health conditions or health actions can be crucial in treatment.

Both client and counselor must be willing to learn from one another and able to communicate with trust and frankness. Both must accept the premise that it is the client alone who is ultimately responsible for his own health and whose decision must be final (except for those instances when a particular decision might endanger others).

The *objectives* of health counseling are all contributory to the development of the client's ability to act wisely on behalf of his own health and that of his family and his community.

First, the individual must have access to the facts (or the best current opinion) on which to base a decision to act. The odds that certain genetic traits or diseases may actually appear, given a specific family pedigree; the impact of positioning on the occurrence of bedsores in a bed-bound patient; the real risks involved in the use of drugs — all of these affect the decision making process.

The individual needs support to *clarify his own beliefs, values, and feelings* about the problem and the choice of several possible actions. To make sensible health decisions, the individual must be informed of all the possible actions that could be taken, the alternatives that are open. For example, there are several choices regarding smoking: the individual may elect to continue smoking heavily, accepting the high risk of shortened life and disabling illness; he may decide to stop completely, and so reduce the risks substantially; he may decide to cut down on cigarettes, to smoke lower tar/low-nicotine brands; or he may choose to turn to cigars or a pipe. Each alternative has variable anticipated reduction of risk.

Grown children, determining care for an elderly and disabled parent, may elect to provide care at home with consequent additional work for family members and possible interruption of social activities; they may employ a helper who can share the responsibility for care; they may opt for institutional care after evaluating degrees of guilt, economic strain, and difficulties of maintaining patient-family contacts.

Health counseling also may help the family to anticipate and mitigate stress, feelings of guilt, and frustrations. An opportunity to ventilate frustrations with a neutral but concerned counselor may in itself limit their impact, or it may result in new alternatives and mitigating action. In sum, counseling assists the client to use sound problem-solving techniques in dealing with his or her health problems.

The *processes* in counseling are generally familiar to community health nurses as part of their on-going practice:

Listening, which is basic to counseling is active rather than passive. It is important to listen with absolute attention to the speaker in an effort to understand as fully as possible the meaning of what is (and what is *not*) said. The tone of voice and the sequence of the ideas or statements put forth all have meaning.

Time limits sometimes help to focus the discussion between nurse and client, encouraging concentration on the concerns in hand. Time limits may be built in by clinic schedules, or by agreement between nurse and client.

The nurse can *demonstrate concern* by her body language, her facial expression, and a comfortable relaxed posture.

Reflecting — repeating or rephrasing the client's statement — may help the individual to explore his problem further, consider whether what he said was truly what he intended to say, and clarify the stance he has taken. It also maintains the neutral position of the counselor and may help avoid hasty or premature decisions. The aim of the counselor is to expose findings, not to impose them.

Questioning is another device for encouraging full consideration of the problem, its demands, and its alternatives. Care must be taken not to indulge in leading questions that may serve to suggest a "right" answer. Rather, it should be clear that the purpose is to ensure consideration of *all* significant factors or conditions and of all available options as a basis for decision. "Have you thought about . . . ?" can open a new train of thought without diminishing the relevance of other approaches.

Reassurances engender a feeling in the client that he *can* handle his problems by strengthening his self-concept and assuring him of the availability of help. For example, the young girl who has contracted syphilis may feel her reputation and personal integrity have been irreparably damaged. The counselor's own respect for the girl is a step toward rebuilding a favorable self-concept — for example, asking about her plans rather than launching into instructions may restore the patient's self-confidence; suggesting that the patient might "rehearse" what she will say to her sexual partner or others who must be told, shows that the nurse feels she has a capacity for facing the issues. Her sense of responsibility in coming for treatments should be commended.

Information giving is an appropriate part of the counseling process, but should be used with caution. The information provided may be related to areas in which the counselor is expert — the nature of treatment, the sources of care, the epidemiologic pattern etc.; however, in providing such information, the counselor must be careful not to imply a decision but rather, to supply a background for decision making. In some cases, information may be needed to outline constraints within decisions — e.g., interpretation of the legal aspects of treatment for syphilis. Sometimes, however, the nurse will be asked what she would do, or which of several courses of action is the "right" or "best" one. In her response she should make clear that *for her* a given course of action was right but might not be for another person, or she may speak of ways in which others with similar problems handled theirs.

Follow-through action is often indicated. The client may call back to report results, or the nurse may "stop by" to be sure all went well. It is essential that the nurse have knowledge of both negative and positive outcomes if the counseling effort is to be effective. For example, one family living in a dangerous environment may have been put on the waiting list for public housing, only to discover there would be no vacancies for at least two years; or a young man may have lost his courage about talking to his parents concerning his need for more independence.

Health counseling is a useful approach to increasing individual and family capability for self-care and the effective use of other care sources. It is a subtle and highly responsive element in community health nursing practice.

Operant Conditioning

The concept of operant conditioning has been widely acclaimed as a breakthrough in behavior modification. It is essentially a method by which the value of behaving in a given way is increased, and the value of alternate behavior is decreased. Operant conditioning is rooted in two concepts: behavior *reinforcement* as a measure for changing behavior (as developed by B. F. Skinner) as well as the "pleasure principle" as a motivator (as developed by Jeremy Bentham.)[5, 6]

The value of a given *behavior* or course of action to the learner is enhanced by providing reinforcement that is consistent with a desired result and failing to give reinforcement for undesired behavior. The *characteristics* of this behavior modifying activity may be identified:

1. The objective is to channel behavior into a preconceived, acceptable pattern. The desired behavior is developed by the change agent, usually based on "models" — behavior characteristic of prestigious individuals or groups. For example, the desired behavior may be control of aggressive behavior, as determined by the society in which the individual lives or as demonstrated by people or institutions that the change agent considers "right." Such desired behavior may range from avoiding smoking or the taking of drugs to exerting physical control over enuresis or promoting regular exercise.

2. Reinforcement of the desired behavior is provided by associating *something the individual wants* with performance of the desired behav-

ior — e.g., parental approval or special privileges such as watching television or using the family car. Reinforcement may also be simply a feeling of progress and accomplishment, as when an obese person brings his weight down through proper dieting. Whatever the reinforcer, it must be valued *by the learner:* the adolescent who loves rock music may place a low value on tickets to the opera.

3. The reinforcement must be *earned* by the learner for displaying the desired behavior (or failing to display undesired behavior). The earning may come as a single response to a single problem — getting home at an agreed upon time may make the older child eligible to borrow the family car. Sometimes the desired behavior involves a number of individual actions, such as refraining from a quarrel with siblings or from a display of excessive temper. In some cases, time is needed to display the desired behavior, such as in reducing cigarette smoking. In this instance, a "token" system may be developed, in which the token is awarded for immedaite satisfactory behavior and then is collected and redeemed for the eventual desired benefit.

The reinforcement is awarded in accordance to rules or methods of computation understood and accepted by both learner and change agent. The strength of the reinforcement is strongly influenced by the immediacy of the reinforcement.

4. When the desired behavior is *not* exhibited, reinforcement is withheld. Care must be taken to avoid any reinforcement that denies the learner his rights as an individual, a child, or a patient (withholding love, for example, or denying the right to choose).

5. Behavioral goals and reinforcement patterns are set by the individual and accepted (whether satisfied or not) by the teacher. The rules — what constitutes compliance, time tolerance, and regulations concerning intermittent compliance — must be fully understood by everyone involved in the change process. The learner always has the right to refuse or agree only partially with the projected change. Sometimes negotiation for changing reinforcers may be required. In some instances, it is desirable to have a formal contract, signed by the individual and the change agent.

6. A record of performance is an important part of the change effort, so that progress can be charted and methods of conditioning re-evaluated.

7. After the desired behavior is well established, the reinforcement is withdrawn. By such time, it is hoped that the learner will have developed a sense of satisfaction from the change or that, at least, will find it difficult to revert to his former behavior. Reinforcing agents may then be applied to different areas of desired change.

Operant conditioning has been found to be useful in a variety of health situations. It may help elderly people to avoid behavior prejudicial to their continuing independence or eliminate distasteful habits that isolate them from other people. It has also proved useful in working with mentally retarded or mentally disturbed individuals and in developing social skills in children.

This approach, used with discretion, is a quick and inexpensive way of changing behavior. There are, of course, those individuals who find the process stultifying or even repugnant because of the reliance on external motivation. They believe it is based on manipulation and a disregard for human self-determination. It cannot be denied that much human behavior is *not* guided by rational consideration of its consequences. Certainly for individuals capable of and accustomed to defining their own problems and acting on their own decisions, this approach would not be indicated at all.

It is not certain, either, that the desired behavior may not be actually harmful for a particular individual. For example, if the desired behavior is based on parental standards of sexuality, without regard to modern attitudes, and if this behavior pattern is embedded through conditioning, the outcome may be a repressed sexuality that is injurious to the learner.

Used with discrimination, however, the results may be highly satisfactory. The mother who pays little attention to undesired behavior on the part of a young child, and who cuddles and comforts him when he exhibits "good" behavior is simply supplying good parenting. For the youngster with a high automobile accident rate and reckless driving habits, the full-scale application of operant conditioning may prove extremely helpful.

Many studies are under way concerning the effectiveness of operant conditioning, and it would be well worth the community health nurse's time to watch its development.

Reducing Family Health Care Tasks to Tolerable Levels

Sometimes, the combined total of family home care tasks seems overwhelming. When problems are encountered one by one, the family can normally cope; when they accumulate, or descend all at one time, these problems can become unmanageable and frightening. For example, it may be physically and technically possible for the family to provide care for a severely impaired senile member; however, if another member falls ill, if emotional problems arise, or if financial conditions worsen, the compounding of problems may raise stress to intolerable levels.

When problems multiply and a danger point is reached, the nurse should seek to *reduce the problem.* Most families can provide *some* of the care, and the additional load may be assumed on a regular basis by a nursing aide or by volunteers from the community or extended family. Husbands should be encouraged to lend a hand with young children by getting up at night part of the time. Day-care services may relieve the hard-pressed mother coping with an intractable brain-damaged child.

The nurse may make periodic visits, combining personal care with reassurance and instruction for the family or primary care giver. Such steps may often save expensive hospitalization, and they are compatible with good care.

Intermittent nursing home care may sufficiently relieve the home-care giver, so that it is possible to continue without hazard to personal health. Institutionalized patients may return home when death is imminent, since the family is often willing to accept an overload at such a crisis but not willing as a continuing practice. The working mother can be relieved of some of her child-care tasks by after-school classes or by cooperative arrangements with other families.

Family tolerance levels may be increased by nursing reassurance and training in required skills. Much of the tension in providing care arises from a feeling of incompetence — of being beyond one's depth. Continuing visits by the nurse (or other member of the nursing staff) serve to alleviate the loneliness of the home care giver, and offer an opportunity for him or her to ask questions or discuss concerns with a knowledgeable ally.

In some instances, the problems can be made tolerable by *redefining the problem* in more realistic terms. The family may feel that they *alone* should provide care for a disabled parent, when in fact the interposition of a paid helper or nurse's aide may offer a very real contribution to the patient as well as the family. Twenty-four–hour care is usually not necessary — except in the exaggerated view of an affectionate and dutiful family member. Most confined patients can and do get along by themselves (properly safeguarded and instructed if necessary), or with a volunteer or paid "sitter." Caring for a well pre-school child does not mean answering *every* question or listening to *every* experience the child wants to share.

Supplementation and realistic assessment of family health care are natural and familiar roles to most community health nurses. The need at present is to explore more deeply the implications and promise of new approaches to this old responsibility.

Finale

There is always more than one way to approach a problem, and in the changing world of nursing the possible directions are many. As the community health nurse looks at the strategies that might be used — choosing thoughtfully, with knowledge of relative values and strengths of the different specific courses of action — her methods of practice will be refined and her energies channeled in ways that are efficient and orderly — and good for both the nurse and the families or communities she serves.

REFERENCES

1. Sehnert, K. W.: *How to be Your Own Doctor — Sometimes.* New York, Grosset & Dunlap, Inc., 1975, p. 641.
2. U.S. Department of Health, Education, and Welfare: *A Conceptual Model of Organized Primary Care and Comprehensive Community Health Services.* Washington, D.C. U.S. Government Printing Office, PHS Pub. No. 2024, 1970.
3. Report of the President's Committee on Health Education. Washington, D.C., U.S. Government Printing Office, 1973, p. 1. (Now out of print.)
4. *Time,* January 17, 1972, p. 67.
5. Skinner, B. F.: *Beyond Freedom and Dignity.* New York, Alfred A. Knopf, Inc., 1971.
6. Wheeler, H.: *Beyond the Punitive Society.* San Francisco, W. H. Freeman & Co., Publishers, 1973.

SUGGESTED READINGS

Ahmed, P. I., and Coelho, G. V. (eds.): *Toward a New Definition of Health.* Psychosocial Dimension, Plenum Press, New York, 1979 (Healthy Family Functioning, Ch. 14).

American Red Cross: *Family Health and Home Nursing.* Garden City, N.Y., Doubleday and Co., Inc., 1979, Chapter 3.

Auger, J. R.: *Behavioral Systems and Nursing.* Englewood Cliffs, N.J., Prentice-Hall, Inc., 1976.

Avila, D. L., Coombs, A., and Purkey, W. W.: *The Helping Relationship Sourcebook.* Boston, Allyn & Brown, 1971.

Bandura, A.: *Principles of Behavior Modification.* New York, Holt, Rinehart & Winston, 1969.

Bates, B.: *A Guide to Physical Examination.* Philadelphia, J. B. Lippincott, Co., 1974.

Bauernfeind, L.: Strengthening a disorganized family. Am. J. Nurs., 75:2198, 1975.

Becker, M. H., Brachman, R. H., and Kirscht, J. P.: A new approach to explaining sick-role behavior in low-income populations. Am. J. Pub. Health, 64:205, 1974.

Becker, M. H., and Maiman, L. A.: Sociobehavioral determinants of compliance with health and medical care recommendations. Med. Care, 13:10, 1975.

Belkins, G. S. (ed.): *Foundations of Counseling.* Dubuque, Iowa, Kendall & Hunt Pub. Co., 1974.

Berdie, R. F.: The 1980 counselor: Applied behavioral specialist. Pers. Guid. J., 50:451, 1972.

Berni, R., and Fordyce, W. E.: *Behavior Modification and the Nursing Process.* St. Louis, Mo., C. V. Mosby Co., 1973.

Berni, R., Dressler, J., and Baxter, J.: Reinforcing behavior. Am. J. Nurs., 71:2180, 1971.

Bessel, R.: *Interviewing and Counseling.* London, Batsford, 1971.

Blocher, D. H. (ed.): *Developmental Counseling,* 2nd ed. New York, Ronald Press, 1974.

Brammer, L. M.: *The Helping Relationship: Process and Skills.* Englewood Cliffs, N.J., Prentice-Hall, Inc., 1973.

Brody, S., et al.: The family caring unit: A major consideration in the long-term support system. Gerontologist, 18:556, 1978.

Campbell, C.: *Nursing Diagnosis and Intervention in Nursing Practice.* New York, John Wiley and Sons, 1978.

Chang, B. L.: Generalized expectancy, situational perception, and morale of the institutionalized aged. *Nurs. Res.,* 27: 316, 1978.

Chang, B. L.: Locus of control, trust, situational control and morale of the elderly. Int. J. Nurs. Studies, 16: 169, 1979.

Christensen, D. B.: Drug taking compliance: A review and synthesis. Health Serv. Res., 13: 171, 1978.

Cormier, W. H., and Cormier, L. S.: *Behavioral Counseling.* Boston, Houghton Mifflin Co., 1975.

Deibert, A. N., and Harmon, A. J.: *New Tools for Changing Behavior.* Champaign, Ill., Research Press, 1970.

Delaney, D., and Eisenberg, S.: *The Counseling Process.* Chicago, Rand McNally & Co., 1972.

Doll, W.: Family coping with the mentally ill. An unanticipated problem of deinstitutionalization. Hosp. Comm. Psychiatry, 27:183, 1976.

Eggebroton, E.: Why not the laundromat? Nurs. Outlook, 21:758, 1973.

Enterline, P. E., Salter, V., McDonald, A. D., and McDonald, J. C.: The distribution of medical care services before and after free medical care: the Quebec experience. N. Engl. J. Med., 289:1174, 1973.

Erickson, M. L.: Assessment and Management of Developmental Changes in Children. St. Louis, Mo., C. V. Mosby Co., 1976.

Fleck, S.: Unified health services and family-focused primary care. Int. J. Psychiatry Med. 6:501(b), 1975.

Fowler, R., Fordyce, W., and Berni, R.: Operant conditioning in chronic illness. Am. J. Nurs., 69:1226, 1969.

Gardner, H. H., and Ouimette, R.: A nurse-physician team approach in a private internal medicine practice. Arch. Intern. Med., 134:956, 1974.

Hackney, H., and Nye, S.: Counseling Strategies and Objectives. Englewood Cliffs, N. J., Prentice-Hall, Inc., 1973.

Henriques, C. C., Virgadamo, V. G., and Kahane, M. D.: Performance of adult health appraisal examinations utilizing nurse practitioners, physician teams, and paramedical personnel. Am. J. Pub. Health, 64: 47, 1974.

Honig, W. (ed.): Operant Behavior. New York, Appleton-Century-Crofts, 1966.

Hulka, B. S., Cassel, J. C., Kupper, L. L., and Burdette, J. A.: Communication, compliance and concordance between physicians and patients with prescribed medications. Am. J. Pub. Health, 66: 847, 1976.

Hyde, N.: Behavior theory and therapy in mental retardation. Am. J. Nurs., 74: 882, 1974.

Institute of Medicine: A Manpower Policy for Primary Health Care. Washington, D.C., National Academy of Science, 1978.

Kane, R. L., and Deuschle, K. W.: How much do patients know and how much do health professionals think they know? Int. J. Health Ed., 11:102, 1968.

Kanfer, I. H., and Goldstein, A. P. (eds.): Helping People Change. New York, Pergamon Press, Inc., 1975.

Kasl, S. V.: Issues in patient adherence to health care regimens. J. Human Stress, 1:5, 1975.

Kitzman, H. J.: Well child care. Am. J. Nurs., 75:1705, 1975.

Krumbholtz, J. D., and Krumbholtz, H. B.: Changing Children's Behavior. Englewood Cliffs, N.J., Prentice-Hall, Inc., 1972.

LeBow, M. D.: Behavior Modification: A Significant Method in Nursing Practice. Englewood Cliffs, N.J., Prentice-Hall, Inc., 1973.

Levin, L. S., Katz, A. H., and Holst, E.: Self Care: Lay Initiatives in Health. New York, Prodist, 1976.

Levin, L. S.: Patient education and self-care: How do they differ? Nurs. Outlook, 26:170, 1978.

Lewis, J. M., Beavers, W. R., Gossett, J. T., and Phillips, V. A.: No Single Thread: Psychological Health in Family Systems. New York, Brunner-Mazel, 1976.

Linn, L. S.: Factors associated with patient evaluation of health care. Milbank Mem. Fund Qtly., 53: 531, 1975.

MacDonald, M. E., Hagberg, K. L., and Grossman, B. J.: Social factors in relation to participation in follow-up care of rheumatic fever. J. Pediatr., 62:503, 1963.

Manciaux, M.: The health of the family. World Health, September 1975, Nos. 4–9.

Marston, M. V.: Compliance with medical regimens: A review of the literature. Nurs. Res., 19: 312, 1970.

Mohammed, M. F. B.: Patient's understanding of written health information. Nurs. Res., 13:100, 1964.

Murray, R. B., and Zentner, J. P.: Nursing Assessment and Health Promotion through the Life Span, 2nd ed. Englewood Cliffs, N.J., Prentice-Hall, Inc., 1979.

Oelbaum, C. H.: Hallmarks of adult wellness. Am. J. Nurs. 74:1623, 1974.

Peplaw, H.: Talking with patients. Am. J. Nurs., 60:964, 1960.

Putt, A. M.: A biofeedback service by nurses. Am. J. Nurs., 79(1):88, 1979.

Redman, B. K.: The Process of Patient Teaching in Nursing. St. Louis, Mo., C. V. Mosby Co., 1976.

Rubin, L. S.: Biofeedback: Medicine's newest cure-all? Fam. Health, 11(3):50, 1979.

Runyan, J. W., Jr.: Primary Care Guide. New York, Harper and Row Pub., 1975, pp. 33–40.

Sampson, E. E., and Marthos, M. S.: *Group Process for the Health Professions*. New York, John Wiley & Sons, 1977.

Schultz, P., and McClone, F.: Primary health care provided to the elderly by a nurse practitioner/physician team: Analysis of cost effectiveness. J. Am. Geriatr. Soc., *25:* 443, 1977.

Schweer, S. F., and Dayant, E. C.: The extended role of professional nursing — patient education. Int. Nurs. Rev., *20:*174, 1973.

Sehnert, K. W. (with Howard Eisenberg): *How to be Your Own Doctor— Sometimes*. New York, Grosset & Dunlap, 1975.

Shanas, E., and Sussman, M. (eds.): *Family, Bureaucracy, and the Elderly*. Durham, N.C., Duke University Press, 1977.

Skinner, B.F.: *Beyond Freedom and Dignity*. New York, Alfred A. Knopf, Inc., 1971.

Tarver, J. and Turner, A. J.: Teaching behavior modification to patients' families. Am. J. Nurs., 74:282, 1974.

Thorpe, H. S., and Werner, E. E.: Developmental screening of pre-school children: A cultural review of inventories used in health and educational programs. Pediatrician, *53:* 362, 1974.

Valett, R. E.: *Modifying Children's Behavior: A Guide for Parents and Professionals*. Palo Alto, Calif., Feron Publishers, 1969.

Ware, J. E., Davies-Avery, A., and Stewart, A. L.: The measurement and meaning of patient satisfaction: A review of the literature. Health Med. Care Serv. Rev., *1:*1, 1978.

Ware, J. E., and Snyder, M. K.: Dimensions of patient attitudes regarding doctors and medical care services. Med. Care, *11:* 669, 1975.

Wheeler, H. (ed.): *Beyond the Punitive Society*. San Francisco, W. H. Freeman and Co., 1973.

Wong, R. Y., and Watson, J.: Contracting for weight reduction — Making the sacrifices worthwhile. Am. J. Maternal Child Nurs., 3:46, 1978.

World Health Organization: *Primary Health Care, Report of the International Conference on Primary Health Care*. Geneva, World Health Organization, 1978.

Yacenda, J. A.: Turning on high schoolers (about health). J. School Health, *42:*597, 1972.

CHAPTER 6

RECORDS, REPORTS, AND INFORMATION SYSTEMS

The general objectives of records and reports in a public health nursing agency are to assist the nurse and the agency to render a better quality of service to the individual family and community; to make available certain information about community health conditions; and to provide a means of measuring the program of the agency in relation to community needs.[1]

The objective stated above is as true today as it was 50 years ago when it was written. What has changed, however, are the accounting requirements and the technology for gathering the required information.

Supplying the data needed, and completing the forms required for the information needs of agencies has proved burdensome, particularly for the community health nurse. Tremendous efforts have gone into developing information systems that continuously and systematically collect needed data and are simple and easy to use. These systems have helped meet the information needs for reporting, billing, and planning of services. Data required for the knowing application of professional services for the improvement of family health — the most important to the practitioner — has been more elusive.

FUNCTIONS OF THE RECORD SYSTEM

The well-organized and maintained recording and reporting system serves several functions.

1. The record system documents the sources and uses of funds. In most local agencies, financing comes from many sources — including local, federal, and state funds; voluntary agency contracts; contributions; research or special project funds; and foundation grants. The administra-

123

tor must report on, and sometimes bill, each of these agencies separately for the services provided. Medicare and Medicaid programs alone have added immeasurably to the amount of accounting required. Information necessary to identify the patient and his eligibility for care must be accurate and complete. Additionally, since some types of care are reimbursable while others are not, information must be supplied about the precise care given and the level of nursing personnel that was required.

2. The record system provides a control mechanism to assure that services are provided according to plan. In the process of setting goals, certain specific outcomes have been identified, often with measurable indicators of accomplishment. When screening measures are planned, for example, some follow-up work is essential to determine just how near the program is in achieving its goals. Contracts with private industries or schools are often based on the provision of a defined number of nursing hours or a defined quantity of service, and there must be a way to assure that these commitments have, in fact, been fulfilled. In most instances, this information must be secured periodically throughout the year, in order to correct any errors of omission or misdirection of effort. The record system must supply the basic data required for making these estimations.

3. The record system provides information for planning and evaluating the nursing service. Identification of the characteristics of the population being served may determine whether or not that population is, indeed, the one most needing care. If nursing care were centered on welfare clients to the neglect of the low-income, non-welfare population, the question might be raised as to whether the program was in fact meeting the needs of the community. The characteristics of the population being served, over a period of time, may provide a valuable clue to anticipated nursing needs. For instance, low-income populations and older populations tend to require more intensive and time-consuming nursing care than that required by the rest of the population; a young suburban group will have problems related to growing families. Changes in the nature of the population being served are of particular significance. Groups that have not hitherto used nursing services may suddenly become frequent users — as occurs when home care for psychiatric or geriatric patients is instituted.

4. The record provides facts, intuitive assessments, and shared judgments necessary for evaluating the nursing situation in the family. It should describe the nature and the impact of the health threat. It should delineate the interacting forces of the health condition of the family and of the community as they function in daily life. The record can afford an opportunity for mutual exploration of the health situation by the nurse and family, so that they can define their respective concerns, expectations, and probable action. Information collected in a specific and systematic manner can provide baseline and periodic data from which to

estimate long-term changes in the impact of the health challenge as related to the service provided and to the family response.

By reviewing her own records and reports, the community health nurse has a basis for deciding the extent to which the things she is doing are relevant to the particular needs of the population she is serving, for judging whether or not the approaches appear to be suitable, for identifying the recurring problems that confront her, for deciding if these problems recur because they are not being handled as effectively as they might be, and for determining whether or not community resources are being used as fully as possible. By reviewing the composite records of a particular service group, the administrator can find the information needed to decide whether or not the level of staffing is appropriate to the work being performed. He or she can find in records the documentation needed for proposing additional staff or a different kind of staff, or for requesting appropriations from the agency's budget committee or the United Fund. The administrator has a basis for considering the degree to which nursing support is contributing to each of the agency programs and whether or not additional support may have to be directed to a particular program that is either new or understaffed.

Criteria for the Record System

Although the staff nurse is unlikely to be responsible for designing the record system, she will make better use of the system in operation if she understands the criteria the system is expected to meet. An effective and efficient record system should meet the following criteria:

Form. The record system should be sufficiently uniform to provide for easy recording, tabulating, and collating, and to permit interunit and interservice comparisons. In general, records prescribe the placement and content of identifying and service data that are likely to be tabulated and compared. Thus, the record may have a space for the insurance carrier, the social security number, the dates of admission and discharge from service, and the type of service provided; space for this information is often identically placed in all appropriate record forms. The purely narrative record does not lend itself to accurate and economic automatic or hand tabulation.

Format. The record system should require the minimal amount of time that is consistent with the record's purpose. It is quite possible to reduce record time at the expense of reducing the effectiveness and efficiency of the service. On the other hand, unproductive record time is probably one of the greatest thieves of scarce nursing time today. Unproductive record time includes time spent hunting for records that should be readily available, making long and neat notations, long-term storing of information that is of transitory value, reading irrelevant or unimportant data, and voluminous recopying of service data for transmittal to another agency when other alternatives (such as photocopy or person-to person contact) are available.

The format of the record affects the accuracy and time required in recording. For example, boxes providing the expected number of digits in a social security or an insurance number help prevent omission or repetition of a digit; uniform location of an item such as an address saves time, since both reader and writer will know where to find it. Dictation of record content may conserve scarce professional time, provided it does not encourage excessively long recording or result in significant errors in transcription.

Access. The record should be quickly available to the user. Both individual service records and compiled data are useful to the degree that they are where they are needed at the time they are needed. The family history that is filed in a central location and cannot be retrieved in time to use for planning care is only half effective. The record that should be immediately available to the school teacher but that is filed in the health department several blocks away is similarly decreased in value as a tool for service planning and implementation. Compiled data, too, need to be easily available. The nurse who would like to know how her use of a home health aide is similar or different from that of other nurses finds it difficult to look at her own performance comparatively if the records are "in the computer" for months before they are available to her.

Accessibility is not always easy to achieve. For instance, it would seem apparent that school health records should be in school and that clinic records should be in the clinic. Yet the same information may also be needed in the general family record that is used by the nurse in providing assistance to the family as a whole.

Compact Storage. The record system should require reasonable storage space. The proliferation of records, as well as the increase in the number of people under care, may create serious problems of record storage and increased demands for clerical time. The period for which records are retained is usually a matter of agency policy; often the period of retention is as low as five years. A short retention period does save space; however, it also presents problems, since community health needs and methods are changing and the period over which care is provided to a family may be prolonged. Microfilming is used in some agencies as a space-saving procedure. In others, a representative sample of records that would normally be retired may be held for comparisons over time. For example, it is conceivable that a full nursing record from the 1970's would be of considerable interest to nurses in the year 2000 as an indication of the general directions taken in nursing practice in an earlier period.

Coordination with Other Records. A good record system can be coordinated with other data. For example, it should be possible to pull out all of the records for a particular service (such as service to crippled children or to industrial plants) or for a given geographic area or population unit regardless of whether the service was provided in the school, the clinic, or the home. When automatic data processing is used, aggregations of record data are more easily secured. When such processing is not available (for instance, in the small population of an individual case load), identification of special records (by color tabs or other distinguishing mark) or the assignment of a single number to all of a specific family's records, wherever they are filed, may help identify special groups quickly.

Security. The record system should provide for confidentiality of record content. The assurance of privacy is one of the big problems in developing community-wide, coordinated health-care information systems, and even in a small service it is not an easy matter to deal with. For example, it may not be appropriate to open to the teaching staff in the school some of the health information held by the nurse. In some agencies, family permission must be secured before releasing information to any other person or agency. In most agencies there are regulations that limit the degree to which information may be shared; often the specific groups in the community that are eligible to have specific data are defined. In the use of data processing systems in hospitals, special keys issued only to those who are entitled to use the information are required to activate the data-issuing mechanism. The community health nurse's individual responsibility in this respect may be limited to careful observation of agency policies regarding release of information and, when necessary, working out special methods for storing and handling "sensitive" information.

The criteria for recording should reflect the purpose and the process of community health nursing practice. Perhaps the easiest way to consider the degree to which recording implements purpose and practice is to raise a series of questions.

1. *Does the record focus on the family and community as the object of care?* If nursing practice is oriented to a family rather than to an individual approach, the record should reflect not only the condition of the members of the family but also the ways in which the family unit is functioning and the impact of the health challenge on the family as a whole. The record should also specify the ways in which a family functions in and with its physical and social environment.

2. *Does the record present the problem in comprehensive, explicit and dynamic terms?* Records frequently appear to be quite specific about the immediate health deficits in a family: illnesses, disturbances in development, and stress conditions that have been diagnosed and that clearly require nursing care. If the record is to serve as a guide for comprehensive care, however, it is important that it also fairly represent those less obvious health threats and health behaviors that have significance for family health. An inadequately immunized family may be

harboring a health threat, as may the family with emotionally immature and impulsive parents. A "well" family may have poor nutritional habits or poor housekeeping practices that invite disease and accidents. A simple medical diagnosis may express a health problem in nondefinitive terms: the term "diabetes," for example, does not identify a specific health problem. The family may be coping with the disease but have an inadequate educational base for decisions that must be made or an immature or unrealistic attitude toward health care. The problem may be expressed too generally (for example, "poor nutrition") and not in terms of the basic or contributing factors (such as an absent, working mother or inadequate family skills in the purchase and preparation of foods). The "problem" in most families is really a complex of many small problems, the bits and pieces of which are constantly changing with the passage of time. It is important that the record show the problem as it develops, so that change can be readily identified.

3. *Are the goals explicitly defined?* Explicit goal statements should clearly indicate the outcomes considered feasible and also the degree to which these outcomes are agreed upon by the nurse, the referring agent, and the family. For a psychiatric patient returning to his home after lengthy hospitalization, a goal of "providing rehabilitative care" is not sufficiently explicit to be helpful as a guide to nursing practice. The goal of maintaining the prescribed therapeutic regimen is explicit and will presumably be one that all three concerned parties agree to. However, the goal of maintaining the family balance in the face of this threat of disruption may create some problems. One family goal may be to keep the patient secluded in order not to embarrass the family's relationship with the neighbors. The desire to secure the maximum progress of the patient in his cure may be equal to or secondary to this limited family goal. The referral agent — the physician or hospital — probably hopes for the best possible treatment of the patient and also for the continued release of the hospital bed, while the nurse's goals may lie somewhere in between. She may wish to facilitate the patient's adjustment to the home without prejudice to either patient or family, and to support vulnerable family members whose emotional or physical health may be threatened by the introduction of this source of family stress. The record should indicate this qualified endorsement of goals.

4. *Is the program of action explicitly stated?* The record should clearly show what specific action is planned; what activities are actually being carried out; and what the distribution of responsibility for action is among the nurse (or nursing group), the family, and other community resources. The action plan should be in an accessible part of the record so that it can be located quickly.

5. *Is family response to the problem and to subsequent nursing action clearly identifiable?* The family response to problems and care is indispensable in the planning and the validation of nursing action. The record should indicate family response in four areas:

Feeling and Value Response: the family's acceptance of the problem, their feelings about its relative importance, their opinion of the adequacy or relevance of available community measures for handling the problem, and their own commitment to its solution.

Therapeutic Response: the family's response to nursing or other treatments for disease and disability.

Behavioral Response: the action taken — either independently or as an outcome of the care plan — by the family in response to the problem.

Conceptual Response: evidence of the family's understanding or knowledge of the problem.

6. *Is there provision for quick reference to periodic comprehensive assessments?* Community health nursing practice proceeds by a series of revisions. The problem is defined, the action is planned and instituted, progress is evaluated, and the problem is redefined; this process is continually repeated. The record must show these revisions in the status of the problem and the plan in a way that is quickly accessible to the user. For example, a family may welcome and support the returning psychiatric patient for a while; then, as the newness wears off and the adjustments required begin to chafe, the general progress of family care may deteriorate.

THE RECORD SYSTEM INCLUDES A VARIETY OF FORMS

The record system in any agency includes a large variety of forms, each presumably serving a particular purpose. These forms may be standard throughout the state (or other political jurisdiction) or developed specifically for each agency. The agency may adopt a record system based on the use of records from a particular source, such as the National League for Nursing, or it may select parts of the record system from many different sources (see Appendix, NLN Record). The system may be highly structured and prescribed or subject to great individual adaptation by the nurse. When computer analysis is part of the record system, certain parts of the reporting must be in standard form, so that they can be easily converted to computer language.

Service Records

Service records document the care provided. They provide a register, usually in chronologic order, of the services given to any population served by the nurse. Ideally, they provide a record of the needs and goals (another facet of the documentation process) on which these services are based. They also supply the data required to describe the characteristics of the population receiving definitive nursing care. The compilation of data from these records answers the question, "In what direction did we place our nursing efforts?"

Accounting Records

Time and Effort Records

Accounting records include time and effort expenditure records and fiscal records. "Time and effort" records center on the nurse's daily report, which may be set up in a variety of ways. In some manner, the agency will maintain daily reports of the time worked and the services provided. Sometimes the daily time sheet provides more detailed information about time spent in various activities (travel, for instance); however, the tendency is to minimize routine daily recording and to substitute a time study based on a representative sampling of the nurse's time.

Financial Records

The need for fiscal accounting is obvious, and the record system will provide vouchers on which to record expenditures made on behalf of the agency; examples of this kind of expense are purchases of equipment, car maintenance, and reimbursement for mileage when the nurse uses her own car. Records may also provide a means for acknowledging receipt of fees when the nurse collects them directly or for validating nursing bills when submitted to the family or to a third party for payment directly to the agency.

Systems

The National League for Nursing and the Division of Nursing of the U. S. Public Health Service have compiled descriptive information about computer systems currently in use or being tested by a variety of agencies that incorporate service and accounting forms.[2] Pressures on agencies to produce documentation of services for third party payers have intensified the need for quickly accessible uniform program and fiscal data.

Control Records

Control records assure that service commitments are met. Requests for service, or referral forms requesting service, are usually kept for a limited time and indicate the source of referral and what disposition was made of the request. A compilation of such requests may be maintained in order to estimate trends in the sources of referral, in the proportion of those referred who are already known to the service, and in the kinds of disposition made of these requests.

Case Control Record

A case control record may be maintained in the service unit or by the individual nurse. This is usually a card containing minimal information that can be filed either by date (when localities are visited at specified times) or location of the case. This helps to assure that return visits will be made as planned. For cases receiving intensive nursing care, this second record may not be necessary, since it is not likely that visits planned on a daily or otherwise frequent schedule will be forgotten. However, for follow-up services and visits that are planned at infrequent intervals, such a control file can be very useful. In some agencies a control file is kept by the supervisor or a program director, when a particular program has a high priority or is under special study; this kind of file may be maintained, for instance, as a control measure to assure return visits to families with tuberculosis.

Special case registers also serve as a control device. The register may be used to secure immediate information about the service status of any one of the cases in the register or as a means of analyzing the service status or progress of the entire group on register.

Index File

An index file identifies all who have been admitted for nursing service, the dates of service, and sometimes the general nature of the service provided. The case may be identified by name or number. This makes it possible to retrieve earlier records and relate the present service to past efforts. It may also yield important information about trends in the general type of service requested and persistence in the use of the agency by families or groups. This information may be stored in and retrieved from a computer, in which case the data may be more inclusive.

Family History and Progress Record

The family history and progress record may be a standard form identical to those of other agencies, or it may be a special form designed to meet the needs of a particular agency. The state health department, for example, may supply prescribed record forms to local agencies, or the local agency may use forms developed by the National League for Nursing. The use of common record forms facilitates interagency and interunit comparisons as well as collation of service data. These forms may be supplemented or modified to meet the needs of a particular agency and still retain enough similarity to provide a common base of comparison.

Prescribed and optional components may also exist in individual record notation as well as in the record forms. Record notations may require highly structured approaches, such as codes or checking boxes for the description of a health situation and the course of care. This type of notation is increasing as agencies come to rely more on the computer for service analysis. In other agencies, great reliance may be placed on the "free-form" type of notation in which the record form consists mostly of blank lines. Notations are usually chronologic and may sometimes assume massive proportions. This method obviously presents difficulties in the quick location of significant data; however, it may serve a useful purpose when records are being used to investigate nursing care or when families are being served by several nurses (as often occurs when a large student nurse contingent is involved).

Most practitioners and agencies use a combination of prescribed and optional approaches, allowing the nurse to make the adaptations she finds useful and consistent with her own style.

The nurse may need to incorporate into the record methods for organizing information necessary for case planning. If the record provides for chronologic recording but not for "quick reference," statements of problems, plans, and action, the nurse may use a system of writing periodic summaries, writing in different colors of ink, or underlining, so that a synoptic reading of long records is possible. Items of general importance, such as the family's pattern of health service utilization, may be located in a specific place on each family record. Such notation procedures can be consistent with the overall records system and meet the particular needs of the nurse. For some families, the nurse may wish to use more extensive data collection measures to supplement the official record, such as the interview schedule developed by Schwartz, Henley, and Zeitz[3] for use with the elderly ambulatory patients, Barnard's Child Health Assessment,[4] or The Patient Classification for Long-Term Care.[5]

PATIENT ASSESSMENT AND COMMUNITY HEALTH SERVICE EVALUATION MODELS

A number of studies have attempted to develop methodologies for measuring patient and family progress or evaluating the effectiveness of nursing services. Elements of each have been adopted for use by nurses in their everyday care and management of families.

Roberts and Hudson developed a method to document patient progress based on the nurse's listing of the patient's needs, which she evaluates in the course of planning patient care, and her periodic assessing of these needs during the time she provides care.[6]

Freeman and Lowe developed a scale to estimate intensity of family health needs along nine parameters, as discussed in the Appendix. For each category of health need, the nurse estimates the family's capacity to cope with this particular type of health problem. Over a period of time, the nurse can determine how the health needs and coping behaviors of families have changed.[7]

The School of Nursing of the State University of New York at Buffalo worked to develop a computerized system that would incorporate nursing assessment of the following: patient transfer summary (such as health/illness status, health goals, and a coping index of the patient and family); basic patient-family information; patient physiologic and psychologic responses to illness and therapy; patient-family roles and activity patterns; medications, treatment and self-care deficits; and patient clinic therapy record.[8]

Other efforts have been aimed at adopting the Problem-Oriented Record (POR) to the Community Health arena developed by Weed.[9] Examples of modified POR systems for community health agencies are the VNS of Burlington, Vermont, the VNA of Omaha, Nebraska, and the Indian Health Service. The record forms are designed to elicit an orderly and problem-oriented analysis of the client's condition and situation. This format does not so much create a new approach as facilitate and strengthen the problem approach that existed before. Basic components of this system are: (1) a problem list defined and identified by number; (2) an integrated multidisciplinary effort, with all workers identifying and refining problems and care plans; (3) problem-specific plans of action; and (4) evaluation of services as related to changes in the problem status.

The nursing audit is a frequently used tool for appraisal of care. Phaneuf has been an outstanding proponent of this method and has made many contributions to its development.[10]

The audit approach to evaluation is based upon a systematic and intensive review of a representative sample of service records; this review is performed by an expert or experts who are not associated with the provision of care being evaluated. The review is based upon a carefully constructed set of categories of care elements and, for each category of elements, a set of criterion measures that are considered to be indicators of the quality of the care provided. Additional criteria measures are developed for the service unit as a whole. Thus, one element of care might be "supervision of others providing nursing care," and the criteria might include such measures as recorded evidence that prescribed treatments were carried out as ordered or that the supervisee was adequately checked on the treatments she was expected to provide. Some of the measures will be objective in character and clearly deducible from the record; others will be based on the judgment of the reviewer or review panel. The evaluations made are combined into scores for each category and the service as a whole.

The reviewers may be professional nurses, or when there is more than one service involved, the review board may include members of other relevant disciplines.

This methodology has several advantages. The use of "outside" reviewers helps maintain objectivity in rating, since those providing the service may have some bias arising from their closeness to the situation. The use of records rather than direct observation as the basis of the rating allows a wide range of recipients of service and types of care to be covered in a relatively short time. The scoring by category makes it possible to pinpoint areas of difficulty.

This is obviously not a method for the amateur, and arrangements for such evaluation will be made by the agency. In the multiservice agency, nursing will often be only one of the audited programs.

Systematic self or self-and-supervisor record review provides an overview of progress. Some of the methodology of the audit can be adapated for use by the community health nurse herself or by the nurse along with her supervisor. This approach does not have the same objectivity or the level of expertise as the audit, inasmuch as judgments of one's own work are always subject to some degree of bias. Despite these limitations, the systematic review of records can be a valuable device for estimating progress.

When such a self-study is used, efforts should be made to avoid the use of general impressions in favor of assembling from the record facts that are indicative of comprehensiveness or quality of care. One way of assuring a systematic review is to develop a schedule as a basis for the review.

Other methods of evaluation based on record reviews are in various stages of development.[11, 12] Some stress nursing process; others stress wellness or outcome criteria for special conditions.[13] Methods of evaluation developed to date have been unable to integrate the individual into his complex family and community system. This is not to say that protocols, criteria, or whatever technology available should not be used; however, they do not as yet provide the information needed about the effect of nursing care on the health of families and communities. Care should be oriented to the family and community — not condition-, protocol-, or computer-oriented.

Efforts have been made to develop a means of measuring the program of an agency in relation to community needs. The Community Nursing Services of Philadelphia (under contract from the Division of Nursing, Department of Health, Education, and Welfare) developed a scheme to answer the following questions:
1. What are the characteristics of the population served in relation to the population for which the agency is responsible?
2. What happens to the health status of persons and families during the period when agency services are given?
3. What resources are utilized at what cost to achieve what outcomes for what population groups?

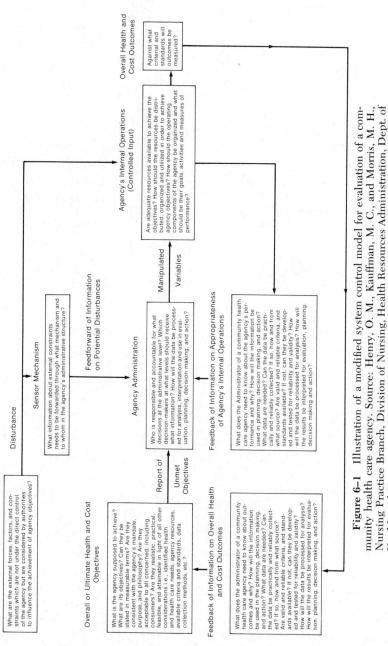

Figure 6–1 Illustration of a modified system control model for evaluation of a community health care agency. Source: Henry, O. M., Kauffman, M. C., and Morris, M. H., Nursing Practice Branch, Division of Nursing, Health Resources Administration, Dept. of Health and Human Services, 1979.

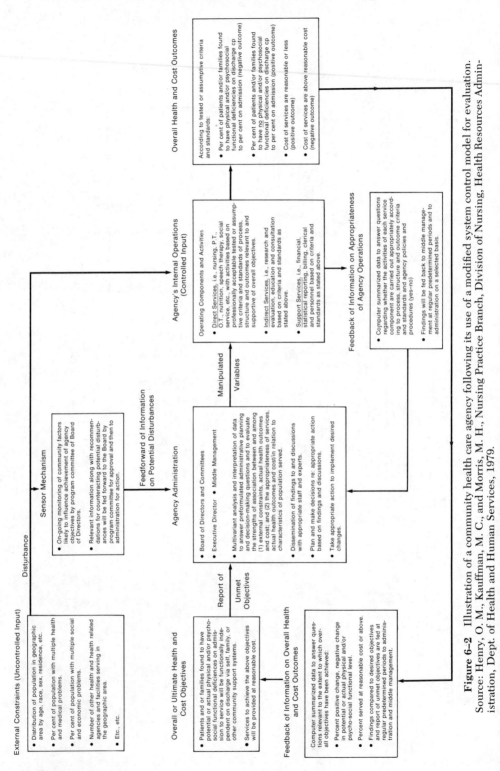

Figure 6–2 Illustration of a community health care agency following its use of a modified system control model for evaluation. Source: Henry, O. M., Kauffman, M. C., and Morris, M. H., Nursing Practice Branch, Division of Nursing, Health Resources Administration, Dept. of Health and Human Services, 1979.

4. What are the different strengths of the association among process, structure and outcome variables in relation to population characteristics?[14]

Charts, adapted from Zemach's[15] system control model to illustrate this approach, are shown in Figures 6–1 and 6–2. These charts show a systems model developed by staff to assist them in examining nursing care in terms of community need. By writing specific objectives directed at high-risk groups in the population and directing resources and services to meet the needs of these groups, staff were able to scrutinize the effect of nursing care in relation to nursing activities and agency structure.

Reporting, recording, explaining, and justifying one's work with families is part of every nurse's responsibility to be accountable — accountable to oneself, the profession, and to the public.

All fact-collectors, who have no aim beyond their reason, are one-story men. Two-story men compare, reason, generalize, using the labors of the fact collectors as well as their own. Three-story men idealize, imagine, predict; their best illumination comes from above, through the skylight.

O.W. HOLMES, 1872

REFERENCES

1. National Organization for Public Health Nursing: *Manual of Public Health Nursing*, 3rd ed. New York, Macmillan Pub. Co., Inc., 1939, p. 76.
2. National League for Nursing: *Selected Management Information Systems for Public Health/Community Health Agencies.* New York, 1978.
3. Schwartz, D., Henley, B., and Zeitz, L.: *The Elderly Ambulatory Patient.* New York, Macmillan Pub. Co., Inc., 1964, p. 299.
4. Barnard, K. E., and Douglas, H. B.: *Child Health Assessment.* Washington, D.C., U.S. Government Printing Office, Department of Health, Education and Welfare, Pub. No. (HRA-75-30), 1974.
5. Jones, E. W.: *Patient Classification for Long-Term Care: User's Manual.* Washington, D.C., U.S. Government Printing Office, Department of Health, Education, and Welfare, Pub. No. HRA 74-3017, 1973.
6. Roberts, D. E., and Hudson, H. H.: *How to Study Patient Progress.* Washington, D.C., U.S. Government Printing Office, Department of Health, Education, and Welfare, Pub. No. 1169, 1964.
7. Freeman, R. B., and Lowe, M.: A method for appraising family public health nursing needs. Am. J. Pub. Health, 53:47, 1963.
8. Taylor, D. B., and Johnson, O. H.: *Systematic Nursing Assessment — A Step Toward Automation.* Washington, D.C., U.S. Government Printing Office, Department of Health, Education and Welfare, Pub. No. HRA 74-17, 1970.
9. Weed, L. L.: *Medical Records, Medical Education, and Patient Care.* Cleveland, Ohio, Press of Case Western Reserve University, 1969.
10. Phaneuf, M.: *The Nursing Audit: Self-Regulation in Nursing Practice*, 2nd ed. New York, Appleton-Century-Crofts, 1976.
11. Wandelt, M. A., and Slater, S. D.: *The Slater Nursing Competencies Scale.* New York, Appleton-Century-Crofts, 1975.
12. Wandelt, M. A., and Ager, J. W.: *The Quality Patient Care Scale.* New York, Appleton-Century-Crofts, 1974.
13. Ibrahim, M. A., et al.: *Assessing the Clinical Skills of Nurse Practitioners.* Springfield, Va., Department of Health, Education and Welfare. Contract No. NO-2400, NTIS No. HRP 0900-601.

14. Kauffman, M. C.: *State of the Art in Management Information Systems for Public Health/Community Health Agencies: Report of a Conference.* New York, National League for Nursing, 1976, p. 42.
15. Zemach, R.: Program evaluation and system control. AJPH, *63*:608, 1963.

SUGGESTED READINGS

Aradine, C. R., and Guthneck, M.: The problem-oriented record in a family health service. Am. J. Nurs., *74*:1108, 1974.
Birkhead, L. M.: Nursing and the technetronic age. J. Nurs. Admin., 8:16, 1978.
Daubert, E.: Patient classification system records and outcome criteria. Nurs. Outlook, 27:450, 1979.
Daubert, E.: A system to evaluate home health care services. Nurs. Outlook, 25:168, 1977.
Freeman, R. B.: Measuring the effectiveness of public health nursing service. Nurs. Outlook, 9:605, 1961.
Guidelines for Review of Nursing Care at the Local Level. Department of Health, Education, and Welfare, HSA, Quality Assurance Bureau, 1975 (for sale by the American Nursing Association).
Hannah, K. J.: The computer and nursing practice. Nurs. Outlook, *24*:555, 1976.
Ibrahim, M. A., et al.: *Assessing the Clinical Skills of Nurse Practitioners.* Springfield, Va., National Technical Information Service (NTIF), DHEW Contract No. 01-NU2400, HRP 0900-601.
Jones, E. W., et al.: *Patient Classification for Long-Term Care: User's Manual.* Washington, D.C., U.S. Government Printing Office, DHEW Pub. No. (HRA) 74-3107, 1973.
Katz, S., et al.: Studies of illness in the aged: The index of ADL, a standardized measure of biological and psychosocial function. J. Am. Med. Assoc., *185*:914, 1963.
Katz, S., et al.: *Effects of Continued Care: A Study of Chronic Illness in the Home.* Washington, D.C., U.S. Government Printing Office, DHEW Pub. No. (HSM) 73-3010, 1973.
Kelly, M. E., and Roessler, L. M.: Development of interdisciplinary problem-oriented recording in a public health nursing agency. J. Nurs. Admin. 6:24, 1976.
Lohmann, G.: A statewide system of record audit. Nurs. Outlook, *25*:330, 1977.
Mayers, M. G.: *A Systematic Approach to the Nursing Care Plan,* 2nd ed. New York, Appleton-Century-Crofts, 1973.
McDonald, C., et al.: A computer-based record and clinical monitoring system for ambulatory care. Am. J. Pub. Health, 67:240, 1977.
Moore, K.: What nurses learn from nursing audit. Nurs. Outlook, *27*:254, 1979.
National League for Nursing: *Selected Management Information Systems for Public Health/Community Health Agencies.* New York, 1977.
National Observer, 13:14, 1974.
Phaneuf, M.: *The Nursing Audit: Self-regulation in Nursing Practice,* 2nd ed. New York, Appleton-Century-Crofts, 1976.
Riedel, D., et al.: Psychiatric utilization review as patient care evaluation. Am. J. Pub. Health, *62*:1222, 1972.
Roberts, D. E., and Hudson, H. H.: *How to Study Patient Progress.* Washington, D.C., U.S. Government Printing Office, DHEW Pub. #1169, April 1964.
Saba, V., and Levine, E.: Management information systems for public health nursing services. Pub. Health Rep., *83*:79, 1978.
Simmons, D. A.: A Classification Scheme for Client Problems in Community Health Nursing. Div. of Nursing, HRA, DHHS, Springfield, Va., National Technical Information Service (HRP-0501501), 1980.
Springer, E. W.: *Automated Medical Records and the Law.* Pittsburgh, Pa., Aspen Systems Corp., 1971.
Sweet, P. R., and Stark, I.: Circle care nursing plan. Am. J. Nurs., *70*:1300, 1970.
Taylor, D. B., and Johnson, O. N.: *Systematic Nursing Assessment —A Step Toward Automation.* Washington, D.C., U.S. Government Printing Office, DHEW Pub. #7417, 1974.

Vincent, P. A.: Developing a mental health assessment form. J. Nurs. Admin., 6:25, 1976.

Visiting Nurse Association, Inc.: *The Problem-Oriented System in a Home Health Agency* — A Training Manual. New York, National League for Nursing, Pub. No. 21-1554, 1975.

Watson, A., and Mayers, M.: Evaluating the quality of patient care through retrospective chart review. J. Nurs. Admin., 6:17, 1976.

World Health Organization: *Statistical Indicators for the Planning and Evaluation of Public Health Programs,* Fourteenth Report of the WHO Expert Committee on Health Statistics. Geneva, WHO Technical Report Series No. 472, 1971.

Zielstorff, R.: Nurses can affect computer systems. J. Nurs. Admin., 8:49, 1978.

RESOURCES/RECORDS

Problem Oriented Record Forms for Home and Community Health Agencies. Available from National League for Nursing, 10 Columbus Circle, New York, N.Y. 10019.

Child Health Record. Available from American Academy of Pediatrics, Ms. Vivian Olson, PO Box 1034, Evanston, Ill. 60204.

Personal Health Record. Available from Metropolitan Life Insurance Co., 1 Madison Avenue, New York, N.Y. 10010.

Family Health Record, National Foundation. Available from March of Dimes, Box 2000, White Plains, N.Y. 10602.

CHAPTER 7

EPIDEMIOLOGY

Community health nurses, wanting to improve the health status of a community, share with others in investigating the health status, disease patterns, and health expectations of people in the community. Epidemiology is a basic tool for looking for the "signs and symptoms" of the communities' health.

Epidemiology, and the statistical and research methods it employs, is focused on comparisons between groups or defined populations — an approach which Cassel describes as the basic strategy of epidemiology. It is a way of studying the distribution (or variation) of a disease or condition in a defined population and examining the factors that influence this distribution. By making these comparisons, it can be determined if there is a relationship between possessing a certain set of characteristics and having the condition or disease. For example, a research group may be interested in knowing whether people who have a particular characteristic, such as maternal deprivation as a child, have a greater risk of developing a condition, such as child abuse, than those who were not deprived.

In the past, the term epidemiology was used to describe the study of acute outbreaks of infectious disease. Today, the epidemiologic method is applied to the study of a variety of phenomena at all levels of organization, with the emphasis on the concept of "excessive prevalence" in comparing one group to another. Knowledge of the distribution of disease in a population has been utilized to acquire an understanding of causal mechanisms, to explain local disease patterns, to describe the natural history of a disease, and to provide information for program planning and evaluation.[2]

AGENT, HOST, AND ENVIRONMENT

One of the most important principles in epidemiology is the host-agent-environment relationship. Whether a person develops a specific

140

disease or condition depends upon the extent of his exposure to a specific agent, the strength of the agent (dose), the individual's susceptibility level (which may be genetic or immunologic), and environmental conditions at the time of exposure, as well as climatic conditions affecting survival of the agent.

Agents or etiologic factors of disease may be such things as chemical agents or poisons, excess nutrition, physical or mechanical agents, and infectious agents such as chicken pox, malaria, or schistosomiasis.

Host factors (intrinsic factors), important to epidemiologic studies, that influence disease include age, sex, ethnic group, genetic factors, physiologic state such as stress or pregnancy, immunologic level, existing disease states, and human behavior — i.e., diet, smoking, and occupation.

Environmental factors or extrinsic factors that influence disease are climate or physical environment, density of populations, food sources, and socioeconomic conditions such as income level and education.

An inquiry into possible cause of disease must consider a variety of possible interactions among these factors. Within the framework of infectious diseases, the agent is clearly specified, but actual disease will depend on a multitude of other factors. For example, the infectious agent for tuberculosis, *Mycobacterium tuberculosis*, is well known. We know that man is the reservoir for this disease, and that it is usually transmitted in airborne droplets from sputum of infected persons. Susceptibility and resistance to the disease vary with age, nutritional state, fatigue, presence of other diseases, exposure, and virulence of the bacilli — to name just a few.

Lead poisoning in children is an example of a chronic disease with a known etiologic agent. The disease varies with socioeconomic status, environment, and season of the year. Most chronic diseases have no single known etiologic agent but a variety of identified factors that, through careful observations, are closely associated with disease states.

COUNTING AND MEASURING

Epidemiology is a study of patterns among groups. To discover the pattern, pieces of information are collected, categorized, summarized, and analyzed. For example, Snow noticed a particular pattern about people who died from cholera and the nature of the drinking water. This led him to a set of observations about the people, the disease, and the environment. Having developed a classification scheme, Snow then gathered the data and summarized it according to those individuals with the disease and those without and those using the contaminated water supply and those not using it. He was then in a position to make some interpretations about what he had observed, based on an analysis of the group's experience and observed pattern of disease'—and then to suggest what should be done about it.[3]

Descriptive and Analytic Observations

Descriptive statistics are for the purpose of understanding the make up of a population or community in terms of age, ethnicity, sex, incidence of various diseases, economic factors, morbidity, and mortality. Frequently used sources of data include vital records (birth and death certificates), surveys, disease registries, and service records. The precision and completeness of data and methods used for the collection of information are very important for future use of the information, generalization from the findings, and possible policy decisions based on these factors. A variety of statistical indices are helpful in measuring a community's problems. Vital rates commonly used in public health to describe a population's health are given in Table 7–1.

Other rates potentially helpful in community nursing services involve abortion, absenteeism from schools or industry, disability, and health resource utilization (to name just a few).[4]

There are many organizations in the community interested in these descriptive statistics, and the community health nurse will find it useful to use their resources. Regional planning agencies, hospitals, and many government programs both at the state and local level need population statistics for program planning and evaluation purposes. For example, the Area Resource File, a computer-based county-specific health information system, collects and updates data in eight categories: (1) health manpower (especially in relation to designated shortage areas); (2) health facilities; (3) health training; (4) population characteristics such as age, race, sex, mortality, infant mortality and birth rate, crime, and housing statistics; (5) economic data, with number of recipients of Aid to Families with Dependent Children; (6) hospital utilization levels; (7) hospital expenditure data; and (8) environmental factors such as elevation, temperature, precipitation, and large animal population.[5]

Analytic statistics are concerned with making an inference about a population. This is where groups are compared, according to well-defined factors, in an effort to identify differences, similarities, and probability of disease. A great variety of statistical techniques are available for evaluating epidemiologic hypotheses, testing the probability of chance occurrence of differences, demonstrating associations or risk factors, and fitting the multiple factors of conditions together. What must be remembered is that complex statistical manipulations are only meaningful if the data on which they are based are accurate, collected systematically to prevent bias or other artifacts, and meet the basic standard of "common sense."[6]

Table 7-1   A POPULATION'S HEALTH AS INDICATED BY VITAL RATES

Crude Death Rate:
$$\frac{\text{Total Number of Deaths}}{\text{Total Population}} \times 1{,}000$$

Crude Death Rate for Specified Cause:
$$\frac{\text{Total Number of Deaths from Cause}}{\text{Total Population}} \times 100{,}000$$

Specific Death Rate:
$$\frac{\text{Number of Deaths in Specific Class}}{\text{Population of Specific Class}} \times 1{,}000$$

Crude Birth Rate:
$$\frac{\text{Total Number of Live Births}}{\text{Total Population}} \times 1{,}000$$

Birth Rate for Women of Childbearing Age:
$$\frac{\text{Total Number of Live Births}}{\text{Number of females 15--44 years of age}} \times 1{,}000$$

Infant Mortality Rate:
$$\frac{\text{Number of Deaths 1 Year of Age}}{\text{Number of Live Births}} \times 1{,}000$$

Neonatal Mortality Rate:
$$\frac{\text{Number of Deaths 28 Days of Age}}{\text{Number of Live Births}} \times 1{,}000$$

Postneonatal Mortality Rate:
$$\frac{\text{Number of Deaths 28 Days to 1 Year of Age}}{\text{Number of Live Births}} \times 1{,}000$$

Maternal Mortality Rate:
$$\frac{\text{Number of Deaths from Causes Related to Pregnancy, Child and the Puerperium}}{\text{Number of Live Births}} \times 10{,}000^{*}$$

Fetal Death Rate:
$$\frac{\text{Number of Fetal Deaths}}{\text{Number of Live Births}} \times 1{,}000$$

Case Fatality Rate:
$$\frac{\text{Number of Deaths from Specified Disease}}{\text{Number of Cases of the Disease}} \times 100$$

Incidence Rate:
$$\frac{\text{Number of New Cases of Specified Disease Occurring During Given Time Period (as During a Year)}}{\text{Estimated Mid-period Population}} \times 100{,}000^{**}$$

Prevalence Rate:
$$\frac{\text{Number of Cases of Specified Disease Existing at Given Time}}{\text{Estimated Population at that Time}} \times 100{,}000^{**}$$

*May be expressed per *100,000* particularly when rate is for some specified cause of maternal mortality, as for toxemia.

**May be expressed per 1,000 or per 10,000 when the number of cases is large compared to the size of the population.

EPIDEMIOLOGIC INVESTIGATION

Surveys

Epidemiologic surveys can provide important information for planning the local nursing program. A survey may be based on a sample (randomly selected) of households to determine needs of families for community health nursing, as in the Mickey study of extra hospital nursing needs,[7] or on community organizations and the groups they serve.

The National Center for Health Statistics uses the survey approach on a national sample of households to answer questions about disease rates, health status, use of health facilities, and a variety of other topics.[8]

Community health nurses can use the survey approach to document specific problems and conditions or needs of the population they are responsible for — be it a census tract, neighborhood, large rural area, or special community. The important elements are the selection of the sample and the formation of the questionnaire or interview. There must be consistency in the way questions are asked; this enables the researcher to generalize findings of the community being described. The special considerations and procedures for epidemiologic surveys are described in Abramson.[9]

Experimental Studies

The experimental method of testing a hypothesis is the deliberate applying or withholding of the supposed cause of a condition and observing for subsequent appearance (or lack of appearance) of the effect of this action.[10] In experimental studies, the factors of interest can be controlled by the investigation, with random assignment of the etiologic factor.

Ethical considerations usually restrict this type of testing on human populations, although there are historical studies that have used the experimental method. Cases implicating the lack of fresh fruit in the diet as the cause of scurvy, Jenner's experiments with cowpox vaccination, and the discovery of high oxygen levels given to premature infants resulting in blindness are examples of such studies.[11] An experiment that was brought to public attention several years ago involved the withholding of penicillin treatment for cases of tertiary syphilis. This was a deeply disturbing example of ethical dilemmas inherent in experimentation on human populations.[12]

Carefully monitored clinical trials, on the other hand, have been used successfully to prove or disprove efficacy of treatment. This method could be applied to test specific nursing interventions but has rarely been used in the community health nursing setting.

Cohort (Prospective) Studies

In a cohort study, people are classified into groups according to whether or not they possess a particular characteristic that is thought to be related to the condition of interest; observations are then made over time to see who, in fact, develops the disease or condition. For example, healthy pregnant women could be classified according to the characteristic of cigarette smoking, followed through pregnancy to see if cigarette smoking was related to birth weight of the infant — or more specifically, to answer the questions: Do pregnant women who smoke cigarettes have a greater proportion of low birth weight babies than pregnant women who do not smoke?

A classic example of a cohort study is the Framingham study of heart disease by the U.S. Public Health Service. A defined community has been followed for many years to see who develops heart disease and who does not. Careful records of eating, smoking behavior, and other risk factors have been kept for many years, resulting in new information about risk factors associated with heart disease.[13]

In community health nursing settings this method has been used to study a variety of problems. For example, Christensen and Lingle studied the effectiveness of team and non-team public health nursing in the health of patients with strokes using the cohort approach.[14]

Sultz and colleagues followed a cohort of nurse practitioners to determine how these nurses function within the health care system.[15] Nurse practitioners and their employers were followed approximately one year after graduation. Information about income, duties and responsibilities, and job satisfaction was obtained by using pretested, self-administered questionnaires.

Studies of this nature are expensive in time and personnel; they are economical only when there is existing information about factors associated with a condition or when the condition under study is relatively frequent. For infrequent conditions other methods, such as case-control studies, are used.

Case-Control Studies

Another approach is to select a population consisting of some individuals with a specific condition (the cases) and some without it (the controls). The researcher tries to determine through accurate interviewing, the frequency of exposure to the particular condition-producing agent. Cigarette smoking was originally implicated as a causative agent in lung cancer by this approach. People with lung cancer and people without lung cancer were interviewed to see how they differed in their smoking patterns in order to determine if a greater proportion of the people with the disease were smokers.

This type of study is also called a case history, or retrospective study, and can often be accomplished through a careful record review. It is less costly than the cohort method but, at best, can only give an estimate of the risk between the condition and the characteristic.

Cross-Sectional and Longitudinal Studies

Epidemiologic studies can also be characterized on whether the hypothesis testing is related to two different points (longitudinal study) or a single point (cross-sectional study) in time. Most cohort and case-control studies are longitudinal. Some nurses have studied the effect of nutritional counseling with a group of families, based on dietary habits over time. A study of the prevalence (number of cases) of gastrointestinal upset in students after a school pot-luck dinner is an example of the cross-sectional approach.

These, then, are some of the techniques frequently used in epidemiology studies. After reviewing the literature, it soon becomes apparent that clever investigators have found a variety of ways of combining these typical methods in their search for causes.

USES OF EPIDEMIOLOGY

The community health nurse will find a great many ways of using the epidemiologic method to ask questions about people and their conditions as she interacts with families and various organizations and works within the community setting. It is a common occurrence for most community health nurses to wonder how some families can cope so well with extensive problems while others have barely enough resources to contend with the common cold. Many nurses have made the observation, as they carefully step through a neighborhood, that a large number of the young mothers needing concentrated care are poor and live in neighborhoods with high crime rates, where illegal drugs are sold freely on the streets. Also, the community health nurse may notice a block of houses that are particularly well kept, with flowers growing in the windows, in an otherwise run-down housing area — and wonder why this is so.

The community health nurse will also use the epidemiologic approach in diagnosing the health of a community and its need for nursing services. (See Chapter 17, Community Diagnosis.)

The nurse will find it useful to obtain descriptive information about the community in the smallest unit possible — such as per household, census track, or block — as well as health and illness data. For example, she will need measures of the physical environment, the social environment, and health attitudes and practices, trends in birth, deaths and disease rates of the poorest communities as well as diseases and problems observed in more affluent groups. There will be special communities, such as small industries with increased risk of exposure to harmful substances, that may need particular attention or vulnerable families in a neighborhood that may need constant support. Part of the diagnostic effort must identify the strengths of the community or neighborhood, so that the nurse can incorporate these into the community nursing effort. If these strengths do not exist, she may need to work to develop a greater sense of community and assist families and groups in helping each other and working together as a community.

Another application of the epidemiologic method is in program evaluation, or the study of how health services in a community are working. Setting specific measurable objectives for a defined population; relating these objectives to the population's needs; and measuring success or failure in terms of observed changes in the population are steps in the basic epidemiologic approach. What needs are the existing health services serving, — and how well? What needs are not being met? Who utilizes what services; when; and for what reasons? These are but a few of the questions that community health nurses, in conjunction with other services, need to continuously ask themselves.

Morris summarizes the uses of epidemiology in the following way:

1. To study the history of the health of populations.
2. To diagnose the health of a community and measure ill-health in terms of incidence, prevalence, mortality, and morbidity from defined diseases.
3. To study the working of health services.
4. To estimate from the group experience what are the individual risks, on average, of disease, accident and defect.
5. To complete the clinical picture of chronic disease and describe its natural history.
6. To identify syndromes by describing the distribution, association and disassociation of phenomena on the population.
7. To search for causes of health and disease by studying the incidence in different groups; to estimate the relative importance of different causes in multiple etiology.[17]

Epidemiology is a strategy for studying man in his total environment. It is a way of developing knowledge about both the earliest beginnings of dysfunction and those characteristics of individuals within groups that predispose them to future problems. These observations can help determine what to assess, what factors present potential problems, and what can be done to help. Epidemiology is a tool for the improvement of public health practice.

REFERENCES

1. Cassel, J. C.: Information for epidemiology and health service research. Med. Care, 2:76(Supplement), 1973.
2. Morris, J. N.: *Uses of Epidemiology*, 2nd ed. Baltimore, The Williams and Wilkins Co., 1964.
3. Terris, M.: The epidemiologic tradition. Pub. Health Rep., 94:207, 1979.
4. World Health Organization: *Statistical Indices of Family Health*, Technical Report Series 587, Geneva, World Health Organization, 1976, pp. 87–92.
5. *The Area Resource File: A Manpower Planning and Research Tool*. Washington, D.C., U.S. Government Printing Office, DHEW (HRA) 78–69, April 1978, pp. 3–5.
6. For a complete description of analysis and allowable interpretations of data from epidemiological studies, see MacMahon, B., and Pugh, T. F.: *Epidemiology: Principles and Methods*. Boston, Little, Brown & Co., 1970, pp. 39–46.
7. Mickey, J. E.: Studying extra-hospital nursing needs: A preliminary report. Am. J. Pub. Health, 48:880, 1958.
8. See National Center for Health Statistics, Scientific and Technical Information Branch, 3700 East-West Highway, Hyattsville, Maryland 20782.
9. Abramson, J. N.: *Survey Methods in Community Medicine*. Edinburgh, Churchill-Livingstone, 1974.

10. MacMahon and Pugh, p. 40.
11. Terris, M.: The epidemiologic tradition. Pub. Health Rep., 94:203, 1979.
12. Brandt, A. M.: *Racism and Research: The Case of the Tuskegee Syphilis Study, The Experiment and HEW's Ethical Review.* Hastings Center Report, December 1978.
13. Dawber, T. R., Meadors, G. F., and Moore, F. E.: Epidemiological approaches to heart disease: The Framingham study. Am. J. Pub. Health, 41:279, 1951.
14. Christenson, K., and Lingle, V. A.: Evaluation of effectiveness of team and non-team public health nurses in health outcomes of patients with strokes or fractures. Am. J. Pub. Health, 62:483, 1972.
15. Sultz, H., Zielezny, M., and Gentry, J.: *Longitudinal Study of Nurse Practitioners: Phase I and II.* Washington, D.C., U.S. Government Printing Office, DHEW (HRA 78–92), September 1978.
16. Morris, pp. 274–275.

SUGGESTED READINGS

Abramson, J. H.: *Survey Methods in Community Medicine.* Edinburgh, Churchill-Livingstone, 1974.

The Area Resource File (ARF). A Manpower Planning and Research Tool. Washington, D.C., U.S. Government Printing Office, DHEW (HRA) 78–69, April 1978.

Baker, S. P.: Determinants of injury and opportunities for intervention. Am. J. Epidemiology, 101:98, 1975.

Bass, F.: *A public health approach to illness-producing behavior; The example of tuberculosis control applied to cigarette smoking.* In *Preventive Medicine, U.S.A.,* New York, Prodist, 1976, pp. 148–162.

Bouchard, J. C.: Childhood accidents. *In* Barnard, K. E., and Douglas, H. B. (eds.): *Child Health Assessment.* (HRA75–30), Washington, D.C., U.S. Government Printing Office, U.S. Department of Health, Education and Welfare, December, 1974, pp. 149–160.

Brandt, A. M.: *Racism and Research, The Case of the Tuskegee Syphilis Study, The Experiment and HEW's Ethical Review.* Hastings Center Report, December 1978.

Cassel, J.: *In* Omran, A. R. (ed.): *Community Diagnosis in Community Medicine in Developing Countries.* New York, Springer, 1974, pp. 345–362.

Cassel, J. C.: Information for epidemiology and health service research. *Med. Care* 2:76(supplement), 1973.

Christensen, K., and Lingle, J. A.: Evaluation of effectiveness of team and non-team public health nurses in health outcomes of patients with strokes or fractures. Am. J. Pub. Health, 62:483, 1972.

Christiansen, K. E.: *In* Hymnovich, D. P., and Barnard, M. U. (eds.): *Family Epidemiology; An Approach to Assessment and Intervention in Family Health Care,* 2nd ed. Vol I. New York, McGraw-Hill Book Co., 1979, pp. 17–30.

Corey, E. J. B., Miller, C., and Widlak, F.: Factors contributing to child abuse. Nurs. Res., 24:293, 1975.

Duncan, B., Smith, A., and Briese, F.: A comparison of growth: Spanish-surnamed with non-Spanish surnamed children. Am. J. Pub. Health, 69:903, 1979.

Elliott, J. E., and Kearns, J. M.: *Analysis and Planning for Improved Distribution of Nursing Personnel and Services,* Final Report. Washington, D.C., U.S. Government Printing Office, DHEW (HRA) 79–16, December 1978.

Given, B., Given, C. W., and Simoni, L. E.: Relationships of process of care to patient outcomes. Nurs. Res., 28:85, 1979.

Goodman, M. B.: Incidence of respiratory infections in full-term and premature infants during their first year. Nurs. Res., 22:160, 1973.

Gresham, G. E., et al.: Residual disability in survivors of stroke — The Framingham study. New Engl. J. Med., 293:954, 1975.

Healthy People: The Surgeon General's Report on Health Promotion and Disease Prevention. Washington, D.C., U.S. Government Printing Office, 1979.

Ibrahim, M. A. (ed.): The case-control study: Consensus and controversy. Special Issue J. Chronic Dis., 32:1 (Special issue), 1979.

Kasl, S. J., et al.: Experience of losing a job: Reported changes in health, symptoms and illness behavior. Psychosomatic Med., 37:106, 1975.

Kauffman, M. C., and Cunningham, A.: Epidemiologic analysis of outcomes in maternal and infant health in evaluating effectiveness of three patient care teams. Am. J. Pub. Health, 60:1712, 1970.

Marshall, H. B., Kabock, M. M., Rosenstock, I., and Ruth, V.: Some influences on public participation in a genetic screening program. J. Comm. Health, 1:3, 1975.

Milio, N. A framework for prevention: Changing health-damaging to health-generating life patterns. Am. J. Pub. Health, 66:435, 1976.

Muller, A.: Evaluation of the costs and benefits of motorcycle helmet laws. Am. J. Pub. Health, 70:586, 1980.

Nursing Digest, editorial staff: *1975 Review of Community Health*. Wakefield, Mass., Contemporary Pub. Inc., 1975.

Pesznecker, B. L., and McNeil, J.: Relationship among health habits, social assets, psychologic well-being, life change, and alterations in health status. Nurs. Res., 24:442, 1975.

Pierce, S. F., and Thompson, D.: Changing practice by choice rather than chance. J. Nurs. Admin. 6(2):33, 1976.

Preventive Medicine, USA: Task Force Report by the John E. Fogarty International Center, NIH, and the American College of Preventive Medicine. New York, Prodist, 1976.

Rouché, B.: *Eleven Blue Men and Other Narratives of Medical Detection.* New York, Berkeley Medallion Books, 1955.

Ruybul, S. E., et al.: Community assessment: An epidemiological approach. Nurs. Outlook, 23:365, 1975.

Sartwell, P. E.: Cohorts: The debasement of a word. Am. J. Epid., 103:536, 1976.

Schultz, P. R.: *Primary Health Care to the Elderly: An Evaluation of Two Health Manpower Patterns.* Denver, Colo., Final Report Medical Care and Research Foundation, May 1977.

Snyder, C., and Spietz, A.: Characteristics of Abuse: A report of five families. *Nurse Pract.* 2:23, 1977.

Starfield, B.: Health services research: A working model. New Engl. J. Med., 289:132, 1973.

Sultz, H., Zielezny, M., and Gentry, J.: *Longitudinal Study of Nurse Practitioners*, Phase II, Washington, D.C., U.S. Government Printing Office, DHEW (HRA) 78–92, September 1978.

Wintermeyer, L., and Myers, M.: Measles in a partially immunized community. Am. J. Pub. Health, 69:923, 1979.

CHAPTER 8

RESEARCH — A TOOL
FOR PRACTICE

The main concern of research is to develop a realistic plan for asking an important question in a way that will yield a reliable answer that can, in good conscience, be shared with others.[1] Approaches to research can be seen as a continuum ranging from the most complex and controlled large scale study to the less contrived systematic observations of human behaviors or phenomena. Whatever methodologies are used, research is essentially a way of comparing — evaluating variation or observed differences and making judgments about the importance of these observed differences, both in terms of statistical significance and clinical (common sense) meaning.

The need to know the "why" of things is an integral part of community health nursing and public health service. Concern for the health of people, the need to know why some people develop disease and others do not, the desire to be more effective and efficient in the delivery of services, and the necessity of providing proof of effectiveness for continued public funding are some of the motivating factors for conducting research.

There are a variety of tools and approaches available to researchers, the choice depending on the problem or types of questions to be answered, the possible or desired amount of control over design, and the creativity of the researchers.

ASKING THE QUESTION

The fun of research is in the intelligent exploration of ideas, problems, and concerns. The process of identifying a specific problem for a study can and usually is a rather messy affair — mixed with profound insights and excitement, equally profound disappointment, and an eagerness to "do it all" when there are so many questions to be answered.

150

Polit and Hungler outline four criteria to be considered in defining a problem for study:

1. Significance of the problem. The research question should contribute to nursing practice or nursing theory.
2. Researchability of the problem. Questions of moral or ethical value cannot be answered by research.
3. Feasibility of the problem. Issues of timing, availability of subjects, cooperation of key individuals, availability of facilities and equipment, monetary requirements, expertise and availability of competent people, and ethical considerations need to be answered.
4. Interest to the researcher.[2]

Many community health nurses have a variety of questions — arising from their everyday activities with families, community groups, or colleagues — that they would like to have answered. All too often, the "wonderlust" is lost in the furor of these usual activities. People who can help the nurse in clarifying the questions being asked are not usually readily available in the busy practice setting. Practitioners, supervisors, and administrators may recognize the existence of a problem of mutual interest in their work, and cooperate in developing a research project idea. The sharing of resources and pooling of ideas are good ways of helping to define ideas, to see similarities and differences, to recognize the unusual, and to determine what is most important for improved practice and worthwhile in terms of time spent. It is easy to get caught in the complexities of research designs and statistical analyses unless the question to be answered is clearly defined and limited at the outset. Practical advice may be obtained from colleagues with previous research experience, through collaboration with researchers in university settings, and less frequently through research centers within the practice setting. Several regional agencies in higher education in the West, South, and Midwest have been developed, partly for the purpose of assisting in nursing research efforts. The Western Council on Higher Education for Nursing (WCHEN) — the forerunner in this type of regional organization — has provided technical assistance as well as research seminars and conferences for sharing information and findings.

Research in the practice setting takes time, managerial support, and access to certain types of expertise and resources. It also requires a pervading atmosphere of inquiry — a belief that identifying problems in the provision of care and solving these problems systematically should be a part of every nurses's practice. Many nurses do take a research stance in their everyday problem solving and ask questions about the practice, the health needs of people in the community, and the ways in which programs might better serve the people. Perhaps the biggest problem is developing a project that is not too broad or too complex to be handled in the practice setting — especially when so many of the problems confronting the nurse who works in the community setting are potentially overwhelming. Projects often start because a nurse is bothered by something and needs to find out the "why of it" in order to satisfy her own curiosity. Talking with others about the problem, documenting the parameters of the question, identifying related issues, and analyzing the literature are first steps in formulating and defending ideas. Once the question is succinctly stated, other steps in the research process, such as developing the best methodology, will follow.

THE IMPORTANCE OF SMALL DISCRETE STUDIES IN THE PRACTICE SETTING

The essence of community health nursing research is contained in the everyday practice of nursing — whether at the family, community, or organizational level. Assessment and problem identification of the individual, family, or community are similar to describing, defining, and explicitly stating the research question. Collecting information and making observations for the nursing assessment are similar to the data collection process essential for research. Developing a care plan is similar to deciding what strategies and methods will be used to answer the research question. The concern for accuracy of measures and the analysis of care results in relation to stated objectives of care are similar to the data analysis and interpretation of results that occur in research studies.

Small studies with well-defined research questions developed by nurses in the practice setting are invaluable for ongoing improvement of patient care. Small pilot studies — the early testing out of the questions "I wonder why . . ." or "What would happen if . . ." — are the prerequisite to larger, more definitive research. Small discrete studies also serve to answer important local questions — such as identifying the problems and needs of groups at special risks, determining local hazards to health, developing different ways of providing nursing services, and measuring the effectiveness of a particular program. Careful scrutiny of various health problems, needs, and characteristics of both served and non-served populations (groups) continues to be an important area for research at the local level.

Descriptive Studies

The purpose of descriptive studies in community nursing practice is to assess the current situation in a systematic way. Circumscribed studies on various aspects of the nursing program and how it is coordinated with other services for families in the community serve as the foundation for a continuing program.

Descriptive studies frequently seen in community health agencies include time studies or activity analysis. Employees may be asked to keep a diary of how the day is spent, or observers may record activities as they occur. Activity analysis can be used to determine cost per activity and distribution of work.

Review of client records is another method frequently used for descriptive studies. Records are not usually kept for research purposes and, for the most part, are deficient in terms of accuracy and uniformity of data; however, when used with care, records can provide useful information about characteristics of families served, types and duration of services provided, or usual sources of referral to nursing services — to name just a few.

Specific questions about nursing services can often be best handled through special surveys designed to provide the relevant descriptive data. Surveys are usually based on a sample of people or families from a defined population, and they make use of questionnaires or structured interviews to increase the likelihood of reliable findings. For example, the nurse may plan a household survey in a given geographic area to determine the needs of families currently not using nursing services. In what ways are families receiving care similar to or different from families not receiving care? What are the high-risk characteristics of families not utilizing antepartum, well-child, or venereal disease clinics or services? Many other questions can be asked, and the answers could help in planning needed outreach services.

Need-assessment studies of special groups in the community can provide vital information for planning nursing services. For example, the needs of families with multiple problems, special industrial or work groups, preschool or school-age populations, and families over 65 years of age have been studied in the past and are known to have different health and social requirements for services as well as different levels of coping with health problems and daily activities. Studies of population needs frequently use a survey method but, depending on the questions asked and the comparisons to be made, may make use of various measurement tools and health indexes.[3]

Evaluation Studies

There is currently some ambiguity in the definitions for the terms evaluation, program evaluation, evaluative research, and quality assurance. The confusion is understandable since definitions overlap and relationships are unclear. Community health nurses participate in some form of evaluation for a variety of purposes. Nurses at all organizational levels vehemently attest to the urgent need for practical evaluation methods that can be productively applied to practice settings.

The American Public Health Association's definition states that evaluation is the process of determining the value or amount of success in achieving a predetermined objective. Four steps are inherent in this process: (1) formulating the objective; (2) identifying proper criteria to be used in measuring success; (3) determining and explaining the program's degree of success; and (4) recommending further program activity.[4]

A working definition of program evaluation provided by Attkisson and Broskowski is as follows:

Program evaluation is:
1. A process of making reasonable judgments about program effort, effectiveness, efficiency and adequacy.
2. Based on systematic data collection and analysis.
3. Designed for use in program management, external accountability, and future planning.
4. Focused especially on accessibility, acceptability, awareness, availability, comprehensiveness, continuity, integration, and cost of services.[5]

Schulberg describes two general approaches to program evaluation — the goal-attainment model and the system model. In the goal-attainment model, emphasis is on measurement of progress toward predetermined objectives. The system model, on the other hand, describes the organization in transaction with the surrounding environment in terms of inputs, processes and outputs having a variety of goals.[6] The open system model of an organization is particularly compatible with the concerns of community nursing agencies interacting with diverse client groups who have changing needs and multiple community service agencies, all of which are also constantly changing.[7]

Because service organizations are constantly changing, program evaluation employs multiple sources of data that vary in detail, source, validity, and scientific and practical merit. The methodologies by which these data are collected vary — ranging from rigorous experimental and quasi-experimental design to systematically collected observations, depending on the degree of current knowledge available about the program under study.

Evaluative research[8] tries to adapt recognized methods and verified measurement tools to the practice setting, using the most rigorous research design possible to test program effort, effectiveness, efficiency, and adequacy. Certain costs in terms of timeliness, expense of data collection, and ultimate usefulness to the operating program need to be considered before embarking into evaluative research. Special studies of this type can aid in the documentation of effectiveness of programs. However, the main purpose of evaluative research is new scientific discovery.

Despite enormous pressures to move quickly, planning for self-evaluation takes considerable effort and time. Participants in this planning effort must be cognizant of the unique information needs of the particular service or organization.

Attkisson describes four fundamental questions that structure the evaluation planning process, regardless of the level of organization:

1. What information does the organization require for internal management and external accountability purposes?
2. What are the basic evaluative tasks?

3. What information collection and processing capacity is required by the organization's informational needs and the related evaluative tasks?
4. What functional and organizational role must evaluators assume to ensure that evaluative information is available and utilized?[9]

The community health nurse, the supervisor or program director, and the agency administration must answer these questions as they develop plans for evaluation activities that will be useful to ongoing planning and documentation of services.

WHAT TO MEASURE AND WHY

Interest in evaluating nursing services provided to families and communities and in proving the efficacy of these services is not new. In the early 1900's people such as Cannon, Gardner, and Tucker were describing community needs for preventive nursing services, advocating the scientific approach to disease and prevention, and emphasizing the social as well as physical determinants of disease.[10] Evaluation activities have progressed from focusing only on adequacy of staff and resources (measures of structures), to counting numbers of families or clients seen (measures of process), and more recently, to the broader focus of documenting changes in family behavior or infant mortality in a community (measures of outcome).

There is an evolutionary process within each agency as experience with evaluation activities grows. Attkisson describes this development as usually beginning at the systems research management level and then progressing to measures of client utilization, outcomes of intervention, and community impact.[11] Table 8–1 describes typical tasks and evaluation activities at each level of evaluation.

Program evaluation activities at every organizational level will ultimately lead back to records and information systems. The community health nurse's documentation of her care to families, including all the elements of the nursing process, and her documentation of local community needs and nursing services designed to meet them are the basis for sound program evaluation.

Quality Assurance Programs

Quality assurance has existed in home care programs for many years. Essentially, it is a peer review of clients, intended to assure adequate and appropriate care, that is based on an evaluation of records. Third-party payers (e.g., insurance and Medicare) have required home health agencies to document that care provided to eligible recipients is essential, adequate, and appropriate. Both quality of care and cost containment have been goals of such assurance programs.

There is much overlap in the activities of program evaluation and

Table 8–1 TYPICAL MANAGEMENT TASKS AND EVALUATION ACTIVITIES AT FOUR PROGRESSIVELY EVOLVING LEVELS OF EVALUATION ACTIVITY

Level of Evaluation Activity	Typical Management Tasks	Typical Evaluation Activities
I. Systems resource management	• Clarify organizational objectives. • Develop program plan and budget. • Establish lines of management responsibility. • Obtain and maintain financial support. • Allocate fiscal resources and staff effort. • Coordinate personnel supervision. • Establish new services and phase out existing services. • Relate to community advisory groups. • Meet external reporting requirements and program standards. • Monitor income and expenditures. • Establish fees and billing rates.	• Review objectives and formulate indicators of attainment. • Meet external reporting requirements. • Clarify roles of evaluator and integrate with management tasks. • Develop improved information capability and integrate data collection systems. • Review mandated services or documented needs. • Establish evaluation liaison with community advisory groups and evaluators from other organizational levels. • Monitor staff effort and deployment of human, fiscal, and physical resources. • Collaborate in establishment of a cost-finding system and determine unit costs of services. • Provide effort feedback to management and service staff.
II. Client utilization	• Make workload projections. • Maintain efficiency of service delivery. • Assure equity of service access. • Assure appropriate client screening and treatment assignment. • Assure adequate treatment planning.	• Monitor unduplicated counts of clients served. • Analyze caseloads and client flow. • Compare client demographics to census data and high risk-need populations. • Analyze reasons for premature dropout and under-utilization of services.

	• Assure appropriate service utilization and integration with other community services at the individual client level. • Assure continuity of care. • Establish quality assurance program.	• Assist in installation of problem oriented client; record and monitor service needs of clients. • Provide technical support for utilization review and other quality assurance activities. • Analyze continuity of care. • Analyze costs per episode of care within specific client groups or service settings.
III. Outcome of intervention	• Provide services acceptable to clients and referral sources. • Detect and correct grossly ineffective service activities. • Assure that services are generally effective. • Improve cost-effectiveness of services. • Reallocate resources to support and enhance most cost-effective services. • Communicate service effectiveness to funding sources and advisory groups.	• Routinely monitor client status. • Study client and referral source satisfaction. • Study post-treatment outcomes. • Compare program outcomes to outcome norms. • Undertake comparative outcome experiments. • Do systems simulation and optimization studies. • Compare cost-outcomes of different approaches to service needs and establish cost-effectiveness of services. • Find cost-outcome per duration of problem or illness within specific client groups and/or service settings.
IV. Community impact	• Participate in regional health planning. • Develop joint interagency services and administrative support systems. • Provide effective primary prevention and indirect services. • Collaborate in integration of services for multi-problem clients and stimulate effective inter-agency referral system.	• Assess community needs. • Undertake incidence and prevalence studies. • Test primary prevention strategies. • Evaluate consultation and education services. • Participate in systematic regional need assessment. • Facilitate and provide technical assistance to citizen and consumer input to need assessment, program planning, and evaluation.

From Attkisson, C. C., et al. (eds.): *Evaluation of Human Service Programs*. New York, Academic Press, 1978, p. 70.

quality assurance. Both are concerned with the need for accountability — i.e., what we do, how we do it, and what it costs — and the need for measuring quality of care; and both share common information needs. In describing their differences, Attkisson makes the following statement:

In contrast to program evaluation, quality assurance activities have more extensive legislative mandates; rely extensively on peer review and less on administrative review; are client- and service-provider specific; are organized to assure adequacy and appropriateness of care and to control costs by preventing overutilization; and rely on methods that focus on specific service plans and service transactions methods that involve minimal data aggregation and focus on service records.[12]

These differences between quality assurance and program evaluation are summarized in Table 8–2.

COMMUNITY HEALTH NURSING AND RESEARCH

Community nursing involves the activities of many people as they interact and cope with life's many events. How behavior promotes health or affects increased risk of disease is a complex area of study — a puzzle needing the strength and intelligence of many disciplines. Community health nurses have a perspective on behavior that provides a natural base for exploration on preventive health problems considered with growth and development of all age groups. When assessing individual, family, and community health, nurses are constantly looking for clues and associations between health behaviors, environmental factors, and potential for illness or exacerbation of existing disease. Gortner recently described the areas of inquiry most essential to human health and illness prevention as lying between the biological and behavioral sciences. Topics outlined as relevant were: genetic endowment, organ/system integrity, family (child rearing) practices, exercise, education, socioeconomic status, environmental hazards, stress management, drug use and abuse, life styles, and culture.[13]

Special studies are needed to determine whether routine practice and procedures are sound. For example, group teaching of young mothers about child care was found to be more effective than teaching the same material on a home visit.[14] Another example is a study that compares three methods of providing nursing care to families with high-risk newborns during the first three months of the infant's life. Nursing process, infant and parent adaptive behavior, and child health and development are assessed and measured.[15]

As the U.S. population of those aged 65 years and over continues to grow, there is a need to understand more about the special nursing needs of the elderly as they live and work in the community. Schwartz reported on a study of this topic in 1966.[16] Sullivan investigated the effect of specific nursing approaches designed to provide extension

Table 8-2 PROGRAM EVALUATION AND QUALITY ASSURANCE: CONTRASTING CHARACTERISTICS ACROSS KEY DIMENSIONS

Key Variables	Contrasting Characteristics	
	Program Evaluation	*Quality Assurance*
Legislative sanctions	Minimal but increasing	Extensive — but only in the past 10 years
Reliance on peer review	Minimal	Extensive
Reliance on administrative review	Extensive	Minimal
Level of analysis	Generalized and program-specific, focused on data-based judgments about program (or service modality) effort, efficiency, effectiveness, and relevance	Client- and service provider-specific and focused on quality of specific service delivery transactions through reliance on service/client records
Basic objectives	• Maintain high levels of effort relative to program capacity for effort. • Assess outcome and select most effective/efficient programs. • Assess relevance and impact of total program effort with regard to service needs in a specified community.	• Assure that individual clients receive appropriate care. • Detect deficiencies and errors in service provider capacity. • Control costs by preventing overutilization and ensuring that needed services are provided in a timely, efficient manner.
Principal methods	• Analysis of resource utilization, capacity for effort, and level of effort. • Assessment of outcomes and the effectiveness of program effort. • Assessment of program efficiency relative to effort and outcomes • Analysis of comparative cost-effectiveness. • Analysis of program adequacy relative to needs for services.	• Concurrent review. — Admissions certification — Continued stay review — Utilization review and "length of stay" analysis • Retrospective review. — Medical (clinical) care evaluation — Profile monitoring

From Attkisson, C. C., et al. (eds.): *Evaluation of Human Service Programs.* New York, Academic Press, 1978, p. 413.

services — to identify the needs of isolated individuals, increase social bonding, and meet specific individual health needs — on the health of well elderly living in high-rise housing units.[17] Contemporary problems of the elderly, from both the client's and the nurse's point of view, need to be addressed by research.

Other age groups; vulnerable families with multiple problems; families' coping skills; culturally derived health practices; and special groups such as those found in schools, industries, and prisons also need special attention. The management and administration of nursing services in various settings, the impact of the setting on nursing practice, and the best utilization of health manpower are examples of additional areas of needed research.

Funding for Research

Monies and support for research activities are available from government sources, private organizations and foundations, and professional associations.

Most research is funded by federal government programs; but smaller awards may be available from state and local governments, if the problem to be studied is important to the local area. At the federal level, each institute within the National Institutes of Health (NIH) system has a research grant program — as do other components of the federal government such as the Center for Disease Control, the National Institute for Occupational Safety and Health, the National Center for Health Services Research, and the Bureau of Health Professions. The major focus for nursing research is centered in the Division of Nursing within the Bureau of Health Professions. A comprehensive listing of research grant programs can be found in the *Catalogue of Federal Domestic Assistance*, and specific information about requirements obtained from the funding organization.

Several foundations have been interested in health issues and have contributed to research efforts related to community health. Major contributors in the past have been the Rockefeller Foundation, W. K. Kellogg Foundation, and the Robert Wood Johnson Foundation — to name just a few. Private organizations such as the American Heart Association and the American Cancer Society also support research related to their goals.

Professional associations such as the National League for Nursing, the American Nurses' Foundation, Sigma Theta Tau, the American Public Health Association, and the American Association of University Women offer limited grants for research. Each group has its own requirements and interests, and information about these may be obtained through direct inquiry; sound advice and consultation are often available along with the funds.

Nursing services to communities are planned on the basis of existing knowledge about the health of the community. Interventions with families are planned on the basis of the nurses' knowledge of family function, behavior, and disease. Sometimes basic research about behavior, family function, community interaction, risk factors, and disease must precede questions of intervention and quality of care.

What is important to remember is that research can be a tool for improving care and that critical thinking, questioning, and problem solving should be part of every nurse's scientific accountability for practice.

REFERENCES

1. Feinstein, A.: *Clinical Biostatistics.* St. Louis, Mo., C. V. Mosby Co., 1977, p. 17.
2. Polit, A. F., and Hungler, B. P.: *Nursing Research: Principles and Methods.* Philadelphia, J. B. Lippincott Co., 1978, pp. 68–73.
3. Morris, J. N.: *Uses of Epidemiology,* 2nd ed. Baltimore, The Williams and Wilkins Co., 1964.
4. American Public Health Association: Glossary of administrative terms in public health. Am. J.Pub. Health, 50:225, 1960.
5. Attkisson, C. C., et al. (eds.): *Evaluation of Human Service Programs.* New York, Academic Press, 1978, p. 24.
6. Schulberg, H. C., and Baker, F.: *Program Evaluation in the Health Fields,* Vol. II. New York, Human Services Press, 1979, pp. 7–10.
7. For further discussion of systems theory applied to community nursing see Hall, J. E., and Weaver, B. R.: *Distributive Nursing Practice: A Systems Approach to Community Health.* Philadelphia, J. B. Lippincott Co., 1977, pp. 42–47.
8. For further discussion of evaluative research, see Suchman, E. A.: *Evaluative Research.* New York, Russell Sage Foundation, 1967; and Weiss, C. H. (ed.): *Evaluating Action Programs.* Boston, Allyn & Bacon, 1972.
9. Attkisson, pp. 60–77.
10. Gortner, S., and Nahm, H.: An overview of nursing research in the United States. Nurs. Res., 26:11, 1977.
11. Attkisson, p. 69
12. Ibid, pp. 411–412.
13. Gortner, S.: Out of the Past and Into the Future. Nurs. Res., 29:204, 1980.
14. McNeil, H. J., and Holland, S. S.: A comparative study of public health nurse teaching in groups and in home visits. Am. J. Pub. Health, 62:1629, 1972.
15. Barnard, K.: *Models of Newborn Nursing Services.* University of Washington. Division of Nursing, Research Section, HRA, BHM, R01-NU00719, 1979.
16. Schwartz, D. R., et al.: *The Elderly Ambulatory Patient: Nursing and Psychosocial Needs.* New York, Macmillan Pub. Co., Inc., 1964.
17. Sullivan, J., and Armignacio, F.: Effectiveness of a Comprehensive Health Program for the Well Elderly by Community Health Nurses. Nurs. Res., 28:70, 1979.

SUGGESTED READINGS

Ailinger, R. L.: A study of illness referral in a Spanish-speaking community. Nurs. Res., 26:53, 1977.
Arminger, B., Sr.: Ethics of nursing research: Profile principles, perspectives. Nurs. Res., 26:330, 1977.
Aydelotte, M.: The use of patient welfare as a criterion measure. Nurs. Res., 11:10, 1962.
Bates, B.: Nursing in a health maintenance organization — Report on the Harvard Community Health Plan. Am. J. Pub. Health, 1972.
Boyd, H.: *Survey of Public Health Nursing in Connecticut.* Hartford, Connecticut State Department of Health, 1918.

Brook, R. H.: Quality of care assessment: Choosing a method for peer review. New Engl. J. Med., 288:1323, 1973.

Brook, R. H., et al.: Assessing the quality of medical care using outcome measures: An overview of the method. Med. Care, 15:(Supplement), 1977.

Campbell, D., and Stanely, J. C.: Experimental and Quasi-Experimental Designs for Research. Chicago, Rand McNally & Co., 1963.

Chambers, L. W., et al.: A controlled trial of the impact of the family practice nurse on volume, quality, and cost of rural health services. Med. Care, 15:971, 1977.

Clearinghouse on Health Indexes Cumulated Annotations, 1976. Washington, D.C., Department of Health, Education and Welfare, No. (PHS 78-1225) Public Health Service, National Center for Health Statistics, September 1978.

Colt, A. M., Anderson, N., Scott, H. D., and Zimmerman, H.: Home health care is good economics. Nurs. Outlook, 25:632, 1977.

Donabedian, A.: Evaluating the quality of medical care. Milbank Mem. Fund. Qrtly., 44:166, 1966.

Donabedian, A.: The Quality of Medical Care: Methods for Assessing and Monitoring the Quality of Care for Research and for Quality Assurance Programs in Health. Washington, D.C., Government Printing Office, 1978.

Downs, F., and Fleming, J: Issues in Nursing Research, New York, Appleton-Century-Crofts, 1979.

Dyer, E., et al.: Improved Patient Care Through Problem-Oriented Nursing, New York, Springer Co., 1974.

East Harlem Nursing and Health Demonstration, New York (City): A Comparative Study of Generalized and Specialized Nursing and Health Services. New York, The Demonstration, 1926.

Feinstein, A.: Clinical Biostatistics, St. Louis, Mo., C. V. Mosby Co., 1977.

Given, B., Given W., and Simoni, L.: Relationships of processes of care to patient outcomes. Nurs. Res., 28:85, 1979.

Gori, G., and Richter, B.: Macroeconomics of disease prevention in the U.S. Science, 200:1124, 1978.

Hain, M. J., and Chen, S. C.: Health needs of the elderly. Nurs. Res., 25:433, 1976.

Hegyvary, S. T., and Dieter-Haussman, R. K.: Monitoring nursing care quality. J. Nurs. Admin., 6:12, 1976.

Hertz, P., and Stamps, P. L.: Appointment-keeping behavior re-evaluated. Am. J. Pub. Health, 67:1033, 1977.

Highriter, M.: The status of community health nursing research. Nurs. Res., 26:183, 1977.

Hoekelman, R. A., and Peters, E. N.: A health supervision index to measure standards of child care. HSMHA Health Rep., 87:539, 1972.

Holliday, J.: Public Health Nursing for the Sick at Home: A Descriptive Study. Visiting Nurse Service of New York, 1967.

Horsley, J., Crane, J., and Bingle, J.: Research utilization as an organizational process. J. Nurs. Admin., 8:4, 1978.

Hoskins, C. N.: Level of activation, body temperatures, and interpersonal conflict in family relationships. Nurs. Res., 28:153, 1979.

Howell, J. R., Osterweis, M., and Huntley, R. R.: Curing and caring — A proposed method for self-assessment in primary care organizations. J. Com. Health, 1:256, 1976.

Ibrahim, M. A.: Epidemiology application to health services. In Resource Book: Health and Behavioral Sciences. Washington, D.C., Association of University Programs in Health Administration, (in print).

Kalisch, P. A., and Kalisch, B. J.: The Advance of American Nursing, Boston, Little Brown & Co., 1978.

Kane, R. L., Woolley, F. R., Gardner, H. G., Snell, G. F., Leight, E. H., and Castle, C. H.: Measuring outcomes of care in an ambulatory primary care population: A pilot study. J. Com. Health, 1:233, 1976.

Katz, S., et al.: Chronic disease classification in evaluation of medical care programs. Med. Care, 7:139, 1969.

Kauffman, M. C.: The dilemma of assessing nursing services in community health agencies. In Assessment of Nursing Services: Report of a Conference. Washington, D.C., DHEW Publication No. (HRA) 75–40, June 1974, pp. 29–47.

Keener, M. L.: The public health nurse in mental health follow-up care. Nurs. Res., 24:198, 1975.

Kessner, D. M., Kalk, C. E., and Singer, B. A.: Assessing health quality, the case for tracers. New Engl. J. Med., *288*:189, 1973.

Kessner, D. M., Snow, C. K., and Singer, J.: *A Strategy for Evaluating Health Services: Contrasts in Health Status,* Vol. 2. Institute of Medicine, National Academy of Sciences, 1973.

Kessner, D. M., Snow, C. K., and Singer, J.: *Assessment of Medical Care for Children: Contrasts in Health Status,* Vol. 3. Institute of Medicine, National Academy of Sciences, 1974.

Krathwohl, D.: *How to Prepare a Research Proposal,* 2nd ed., Syracuse University Bookstore, 1977.

LeBow, J.: Evaluation of an outpatient pediatric practice through the use of consumer questionnaires. Med. Care, *13*:250, 1975.

Leonard, R. C., Skipper, J. K., and Wooldridge, P.: Small sample field experiments for evaluating patient care. Health Serv. Res., *2*:46, 1967.

Levine, S. (PI): Nurse Characteristics and Patient Progress. (Terminal Progress Report, PHS Research Grant N000128), May 1969.

Lewis, C. E., and Resnick, B.: Nurse clinics and progressive ambulatory patient care. New Eng. J. Med., *277*:1236, 1967.

Logan, R.F.L.: Assessment of sickness and health in the community: Needs and methods. Parts I and II. Med. Care, *2*:173 and 218, 1964.

Maddox, G. L., and Douglass, E. B.; Self-assessment of health: A longitudinal study of elderly subjects. J. Health Soc. Behav. *14*:87, 1973.

Managan, D., et al.: Older adults: A community survey of health needs. Nurs. Res., *23*:426, 1974.

McNerney, W. J.: The quandary of quality assessment. New Eng. J. Med., *295*:1505, 1976.

National Health Council: *An Introduction to Grants and Contracts in Major HEW Health Agencies.* Washington, D.C., National Academy of Sciences, the National Research Council.

National League for Nursing: *Community Health Agency Evaluation.* New York, 1976.

Notter, L. E.: *Essentials of Nursing Research,* New York, Springer Publishing Co., 1974.

Nuckolls, K. B., et al.: Psychosocial assets, life crises and the prognosis of pregnancy. Amer. J. Epidemiol., *95*:431, 1972.

Padilla, G.: Incorporating research in a service setting. J. Nurs. Admin., *9*:44, 1979.

Phaneuf, M.: Quality assurance — a nursing view. Qual. Assur. Med. Care, February 1973.

Phaneuf, M. C.: Quality of care: Problems of measurement. Am. J. Pub. Health, *59*:1827, 1969.

Polit, D., and Hungler, B.: *Nursing Research: Principles and Methods.* Philadelphia, J. B. Lippincott Co., 1978.

Prescott, P. A.: Research issues in program evaluation. Nurs. Admin. Qrtly., *2*:63, 1978.

Prescott, P. A., and Sorensen, J. E.: Cost-effectiveness analysis: An approach to evaluating nursing programs. Nurs. Admin. Qrtly., *3*:17, 1978.

Reid, E. L., and Morgans, R. W.: Exercise prescription: A clinical trial. Am. J. Pub. Health, *69*:591, 1979.

Rogheb, S., and Smith, E.: Beliefs and customs regarding breast feeding among Egyptian women in Alexandria. Int. J. Nurs. Studies, *16*:73, 1979.

Sackett, D. L., et al.: The development and application of indices of health: General methods and a summary of results. Am. J. Pub. Health, *67*:423, 1977.

Schulbert, H., and Baker, F. (eds.): *Program Evaluation in the Health Fields.* New York, Human Sciences Press, 1979.

Seffrin, J. R., and Schafer, R. W.: A survey of drug use beliefs, opinions and behaviors among junior and senior high school students. J. School Health, *46*:263, 1976.

Shorr, G. I., and Nutting, P: A population-based assessment of the continuity of ambulatory care. Med. Care, *15*:455, 1977.

Stephenson, G. R., Smith, O.P.B., and Roberts, T. W.: The SSR System: An open format event recording system with computerized transcription. Behav. Res. Meth. and Instr. *7*:497, 1975.

Stillman, M. J.: Women's health beliefs about breast cancer and breast self-examination. Nurs. Res., *26*:121, 1977.

Suchman, E. A.: Preventive health behavior: A model for research on community health campaigns. J. Health Soc. Behav., *8*:197, 1967.

Suchman, E. A.: *Evaluation Research, Principles and Practice in Public Service and Social Action Programs.* New York, Russell Sage Foundation, 1967.

Terris, M.: Approaches to an epidemiology of health. Am. J. Pub. Health, 65:1037, 1975.

Tetreult, A. I.: Evaluation of development health counseling: healthfulness of self-support behavior. Nurs. Res., 26:386, 1977.

Thomas, D. B., and Hansen, A. C.: Role group differences in assignment of priorities: A variable perspective interpretation. Nurs. Res., 15:12, 1966.

Verhonick, P.: *Descriptive Study Methods in Nursing.* Washington, D.C., Pan American Health Organization, WHO (Pub No. 219), 1971.

Vincent, P., and Price, J. R.: Evaluation of a JNA mental health project. Nurs. Res., 26:361, 1977.

Weissert, W.: Costs of adult day care: A comparison to nursing homes. Inquiry, 15:10, 1978.

Werley, H. H.: *Health Research: The Systems Approach.* New York, Springer Publishing Co., 1976.

White, K. L.: Teaching epidemiology concepts as the scientific basis for understanding problems of organizing and evaluating health services. Int. J. Health Serv., 2:525, 1972.

Williams, C. A.: Nurse practitioner research: Some neglected issues. Nurs. Outlook, 23:172, 1975.

World Health Organization: *Statistical Indicators for the Planning and Evaluation of Public Health Programs.* Fourteenth Report of the WHO Expert Committee on Health Statistics. Geneva, World Health Organization Technical Report Series No. 472, 1971.

Yankauer, A., et al.: The outcomes and service impact of a pediatric nurse practitioner training program. Am. J. Pub. Health, 62:347, 1972.

Yauger, R. A.: A program evaluation in community health nursing: Does family centered care make a difference? Nurs. Outlook, 20:320, 1972.

Zemach, R.: Program evaluation and system control. Am. J. Pub. Health, 63:607, 1973.

CHAPTER 9

COMMUNITY
HEALTH NURSING
IN THE COMMUNITY
STRUCTURE

In order to guide her own work effectively, the community health nurse, whether a beginner or a seasoned administrator, must understand how community health nursing fits into the various parts of the community health care system.

The health care system may be defined as the complex of people, structures, facilities, and relationships that has been developed within a community to provide health care to individuals, groups, special populations, or to the community as a whole. Thus the system would include health professionals of all types; other individuals and groups, including consumers of health care, who are taking health action for themselves or on the behalf of others; the health and health-related institutions, including hospitals, health and welfare departments, school health services, and voluntary agencies; and the mechanisms through which they all interrelate.

GENERAL CONSIDERATIONS

Community health nursing operates under a variety of sponsorships: government authorities, ranging from local to international in coverage; voluntary agencies; and private industry or health groups. Each type of sponsor has particular commitments and ways of organizing to meet these commitments. Within this total system, community health nursing is involved at three levels: the direct-care (operational or practicing) level, the institutional or agency level, and the community level. Each level has its own particular condition, opportunities, and constraints.

PROVISION FOR HEALTH CARE THROUGH THE GOVERNMENT STRUCTURE

Government concern with health is a worldwide phenomenon; virtually every country has some provision for health care under government sponsorship. Community health nursing within a government agency may be placed in departments of health, welfare, or education or, in smaller numbers, in many other government units. Although government agencies do not provide all, or even most of, the health care of the people of the United States, they do have a broad mandate. It is generally accepted that with respect to health, the government is obligated to assure as far as possible that adequate and safe care reaches all segments of the population in amounts and quality calculated to preserve and promote health. Sharing the same broad obligation, community nursing in the government setting is also geared to the public as a whole.

Community health nursing is represented in the health efforts of all three tiers of government: local, state or provincial, and national. In each of these three levels, nursing is adapted to the degree of responsibility characteristic of that particular government level.

The Local Governmental Health Structure: Where the Action Is

In contrast to the federal and state governmental health structures, which are largely supportive and enabling, the local structure is primarily concerned with direct services to people and communities. As in the state and national structures, the local governmental health effort is widely dispersed among other units of government. Of particular interest to nurses is the large health component in the local school system.

The local governmental health structure is anchored by the local health department, which in turn may be organized on a city, city-county, county, or multicounty basis.

The role of the local health department is changing rapidly; and local circumstances such as financial capability, availability of care providers, public commitment to health, and nature of the population will determine the pattern. A position paper of the American Public Health Association spells out, in some detail, the basic services expected of local health departments.[1]

As a delegate of the state health department, the local agency is obligated to implement the basic responsibilities of the state agency. As a figure in local social and political action, the local health department is obligated to be responsive to local desires and need, and to take all possible action in promoting and preserving the health of the total population.

While the primary areas of concern of the local health department — i.e., disease prevention and control; assurance of safe environments in the community, industrial plants, schools, and homes; and promotion of health of the public — echo the concerns of other levels of government, the activities by which these responsibilities are met will differ.

Representative activities of a local health department might include:

1. Surveillance and counseling of well population groups that are at risk — such as families of diabetic patients, adults with high blood pressure (although still within the normal range), or groups that need developmental guidance (mothers and infants, or elderly groups).
2. Therapy and counseling for groups of the population with behavioral disorders — such as drug addiction, alcoholism, obesity, and aggression toward others.
3. Screening for specific diseases — such as sickle cell anemia (inherited), glaucoma (in older age groups), and hearing loss (in school children).
4. Epidemiologic investigation of disease.
5. Inspecting, ensuring compliance with regulations, and advising on improvement of specific environments — such as the home, industry, food establishment, or recreational center.
6. Person-to-person or mass media health education programs.
7. Collection of essential health data.
8. Providing personal health care to the general population or to selected groups — such as Medicaid recipients, individuals with a communicable disease, or special beneficiaries (welfare recipients or members of the agency staff).
9. Planning on an agency or community basis for health care of the population.
10. Studying and acting to improve the health manpower supply.

In all of these activities there is a part for the community health nurse to play.

Local departments of education also conduct substantial health programs; virtually all have some nursing personnel either employed directly by the school system or assigned by the local public health agency. In 1974, 21,183 nurses — representing 35.7 per cent of the total community health nursing population — were working in school health nursing service. Of those, 81.6 per cent were employed by Boards of Education.[2] The purposes of the health program in the school situation are identical, whatever the sponsorship. Working in coordination with the teaching, special service, and administrative personnel of the school and with appropriate community health agencies, these objectives are:

1. To contribute to the health of the school population by early recognition and treatment of any health impairment, and by health counseling.

2. To contribute to the health education of the school population by serving as a resource or in selected situations participating in teaching.
3. To contribute to the general educational program by alerting instructional staff of physical or emotional problems that might interfere with learning.
4. To contribute to the improvement of the physical and social environment of the school.
5. To contribute to the general community health program by using the child as a channel for health education of the family, by reporting unusual patterns of disease occurrence in the school population, and by re-enforcing the efforts of the community agencies through appropriate in-school action.

As is true of other local agencies, the school nurse's work is largely in direct care. Many school nurses work with little or no direct nursing supervision. While there may be certain prescribed activities or general program requirements, it is often possible to adapt programs to fit individual situations.

The State Government Health Structure

The state may, and usually does, delegate considerable power to local units of government; however, it retains the ultimate responsibility and authority for the public's health. In the early 1800's, Shattuck described this responsibility as "to take cognizance of the people." The legal charge is as broad today.

The organization structure of state health departments varies considerably among the many types of state agencies that contribute, in some way, to health programs — e.g., the Departments of Welfare, Mental Health, Education, Agriculture, Labor, and the Environmental Protection Agency. However, every state has a department of health that has the primary legal responsibility for the public health program.[3] It is in this agency that most of the public health nursing effort is found.

A tremendous variety of activities are reported by state health departments, most of them needing nursing support. Primary responsibilities are:

1. To speak for public health interests and goals in planning groups and before elected officials.
2. To promulgate and enforce rules and regulations, and to propose and justify needed legislation.
3. To generate a coordinated and comprehensive planning and policy base for health care, directly or through others, with full representation of consumers.
4. To delegate to and supervise health agencies in their provision of health services best rendered locally.

5. To support local health units and needed nongovernmental services through financial aid grants and consultation.
6. To conduct or arrange for such direct care programs as are required but cannot be provided for locally.

In general little direct care is rendered by state health departments, although some diagnostic clinics or highly specialized services may be provided.

Nursing is most often organized by program, with the nurse acting in an advisory capacity to local groups and in a consulting capacity to administrative heads of specialized programs within the state system. Typical responsibilities of community health nursing in state health departments are:

1. To study and recommend, in conjunction with other groups concerned, action relating to the overall nurse manpower supply. This involves activities such as arranging for nurse manpower surveys; evaluating the adequacy of training facilities and making recommendations for change; helping communities to adapt to change in the nurse manpower supply; and working with professional associations, hospitals, and others to develop required data.
2. To relate nursing to the larger health effort of the state by consulting with other health or health-related bureaus, departments, agencies, or organizations on nursing phases of their work, so as to ensure coordination and effective utilization of the available nurse supply. This includes participation in the development of the overall plan and administration of the total health programs, including administration of grants to local communities.
3. To assist and supplement the efforts of local government and voluntary and private groups engaged in nursing. This involves activities such as providing supplementary general or specialized staff to advise on professional or administrative problems in nursing, establishing uniform record systems, and providing computer services for reporting.
4. To improve the quality of nursing efforts within the state. This will include activities such as developing criteria or guidelines; establishing recommended or required personnel standards for employment or for certification or licensing, and engaging in, or arranging for, ongoing educational programs for employed or to-be-employed nursing staff.
5. To promote coordination of all state-wide efforts for nursing, whether sponsored by government, voluntary, professional, quasi-professional, or private agencies.

Because of the nature of these tasks and responsibilities, when local health services are well established, the nursing staff at the state tier is apt to consist primarily of specialists or consultant personnel. In a few states where local services have not been developed, the state-employed staff may include a larger number of direct-service personnel.

Nursing concerns in a state or provincial health department are not limited to community health nursing. Labor disputes in state hospitals and supervision and regulation of nursing homes are major problems involving nursing at the state level. Nurses are also important members of state and regional planning bodies. They may be assigned as staff workers or serve on a periodic basis as members of planning committees.

The Federal Government Health Structure

Health agencies in the federal tier of government have two types of responsibility: the first is concerned with acting on problems that cannot be logically or feasibly dealt with by the states, and the second is concerned with supporting and improving the health care provided through state and local health authorities. This responsibility is met through the following activities:

1. Maintaining a health intelligence system for the nation as a whole in coordination with the states and with international health sources. This includes the collection of data by the National Center for Health Statistics and the maintenance of interstate and national data required for the control of communicable disease, air pollution, and similar problems that transcend state boundaries.
2. Setting national health policy and providing the legislative arm of government with information and technical assistance required for developing adequate and appropriate legislation. Most health professionals feel that the national health policy is, as yet, not very clearly defined.
3. Providing financial aid to state and local health groups through grants-in-aid, contracts, project grants, and other funding mechanisms.
4. Supporting state and local health efforts through a system of continuing technical consultation to the states; allocating highly specialized personnel to deal with exceptional state or local problems that require a degree of expertness not available in the states; and developing standards and supportive guides, criteria, and other materials for use by the state and local agencies.
5. Providing direct services to groups — for example, Indians, Eskimos, members of the armed forces, and veterans — to which the federal government has a specific commitment.
6. Conducting or supporting research in health care.

In many countries, there is a ministry of health at the national level, with direct responsibility for planning and providing health services. A ministry for health has the advantage of promoting and coordinating health issues at the cabinet level of government and can more easily assure that national health needs are met.

In the United States, many agencies of the federal government have responsibility for some aspect of the public's health. The Bureau of the Census, the Department of Agriculture, the Department of Defense, the State Department, the Veterans' Administration, the Social Security Administration, the Environmental Protection Agency, and the Department of Health and Human Services (DHHS) have major health programs (see Fig. 9–1). Of these, the Public Health Service in the Department of Health and Human Service has the major responsibility for improving the health of the American people. The Center for Disease Control, with the National Institute for Occupational Safety and Health; the Food and Drug Administration; the Health Resources Administration, with the Bureau of Health Manpower and the Bureau of Health Planning and Resources Development; the Health Services Administration, with the Bureau of Community Health Services, Indian Health Services, and the Bureau of Medical Services; the Alcohol, Drug Abuse, and Mental Health Administration; the complex of National Institutes of Health; the Health Care Financing Administration; and the Office of Health Research, Statistics and Technology are all part of the Public Health Service. (See Fig. 9–2).

Within the federal government structure, nursing is integrally related to virtually every unit and program having substantive health content. There is a chief nurse officer, currently located in the office of the Assistant Secretary for Planning and Evaluation, who is concerned with broad policy and program development. The Division of Nursing in the Bureau of Health Manpower serves as the Federal focus for nursing with regard to nursing education, practice, and research. There are also strong nursing components in the Bureau of Community Health, the Veterans' Administration, National Institutes of Health, and the Mental Health Administration (ADAMHA).

In the direct-care services (such as services to special population groups or to employees) afforded under federal sponsorship, community health aspects of health care correspond to those at a local level. For instance, although federally supported, the army health nurse assigned to an army post is expected to relate not only to the army preventive medical service but also the community in which the post is located.

Typical responsibilities of the combined nursing effort in the national government structure include:

1. To document the needs of people for nursing care and incorporate these into national health policy, plans, and action. This involves anticipating nursing implications of national developments — for example, anticipating the nursing impact of National Health Insurance legislation and new approaches to health care delivery or answering the demand for nurses with particular skills. New plans and policies regarding manpower development, support of research, foreign aid, or civil defense are other examples of action that has distinct nursing implications. This requires that nursing provisions be built into legislation or policy statements. It may also require the mobilization of national resources to brief, train, or advise state and

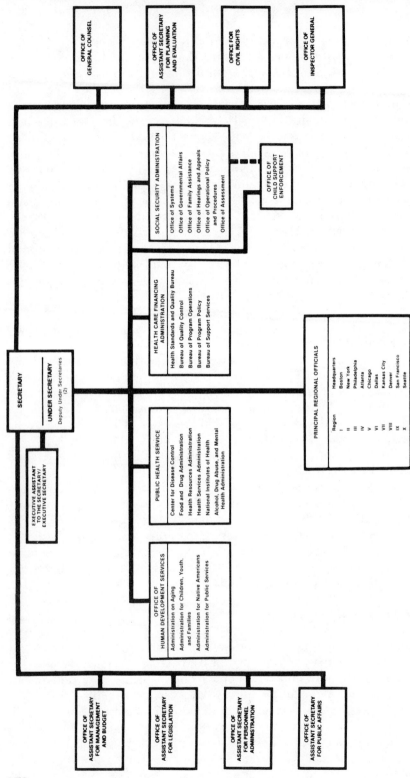

Figure 9–1 U.S. Department of Health and Human Services.

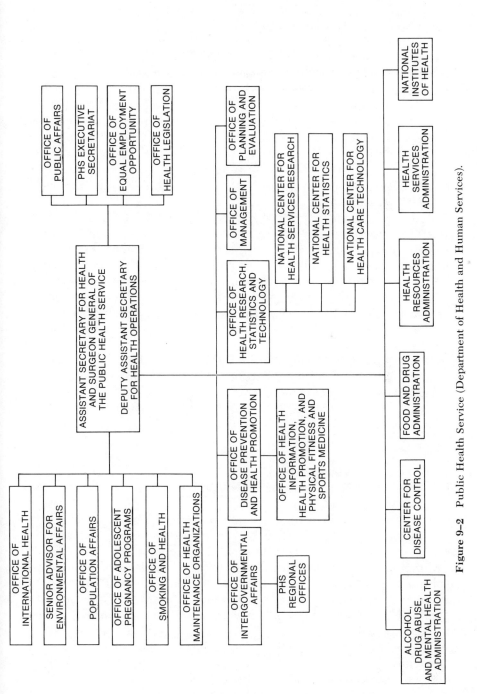

Figure 9–2 Public Health Service (Department of Health and Human Services).

local nursing groups, and also the development of criteria, manuals, or supportive educational materials.

2. To provide consultation, advice, and training. Federal agencies working with the regional offices of the Department of Health and Human Service and through special institute-like structures, such as the Communicable Disease Center, offer continuing or *ad hoc* consultation and training services to the states and to local health, education, and welfare groups. The nursing advisors of the regional offices maintain a continuing relationship with the states in their region.

3. To administer nursing aspects of national programs authorized by legislation. Noteworthy are the programs developed under provision of the National Nurse Training Act.

4. To coordinate and support research pertinent to nursing. This includes supporting "internal" research essential to the agency's work, administering various research grants programs, and providing for scientific review panels for grants falling within the nursing sphere and for a continuing surveillance of supported projects.

5. To provide health services to groups to which the federal government has a special commitment. This includes nursing services to the military forces, veterans', special groups such as Indian or Alaskan populations, and government employees. Also provided for is the nursing support in surveillance and action of health problems that are of interstate or international scope. Migrant health problems have long been a matter of national concern, and nursing has a strong part to play, in both technical and administrative consultation, in meeting the national obligation to this group.

HEALTH PLANNING: A QUASI-GOVERNMENTAL ORGANIZATION

The National Health Planning and Resources Development Act of 1975 (PL 93–641) requires state governors to designate health service areas (HSA's) or regions in their state and to create statewide health coordinating councils. The law also provides for a National Council on Health Planning and Development, a national planning information center, and financial assistance to states and regional HSA's to facilitate planning for health services, manpower, and facilities. A majority (but not more than 60 per cent) of the governing body of each planning agency must be consumers who reside in the area. (Consumer is defined as someone not directly involved in providing health care services or with a fiducial relationship in health care services.)

A planning network to coordinate local areas with state and national efforts is evolving — setting priorities for action and standards and guidelines for a variety of facilities and health services. This effort has not been without controversy, however, at every level of application.

Planning guides at the local, state, and federal levels require the constant attention of the public and health professionals.[4]

Nurses are important members of these planning bodies; they may be either employees of the group (staff assigned to special projects or geographic areas) or nursing leaders who serve periodically as members of committees.

Congress identified ten priorities for consideration in health planning goals and development of resources. These are:

1. The provision of primary care services for medically underserved populations, especially those which are located in rural or economically depressed areas.
2. The development of multi-institutional systems for coordination or consolidation of institutional health services (including obstetric, pediatric, emergency medical, intensive and coronary care, and radiation therapy services).
3. The development of medical group practices (especially those whose services are appropriately coordinated or integrated with institutional health services, health maintenance organizations, and other organized systems for the provision of health care).
4. The training and increased utilization of physician assistants, especially nurse clinicians.
5. The development of multi-institutional arrangements for the sharing of support services necessary to all health service institutions.
6. The promotion of activities to achieve needed improvements in the quality of health services, including needs identified by the activities of professional standards review organizations.
7. The development by health service institutions of the capacity to provide various levels of care (including intensive care, acute general care, and extended care) on a geographically integrated basis.
8. The promotion of activities for the prevention of disease, including studies of nutritional and environmental factors affecting health and the provision of preventive health care services.
9. The adoption of uniform cost accounting, simplified reimbursement, and utilization reporting systems and improved management procedures for health service institutions.
10. The development of effective methods of educating the general public concerning proper personal (including preventive) health care and methods for effective use of available health services.

The Voluntary Agency Supplements and Enhances Government Effort

Unlike governmental agencies, voluntary efforts are not bound to serve the entire population or to concern themselves with the entire spectrum of health care. As demands for health care become more massive, the question of the viability of voluntary effort is being raised. As early as 1939, Marquette raised the question, "Is the private agency on the way out?"[5] However, the voluntary health movement appears to be deeply entrenched as a method of getting a health job done and, for those who serve as volunteers, as a means of expressing social concern and personal commitment.

Three types of voluntary agencies may be identified:

1. The *foundations*, which are established and financed by private philanthropy, come in assorted sizes and styles. Many have strong interests in nursing, such as the Kellogg Foundation and the Rockefeller Foundation.
2. The *professional* associations.
3. *Service* organizations, which may focus upon direct services to people or on backup service to other operating groups. For example, the Visiting Nurse Association is a direct service organization. The American Heart Association and the National Safety Council provide valuable information about the problems of their special concern and resource materials for health and educational workers.

The voluntary agency derives its authority from a board of directors. It functions within the legal restrictions regarding incorporation and fund raising and within the general welfare and public health laws of the particular state. The board of directors sets policy, provides broad directional leadership, and takes final responsibility for the conduct of the agency's business. Boards of voluntary health or nursing agencies are usually made up of representative citizens who serve as volunteers; members of the health professions constitute a minority in the total membership. In the past, these boards have failed to secure adequate representation from certain segments of the population; in particular, representation from the low-income or minority groups. However this situation is being remedied in most instances.

The voluntary agency is expected to work within the framework of the total health effort: to relate its work to the work of others, to avoid unnecessary duplication, and to recognize all needs that fall within the purview of its commitment. This relation to the total health effort is essential if the voluntary agency is to meet its obligation to spend prudently and for the purpose intended the money it receives from contributions or contracts.

Voluntary organizations in the United States may be local, regional, or national in coverage. The major voluntary nursing services are organized on a local level. (However, in Canada and Great Britain, the major voluntary nursing services are organized on a national level.)

The great majority of community health nurses in voluntary agencies are found in locally based visiting nurse associations or home health agencies. In the past, home health agencies have been either governmental or voluntary agencies, with a small number located within hospitals. In 1974 there were 5984 nurses employed by voluntary agencies — about 10 per cent of the total full-time equivalent nurses employed by community health agencies. Medicare payment and interest by other third-party payers in care for the sick at home have resulted in substantial increases in the numbers of certified home health agencies other than those traditionally involved.[6] These new programs are sponsored by hospitals, private nonprofit organizations and proprietary home health agencies. Data from a 1979 survey of Medicare[7]-certified home health agencies show 512 VNAs, 50 combined agencies, 1,290 official agencies, 351 hospital-based programs, and 603 private nonprofit and proprietary agencies.

Voluntary nursing and home health agencies are in the process of massive change arising from the rapid expansion of government commitment to personal health care and the expansion of new programs now competing for limited dollars. Use of voluntary facilities for implementation of governmental programs establishes new conditions. Availability of funds for support of home health care leads to reconsideration of the local program as a whole; the requirement that home health care agencies have at least one service in addition to nursing has changed the staff composition and, indeed, has broadened the overall thrust of the local agency. The requirement that certification be a prerequisite for Medicare payments has created a new concern for supervisory and administrative controls in the small agency. Quality assurance requirements have also prompted a deeper look into the practice aspect.

State nursing units have moved to stimulate the development of new resources for home health care, establish standards and procedures for certification, and provide intensified consultation to local unofficial agencies.

The National League for Nursing, through its Council of Home Health Agencies and Community Health Services, has provided a mechanism for concerted action by the agencies themselves. Through consultation on program and organization, intervention and explanatory efforts with planners and legislators, and development of guides and criteria, the Council has provided a valuable action base. The agency accreditation program, cosponsored by the American Public Health Association and the League, provides a strong incentive for change.

It is not difficult to predict the likely directions of change for voluntary nursing agencies — a movement toward multiprofessional staff and services; much greater concern with serious illness and long-term care; greater nursing responsibility in diagnosis and treatment of illness; and merging of agencies into larger and more sophisticated administrative entities.

Combination Voluntary/Official Home Health Agencies

One possible effective local public health structure is the combination agency — that is, two or more agencies under official and voluntary

Table 9-1 MEDICARE-CERTIFIED HOME HEALTH AGENCIES (1966 to 1979)°

	Official		Visiting Nurse Associations		Combination		Hospital-based		Private-nonprofit		Proprietary		Other†		
	No.	%	No.	%	No.	%	No.	%	No.	%	No.	%	No.	%	Total
1966	579	45	406	40	83	7	81	6					26	2	1275
1977	1240	50	504	20	43	2	282	11	293	12	98	4	36	1	2496
1979	1290	45	512	18	50	2	351	12	440	15	163	6	67	2	2873

°From Social Security Administration, Office of Research and Statistics, Washington, D.C., 1966, U.S. Government Printing Office Health Care Financing Administration, Office of Policy, Planning and Research, Washington, D.C., 1977, U.S. Government Printing Office, Preliminary Data 1/30/80.
†Including private nonprofit and proprietary agencies in 1966.

auspices that have joined forces in order to provide more economical and more effective public health nursing. In 1966 there were 83 combination agencies; by 1977, this number had decreased to 43. (See Table 9–1).

In such situations, the combination agency absorbs the general responsibilities of all its constituents. Funds come from some combination of taxes, fees, voluntary contributions, endowments, or joint fund raising efforts (such as the Community Chest). Authority for the various functions in the combined agency is drawn from the same sources as pertain to the constituent agencies. The boards of directors of the voluntary agencies and the appropriate government authorities draw up agreements to define the respective responsibilities and coordinate planning and action. Problems in accounting and ambiguous lines of administrative authority are major causes for the decrease in the number of combined agencies. The increased variety of programs offered by home health agencies and the organized nursing service by program in official agencies have also been contributing factors.

Many combined programs continue to exist, saving valuable nursing time and dollars. The pooling of resources enables agencies to respond more readily to the communities' need for nursing services.

Professional Organizations

The professional association has special responsibility for increasing the societal contribution of the profession, for improving the quality of professional practice, and for representing the practitioner as a negotiator or interpreter. There are many professional groups and associations with pertinence to public health and public health nursing, but the major responsibility is assumed by the American Nurses' Association, the National League for Nursing, and the American Public Health Association. Each offers educational programs, publications and journals, and efforts toward the development of standards of practice.

NURSING AT THE INTERNATIONAL LEVEL COMBINING GOVERNMENT AND VOLUNTARY ACTION

Programs of health aid between nations have broadened in the past decade along with developments in world politics, economics, and transportation. World health efforts may be bilateral (independent arrangements between two countries), or international (developed by an international body such as the World Health Organization or the International Council of Nurses), or sponsored by voluntary private organizations (such as Catholic missions or the Rockefeller Foundation).

The World Health Organization provides overall coordination of health work and technical assistance on a wide variety of problems; most important, it helps member countries strengthen their own health services.[8] Nursing has been an integral part of the World Health Organization (WHO) since the creation of the organization in 1948. WHO is headquartered in Geneva, Switzerland, with regional offices in several locations: Brazzaville (for Africa), Washington, D.C. (the Pan American Health Organization — for the Americas), New Delhi (for Southeast Asia), Copenhagen (for Europe), Alexandria (for the eastern Mediterranean), and Manila (for the western Pacific). Nurses are assigned as nurse advisors on programs or special projects in each of these regions. Major efforts are directed toward long-range planning, the establishment of sound country plans for nursing, and the education of local community outreach workers and traditional "healers" in providing primary health care. The nature of the nursing aid supplied has ranged from direct nursing services at the staff level in some projects to consultation with a country's government. The trend is toward more advisory support on issues and problems defined by the host country, with less direct service.

In the United States, the Office of International Health of the Public Health Service and the Agency for International Development of the Department of State work jointly in bilateral international health activities. The official U.S. involvement in international health is difficult to assess because it involves 23 different Federal agencies.[9] Typical nursing programs are: developing nursing education programs, educating special groups, especially those likely to become leaders; and assisting in the development of nursing legislation and national standards.

The Peace Corps, established in 1961, is a government agency designed to give citizens of the United States an opportunity to serve as volunteers in a people-to-people assistance program. Nurses serving in the Peace Corps are paid only travel expenses and a living allowance. They serve primarily in direct service capacities in countries whose health services are poorly developed or very much understaffed.

The International Council of Nurses, the League of Red Cross

Societies, and various foundations, such as the Rockefeller and the Kellogg foundations, have sponsored international nursing activities. These activities vary as the agency's or foundation's program goals change to adjust to new developments and new problems.

Missionary societies throughout the world contribute much to the development of both community health nursing and nursing in general. The consolidation of missionary operations has allowed for more substantive approaches in many countries.

Whatever the sponsorship, certain threads appear consistently throughout reports of international nursing actions. These may be summarized as follows:

1. The recipient country must have the final decision regarding the action to be taken.
2. Emphasis is upon long-term development of the country's own resources. Thus, the stress is on developing leaders and teachers rather than on meeting only immediate needs. These leaders are selected by the local community.
3. Nursing must be related not only to the overall health plans and needs but also the general development of the country. Nursing efforts must therefore reinforce and support efforts to upgrade the food supply or to promote local (village) development or rural health centers.
4. The nurse from the "provider" country must be prepared to make the adjustment to the host country — and not expect the host country to adopt her cultural patterns. The nurse in international work must be prepared to work with differences in language, methods of medical treatment, interprofessional relationships, and social customs.
5. Programs must be flexible to adapt to rapid change in the situation, since many countries are concentrating 50 years of advancement into a 10-year time period.
6. Although not frequently mentioned, of primary importance is the fact that the efforts of all "provider" countries for a particular country should be coordinated to unify and maximize the contribution. This is currently one of the weakest links in the provision of intercountry assistance.

THE ROLES OF HEALTH-CARE SOURCES ARE BLURRED

The traditional roles of the many partners in organized health care are becoming more and more blurred. Private or voluntary sources, such as universities or groups of physicians, undertake responsibilities that were formerly considered the province of government. Federal agencies, at one time restrained from by-passing the state health structure, now deal directly with local governments or voluntary groups. Projects under voluntary agency management may have responsibility that has traditionally rested with the public authorities.

Realignment of responsibilities and programs is a continuous process. Interposed among these structures is a relative newcomer to the organization family: the community-based citizen advisory or controling group. Nursing agencies, especially voluntary agencies, have traditionally leaned on citizen advisory groups. However, in the past these groups have been represented by boards, committees, or advisory bodies that dealt with a particular agency or phase of the health effort. Recently, though, citizen groups have become much more powerful and involved in larger spheres of responsibility. Implementation of the National Health Planning and Resources Development Act of 1975 requires that planning and evaluation of health programs in the public sector be undertaken by a representative group from the general public (consumers) as well as professional personnel (providers). To the degree that the private and public sector work together in these agencies, a more rational system for providing services may be effected.

At present, problems of health care are being dealt with largely on an expedient *ad hoc* basis. Any accredited agency or care source is free to move into any program in which it is interested and for which it can mobilize the necessary money and personnel.

This convenient "no system" approach is understandable. The public, impatient with any delay, is demanding that its institutions apply quickly what is known about health. Thus, there is often a failure to consider at what level of organization or through what type of structure the most effective and economical total result could be achieved.

Furthermore, health problems refuse to stay put within given geographic boundaries or service units: Often a safe and plentiful water supply cannot be assured by a single state authority; nor can a single agency, such as a hospital or a health department, deal with the multiple social and health problems families face. As Lewis Thomas states:

> These days, with the increasing complexity of organizations in which we live and the great numbers of us becoming more densely packed together, the work of committees can be a deadly serious business. This is especially so when there is need to forecast the future. By instinct, each of us knows that this is a responsibility not to be trusted to any single person; we have to do it together.[10]

REFERENCES

1. American Public Health Association: The role of official local health agencies. Am. J. Pub. Health, 65:189, 1975.
2. Division of Nursing, BHPr, DHHS: Survey of Community Health Nurses: 1974. Springfield, Va., National Technical Information Service (NTIS), (HRP-0900628) (unpublished), 1979, p. 139.
3. Hanlon, J.: *Public Health Administration and Practice.* St. Louis, Mo., C.V. Mosby Co., 1974, p. 298.

4. Zwick, D. I.: Initial development of national guidelines for health planning. Pub. Health Rep., 93:407, 1978.
5. Marquette, B.: Is the private agency on the way out? Am. J. Pub. Health, 29: 46, 1939.
6. Division of Nursing, BHPr, DHHS: Survey of Community Health Nurses: 1974. Springfield, Va., National Technical Information Service (NTIS), (HRP-0900628) (unpublished), 1979, p. 221.
7. Preliminary Data, Medicare Certified Home Health Agencies, Health Care Financing Administration, Office of Policy, Planning and Research, Washington, D.C. 1980.
8. Division of Information; World Health Organization, Geneva, 1967.
9. Bourne, P. G.: A partnership for international health care. Pub. Health Rep., 93:116, 1978.
10. Thomas, L.: The Medusa and the Snail, More Notes of a Biology Watcher. New York, Viking Press, 1979, p. 117.

SUGGESTED READINGS

Abrams, H. K.: A community perspective on health care: Nurs. Outlook, 19:92, 1971.
American Public Health Association: A national program for personal health services: Resolution adopted at 98th American meeting October 28, 1970. Am. J. Pub. Health, 61:191, 1971.
American Public Health Association: The role of official local health agencies. Am. J. Pub. Health, 65:189, 1975.
Archer, S. F., and Fleshman, R.: *Community Health Nursing.* Belmont, Calif., Duxbury Press, 1975.
Arndt, C. and Huckabay, L.: *Nursing Administration.* St. Louis, Mo., C. V. Mosby Co., 1975.
Bryant, J.: *Health and The Developing World.* Ithaca, N.Y., The Rockefeller Foundation. Cornell University Press, 1969, p. 95.
Bryant, J. H., Ginsberg, A. S., Goldsmith, S. B., Olendzki, M. C., and Piore, N.: *Community Hospitals and Primary Care.* New York, Center for Community Health Systems, Columbia University.
Collier, D. J., and Segall, M.: *Analysis and Planning for Improved Distribution of Nursing Personnel and Services: A Blueprint and Recommendations for Improved Nursing-Related Data.* Boulder, Colo., Western Interstate Commission for Higher Education, 1977.
Cuninggim, M. *Private Money and Public Service,* New York, McGraw-Hill Book Co., 1972.
DeHoff, J.: Health care consortiums — new role for local health departments. Am. J. Pub. Health, 63:672, 1973.
Department of Home Health Agencies and Com. Health Services: *The Board Member in the Community Agency.* Proceedings of the Board Members Forum at the NLN Biennial Convention. New York, National League for Nursing, 1972.
Donabedian, A.: *Aspects of Medical Care Administration: Specifying Requirements for Health Care.* Cambridge, Mass., Harvard University Press, 1973.
Hasse, P. T., Smith, M. H., and Reitt, B. B.: *A Workbook on the Environments of Nursing. Pathways to Practice.* Nursing Curriculum Project, Vol. 3. Atlanta, Ga., Southern Regional Education Board, 1974.
Hanlon, J. J.: *Public Health Administration and Practice,* 6th ed. St. Louis, Mo., C. V. Mosby Co., 1974, pp. 309–318.
Haughton, J. G.: The role of the public general hospital in community health — 1974 Rosenhaus lecture. Am. J. Pub. Health, 65:21, 1975.
Klarman, H. E.: Health planning: Programs, prospects and issues. Milbank Mem. Fund Q., 36:78, 1978.
Mahler, H.: Promotion of primary health care in member countries of WHO. Pub. Health Rep. 93:107, 1978.
Myrdal, G.: *Asian Drama — An Inquiry Into the Poverty of Nations,* New York, Pantheon, 1968.

Organization of Local and Intermediate Health Administrators. WHO Technical Report Series No. 499. Geneva, 1972.

Paine, L. (ed.): *Health Care in Big Cities.* London, Croom Helm, 1978.

Pan American Conference on Health Manpower Planning: *The Health Manpower Planning Process,* Vols. I–III. Ottawa, Canada, 1973.

Reitt, B. B.: To serve the future hour: An anthology on new directions of nursing. Atlanta, Ga., Southern Reg. Ed. Bd., February 1974.

Roemer, M. I.: Health care — financing and delivery across the world. Am. J. Nurs., *71*:1158, 1971.

Rosenkrantz, B. G.: *Public Health and the States Changing Views in Massachusetts, 1842–1936.* Cambridge, Mass., Harvard University Press, 1972.

Smith, K. R., and Trager, B.: In-home health services in California: Some lessons for national health insurance. Med. Care, *16*:473, 1975.

Stiles, S. J., and Johnson, K.: Regulatory and review functions of agencies created by the act: National Health Planning and Resources Development act of 1974. Pub. Health Rep., *91*:24, 1976.

Taylor, C. E.: Changing patterns in international health: Motivation and relationships. Am. J. Pub. Health, *69*:803, 1974.

U. S. Department of Health, Education and Welfare, Public Health Service. *Forward Plans for Health.* Washington, D.C., U.S. Government Printing Office, FY 1978–82, August 1976.

Velimirovie, B., and Velimirovie, H.: Utilization of traditional medicine and its practitioners in health services: A global overview. *In Modern Medicine and Medical Anthropology in the United States-Mexico Border Population.* Washington, D.C., Pan American Health Organization, 1978, p. 172.

WHO/UNICEF: *Report of World Conference on Primary Health Care at Alma Ata, Soviet Kazakhstan, September 1978.* Geneva, WHO; New York, UNICEF, 1978.

RESOURCES

American Nurses' Association
1030 15th Street, N. W.
Washington D.C. 20005

American Public Health Association
1015 18th Street, N. W.
Washington, D.C. 20036

Association of State and Territorial Health Officers
302 5th Street, N. E.
Washington, D.C. 20002

National Association of Home Health Agencies (NAHHA)
Suite 200, 426 C Street, N. E.
Washington, D.C. 20002
(202) 547–1717

National Center for Voluntary Action
1785 Massachusetts Avenue, N. W.
Washington, D.C. 20036

National Council of Homemaker–Home Health Aide Services, Inc.
67 Irving Place
New York, New York 10003
(212) 674–4990

The National League for Nursing
10 Columbus Circle
New York, New York 10019
(212) 582–1022

World Health Organization
Headquarters: Geneva, Switzerland
Publications distributed by: Q Corporation
49 Sheridan Ave.
Albany, New York 12210

CHAPTER 10

COMMUNITY HEALTH NURSING IN THE AGENCY STRUCTURE

Community health nurses function in many different types of organizations and settings and, more rarely, in independent practice. Each system sets both opportunities and constraints that influence the way nursing operates. The scope and nature of community health nursing practice are strongly affected by agency or institution policies that — for medical, legal, financial, and administrative reasons — are considered essential. It is useful to look at some common types of employing agencies and any characteristics of these agencies that may influence community health nursing practice.

NEEDS AND GOALS OF THE EMPLOYING AGENCY

When individuals accept employment in an agency, they imply a willingness to accept or reconcile the goals of the agency with their own personal and professional goals and values. Professional workers maintain a fundamental right to be accountable for their own practice. At the same time, they are committed to the obligation of furthering the work of the agency through the application of their professional skills.

THE AGENCY COMMITMENTS

Agency commitment will vary with sponsorship, sources of authority, financial sources and mechanisms, and formal or "understood" agreements with planning or administrative groups in the community.

For example, the health department, by virtue of its legislative authorization, must concern itself with the health of the population as a whole. The school health unit, on the other hand, is specifically concerned with the health of school children, sometimes with the health of school personnel, and with certain specified services for pre-school–age children. The voluntary or private agency involved in nursing services may limit its concerns, acting within the purpose stated in its articles of incorporation.

In government agencies, these commitments are explicitly or implicitly stated in either the legislation that authorize the agency or the regulations that supplement this legislation. The commitment of the health department, welfare department, or school health service is to be found in state or federal health, education, and welfare legislation. In addition, there is likely to be a set of regulations that further defines the nature of the agency commitment. For example, the authority under which the federal health services in the United States operate emanates from the basic mandate of the Preamble to the Constitution: the federal government is obligated to "promote the general welfare." This authority is further defined by other powers specifically reserved for the federal government — by the Constitution such as the authority to regulate interstate and international commerce and the power to levy taxes. The implied commitments in these legislative statements are realized through many specific legislative enactments, such as the Social Security Act and the Public Health Service Act.

Other health or health-related legislation and regulations may further define the commitment of the agencies and their various subunits. For instance, in the Community Mental Health Centers Act (which provides for the development of comprehensive mental health services), there is specific reference to the groups to be served (or catchment areas) and to the involvement of community residents on the governing boards that make the decisions relating to general policy. State education laws may specifically require medical examinations, hearing tests, or vision tests at prescribed intervals; or they may define the relationship that must obtain between the health and education authorities, with respect to the school health program.

The commitments of a particular agency are further clarified in policies, regulations, and agreements or contracts that specify conditions to be met. For example, a school health manual, prepared jointly by the schools and the health department, may spell out the responsibilities of each agency. The home health agency must provide certain services, in addition to nursing, to be eligible for certification of third party payment.

Sometimes there are commitments that have evolved informally. These commitments have never been put into writing or explained in conference; nevertheless, they are binding as a result of custom. A Visiting Nurse Association, for instance, may have an informal understanding with a local hospital to provide certain supportive services to clinical patients who are required to carry out prescribed therapeutic measures at home.

The community health nurse should familiarize herself with the conditions under which the agency is authorized to function. She should also be aware of the commitment that the agency has undertaken — as shown in reports of the governing board, in the agency's legislative or board authorization, in the agency's by-laws and annual reports, and in policy statements or informal agreements. The community health nurse will then be able to better understand her own place in the agency structure and will have a basis on which to project her own particular contribution for those activities involving more selective flexible development.

Agency Operating Policies and Patterns Also Influencing Nursing

Within the general framework of the agency's commitments, each agency further develops certain operating policies and patterns that will affect the nature of the community health nurse's responsibilities.

Staffing may be multilevel or single-level; the staff may include only community health nurses or a variety of nursing personnel (including nurse specialists, aides, or other special groups). The staff may include a generous or meager supervisory and consultant component, which places different levels of responsibility upon the individual staff member. The staff may be organized into teams (or clusters) or act as individual practitioners, each with a separate set of responsibilities. Personnel may be centralized, with everyone working from a central office, or decentralized according to service areas.

There may be an operating principle dictating that nursing services will be generalized — i.e., the assignment of each nurse or nursing group is in terms of *families* to be cared for rather than *specified patient groups*. For example, if 20 nurses are functioning in the agency, each of the 20 is expected to care for the families assigned to her whether the primary problem concerns maternal and child health, long-term or acute illness, psychiatric or behavioral disturbance, or a communicable disease. Each nurse or nursing group would function as a generalist in the health field.

The community health nurse may also be assigned to specialized functions. The nurse on a special tuberculosis project may serve only those requiring diagnostic, preventive, or curative care. A pediatric nurse specialist may handle a defined case load made up of those whose pediatric problems require unusual depth in nursing care. School nursing may be provided on a specialized basis, with only some nurses assigned to this service; or it may be provided as part of a generalized program, with all nurses participating.

Recently there has been intensive development of nurse specialists in various fields. This development is based on the premise that the increasing complexity of care justifies the use of one whose expertise is deeper, but narrower in range. This is undoubtedly true in certain settings, especially in the hospital or in the special intensive care clinics. For example, in an "all-out" type of clinic, dealing with high-risk mothers and infants, the nurse-midwife may be able to accomplish more with some families than could the generalized nurse. Furthermore, the introduction into the case load of the community agency of large numbers of older patients needing relatively simple care over a long period of time suggests the need for a specialized staff that is temperamentally and technically adapted to this kind of work.

Most feel, however, that it is important not to lose the family-oriented approach, even though the service is rendered by a specialist. Through group planning and shared visiting, the generalist may "back stop" the specialist (and vice versa) to allow the care to be truly family centered and as comprehensive as possible.

Other agency policies may also define the kinds of groups admitted to care and the types and extent of care rendered. For example, agency policy may dictate that no family may be admitted unless it is under some kind of medical supervision, or certain treatments may be deemed by a medical review or advisory committee as unsuitable for administration by nurses in the home setting. These policies are usually clarified during the nurse's orientation to the agency.

Concepts of the Supervisor's Role Will Also Affect Practice

In some agencies, the level of staff responsibility will rest upon the supervisor's estimate of the readiness of a particular nurse to carry out a given task. For example, the supervisor may decide when a community health nurse will head a nursing team or assume the responsiblity for certain community organization or group teaching duties. Such judgments in other agencies may be made by the nurse herself, or jointly by the nurse and the supervisor, and may be based on the training and experience of the nurse and the complexity of the immediate situation.

CHANNELS OF ACCOUNTABILITY DEFINED BY AGENCY'S ORGANIZATION

In any professional activity, there are two kinds of action for which the nurse must be accountable: (1) the action taken to accomplish a *function* and (2) the action taken in carrying out professional *practice*. The latter is generally conceded to belong within the sphere of the professional worker and his peers. Accountability for the function, on the other hand, is a concern of the agency as a whole — and, in particular, of the administrative staff. Thus, the nurse must account for the way in which she contributes to the management of the prenatal patient and her family during the maternity cycle, in terms of the degree to which the agency's program objectives are realized. At the same time, the nurse must account for the way in which she has exercised her professional practice in the accomplishment of this responsibility — that is, she must be aware of the relevance, effectiveness, and safety of the nursing process itself. It is important to understand the dyadic nature of this accountability; it is reflected in the ways that the community health nurse reports on what she has done, while it also determines the person to whom she looks for the direction and evaluation of her work.

All-Nurse Hierarchy

Nursing may be organized within an agency into an essentially professional hierarchy. The members of the nursing-care group may report to and be guided by a nursing supervisor in all aspects of work; the supervisor may, in turn, report to a nurse director. The nurse may plan and work with a multidiscipline group in carrying out her work; however, for the effectiveness and quality of her work, she is accountable only to a nursing line of authority. This is the usual pattern in voluntary agencies where function is restricted to nursing and some additional personal care services (such as physical or occupational therapy).

With such organizations, it is usual for each supervisor to have a designated number of staff nurses under her supervision. In general services in the United States, the number of staff nurses is most often somewhere between six and eight. This ratio of supervisor to staff nurse tends to vary in specialized service such as school nursing, where it may be lower, or in highly specialized projects, where it may be higher. The average ratio in the United States is considerably above the level found in some other countries; in Great Britain, for example, the ratio is usually one supervisor to 20 staff nurses.

Multidiscipline Hierarchy

In other instances, nursing may be organized primarily around a multidiscipline functional area under the direction of personnel other than the nurse. Many health department activities and special projects follow this pattern. This functional pattern may also appear in agencies where the nursing service provided is more advisory in function rather than direct. Such is the case in a state health department where the nurse advisers may work most directly with the chief of the service for which she is an advisor. Thus, the nursing consultant in mental health may be assigned to the bureau of mental hygiene; and the nurse in maternal and child health may be assigned to the bureau of family health. The nurse reports directly to the director of the service unit, and her work is directed and judged by him or her, in regard to its program effectiveness.

When this pattern of organization exists, it is important that there also be a channel through which the nurse can secure guidance and evaluation of the nursing *practice* facets of the work. She needs a method of accounting for the pertinence, safety, and currency of nursing itself. Professional guidance of this nature can be provided only by a member of the particular profession involved — be it nursing, engineering, medicine, or administration. The agencies generally provide a nurse advisor or a director of nursing services who works directly with the nursing staff and also with the non-nurse service leader to ensure the quality of nursing performance.

In addition to accounting for the work she is doing with respect to a given program or agency, the community health nurse must constantly evaluate and expand her general professional competence. As previously noted, she needs the support of a member of her own profession, more qualified by training and/or experience, who can help in this evaluation and growth process.

This presents no particular problem when the channels of accountability go through an all-nurse hierarchy. Since the program accounting and staff developmental measures tend to merge. When there is an established nurse consultant or nurse advisory system that provides for consistent and continuing professional review and counseling, there is likewise little difficulty. When neither of these situations exists — for example, when an occupational health nurse is working alone — it may be necessary for the nurse to identify a source for such help on her own initiative. The occupational health nurse may request to be included in the staff education activities of the local health department; she may request advice from the supervisory staff in that agency; or she may find a state consultant nurse in the field of occupational health who can provide some help. When such help is requested, the administrator should be informed and should understand that securing assistance with professional practice problems does not in any way interfere with usual administrative channels of responsibility.

PATTERNS OF COMMUNICATION ARE USUALLY BASED ON CUSTOM

Although an organization chart shows channels of reporting and responsibility, the patterns of communication within an agency rarely follow the same channels. It is important to know how people communicate in a particular agency. For instance, do nurses tend to go directly to specialized consultants in an agency, or do they first go to their own supervisor? Does the staff nurse consult freely with a physician responsible for service, or does information generally go through the supervisor? Are there multidiscipline meetings or case conferences to which the nurse may go? Are there regular nursing staff meetings?

The general trend is definitely toward the greatest possible freedom in communication, with the problem (rather than the organization chart) as the deciding factor in agency organizational patterns within which nursing functions. However, there are four general conditions that the agency organizational structure should assure:

1. Recognition of accountability of the individual professional worker for his professional practice.
2. An opportunity for the community health nurse to identify herself with the functional or service group and also with those in her own profession.
3. Freedom to communicate with the many agency and community groups that have some concern with the work of the nurse.
4. Professional guidance for continued professional growth.

EXAMPLES OF COMMUNITY AGENCIES

In 1946 the former National Organization of Public Nursing (since incorporated into the National League for Nursing) issued a statement (reaffirmed at a 1952 conference on the home care of the sick) suggesting three types of community organization for public health nursing:

1. All public health nursing services, including care of the sick at home, administered and supported by the health department. This is the usual pattern for rural communities.
2. Preventive services carried by the health department with one voluntary agency working in close coordination with the health department carrying responsibility for nursing care of the sick and for some special fields. This type of organization is the most usual one found in large areas.
3. A combination nursing service jointly administered by official and voluntary agencies with all field service given by a single group of public health nurses. Such a combination of services is especially desirable in small cities.[1]

These recommendations were designed to reduce the proliferation of community nursing services; they were based on the concept of providing service solely by public health nurses, each of whom carried a generalized program and served a designated population group. Subsequent developments, legislation, special programs, and regulations made these recommendations unlikely, however logical they may have been. There are currently a variety of organizations other than the traditional official and voluntary agencies that are involved in some aspects of community nursing.

Urban and Rural Decentralized Health Centers

In many areas, especially in defined underserved areas such as inner cities or geographically remote rural areas, health centers are being established in an effort to bring health care closer to the people served. In this setting, it is felt that nursing service may be more quickly responsive to the needs of people and close enough to get the kind of feedback from the population that is essential for planning the health program. The community health nurse is frequently seen as the primary health care provider, as demonstrated in policy statements describing the expected scope of practice and protocols that define usual activities and responsibilities. Organization goals and operating policies should be specific to the population served.

Nursing Clinics or Centers

Nursing clinics and centers may be associated with universities, other official organizations, or are free standing. They frequently work with a defined population and function such as education of prospective parents, rehabilitation of workman's compensation cases, or care of university students. Nurses in these centers have considerable latitude in defining the organizational goals and working out their mutual responsibilities.

Hospital-Based Home-Care Programs

The hospital-based home care program may purchase nursing service from existing agencies or establish an independent home visiting service. In this setting, the community health nurse may deal directly with families in the home, hospital, and clinic setting; or she may serve as a liaison with other community nursing and health services. There is usually a clearly defined commitment to a geographic area, with specifically stated policies describing those services provided. There is a hierarchy of function within the hospital as well as with other community organizations.

Hospice Programs

The "Hospice Movement" — well established in Great Britain, yet a fairly new concept in the United States — has as its goal the care and comfort of families during the process of terminal illness.[2] The community health nurse is a member of an interdisciplinary team that considers the changing needs of the dying person and their families, helping the terminally ill person to lead a full and complete life free of pain. The patient and family are the key decision-makers. The nurse has primary responsibility for the coordination of a broad spectrum of community services and works with a wide range of professional and non-professional workers. Hospice service may be organized as a free-standing unit within the community, as part of a hospital service or other facility, as a home care program, or simply as a group of professional and non-professional people having special concern for the dying person's quality of life. Whatever the organizational structure for hospice, the integration of home care, outpatient care, and an inpatient unit is essential.

Group Practice and Health Maintenance Organization

It is not known how many private group practices employ nurses for health maintenance, or preventive care practices that would require community health nursing skills. In England there has been, for some years, an "attachment" program, in which health visitors are assigned to a physician group. The nurse is employed by the government health agency, but her "population" becomes the families on the group's role.[3] A similar plan exists in Canada, and there have been occasional references to this idea in the United States. The rationale behind such an arrangement is that the physician's case load provides a convenient work unit for the community health nurse, promoting continuity of care and strengthening the team approach.

Prepaid group health care is growing rapidly in all areas and is a popular model for governmental and professional planners. Frequently, these group care facilities are large and provide a wide range of services. Plans such as the Health Insurance Plan of New York City, or the Kaiser-Permanente plan are examples of large prepaid groups. The Health Maintenance Organization (HMO), described in Chapter 1, is based on the prepayment principle, but allows for development of small as well as large and comprehensive organizations.

It is not known how many nurses are employed in such groups or to what extent their practice would fall within the area of community nursing. There has been emphasis on care of the well and worried well in some groups, but descriptions of these programs suggest that a medical rather than nursing model is being followed in care. Some plans have used nurse practitioners in providing primary care with success, or may use nurses in health teaching and health promotion efforts.

Regulatory Agencies

The amount of health legislation enacted by Congress since 1965 has been tremendous, accompanied by more money, more regulations, and more agencies to oversee how the public monies are spent.[4] These agencies for administrative regulation are the foremost institutionalized advocates of the public interest. Regulatory agencies are involved in pure foods, safe water, product safety, safe working conditions, fair wages and labor relations, and quality of health care in institutions and agencies receiving government monies. The agencies may be organized at the federal or state level (as in the case of nursing homes). They may also be in the private sector or quasigovernmental (as is true of the Professional Standards Review Organizations, or PSRO's).

Community Health Nurses are frequently employed by regulatory agencies interested in public health issues, in a broad range of activities:

1. Advising others or writing regulations for specific legislation.
2. Promulgating the rules with involved agencies and the public and assisting affected agencies in meeting the stated requirements.
3. Assisting in development of standards and criteria against which practice will be judged.
4. On-site evaluating and collecting data about conditions and practices.
5. Evaluating the feasibility and usefulness of the stated requirements in assuring the public good.

Enforcement of regulations, essentially laws, has been an important factor in improving health in the past. It can be a valuable tool in assuring a minimum level of care as well as assisting efforts to control mounting costs, especially for Medicare and Medicaid.

Industrial Health Programs

Health care is an important fringe benefit in industry. Many industrialized concerns and privately sponsored health or welfare services provide nursing services to their employees or their members. Such services may be included because of job considerations; that is, they may reduce compensation insurance costs, increase productivity by caring for minor health problems, or reduce absenteeism. These services are often considered to be a fringe benefit and a point for negotiation between industry and labor unions.

Authority for such health service is provided by the board of directors of the organization, either directly or through delegation to the executive or management officers of the corporation. This authority may be written into the directives of the company, or it may be incorporated into the bylaws or regulations of an organization.

Programs vary widely from industry to industry, and occupational health nursing reflects this. The health service may be primarily a first-aid station effort, or it may be a comprehensive and carefully planned health-care program with intensive counseling and preventive services for workers and their families.

Private Non-Profit and Proprietary Nursing Agencies

A prolific movement has been the development of private non-profit and proprietary nursing agencies providing services for home care patients. These agencies usually focus on specific procedures of skilled nursing care, which can be reimbursed by Medicare and other third-party payers. Nurses may find these agencies attractive because they offer more flexible working hours. Problems have evolved in terms of overall commitment of these agencies to serving the total community and family needs. Competition between the voluntary agencies and private commercial agencies for resources, and differences in philosophy have added to public confusion about home care, making coordinated efforts more difficult.

Criteria for Nursing Services

The work environment is an important factor in molding community health nursing practice. The nurse in a government agency, for example, is not free to practice so that only certain segments of the population receive care; rather, she must consider the needs of the total population. On the other hand, she may have access to multidiscipline deliberation and action to a degree not available to her in other settings. In the current widespread reassessment of obligation and direction and of change in structure and methods, agencies and community planners are struggling to develop innovative, responsive, and affordable patterns of action that will provide a reasonable level of care for all the people. The community health nurse is looking to the work environment to provide her with an opportunity to apply her professional skills in ways that will benefit the consumer and the community. Within the general framework of government, voluntary, and private responsibility, each agency must be seen as a unique work situation. Whatever the pattern of organization of nursing within the agency structure and the relation of the agency program to other agencies providing nursing care, certain criteria should be met.

1. Provide, within the limits of available resources, comprehensive and continuing nursing care to all who need it through the integration of nursing with all appropriate health and medical-care services.
2. Recognize the fundamental obligation of the government health authority to concern itself with the total health care of the population regardless of the auspices or financing under which the various segments of care are provided.
3. Provide for a planned combined approach of all involved in care to assure the provision of basic health services, to avoid unnecessary duplication or confusion in the services provided, to hold ineffective time to a minimum, to encourage experimentation, and to make full use of voluntary, private, and government resources.

4. Provide a "closeness" in services to people, allowing for ready access, easy communication, and prompt responsiveness to the needs of the consumer.
5. Recognize not only the responsibility and the right of the public, including users of community services, to share decisions regarding health planning and action but also the importance of having representation from all segments of the population in decision-making bodies.
6. Assume economical and appropriate utilization of the varying skills of each level and unit of nursing in order to conserve nurse resources.
7. Permit the nurse to work as a close member of functional health teams while at the same time maintaining identification with nursing as a whole in the agency or community.
8. Provide for medical direction in all work involving medical care.
9. Provide for nurse leadership of nursing phases of the work, including nursing direction of nursing practice.
10. Allow sufficient flexibility and adaptability to meet changing conditions or special needs.

Although the community health nurse may not be able to change the organizational structure within which she works, fully understanding this structure may enable her to work to the best advantage with the opportunities and limits it imposes. It may also be possible to develop compensating mechanisms: for example, if the agency does not provide professional nursing direction, a nurse advisory committee or a state nursing consultant or a supervisory nurse from another agency may serve as a substitute.

In addition to adapting to the existing structure, the alert community nurse may find opportunities to influence the structure by trying out new ideas in her own area and by participating in committees of the agency, professional associations, and other community groups that are in a position to make recommendations or to effect change.

REFERENCES

1. Desirable organization for public health nursing for family service. Pub. Health Nurs., 38:387, 1946.
2. Kohn, J.: Hospice movement provides humane alternative for terminally ill patients. Mod. Health Care, 6:26, 1976.
3. Lamb, A. M.: Community nursing developing within a national health service. Int. Nurs. Rev., 16:353, 1969.
4. For a partial listing of health legislation, see Hanlon, J.: *Public Health Administration and Practice*, 6th ed. St. Louis, Mo., C. V. Mosby Co., 1974.

SUGGESTED READINGS

Accreditation of Home Health Agencies and Community Nursing Services: Policies and Procedures. New York, National League for Nursing, 1976.

Ahmed, M. B., and Young, L.: The process of establishing a collaborative program between a mental health center and a public health nursing division. Am. J. Pub. Health, *64*: 880, 1974.

Archer, S. E.: Community nurse practitioners: Another assessment. Nurs. Outlook, *24*:499, 1976.

Archer, S. E., and Fleshman, R. P.: Doing our own thing — community health nurses in independent practice. J. Nurs. Admin., *8*:44, 1978.

Arndt and Huckabay: *Nursing Administration.* St. Louis, C. V. Mosby Co., 1975.

Bates, B.: Nursing in a health maintenance organization. Am. J. Pub. Health, *62*:991, 1972.

Bermal, H.: Power and interorganizational health care projects. Nurs. Outlook, *24*:418, 1976.

Brown, B. I.: Realistic workloads for community health nurses. Nurs. Outlook, *28*:233, 1980.

Brown, D. R.: Community health planning or who will control the health care system? Am. J. Pub. Health, *62*:1336, 1972.

Bullough, B.: The law and the expanding nursing role. Am. J. Pub. Health, *66*:249, 1976.

Clark, C. C., and Shea, C. A.: *Management in Nursing:: A Vital Link in the Health Care System.* New York, McGraw-Hill, 1979.

Combs, P. A.: A study of effectiveness of nursing referrals. Pub. Health Rep., *91*:122, 1976.

Coordinated home care program saves $13 million. Consumer Report, Blue Cross Association, 1975.

DeHoff, J. B.: Health care consortiums. Am. J. Pub. Health, *63*:672, 1973.

Edelstein, R.: Self-management in American nursing. Int. Nurs. Review, *26*:78, 1979.

Fox, John and Zatkin, Steven. Third party payment for nonphysician health practitioners: Realities and recommendations. Fam. Comm. Health, *1*:69, 1978.

Freeman, R.: Nurse practitioners in the community health agency. J. Nurs. Admin., *4*:21, 1974.

Gaus, C., Morris, S., and Smith, A.: The Social Security Administration Physician Extender Reimbursement Study: Anatomy of a quasi-experimental design. *In* Bliss, A., and Cohen, E. (eds.): *The New Health Professionals.* Germantown, Md., Aspen Systems Corp., 1977, pp. 341–352.

Hanlon, J.: *Public Health Administration and Practice*, 6th ed. St. Louis, Mo., C. V. Mosby Co., 1974, pp. 174–179, and 292–308.

Heyssel, R. M.: The Columbia Medical Plan and the East Baltimore Medical Plan. Hospitals, *45*:69, 1971.

Institute of Medicine: Controls on Health Care. Washington, D. C., National Academy of Sciences, 1975.

Kinlein, M. L.: *Independent Nursing Practice with Clients.* Philadelphia, J. B. Lippincott Co., 1977.

Leone, R. Public interest advocacy and the regulatory process. Ann. Am. Acad. Pol. Soc. Sci., *400*:46, 1972.

Levenson, G.: *Type, Length and Cost of Care for Home Health Patients: A Report of the Discharge Summary Feasibility Study.* New York, National League for Nursing, 1975.

Mantis, C. A.: PSRO coordination — is it nursing? Am. J. Nurs., *78*:1534, 1978.

Manual of Standards, Council of Home Health Agencies and Community Health Services, New York, National League for Nursing, 1980.

Morrill, R. G.: A new mental health services model for the comprehensive neighborhood health center. Am. J. Pub. Health, *62*:1108, 1972.

Mullan, F. S. M.: The National Health Service Corps. Pub. Health Rep., *94*: (Supplement), 1979.

Murata, J. E.: The nurse as family practitioner. Am. J. Nurs., *74*:254, 1974.

Quinn, J. L.: Triage: A cooperative experiment in community home health. In *Why Experiment with Health Care Delivery?* New York, National League for Nursing, 1976.

Reines, M. O.: A visiting nurse in a problem-oriented group practice. Am. J. Nurs., *79*:1224, 1979.

Ryder, C. F., and Ross, D. M.: Terminal care — Issues and Alternatives. Pub. Health Rep., *92*:20, 1977.

Sherwin, D.: Management of objectives. Harv. Bus. Rev., *54*:149, 1976.

Stevens, B.: Nursing division budget: Generation and control. J. Nurs. Admin., 4:16, 1974.

Stevens, B.: The use of consultants in nursing service. J. Nurs. Admin., 8:7, 1978.

Stevens, B. J.: Nursing management and the sense of structure. J. Nurs. Admin., 4:57, 1974.

Stewart, J. E.: *Home Health Care.* St. Louis, Mo., C. V. Mosby Co., 1979.

Sullivan, J. A., and Warner, J. S.: Economic perspectives for nurse practitioners. Pub. Health Rep., 94:142, 1979.

Sullivan, J. A., Dachelet, C. Z., Sultz, H. A., and Henry, M.: The rural nurse practitioner: A challenge and a response. Am. J. Pub. Health, 68:1097, 1978.

Trager, B.: *Home Health Care and National Health Policy.* New York, Haworth Press, 1980.

U.S. Department of Health, Education, and Welfare: *Hospices and Related Facilities for the Terminally Ill: Selected Bibliographic References,* Washington D.C., U.S. Government Printing Office, DHEW Pub. No. (HRA 79–14022), January 1979.

Ward, B.: Hospice home care program. Nurs. Outlook, 26:646, 1978.

Weston, J. L.: Whither the "nurse" in nurse practitioner? Nurs. Outlook, 23:148, 1975.

White, P.: Resources as determinants of organizational behavior. Admin. Sci. Qrtly., 366, 1974.

Widmer, G., Brill, R., and Schlosser, A.: Home health care: Services and costs. Nurs. Outlook, 26:488, 1978.

Zwick, D I.: Some accomplishments and findings of neighborhood health centers. *In* Zola, I., and McKinlay, J. B. (eds.): *Organizational Issues in the Delivery of Health Services.* New York, Prodist, 1974, pp. 331–364.

CHAPTER 11

THE HEALTH CARE
TEAM

A belief in the team approach is a basic part of health care philosophy today. Certainly it is widely believed that contemporary health problems cannot be solved by unilateral or uncoordinated efforts — that some form of concerted action is required.

WHAT IS IT?

A health group or team is more than an accidental assemblage of workers. It is an *organized* group of individual practitioners and consumers who *identify* themselves with a problem or problems, *commit* themselves to joint effort to solve or ameliorate the problems across the entire spectrum of care-planning action and evaluation of outcomes, and share *common goals* with respect to those problems.

Bergman identifies three categories of teams: the *basic* team which is engaged in day-to-day provision of care; the *extended* team, which adds members who can contribute to selected aspects of the total care; and the *consultative* team, consisting of the extended team enriched by specialists who provide help for a limited time with specific problems or aspects of cases.[1] The community health nurse may use any or all of these types of collaboration.

In practice, team care may take many forms. It may be no more than a systematic exchange of information — e.g., the nurse informs the physician of her observations and services provided to a client, and the physician in turn informs the nurse of the diagnosis and medical progress; or a hospital outpatient service may refer individuals for care by a visiting nurse service, with a plan for continuing interchange.

In a second form, the operation may be essentially a definition of specialized inputs and a plan for allocation of functions and responsibilities. In such instances, there is a designated leader who exercises

199

general control, and each member has a defined role and limits. A nursing team, for instance, may consist of a community health nurse who is responsible for the overall care provided, registered or practical nurses, and nursing aides or students who participate in the care as delegated by the nurse. A physician may carry primary responsibility and delegate to the nurse certain aspects of care.

A third possibility is the integrated or merged team, in which roles are blurred, and leadership is often shared or rotated to adapt to particular situations. For example, when the primary problem is illness, the physician may act as leader and be responsible for coordination of care. When the problem is one of self-inflicted behavior, the team member most likely to relate well to the individual may take leadership — in dealing with a young addict, for instance, a parent or athletic coach may be a member of the team, and may even assume temporary leadership. Depending on the situation and the estimate of relative impact of one or another member, the one most likely to succeed *in this area* would assume leadership to coordinate the efforts of all. When the situation changes, the leadership may change. An integrated, fluid approach that is designed to use most effectively the special skills of each member of the team appears to be exceptionally compatible with the most common types of health problems faced today; and, for this reason, this pattern will be discussed more fully.

The team may be large or small. In the absence of a *medical* problem, and when the situation is amenable to self-care by the affected individual, the care group may consist solely of the nurse and client (e.g., middle-aged person living alone may need help in changing unacceptable living habits such as dangerous eating patterns, poor management of stress, or overdependence on over-the-counter drugs. In other instances, the team will be larger. Various levels of nursing or medical personnel may be used. The physician is almost always involved; the team may also include a teacher, social worker, or environmentalist who has some relationship to the problem. Some of the more frequently utilized collaborators will be discussed in the following pages.

The team may function in a structured and tightly organized manner, or act together informally. Teams in action are usually multidisciplinary and increasingly multiagency.

What Distinguishes Team or Group Care from Fragmented or Unilateral Service?

1. *Common action goals*, for care in a specific situation, may be the result of negotiation. For example, the personal goal of a drug abuser may be to find relief after a "bad trip," then to return to drugs. The goal of the professional may be to have the client stop taking drugs. This, however, requires motivation on the part of the user — a factor involving

time that may not be available. The *action* goal may be to meet the client's immediate needs through safe and knowledgeable care and to assure that he has the best available information about drug use. Another action goal would be to enlist the user's help in preventing addiction of a younger sibling — a preventive measure for the sibling and a boost to the self-image of the user. Thus, the action goal becomes one all participants accept as a basis for their collective efforts to ameliorate the situation.

2. *Shared leadership* is characteristic of care teams. Group leadership is most effectively used in a dynamic rather than static framework. The leadership may rest in one situation with the physician (as in discussing particular medical therapy and the demands this places on the client and family; in another situation, the client or family member — or sometimes the nurse acting as patient-advocate — may take the lead, as in deciding how much change the client can tolerate. In yet another situation, a teacher may be called upon to evaluate to what degree school failure contributes to general behavioral problems such a client's agressive behavior, and whether failure could be avoided.

3. One person usually takes responsibility for the *management* of the team. This includes making sure that any agreement on exchange of information is proceeding as planned, that team members are used appropriately as the care progresses, and that the exchange of information is economical of time. These enabling measures must be distinguished from making decisions for the group.

4. *Roles are interchangeable.* While each participant will have a special role because of particular experience or professional knowledge, roles in a care team are often interchangeable. For example, administering immunizing agents may be the job of the physician, but may be provided by the nurse or physician's assistant or, in resource-poor areas, by specially prepared immunizers, depending on the special conditions that pertain. A very anxious child may be more amenable to nursing than to medical intervention; an older primigravida may be better served by medical intervention than by the usual nurse-midwife care. It is assumed that such shifting of roles will be based on the ability of the assignee to carry out the "borrowed" role. Each member of the team should be sensitive to the *role expectations* of the various members, and to their readiness for such sharing.

5. *Resources are merged* rather than added up. In dealing with a badly disabled child who is receiving psychiatric care to improve his adaption to irreversible damage, an uncle may have been co-opted as a care agent because he has a very close relationship with the child. With professional coaching, the uncle can strengthen the psychiatrist's efforts in a variety of ways. All members of the team should understand and be ready to support the medical regimen that has been established.

6. Relationship among members of the team is *collaborative* rather than hierarchical. The leader of the team does not enlist others to

support a preconceived course of action but rather to cooperate in establishing goals, actions, and evaluative measures that are based on the thinking of the group as a whole. The team rather than the individual develops the overall plan.

Some have referred to teamwork as a philosophy rather than a method. Certainly, unless the philosophy of communal and egalitarian decision making is accepted, true teamwork cannot exist.

MEMBERS OF THE CARE TEAM

There are three general types of members of the direct-care team in which the nurse is working:

1. Recipients of service and other members or representatives of consumer groups who may have prescribed or elective responsibilities for certain aspects of the program. For the community health nurse, the family is, of course, the most frequent example of this type of membership. In addition there may be citizens' committees or volunteer workers who are officially appointed or who serve as informal advisors or helpers.

2. Personnel employed by the agency who are responsible for implementation of agency goals and programs. In a school health program, for example, the sanitarian deals with matters relating to hygiene of the school environment, safety, and accident prevention; in a health department, the nutritionist and the social worker have certain responsibilities in the care of the geriatric patient and his family.

3. Professional or other representatives not within the agency but integrally related to its purpose: the family physician who is responsible for the medical supervision of the family receiving nursing care at home; the physician, hospital nurse, or medical social worker involved in the post-hospital care of patients who are also under the care of the community health nurse; the representative of a parent-teacher association who is helping to plan for an educational accident-prevention program in the school.

The focal place of the *family* in decisions about and rendering of care has already been emphasized. In the development of a care team, the nurse may look beyond the nuclear family for sources of help — an uncle or a grandmother can provide various forms of support and care, and older siblings are a resource often overlooked. Neighbors or fellow church members can serve in a variety of ways.

Nursing staff (members of the agency or another agency) may also be team members. They might include other staff with special knowledge or preparation — a nurse specialist consultant in cancer nursing or in public health, a nurse practitioner in pediatrics, a supervisor with special interest in evaluation. Licensed practical nurses or nurses' aides can often take considerable responsibility for direct care, and may serve as the primary link between family and agency in some situations. Registered and practical nurses from other agencies may also be included: the nurse in school or industry may extend and strengthen the services available or, more importantly, may deepen the understanding of the problems of the client.

Frequent Coworkers

The family physician, sometimes a Board-certified specialist in family medicine and sometimes a generalist in practice, is in many instances responsible for the medical management of patients receiving nursing care from a community agency, forming the basis for a three-member team of physician, nurse, and family care provider. In this instance, the nurse will plan with the physician for the care of his patients and work within the framework of his orders for therapy; at the same time, she must be mindful of the guidelines of agency policy with regard to her own responsibilities.

For example, a patient may need injections of a drug, which is not suitable for administration by the patient or by a family member but which the physician feels could be safely administered by the community nurse from a Visiting Nurse Association. The nurse would provide such treatment only upon specific written orders of the physician. The Visiting Nurse Association may have a policy regarding administration of drugs by its staff, or it may require that a special medical committee of the agency review and advise the staff regarding the safety of administering this particular drug in the home. Thus, both the doctor's prescription and the agency's policy determine exactly what will be done.

The *physician's assistant* is a relative newcomer to the health care profession. Working with doctors, ambulatory and hospital services, and some public health agencies, they serve to extend the physician's capabilities. Most have had substantial training in a medical school or other organized educational unit. They relieve the physician in many ways — such as attending to minor injuries, conducting tests, or explaining routine procedures to the patient. The functions of nurses and physician's assistants overlap quite frequently in hospitals and clinics, less so in the area of public health.

The *public health physician* fills many roles. He may serve as an administrator, directing the total or partial health program of an agency; as a provider of preventive or curative services in schools, industry, or clinics; or as an epidemiologist investigating conditions related to the occurrence of disease or accident. He may serve also as a consultant to other professional workers in the agency or in the community; a psychiatrist, for example, may advise general practitioners, nurses, or comprehensive clinic personnel on matters relating to mental health. The public health physician usually has special training in both public health and preventive medicine.

In public health work, *sanitarians* or *sanitary inspectors* form a group that is second in size only to that of nurses. The sanitarian works closely with individuals and communities to promote and protect public health by controlling environmental hazards. He investigates domestic waste, sewerage systems, and sanitary conditions in private dwellings and locations such as mobile home parks, restaurants, motels, nursing homes, and, sometimes, schools. He interprets and enforces sanitary regulations, serves as a public health educator in matters relating to his field, and supports and promotes many programs in public health. The public health sanitarian is a professional with preparation in biologic and sanitary sciences and in public health. The sanitary inspector often has less formal education.

The *social worker* has long been recognized as an important contributor to health care, and in recent years the number of social workers employed in community health agencies has increased markedly. The boundaries between social work and nursing in the community setting are not always easily defined; it is usually possible, however, for social worker and nurse to delineate those areas which are most readily handled by the one or the other. In addition to sharing in direct care, the social worker may serve as consultant to the community health nurse in those areas in which the social worker is particularly expert, or she may help in determining the need for social services for specific families.

As problems concerning environmental conditions require more and more awareness on the part of the family and the community, the *health educator* has become an increasingly important member of the health-care team. The health educator is usually trained in behavioral sciences and education as well as in public health. He helps the community mobilize for health action by motivating families and groups and organizing instruction. In some countries, short-trained health educators who have had six or nine months of preparation may be used to deal with limited areas of health education. As with the social worker, the boundaries between the work of the health educator and the nurse in direct service to families and groups are seldom clearly drawn. The distinction lies in the degree of expertise required in a given situation rather than on the delineation of different areas of action or responsibility.

The *public health nutritionist* contributes to the appraisal of the nutritional problems of a family or community and to dietary management of those problems. She may provide direct services to individuals or groups, or she may serve primarily as an advisor to other staff members. The community health nurse will have frequent need for such assistance.

The *physical therapist, occupational therapist,* and *speech therapist* also generally serve in a dual capacity, providing services to families and groups and advising others on the staff. In the care of the long-term patient and his family, the physcial therapist assumes an especially important place. In some instances, the physical therapist may be the leader of the team, with the nurse providing only supportive assistance.

Other frequently encountered members of the health team include the lay administrator, the public health engineer, the public health dentist (who is usually a specialist in preventive dentistry), and the psychologist or behavioral scientist.

WHAT MAKES IT WORK?

The team approach to care is not always successful. Team work must be learned and earned — it doesn't automatically happen if one's heart is pure! The following are some factors which have been identified with successful team operation.

1. The members must respect and trust one another. Group meetings and activities cannot be used for damning past failures or as a battleground for protecting the turf of one professional group or another. It is particularly important not to belittle the contribution of nonprofessionals who may need assistance in making their points clear.

2. Goals must be explicit and believable and must be stated in such a way that their intent is clear to all. (It may be necessary to encourage less aggressive members of the team to express their feelings and expectations. The team should agree that the goals are indeed achievable. (The problem-oriented interdisciplinary record may be helpful here; see Chapter 6.)

The sharing of goals is not likely to be achieved by chance, and sometimes the establishment of goals within the team is undertaken in rather formal terms. In an agency which has accepted a "goal-oriented" management or in community groups that have a similar approach, great stress is apt to be laid on goal setting at all levels of care. On the other hand, in dealing with a busy family physician or an anxious community representative, goal sharing may be approached informally by agreement on a joint course of action that implies, rather than defines, a particular goal.

3. There should be clear allocation of responsibility for the action agreed upon: Everyone should be clear as to who does what in a specified situation.

4. Adaptive role interchange should be possible if indicated. While allocations of care will vary from case to case and from agency to agency, allocation decisions need not be hard and fast but should allow for role adaptation and planned coverage. For example, maternity patients and their families registered for care in a specific hospital may reserve "x" type of support from the community nurse. Those registered in different hospitals or planning for home delivery may reserve "y," depending on the pattern of care in the individual hospital or medical group. This

saves planning time while assuring an adaptive scheme for use of team members. A social worker may agree to undertake (during a home visit to a family, which is also under nursing care) checking up on the immunization status of the family, thus saving the nurse a visit. Similarly, the nurse may volunteer to give support to the efforts of a school counselor working with a youngster who is experimenting with marijuana. Such interchanges strengthen the effort, and may save professional time.

5. Team planning efforts must be economical of time and of costs. It might be possible for interdisciplinary team efforts to absorb so much time that they interfere with actual care activities. Through telephone reporting and exchanging information through standard forms or informal notes, it is possible to clearly differentiate between situations that demand discussion and decision and those that fall into already-developed patterns of care.

Barriers to Communication

Open and comfortable communication permits the kind of sharing of ideas and opinions that makes for productive joint effort. Communication is a skill integral to all of the helping professions, but these skills are all too often applied in a much more consistent and thoughtful way in relationships with clients than in relationships with coworkers. It is important to recognize and overcome the barriers to communications as they arise within the team.

Perhaps no barrier is more important or more pervasive than the limitation of time. It takes time not only to find out what another worker has already done with a family, but also to keep others informed in turn. One must be convinced that this time is well spent.

Interprofessional barriers may also interfere. For instance, the nurse (or the physician) may consider the physician to be the final authority on all health matters, which may be interpreted to mean that he makes all of the decisions regarding care. This perception might lead the nurse to withhold her own contributions in favor of ascertaining the physician's wishes, or it might cause the physician to believe that it is not important for others to understand why he wants to establish a particular course of action. This could be called the "single source of decision fallacy." Another fallacy is the attitude that no member of a professional group should "interfere" with the work of other professions. Thus, a social worker might feel that it is not her prerogative to suggest that a family, whose care is primarily the responsibility of the community health nurse, could benefit from being pushed toward more self-help in the nursing phases of care. Such interprofessional barriers must be diminished.

Barriers may be created by the very mechanisms that have been developed to facilitate the interchange of information. The impersonal form; the required, but unnecessary, approval for referral; the use of formal abstracts as a substitute for the telephone call or a personal visit; the substitution of written procedures for face-to-face joint decisions about care — all of these may seriously impede intra-group communication.

Some community health nurses develop their own means of informal communication. The nurse may make it a habit, for instance, to drop in at physicians' offices occasionally to say hello and to ask whether there is any patient-care problem with which she might help. In the course of this friendly visit, the nurse can acquaint herself with the physician's feeling about prenatal care or the handling of adolescent behavior problems. The nurse would probably not obtain this information if her contact with the physician were limited to strictly formal reporting channels. Informal communication devices may be equally effective in relationships with nurses in doctors' offices or in other agencies, with the social case worker, or with the counseling staff in the school.

A TEAM IS MADE, NOT BORN

The importance of the team concept to the amount and quality of health care cannot be overestimated. Not only does it bring rationality to a chaotic care system and a better use of available resources for care, but also it can have many desirable side effects. An effective care team provides an informal interdisciplinary group of consultants who can be called upon for information and assistance in areas of major or minimal concern. For consumer members, it may increase confidence in the desire and the capability of the community to deal with its human problems as well as experience in decision making in the health field.

Special knowledge, commitment, and good will are essential elements, but they are not enough. A group of health workers does not become a care team by good intentions alone. Jacobson describes eight developmental phases in one situation, and the ways in which the need for control, security, and expression influence group cohesion and action.[2]

Not all members will have the same concept of a team. Some members, used to taking quick and independent action, may grow impatient at the "waste of time" required to gain a broader understanding of the action that is indicated. Group organizers may find the process of building a team too frustrating or upsetting. "Bossy" members are unlikely to change quickly, and may be capable of only grudging admission of the validity of the ideas of others.

But, to quote an old country expression, "The juice is worth the squeeze."

REFERENCES

1. Bergman, R. Typology for team work Am. J. Nurs., 74:1618, 1974.
2. Jacobson, S. R.: A study of inter-professional collaboration. Nurs. Outlook, 22:751, 1974.

SUGGESTED READINGS

American Public Health Association: Educational qualifications of social workers in public health programs. Am J. Publ. Health, 52:317, 1962.
Arnstein, S. R.: Eight rungs on the ladder of citizen participation. In Cahn, E. S., and Cahore, J. C. (eds.): Citizen Participation: A Casebook in Democracy Trenton, N. J., Community Action Training Institute, 1970.
Bartlet, H. M.: Social Work Practice in the Health Field New York, National Association of Social Workers, 1961, Chapter 2.
Bartlet, H. M.: The Common Base of Social Work Practice. National Association of Social Workers, 1970.
Bates, B.: Doctor and nurse: changing roles and relations. New Engl. J. Med. 283:129, 1970.
Bates, J. E. Lieberman, H. H., and Powell R.: Provisions for health care in the ghetto: The family health team. Am. J. Pub. Health, 60:1222, 1970.
Bellin, L., Kovaler, R., and Schwartz, A.: Phase one of consumer participation in policies of 22 volunteer hospitals in N.Y.C. Am. J. Pub. Health, 62:137, 1972.
Bellin, L. E., Killeen, M., and Mazuka, J. J.: Preparing public health subprofessionals recruited from the poverty group: Lessons learned from an O.E.O. work study program. Am. J. Publ. Health, 57:242, 1967.
Bergman, R.: Education of paramedical personnel. Int. Nurs. Rev., 16:161, 1969.
Bergman, R.: Typology for team work. Am. J. Nurs., 74:1618, 1974.
Bliss, A. A., and Cohen, E. D. (eds.): The New Health Professionals: Nurse Practitioners and Physicians Assistants. Germantown, MD, Aspen Systems Corp, 1977.
Christensen, K., and Lingle, J. A.: Evaluation of effectiveness of team and non-team public health nurses in health outcomes of patients with strokes or fractures. Am. J. Pub. Health, 62:483, 1972.
Collins, A. H.: The Human Services: An Introduction Odyssey Press, distributed by Bobbs-Merrill Co., Inc., 1973.
Corwin, R.: Some new dimensions of social work in a health setting Am. J. Pub. Health, 60:860, 1970.
Cunningham, R.: Team nursing in a generalized public health nursing program (that does not inlcude bedside care) Can. J. Pub. Health, 62:242, 1971.
Dammann, G. L. A.: Interprofessional aspects of nursing and social work curricula. Nurs. Res., 21:160, 1972.
Derryberry, M.: Health aides. Introduction to a series of papers by authors who have worked with paraprofessionals. Pub. Health Rep., 85:753, 1970.
Dorozynski, A.: Doctors and Healers. Ottawa, International Development Research Center, 1975.
Golden, A., Carlson, D. G., and Harris, B.: Non-physician family health teams for HMO's Am. J. Publ. Health, 63:732, 1973.
George, M., Kazuyoshi, I., and Vambery, C.: The comprehensive health team: A conceptual model. J. Nurs. Admin., 1:9, 1971.
Grass, C. and Umansky, R.: Problems in promoting the growth of multidisciplinary diagnostic and counseling clinics for mentally retarded children in non-metropolitan areas. Am. J. Pub. Health, 61:710, 1970.
Heath, A. M.: Health aides in health departments. Pub. Health. Rep., 82:608, 1967.
Hoff, W.: Role of the community health aide in public health programs. Pub. Health Rep., 84:998, 1969.
Horwitz, J. J.: Team Practice and the Specialist Springfield, Ill., Charles C Thomas, 1970.
Ingles, T.: A new health worker. Am. J. Nurs., 68:1056, 1968.
Jacobson, S. R.: A study of interprofessional collaboration, Nurs. Outlook, 22:751, 1974.

Kane, R. A.: Competency for collaboration. *In* Reinhardt, A., and Quinn, M.: *Current Practice in Family-Centered Community Nursing.* St. Louis, Mo., C. V. Mosby Co., 1977, pp. 318–333.

Lambertson, E. E.: *Team Organization and Functioning.* Toronto, T. C. Publishers, 1969.

Lenzer, A.: New health careers for the poor. Am. J. Publ. Health, *60*:45, 1970.

Levin, L. S., Katz, A. H., and Holst, E. (eds.): *Self-Care: Changing Roles of the Individual in Health Service.* New York, Neale Watson Academic Publications, Inc., 1975.

Lippard, V., and Purcell, E. F.: *Intermediate Level Health Practitioners.* New York, Josiah Macy Foundation, 1973.

McNerney, H. B.: Interdisciplinary collaboration of health care workers. *In* Reinhardt, A., and Quinn, M.: *Current Practice in Family-Centered Community Nursing.* St. Louis, Mo., C. V. Mosby, Co., 1977, pp. 331–340.

McTernan, E. S., and Hawkins, R. O.: *Educating Personnel for the Allied Health Professions and Services: Administrative Considerations.* St. Louis, Mo., C. V. Mosby, Co., 1972.

Moodie, A. S., and Rogers, G.: Baltimore uses inner-city aides in a tuberculosis control program. Pub. Health Rep., *85*:955, 1970.

Morrill, R.: A new mental health services model for the comprehensive neighborhood health center. Am. J. Pub. Health, *42*:1108, 1972.

Mullaney, J. W., Fox, R. A., and Liston, M. F.: Clinical nurse specialist and social worker: Clarifying the roles. Nurs. Outlook, *22(11)*:712, 1974.

Randar, M. A. T.: Expanding the role of the social worker in the health field, Am. J. Pub. Health, *62*:1102, 1972.

Richan, W. C., and Mendelsohn, A. R.: *Social Work — The Unloved Profession.* New Viewpoints, a Division of Franklin Watts, 1973.

Richter, R. W., Beneen, B., Alsup, P., et al.: The community health worker: A resource for improved health care delivery. Am. J. Pub. Health, *64*:1056, 1974.

Roberts, P. R.: The etiology of a new careers program in public health. Am. J. Publ. Health, *63*:635, 1973.

Rogers, M. E.: Nursing is coming of age through the practitioner movement. Am. J. Nurs., *75*:1834, 1975.

Rubin, I. M., and Beckhard, R.: Factors influencing the effectiveness of health teams. *In* Zola, I., and McKinlay, J. B. (eds.): *Organizational Issues in the Delivery of Health Services.* New York, Prodist, 1974.

Rubin, I., Fry, R., and Plovnick, M.: *Improving the Coordination of Care.* Philadelphia, Ballinger Publishing Co., 1975.

Sehnert, K. W.: *How to Be Your Own Doctor — Some of the Time.* New York, Grosset & Dunlap, 1975.

Sheps, C. G.: The influence of consumer sponsorship on medical services. *In* Zola, I., and McKinlay, J. B. (eds.): *Organizational Issues in the Delivery of Health Services.* New York, Prodist, 1974.

Sobey, F.: *The Nonprofessional Revolution in Mental Health.* New York, Columbia University Press, 1970.

Souielle D. A.: Implementation, the delivery of dental services by auxiliaries: the Philadelphia experience. Am. J. Pub. Health, *62*:1077, 1972.

Theis, G.: A change from team nursing. Nurs. Outlook, *22*:258, 1974.

Williams, M. A.: The myths and assumptions about team nursing. Nurs. Forum, *3*:61, 1964.

Wilson, P., and Fabric, D. T.: Teaching community health workers. Nurs. Outlook, *19*:337, 1971.

Wise, H. B., et. al: Family health worker. Am. J. Pub. Health, *58*:1828, 1968.

Yodfat, Y.: A new method of teamwork in family medicine in Israel. Am. J. Pub. Health, *62*:953, 1972.

CHAPTER 12

FAMILY HEALTH NURSING CARE: THE YOUNG FAMILY

FAMILIES ARE THE TRADITIONAL FOCUS OF COMMUNITY NURSING

The nursing of families has been traditionally the major focus of public health and community nursing. It serves not only as a means of providing and extending medical support for the sick, but also as a strong force in developing attitudes, knowledge, and skills that are conducive to voluntary, self-disciplined action by families on behalf of their own health.

Family health nursing comprises a broad program of therapeutic, educational, and supportive services afforded to families by a single nurse or by a nursing team, provided within the multidiscipline framework of the health care system as a whole. It is characterized by a partnership between nurse and family based upon the sharing of decisions and actions. It is characterized also by equal concern for wellness as for illness or impairment, and for the development as well as for the nurturance of the family. Thus family health nursing provided to a family including a very elderly member would be concerned as much with the quality of life for the entire family as with the survival of the individual patient. In general, family nursing services (as contrasted to acute care) extend over a substantial period of time.

While these concepts of family health nursing are widely accepted, in practice the services fall far short of their goals. Health care does not always reach those who need it, and comprehensive services are not always provided. Nursing care may be available to women and infants, but may not be available to children during the crucial pre-school period. Medicaid or Medicare patients may receive care, while middle-aged well populations receive only cursory attention. Families themselves may exhibit little enthusiasm for preventive care of any sort.

However, the interest of community health nurses in comprehensive family health care is being fostered and extended. There are more short courses available, and opportunities for postgraduate preparation in family health nursing or for on-the-job training have increased. Even more important is the "quiet revolution" in nursing — the continuing expansion of concern and capability of all nurses, which enriches family health nursing as well as all other branches of the profession.

Chapters 12, 13, and 14 are concerned with the application of community health nursing to various phases of family growth and development. We discuss the health care needs of the young family (especially in relation to the needs of children) in this chapter, those of families in the middle years in Chapter 13, and those of aging families in Chapter 14.

THE GOALS OF COMMUNITY HEALTH NURSING FOR THE YOUNG FAMILY

Of all groups served by the community health nurse, the young family affords the most opportunity for her to promote and improve health. Young people are responsive — indeed, committed — to change. Young adulthood is a period of taking on new responsibilities, re-examining values, and changing life styles. Young families are under a barrage of statements by many groups that hope to mold their ideas and behavior — i.e., governmental, religious, and special interest organizations; manufacturers and their advertising representatives; and health professionals, with their own agendas and values. Families must develop good judgment to make the health decisions required of them. The young family may be seen as a "good market" for community health nursing care — with an emphasis on teaching, counseling, and early detection of potential problems and risk factors for disease.

The overall goals of community health nursing care for young families will intersect with those of other agencies or professions. These goals provide a necessary framework, within which more specific goals and courses of action may be developed.

Working in concert with the family and with other care givers, the community health nurse addresses herself to the goals that follow.

1. To foster and strengthen the family as the major instrument for family health care.
2. To prevent or minimize effects of adverse health conditions common to the age groups involved.
3. To ensure a safe and satisfying reproductive experience.
4. To provide each child with an environment conducive to safety and growth, with adequate and knowing parenting and child rearing practices.
5. To stimulate and support community response capability on behalf of young families.

Health Problems of Young Families: The Merging Couple

The health problems of young families are rooted in age-related vulnerability; in physical and psychosocial environmental forces in the home, workplace, and community; and in the special demands and stresses associated with marriage or other long-term commitment — and, for those who elect parenthood, the pressures of childbearing and rearing.

The Young Couple: Causes of Death and Disability

On the whole, young adults are a healthy group in terms of death and disability. In 1973 when the overall death rate was 942.2 per 100,000 of the general population, the rate for those aged 15 to 24 was 128.3 and for those aged 25 to 44 years, 216.8. The principal causes of death among 15- to 24-year olds were accidents, homicide, suicide, and cancer and for 25- to 44-year olds, cancer, heart disease, and homicide.[1]

Disability, too, is lower than in older age groups. In a 1973 survey, men aged 17 to 44 years reported 11.4 days of restricted activity per year, 3.8 bed disability days, and 5.8 work days lost. In the same time period, 151.8 acute conditions were reported per 100 men, and 186.3 per 100 women.[2] Respiratory conditions were by far the most frequent cause of disability. Injuries accounted for 43 episodes of illness for each 100 men, and for 25.3 episodes among women. Studies of chronic illness in this age group indicate that the most common conditions were hearing impairments, vision impairments, asthma, heart disease, and chronic bronchitis. Minor ills, not in themselves life-threatening or disabling, may have strong adverse effects if they occur frequently or are left untreated.

Sexually transmitted disease — especially syphilis and gonorrhea — are relatively common in this age group at all social levels. Misuse of drugs — especially marijuana and alcohol — is also very common among young couples. The drug habit, started in the early part of the family-building period, may not become a serious problem for some time, but then suddenly may grow out of control.

Disregard of health needs is common among young adults, especially among the strivers or overachievers whose primary interest is "getting ahead." For many couples, the high cost of housing today requires that both husband and wife work if they are to have a home of their own. The sandwich lunch at the desk; the work taken home at night; the moonlighting job; the long commute, which provides the family with living style and space but may deprive them of time together as a family; the frustration and fatigue of the career wife; or, even more often, the working wife whose salary is necessary to make ends meet are all common precursors to excessive stress that may lead to emotional and/or physical illness.

The young adult is faced with a society that expects and rewards risk taking in his or her age group. "Getting ahead" is often associated with trying out new and experimental ways of doing things, moving to a new community or new field of work as opportunities change, and disrupting the established system. At the same time, the health professions are urging young adults *not* to take chances with their health, to "play it safe" by defensive driving, to follow a prudent diet, and to maintain a proper work/rest/recreation balance.

Developmental Stress: A Predictable Concern

Recent research has identified predictable points of stress in adult life, each demanding to be resolved before the adult can move on to new pursuits.[3] The pattern and timing of these crises may vary between men and women and among different social settings, but the essential adaptive demands are constant. Thus, young couples face common problems: breaking away from their families, setting their own patterns of independence without losing a sense of belonging, channeling the tremendous energy and optimism of youth while searching for values in life (even when the striving seems unrewarding), moving when the time comes to acknowledge limitations that are inescapable, and moving to less competitive and more serene patterns. This struggle is a necessary and major task of young people.

Virtually every young couple experiences some stress in the early years of marriage. Balancing one's own need for privacy and the compelling urge to merge with the partner, dealing with changes in employment and uncertainties when relocation is required may erode confidence and savings. The wider options of modern marriage — i.e., the challenge of the liberated woman, the relative ease of dissolving marriage, and career conflicts when both work — take a lot of adjustment. An increasing number of young people are electing to have a period of cohabitation preceding marriage (shades of the "trial marriage" of the 1930's) — not in defiance of propriety but as a means of evaluating the strength of a mutual attraction.

Young persons need to be alert to the common threats to health and be able to deal with them. For example, young populations should be able to recognize and deal with sexually transmitted disease; to be alert to evidence of depression or suicidal behavior, and to be aware of the usual causes of accidents and know how to prevent them. The young person needs to learn how to deal with common ills and injuries, to be able to evaluate symptoms of illness, and to know where and how to obtain help if necessary.

Young adults also need to know and accept the validity of prudent health practices — such as balanced nutrition, limited drinking and smoking, and rational exercise — and learn how to incorporate these into daily living. Young people in a family need to understand their own and each other's developmental needs and those of other members and must learn how to give each other support. Above all, they need to develop, first, the ability to communicate with one another freely and openly and, second, the habit of facing problems together.

As the young family matures, the scope of concern should broaden to include the community. The family is the base for community development, health action, and supportive habits. Family members who can meet their own needs may reach out to the neighborhood, the work place, or the school — and, thus, support community development.

TYPICAL COMMUNITY HEALTH NURSING INTERVENTIONS

The type of nursing intervention with this age group will differ widely from one situation to another and will frequently be opportunistic. Because increased health care coverage is normally part of a job-benefits package, most employed adults have the opportunity for continuing medical surveillance. These services, though labeled "comprehensive" or "health maintenance," are episodic. They focus on the individual rather than the family, are short on self-help approaches, and largely ignore the effect and potential of the community to care for its own. Most nursing services are not equipped or designed to provide comprehensive family and community based care. The community health nurse will need to adapt case loads and time allocations to the realities of the situation, coming as close as possible to comprehensive care for those families most in need of these services.

Some typical approaches to reaching the young family may be identified.

1. In the "piggy-back" approach, encounters for any problem are used as a channel for positive health counseling. For example, the industrial worker who makes frequent visits to the health office for minor ills may really want to talk about depression; the worker's accident that required a visit to the health office might reflect the effect of marital discord rather than a dangerous environment. Preventive content may be "tacked on" to periodic medical check-ups; and family health content added to the nursing visit for a minor injury. Thus, every nurse-client encounter may become a potential for family health education.

2. The nurse can organize, plan, and/or participate in adult screening or diagnostic procedures. For example, a health department screen-

ing for hypertension may be used by the visiting nurse to discuss stress or health-threatening life styles.

3. Referral to some health services may be extended. For example, an asthma patient may be referred for evaluation of the environment and assistance with medication, but the alert nurse will also be receptive to problems of poor husband-wife communication or sexual incompatibility.

4. Through epidemiologic analysis of her own case load or clinic records, the community health nurse may document specific problems, identifying high-risk groups as a basis for program planning.

5. Family visits or encounters may provide an opportunity to estimate the general level of family coping — i.e., how the family manages money, sexuality, unemployment, relationships with in-laws or members outside the immediate family, and division of family work.

6. Provide support to individuals who have problems with illness or family relationships — directly, if within the scope of the nurse's capability, or by referral to marriage counseling service or other resources.

7. Find and use professional or lay supportive services — such as churches, clinics, library or educational agency group work in adult education programs, family physicians with an interest in and flair for helping families, and self help groups (such as Alcoholics Anonymous, ostomy society group sessions).

8. Encourage couples to discuss their feelings about children and their plans for a family before pregnancy occurs. Most young people need to examine their feelings and motivations in deciding to marry or to have children, to think through the changes such action entails and to study the specific actions they are expected to take. Schools, churches, or welfare groups may offer courses or counseling to young people contemplating (or suddenly faced with) childbearing and child rearing. Examination of the reasons for wanting a child (A lovely animated doll? An extension of one's self? An object to love? Something to provide the love a family did not provide?) may help to evaluate their readiness for this experience. If a young couple decides to not have children or to postpone childbearing, they may need nursing support in interpreting this decision to family and friends.

9. The community health nurse may participate in controlling sexually transmitted disease (see Chapter 18); identifying sexually active young people; and mobilizing all possible sources to inform them regarding how to minimize risk, sources and nature of treatment, and regulations regarding requirements to notify parents.

The "**young couple**" period is a magical time in itself; it is also an effective period for developing good health behavior and minimizing risk of preventable disease. The ingenuity of the community health nurse may help create a network of support, information, and care that can maximize the impact of this period on future health of this important segment of the population.

THE CHILDBEARING EXPERIENCE

The bearing of children is one of the most basic of human experiences, and the obligation of society to assure safe passage of child and parents through this experience is accepted through the world. The community health nurse can play an important role in implementing this commitment.

The Problem

For most adults in the United States, the reproductive experience is safe and satisfying. In 1975, maternal deaths associated with childbearing had dropped to 2 per 10,000 live births from 8 per 10,000 live births in 1950.[4] Infant mortality (deaths of children under 1 year) has also decreased — from 24.7 per 1,000 live births in 1945 to 14.0 per 1,000 live births in 1977.[5] However, this progress cannot be viewed with complacency when compared with other "developed" countries. The figure for infant deaths in Sweden, for example, was 8.0 per 1,000 live births in 1977 and, in Japan, 9.3 per 1,000 live births.[6] Within the United States, there are wide differences in maternal and infant mortality associated with various socioeconomic groups, and a substantial increase in risk exists for non-white populations and for those living in poverty.

By far the greatest threat to the infant occurs during the prenatal and perinatal period. Almost 75 per cent of infant deaths occur during the first month of life, and about 44 per cent occur in the first day of life. The major causes of early death are respiratory distress, immaturity, complications of labor, and congenital anomalies.

While much is still unknown about the causes of these conditions, there is an increasing amount of data on which to predict problems and base a preventive program. Predictive factors associated with greater risks of difficulty during the pre- and postpartum period include maternal age, marital status, race, adequacy of prenatal care, social class, disease or malnutrition during pregnancy, and prior history of obstetrical problems and maternal stress.[7] For example, the very young mother, below age 20, is more likely to deliver prematurely, while women over age 40 have an increased probability of fetal anomalies. Reduced infant death rate seems to be related to early and periodic assessment throughout pregnancy.[8]

Essential to the control of complications is the availability of high-quality preconceptional, prenatal, intranatal and postnatal care, especially for those at special risk. Achievement of high-level preventive care and comprehensive care to women during the childbearing years will involve the cooperation and coordination of health care in schools, religious institutions, hospitals, health centers, occupational health services and community action groups. The community health nurse should be a key partner in this effort.

High-Risk Families

Health care of the growing family must be viewed as more than maternal and infant care. The health challenge implicit in childbearing and child rearing affects every member of the family as well as the community at large. The addition of a child to the family may create problems of emotional security for the siblings, economic concern for the father, and physical and management problems for the mother. The additive effect of family size may create serious economic developmental problems for a community or for a country.

High-risk families include:

1. Families more vulnerable due to socioeconomic risks
   a. Low-income groups and those living in poverty
   b. Immature families
   c. Incomplete families
   d. Families with an adverse genetic history
   e. Families with a history of emotional stress and inability to cope
   f. Families in which the baby is unwanted or in which the pregnancy has been undertaken for secondary reasons.
2. Families more vulnerable due to special obstetrical risk of the mother.
   a. Women under 16 or over 40 years of age
   b. Women having nutritional problems and poor nutritional habits, particularly women who have anemia, or are substantially underweight or overweight
   c. Women with pre-existing disease such as hypertension, cardiac or metabolic disorders, infectious disease or gynecologic abnormalities
   d. Women with a previous history of obstetrical complications
   e. Women who are heavy smokers or alcohol/drug abusers
3. Families more vulnerable due to special risk of the infant
   a. Infants with low birth weight (under 2500 gm) and infants with high birth weight (over 4000 gm)
   b. Infants with a low Apgar score or those whose mothers have undergone prolonged or difficult labor
   c. Infants with congenital malformations or birth injury
   d. Infants whose parents are immature or inadequate with a history of addiction to drugs or alcohol, a history of child neglect, or a history of mental illness.

Early Identification is Important

The health of the infant is very much affected by the conditions found during the intra-uterine period of his life, and these in turn are dependent upon the nutrition and general health of the mother. Furthermore, both the growth and development of the child after birth are dependent in large measure upon the quality of nurturing the family is able to provide. Many investigators have been concerned with the study of parent-infant bonding and the role it plays in child development.[9] Bonding is influenced by early close contact between infants and parents at birth, the parents' experience during the pregnancy, and the quality of mothering or fathering the parents themselves experienced. Parents must derive satisfaction from their family roles and be able to meet their parental obligations. If the mother is grossly malnourished, whatever the reason, or if her ability to mother (or the father's ability to assume the fatherhood role) is endangered by emotional or social inadequacies or stress within the family, both the parents and the child will be jeopardized. Stresses within the family can result in abuse of the children and abusive behavior between the spouses (see Chapter 21).

Multiple Approaches are Required

The early identification of high-risk pregnant groups is not always a simple problem, inasmuch as the family itself must most often take the initiative in reporting early pregnancy and in seeking help.

It would be desirable to identify high-risk groups in the prepregnancy period in order to encourage early and comprehensive use of the services available. When the incidence of multiple adverse conditions is known to be high, it may be best to consider whole populations in certain low-income areas as operating at special risk.

The importance of a careful and probing nursing history in identifying undisclosed or covert risk factors cannot be overemphasized. The informal setting of the home visit and the one-to-one and usually close nurse-family relationship, combined with the opportunity for observation of the family in its own setting, give the community health nurse an unusual advantage in seeking out these important data.

Records of high-risk mothers should be clearly identified, both during the period they are in the active case load and after they are put in the closed or inactive file; a notation in red ink in an obvious place on the record, a tab, a special sticker, or any other device that will make the record stand out from the others will serve. In this way the family does not get "lost" in the file or fail to be identified as a high-risk family immediately upon readmission to service.

Prepregnant groups may be reached through health and education programs in schools, community action centers, or other community health educational activities. Some nurses have used the "every one teach one" approach, asking pregnant mothers who are receiving care to help locate others who should receive care and to talk with prepregnant friends. In some settings, indigenous short-trained paid or volunteer workers may be used to inform people of the urgency of early care and to explain the availability of health services to the community.

The Mother and Family Need Intensified Care

For the most part, high-risk mothers need just what other mothers need, but more acutely. In only a few instances will there be special medications, diets, or treatments that create unusual care patterns. The intensity of the care required is the main difference in caring for high-risk mothers.

More frequent nurse-family visits are usually needed to provide for intensive monitoring of the mother's condition and to assure concentrated and inclusive teaching, support, and referral. The crucial need for mustering the support and assistance of the patient's husband, mother, or "important others" may require special efforts on the part of the nurse. Furthermore, increased risk in childbearing is frequently accompanied by other adverse conditions in the family as a whole, including a low level of family functioning. These related problems must be equally the responsibility of the community health nurse. For these reasons, families designated "high-risk" may require from a third to a half more nursing time than that needed for a family from a low-risk population.

The identification of high-risk groups is an area of community nursing care peculiarly dependent upon the efforts of those in the community for the effective administration of the nursing program. Thus, the nurse must plan for the education of volunteer or paid aides; for general educational efforts in school, industry, and other ready-made groups; and for constant liaison with health, welfare, and social organizations that are likely to be in contact with those who should know about the need for and availability of care services. This is one nursing task that "can't be done by one"!

NURSING SUPERVISION DURING THE MATERNITY CYCLE: MONITORING

Community health nursing operates in two ways to maintain or improve health during the maternity cycle:
1. *Monitoring:* continually evaluating the condition or environment of the patient and her family for evidence of need for special care; and
2. *Anticipatory Guidance:* preparing the family to deal with the physical, emotional, and social changes incident to childbearing.

Monitoring is Shared with the Entire Care Group

Monitoring is a task shared with the physician, other nurses, nurse-midwives, and the family. Early and continuing medical supervision is an essential element in prenatal care and has been shown to be associated with favorable obstetric outcomes. The physician's observations and evaluations are supplemented by the observations of others, particularly the nurse and the family. Unless these additional observations can be communicated, the physician may miss many important clues, either because time with the patient is so limited or because the patient may not be able to recognize her problems and verbalize her concerns to the physician during her visit.

The ways in which the community health nurse will share responsibility with the physician and with nurses in other settings will differ. Nurse-midwives or obstetric nurse specialists may take great responsibility in case management, as may the community health nurse working in isolated areas where there are few physicians available and where the distances to medical care are great. Some physicians will take the major responsibility for counseling the expectant mother and leave little for the community health nurse to do, other than to support his instruction and perhaps concern herself with other family members who may be affected by the pregnancy but are not being seen by the physician. When comprehensive maternal and infant projects extend into home care as well as clinic care, new patterns of coordination may be required of the community health nurse.

Most often neglected is the support of the private family physician, who often works without the social work, nutrition nursing, and other technical support the clinic physician takes for granted. The community health nurse may work directly with the private physician's patients (either individually or in groups), or she may work through the physician's office nurse or receptionist. There must be plenty of opportunity for communication among the various individuals or groups caring for a particular family in order to ensure continuing relevant and coordinated care.

Monitoring must involve the family, too. The nurse cannot expect to be present when changes occur that suggest a need for immediate care or for further study. Therefore, she must depend upon the family's ability and willingness to recognize and report symptoms or concerns that have health significance. In some instances, the expectant mother herself may take most of the responsibility; in other situations, she may seek the help of her husband, her mother, or a friend who has had childbearing experience. For example, the husband may help monitor his wife's food intake or a trusted friend may check with the patient who has missed a clinic appointment.

The Monitoring Process

The frequency of direct contact with the family and the actual content of the monitoring will vary considerably with the style of medical practice, the capability of the family, and the condition of the patient.

Provision of Early Medical Supervision

Assuring early and adequate medical supervision is the first and basic step in the monitoring process. Certain screening and diagnostic procedures for known or usual complicating conditions are essential. A usual "preventive package" of such procedures is shown in Tables 12–1 and 12–2.[10]

Recognition of Adverse Conditions in Mother or Baby

Obviously, the focal concern in the monitoring task is the early recognition of adverse conditions in the mother: finger or ankle swelling; excessive weight gain before 30 weeks' gestation, which may presage hypertension; too nonchalant an acceptance of an unplanned pregnancy, which might indicate mental distress or contemplated abortion; listlessness or apathy; or undue prolongation of prenatal nausea and vomiting. These are areas in which the physician takes the major monitorial responsibility.

Evaluation of "Normal" Discomforts

Because such discomforts as backache, nausea, vomiting, and occasional depression are so common during pregnancy, they may tend to be discounted by the patient. As a consequence, she may suffer unnecessary discomfort; or even worse, she may not realize the importance of reporting when these conditions are persistent or unusually severe. The physician, too, may tend to minimize the discomforts, especially when the patient is shy and takes a rather fatalistic attitude toward her own well-being. The nurse may need to interpret the patient's responses to the physician. She must remember that one mother will discount or disregard her symptoms, whereas another will tend to over-react. The community health nurse serves as the link between family and doctor. She can alert the family concerning things to watch out for, and she can aid the busy doctor in diagnosing and treating the patient who seeks treatment.

Attention to Other Health Threats

Exposure to rubella or other infectious diseases or to x-rays in early pregnancy, contact with a family member who has tuberculosis, or history of genetic problems are all important indices of need for more intensive medical surveillance and study.

Deleterious health practices — such as grossly inadequate diet, exercise or recreational habits that require great physical effort or interfere with sleep or unsuccessful attempts to terminate the pregnancy — represent another important area of monitoring.

Table 12-1 RECOMMENDED PREVENTION PACKAGE FOR MOTHER AND FETUS°

Procedure	Condition	Type of Prevention†	Intervention
History of menarche	Unplanned pregnancy (before pregnancy)	1	Contraception
Serological Exam	Lack of Rubella antibody (before pregnancy)	1	Immunization
Pregnancy Test	Unwanted pregnancy	2	Abortion
History of pregnancy	Unsuccessful prior pregnancy	2	Counseling
History and Counseling	Inadequate preparation for pregnancy	1	Counseling
History and Counseling	Inadequate preparation for delivery	1	Counseling
History and Counseling	Inadequate preparation for parenthood	1	Counseling
History and Counseling	Smoking and other risks to developing fetus	1, 2	Counseling
History and Counseling	Inadequate recognition of signs and symptoms of abnormalities	1	Counseling
Anthropometric Examination and Counseling	Nutritional abnormality	2	Counseling and Diet
Hemoglobin/Hematocrit	Anemia	2	Diagnosis and therapy
Urine albumen	Toxemia	2	Diagnosis and therapy
Pap smear	Genital tract malignancy	2	Diagnosis and therapy
VDRL	Syphilis	2	Diagnosis and therapy Counseling and contact finding
G. C. culture	Gonorrhea	2	Penicillin, Counseling and contact finding
Blood grouping and Rh determination	Rh iso-immunization and other blood abnormalities	1	Antibody
Casual blood sugar	Abnormal glucose tolerance	2	Diagnosis and therapy
Blood pressure measurement	Hypertension	2	Diagnosis and therapy
Examination	Organic heart disease	2	Diagnosis and therapy
Physical Exam	Pelvic inadequacy	2	Diagnosis and therapy
Physical Exam	Reproductive organ abnormality	2	Diagnosis and therapy
Urine culture	Bacteriuria (after third pregnancy)	2	Diagnosis and therapy
Amniocentesis	Genetic disorders (women over age 40)	2	Diagnosis and therapy
Blood Test	Sickle Cell trait (High risk groups only)	2	Diagnosis and therapy

°From Fogarty International Center for Advanced Study in Health Sciences, NIH, and The American College of Preventive Medicine: Preventive Medicine, New York, Prodist, 1976, pp. 296 and 297.

†1 = primary prevention; 2 = secondary prevention.

Table 12-2 RECOMMENDED PREVENTION PACKAGE FOR THE INFANT°†

Procedure	Condition	Type of Prevention‡	Intervention
History and Counseling	Inadequate preparation for infant care (newborn)	1	Parent Counseling
PKU	Metabolic disorders (newborn)	2	Diagnosis and therapy
Silver nitrate prophylaxis	Gonorrheal ophthalmia (newborn)	1	Prophylaxis
Observation and measurement	Congenital malformations (newborn)	2	Diagnosis and therapy
Vaccinations	Diphtheria, Tetanus and Pertussis	1	Immunization
TOPV	Poliomyelitis	1	Immunization
Vitamin K	Hemorrhagic disease	1	Prophylaxis
Hematocrit	Anemia	2	Diagnosis and therapy
Development assessment including height and weight	Growth and development disorders	2	Diagnosis and therapy
Counseling	Accidents	1	Parent Counseling

°Newborn plus four visits after discharge.
†From Fogarty International Center for Advanced Study in Health Sciences, NIH, and the American College of Preventive Medicine: Preventive Medicine, Prodist, 1976, pp. 296 and 297.
‡1 = primary prevention; 2 = secondary prevention.

Unusual stress — the death of a family member, marital difficulties, economic problems, or an overanxious and ubiquitous interfering mother or mother-in-law — may start a series of reactions that can be harmful to mother and baby.

Adverse effects of the situation on other family members may pose a health threat. The embarrassed adolescent whose mother is having a "menopause baby"; the somewhat resentful ambitious husband who believes the pregnancy could and should have been averted; the about-to-be-displaced sibling who has mixed feelings about "this little brother or sister"; and the parents of an unmarried mother who feel "disgraced" — all have very real problems and may need help. Failure to handle these problems effectively may lead to more serious manifestations and present a threat not only to the individual who faces them but to others in the family as well.

PREPREGNANCY AND INTERPREGNANCY CARE: ANTICIPATORY GUIDANCE

As noted previously, the term *anticipatory guidance* refers to the preparation of the family to deal with the physical, emotional, and social changes incident to childbearing.

Preparation for childbearing and parenthood begins long before a baby is born. Ideally, the expectant parents should have experienced a satisfying relationship with their own parents, achieved good physical and emotional health, benefited from family-life education during their school years, and had adequate family counseling before marriage. The couple should have received information about methods of controlling family size and taken steps to correct any reproductive disorders before marriage. When the wife becomes pregnant, the couple should ideally seek early and continuous medical supervision throughout the period of pregnancy and early infancy. The community nursing care provided throughout childhood may serve to improve maternal and infant care to a degree not now possible.

Preconceptional and interconceptional care is the trend of the future. Even though today there is little in the way of an organized program for preconceptional and interconceptional care, the community health nurse may find many ways of interjecting such care: for instance, prolonging the supervision of high-risk patients and their families beyond the usual postpartum period, or integrating material into the ongoing programs of health education provided to parent discussion groups.

Preconceptional and interconceptional care might include the following:

1. Instruction in reproductive processes
2. Training in child care
3. Orientation to family planning and family planning resources
4. Discussion of the effect of parental attitudes on child development
5. Marriage counseling services (nurse would refer applicants)
6. Study of growth and development throughout the life span
7. Effect of physical and social environment on health and development
8. The nature and importance of health maintenance
9. The nature and services of the health-care system and the problems in utilization
10. The importance of correcting "small" defects.

Obviously, this would not all be the responsibility of the community health nurse, nor is it likely that this content can be offered in formal courses to individuals or groups; but the community health nurse may work to enrich the services she offers to those presently in her case load and to reinforce the care provided by other individuals.

THE NURSE'S RESPONSIBILITY

During the months before delivery, there is an opportunity to help the mother and her family safeguard the mother's health and that of the infant *in utero*, to prepare the parents to be intelligent collaborators in the birth process to anticipate the period of physical and mental readjustment following delivery; and to plan for the responsibilities of caring for the new baby.

This "nine months to get ready" period is valuable, since it is a time when there is unusual motivation in general matters relating to family health. The nurse's help is directed toward enabling the family to:
1. Provide any special care that has been ordered by the physician
2. Learn their respective roles in the maternity health-care program
3. Develop skills required in childbearing and child rearing
4. Improve general health practices in order to assure a better maternity experience and also to provide a long-term investment in better health care.

Providing Special Care

For some mothers — those with anticipated complications or those at special risk in other ways — treatments, medications, exercises, periodic tests or measurements, or special rest may be prescribed to relieve an existing condition or to prevent later difficulties. The nurse may be responsible for carrying out certain tests — blood pressure and urine determinations, for example — in intervals between clinic visits. Sometimes the actions required of the family, such as taking iron pills or vitamins daily, are in themselves simple but are hard to maintain because they require regular and continuing attention. At other times conformity to the regimen ordered may be much more difficult, as when recommended procedures are in direct conflict with strongly held cultural taboos. Here the nurse's responsibility is to be sure that the patient and the family understand the reason for the recommended action, that they know how to carry it out, and that they are sufficiently convinced of its importance. It may take considerable effort by the nurse and her coworkers to help the family make the necessary adaptation.

It is helpful, also, to suggest simple homely aids to combat the possible discomforts of pregnancy: the dry cracker in the morning, the small frequent meals for nausea, the changes in posture to help relieve backache. The patient needs the assurance that the nurse does indeed know of these measures and is aware of their importance.

Helping Family Members Realize Roles and Skills

Because childbearing requires a considerable amount of adjustment and change, it may leave prospective parents open to anxiety and self-doubt, and lacking in adaptive mechanisms for coping with their new roles. For the most part, the problems are fleeting and respond well to what might be called "common-sense" measures.

The objective of family monitoring (that is, early recognition of conditions adverse to health of mother or child) has already been discussed. To be effective at their task, however, family members must have at their disposal the authority and the required knowledge.

Development of Confidence. First, the parents are expected to develop commitment to and confidence in their ability to handle parental tasks. Fathers as well as mothers may have serious doubts about their ability to fulfill this role. They may remember their own resentment toward inadequate parenting, and they may fear continuing the process with their own children. They may worry about the financial obligations of parenthood, or they may fear that a happy marital relationship will end with these new responsibilities. These anxieties can be heightened by the wife's adaptive mechanisms — such as her retreat to her own mother for advice and support — that seem to separate her from her husband. She may become depressed. Although usually very independent, she may suddenly take a highly dependent stance, especially if the pregnancy was unplanned or requires a sharp change in her usual mode of living (such as leaving her job). She, too, may worry about whether she can be a "good" mother. An understanding of the interrelated physical, emotional, and psychologic changes that occur with pregnancy can help the young family to deal with them effectively.

Alternatively, young parents, especially teenagers, may seem to comprehend nothing of the responsibilities they will be expected to face. The young expectant mother, looking forward to the "living doll" she will have, may not realize that this doll will require much more care than the inanimate variety. Teenage parents may not recognize the need to adapt their unsuitable living conditions to the baby's needs and may expect to be able to continue with such habits as late-night dancing and drinking parties. Siblings, too, will need help in getting ready for the new baby.

Marital Sharing. The habit of marital sharing may be developed or strengthened during the childbearing period. The wife's tendency to withhold information from the husband (the "I-don't-want-him-to-worry" or "I-don't-want-him-to-think-I'm-a-baby" attitude), the husband's possible guilt about the pregnancy, or his probable shyness about discussing it (the "it's-your-problem-so-you-handle-it" attitude) may lead to later, more serious breaks in marital communication. The community health nurse can do much to help avoid this by her own planning, scheduling some visits at a time when the father can be present, advising the mother to discuss certain aspects of care with her husband, or encouraging the wife to include little details when she writes to a husband on military duty. The couple must realize that the wife's tendency to go back to her own mother at this period may put a strain on the husband-wife relationship, and they must learn to deal wisely with the wife's need for this security.

The nurse may act directly or indirectly in dealing with these problems of support. By being available and visible to the prospective parents and by listening and appearing to be genuinely interested, she can encourage the family to express their concerns — which is, after all, the first step in dealing with problems. Sometimes leading comments by the nurse — such as "Lots of times after starting a pregnancy, mothers wonder if they did the right thing," or "I guess we all worry about things like this; it's such a big step to take!" — will start the discussion.

Enlist the Help of Others. It may be helpful to enlist others in the job of support. A wise older neighbor, the grandmother-to-be, the physician, the aide in the agency, and the school counselor are possible helpers.

Parents must understand that they will continue to be themselves in addition to being parents — that as parents they will still be permitted to "do their own thing." There are many parental styles; not every mother looks like the Whistler portrait!

Skills Practice. Skills practice can also increase parents' confidence and make it easier for them to assume their new roles. Practicing how to bathe a small baby and how to deal with simple emergencies is valuable preparation for the expectant mother and, in some instances, for the father and for others who will be involved in child care.

Young mothers may also bring their babies to a prenatal study group and demonstrate how to handle the infant while the inexperienced mother-to-be practices with the model. Mothers may join parents' classes to discuss what can be expected at the hospital and during the delivery process.

Helping Families Prepare for Labor and Delivery

The ability to be an intelligent participant in the birth process requires that the patients have an understanding of the process of labor and delivery and of the part played by the physician, drugs, and themselves in this process. "Understanding," in this context, is more than knowing about the process; the young mother who knows the physiologic facts about delivery may still have little confidence in her own ability to deal with the phenomenon of birth. She may be afraid of "making a fool" of herself, or she may have great fears about the actual process of birth. Husband and wife need to know about the conditions influencing the doctor's decision whether to intervene in the birth process or to use drugs.

In many communities, there are a variety of resources available for maternity care, including nurse-midwife services, neighborhood clinics, birthing centers, as well as private physicians and hospital delivery services. Many facilities have developed delivery services offering prospective parents choices on delivery that may include active participation of the father, natural childbirth, different levels of anesthesia, infant rooming-in facilities, and planned short stay after delivery (less than 24 hours).

A growing number of couples have wanted labor and delivery to occur in their own home, where the entire family may participate with assistance from a physician or nurse-midwife.

A few areas have developed "birthing centers," staffed by nurse-midwives with medical and hospital back-up for emergency problems, that emphasize a family-oriented approach to delivery. Young families leave the facility about 12 hours after delivery and are referred to the visiting nurse service for general postpartum supervision. Satisfaction, economy, and the "plus" of a supportive family environment during this exciting time, make the birthing center a successful alternative for healthy, normal pregnant women.[11]

Special Problems of Teenage Mothers

Births to teenagers under 16 have risen dramatically in the U.S. from 7,900 in 1950 to 48,000 in 1973. Approximately 780,000 teenage women experience a premarital pregnancy each year, accounting for about one-third of all abortions and 17 per cent of live births.[13]

The physical risks to mother and infant are high, especially for those mothers aged 15 years and younger. There are more complications during pregnancy and childbirth, more premature deliveries, and increased rates of prenatal and infant mortality for women aged 15 to 19 years. The social and economic outlook for many of these babies and their parents is also bleak.[14]

Recent studies show that exposure to possible pregnancy among teenage groups is high. For example, one study found that 35 per cent of adolescent never-married women were sexually experienced and that five in ten of this group reported sexual relations with more than one partner.[15]

In spite of more available information on contraceptives and sexual counseling, reports show that many young people are not taking advantage of available information and services, and lack substantial knowledge about basic anatomy and other factual information normally put under the heading of sex education. On the other hand, information from peers, friends, and the street (language) abound.

There are a variety of social and emotional issues that must be confronted when an adolescent becomes pregnant. This is most often a time of stress — a time when parents and children need special support. Problems that must be resolved may be identified.

1. Does the young woman ignore the problem until the last possible moment, or does she take decisive steps when options are greater? Delay in seeking care increases the risks.

2. What is the desired relationship between the young woman and her sexual partner — i.e., willing or forced marriage, a shared knowledge of the pregnancy with shared decisions, or no further contact or father unknown?

3. How does the young woman relate to her parents — i.e., will they be informed, and will they share in the responsibility and decision making?

4. What are the young woman's feelings about the pregnancy and what are realistic options from her viewpoint — i.e., delivery and keeping the baby, delivery and adoption, or interruption of the pregnancy?

There are no "good" answers to these questions. For some women, the physical and emotional stresses of abortion may be little better or even worse than the prospect of managing a fatherless home or living in an unwanted marriage.

COMMUNITY HEALTH NURSE INTERVENTIONS

The community health nurse can do much to identify early teenage pregnancies and to assure early and understanding maternity care. In a variety of settings (such as schools, social gatherings and street corners), it is possible to identify young people at risk. Often it is the nurse who can reach out to take the initiative in preventive programs and arrange for necessary services.

Once pregnancy is a fact, the community health nurse may provide or arrange for medical and social support for the young parents. A helping network may be identified, or in some cases built, to help the pregnant girl and her partner consider their alternatives as fully as possible.

Sometimes young people will want to have the pregnancy terminated without informing their parents. It is important to know the legal regulations regarding care of minors. There are a variety of organizations and advisors that may be potentially helpful here. Strangely enough, grandparents may be more matter-of-fact and constructive in their approach to these problems than a host of other helping groups.

The community health nurse, especially those with special preparation in maternal and infant care, may serve as the principal advisor to young girls and couples. Nurse-midwives have been found to be very effective in working with adolescents.[16]

For the community health nurse, especially if she is young herself, there is danger of manufacturing problems that do not exist. Not every young mother is immature, unwilling, or unable to carry out parental obligations. Having children at a young age can be an important and usual part of life.

Social support and protective measures for young people who do need help seem to be far below the level of what is essential.[17] The community health nurse, in conjunction with others, can be helpful in defining those needs and in encouraging institutional and social responses to meet them.

Care of the Family with Infants and Young Children

Mothering and fathering are important social skills. The quality of mothering, fathering and the parents' child-rearing practices is increasingly recognized as crucial to the physical and social development of children. Normal parent-child interaction is influenced by early and sustained contact between parents and the infant soon after birth.[18] Lack of this early bonding and attachment has been implicated in later emotional and developmental problems of young families.[19] Public health action directed toward preventing parental deprivation in its varied forms is thus a fundamental part of the program for protecting the health of the growing family.

Although the needs of children must entail community action in terms of providing adequate family incomes, decent housing, preventive and illness care, and a sound education, social action will be less than successful if the parents, as the leaders in family development, are incapable of assuming (or are unwilling to assume) their parental responsibilities. If the family is to carry its share of this responsibility, there is a need for the systematic preparation for parenthood and family living.

Jointly, the family and the community should assure each child of:
1. A secure and stimulating environment in which to grow
2. Protection from avoidable disease or disability
3. Assistance in the recognition of the child's own individuality and an appreciation of the rights of others
4. Prompt and adequate care when the child is ill or injured

In order to carry out these responsibilities in child rearing, the parents will need:
1. Knowledge of what to expect as children grow and develop
2. A relaxed confidence in their ability to fill the parental role
3. Proficiency in the homemaking skills required for the daily management and care of children
4. Confidence and judgment in the use of available health resources
5. The ability to understand and control their own behavior.

Monitoring the Care Plan Is A Shared Responsibility

The needs of children are unlikely to be met by chance. It takes persistent and planned action on several fronts to achieve proper care. The *family* must take the primary responsibility of planning for child rearing. The parents, especially the mother, are expected to take appropriate action when it is time for a preschool medical checkup or immunization. Fulfillment of the immunization schedule is one job that is often undertaken rather haphazardly: immunization during infancy is usually secured because it is an integral part of the infant care program;

booster shots, on the other hand, may be forgotten, especially if they are not tied to the requirements for going to school. There is need for some practical systematic approach for families planning for health care and also for someone to monitor the overall care plan to be sure that the various parts are carried through at the right time and by the right methods.

The use of a family health record (kept with the other family records such as birth certificates) may prove invaluable in completing history forms or in checking dates (for instance, the date of the last tetanus immunization). If every family kept such a record, it would provide a guide for family health planning, supply needed information in time of emergency, and encourage positive health action.

Monitoring responsibility may be assumed by the family physician, who reminds the families under his care when certain procedures are due and who (either individually or in coordination with his office staff) develops a systematic assessment and counseling program. The physician in the well-child center may assume the same kind of responsibility, with the nurse in the center or in another community health agency supporting his activities; or the nurse may be the principal monitor, referring the family to the physician when necessary. Sometimes the community health nurse is the principal monitoring force; and through systematic recording and case management, she guides the family in securing the necessary care.

Unfortunately, the community health nurse's case load is not developed, for the most part, on a population base but rather on a selected group of families or individual patients requiring specific care. As a result, family health planning surveillance for the population as a whole would require substantive restructuring of the organizational patterns under which nursing is provided; moreover, this program of health surveillance would probably go beyond present nurse manpower capability. Recent efforts to increase surveillance of children of medically indigent families (Title XIX of the Social Security Act; Early and Periodic Screening, Diagnosis and Treatment Program [EPSDT]) have been uneven in their application and in conditions screened for across the country, due to lack of adequately trained manpower as well as the current state of the art in screening measures.[20]

It is not the responsibility of the community nurse, then, to personally monitor the general health-care plan of every family but rather to try to see that every family has some provision for such systematic, sequential, and continuing health action on behalf of children.

Knowing What to Expect As Infants and Children Grow

The community health nurse improves the family's capacity to make meaningful observations of its children by *teaching parents what to look for* at given developmental points and how to recognize deviation from expected behavior. The instruction may be bolstered by printed guides or informational pamphlets to which the family may refer. It is helpful if it is possible to prepare for developments in advance of their probable occurrence.

There are many books and popular magazines written about growth and development that the community health nurse can use to help families appreciate the ups and downs of usual growth patterns. (See list of popular publications at end of chapter.) Brazelton and associates have developed a tool for the assessment of the newborn and how he interacts with his environment that nurses can use in helping parents appreciate the individual behavior of their baby and to consider more effective measures to use in responding to the infant's needs and their own.[21] The Denver Developmental Screening Test[22] and the Home Observation for Measurement of the Environment[23] are other examples of tools used by nurses that serve as a screening device as well as providing encouraging information for parents about progress in achieving certain developmental tasks.

It is important for parents to realize that each child will grow in his own way. Anticipatory guidance should not lead to a kind of scoring system in which the game is to keep the child on, or ahead of, the scientists' schedules.

There are predictable problems of growth or behavior for which the parent and professional worker should be prepared. For example, most very young babies will experience some difficulty with eating and sleeping, which they show by crying or wakefulness. The danger of accident or poisoning resulting from the preschool child's characteristic tendency to explore and test may also be expected and, with care, circumvented. The first experience in school is another predictable maturational crisis for many children.

To observe accurately, the parents must recognize and evaluate the cues that the child is giving them; the parents must learn to communicate despite a semantic gap that arises from the age difference. With infants who have not yet learned to speak, parents can usually understand the meaning of the infant's crying — whether it denotes anger, pain, or just a healthy desire for exercise. It is sometimes more difficult for parents to realize that communication with children who *can* verbalize may also be difficult; the child who "lies" when asked about a broken toy may be saying he has learned that honesty brings punishment. Similarly, parents may not be aware that the child who "does not obey" may, in fact, have missed the parents' direction either because of a short interest span or absorption in another task. Frequently, the nurse will be required to do little but bolster the parents' sensitivity to cues and specific danger signals.

However, in the case of the child at special risk — for instance, when a child is failing to thrive or when parents appear inadequate to their task — the action of the nurse may become more direct. In these instances, the nature of the observation involves evaluation of complex psychosocial aspects, as well as physical aspects, that are beyond the capacities of most parents. Moreover, the attitudes and practices of the parents themselves may be implicated in the etiology of the situation, and their interest in the child's welfare may be low.

Confidence in Parental Capability

Parents, as well as children, have their own developmental styles. The patterns of mothering (and of fathering) will differ widely among subcultures in the population and, of course, from family to family. The parental style may be one of stern control or of easy participation; of tightly organized action or of highly casual action. There is no way to characterize a style as being "good" or "bad." Each couple must learn for themselves how best to meet the responsibilities that occur. The nurse who is providing guidance in the development of parental skills must be careful not to be influenced by her own experience as a child or as a parent, or by her theoretical concept of what "good" parents are like. Rather, she should be sure that the parents are helped to recognize the importance and the nature of their role and that they are aided in gaining confidence in the skills and techniques required in child care.

Confidence in parental competence (or capability) depends upon both a sense of personal worth and an assurance of technical skill. If parents are to be relaxed and confident in the care of their children, technique alone is not a sufficient guarantee. Each parent must feel he is important to his children and to his spouse, and that what he does as a person and as a parent is important to his family and to the community.

In some situations, the lack of a sense of personal worth may be the primary barrier. The unmarried mother may feel she does not merit marriage and the respect of others, and she may expect that she cannot be a good parent because she is not a "good" person. The unemployed or alcoholic father may feel inadequate because he cannot provide for the family and, as a consequence, may feel that his contribution to child development is worthless —he may feel, as one man poignantly stated, "You think he'd want to be like me?" or he may vent his frustration through child abuse. Obviously the community health nurse cannot expect to remold personalities formed over many years. However, she can use every nursing contact to help support self-esteem in family members, and she can be alert to the effect of personality problems upon parental functioning. Thus, one arm of the program of building confidence must be sustaining and strengthening a self-image that is consistent with the parental role.

The second facet of parental confidence lies in a feeling of control over the skills and knowledge required; in knowing where help and advice may be secured if they are ever needed. For that reason, whether undertaken by the community health nurse herself or by other groups, the nurse should encourage a systematic educational program which will reach both parents and provide them with the essential knowledge needed to make wise decisions. This might take the form of seeing that the content of the family life course in the local high school supplies the needed information, of teaching individual families directly in their own homes, or of arranging for adult classes in child care and management.

The "Quiet" Need for Skills and Reassurance

The daily tasks of child care perplex many parents, especially the parents of a first child, or of a "caboose baby" born many years after siblings, or those parents considerably younger or older than the norm.

When mothers are asked what help they want to receive from well-baby care, the most frequent request is for reassurance in the simple aspects of care. The nurse can provide some instruction in child care during the prenatal period, either at parents' classes or through individual visits to the home or office. In such a setting, there is an opportunity for leisurely practice in skills and, in the case of group work, for sharing ideas and worries with other expectant parents. In the hospital, instruction may be provided concerning, in particular, bathing and feeding of the new baby and the mother's need for safeguarding her own health. However, the hospital setting and the very short hospital stay limit what can be done. As the child develops, many mothers will feel the need for continued instruction in such simple matters as bathing the baby, feeding schedules, and coping with crying.

The decision to breastfeed the infant is one in which the mother may need considerable help and support. If the mother elects to breastfeed, she will usually have many questions about leakage, diet, the mechanics of positioning the baby, and the problems of reconciling breastfeeding with social obligations.[24]

Obviously, families will differ greatly in the amount and type of support they need and want. Nurses, too, will differ in the amount of help they are able to give because of a lack of time or confidence in this aspect of nursing practice. It will be necessary for the community health nurse to find new and ingenious means in order to meet this "quiet" need. She can find ways to include instructional components into the usual well-baby clinics or in the visit to the doctor's office; she may restrict home visiting to those families whose problems seem move overwhelming and use telephone conferences for those whose needs are not so great. She may mobilize volunteer instructors under the Red Cross teaching program or in the adult health activity sections of the public schools. She can work through individuals, such as the experienced mother in the same block who may become a source of reference, the school nurse, or the nurse in the physician's office.

Because it is not a spectacular need, this need for reassurance and skill may be considered "frosting on the cake." Actually, it is an important factor in increasing the mother's satisfaction in her role and the father's ability to provide support to his wife in many areas other than child care. It improves the parent-child relationship, and it is an important arm of prevention.

Confidence in the Use of Health Resources

Despite the availability of resources for care directed toward health promotion and prevention, many facilities are underused. For example, in 1976, more than one third of all children under age 15 were not adequately immunized. The following year rubella cases increased by 63 per cent, measles cases by 39 per cent, and whooping cough cases by 115 per cent.[25]

The community health nurse can do much to encourage adequate use of available services. She may organize the nursing effort in the clinic to provide reminders, to make the clinic experience a pleasant one, and to build up the parents' sense of pride and accomplishment in child care. She can also study and act on the barriers to care. She can use volunteer or short-trained paid workers to supplement her efforts. She can alert planners to the need for extended or different kinds of facilities, so that the facilities and the needs and the expectations of the users are congruent. Most important, the community health nurse can communicate her own conviction that the quality of early child care is an important factor in the child's future development.

Child Care Outside the Home

Child care in settings other than the home is increasing and may present special problems. Day care centers, foster homes, extended school care, and many types of informal arrangements are being used to provide care for children whose parents work or who need an antidote or supplement for an inadequate home environment.

With any type of day care, there is the obvious problem of assuring that the out-of-home environment is indeed safe and conducive to the health and development of the child. Nursing activities directed toward such institutions are similar to those involved in providing services to nursing homes. Parents may need substantial support when children are placed outside the home. Out-of-home care is often associated with the inadequate or incomplete family, so that the responsible parent may be troubled with loneliness arising from lack of a partner, a sense of bereavement or helplessness at not being able to stay close to the children, or of guilt and anger that the children "have been taken away."

Informal sources of substitute care for children require careful evaluation. It is important to know just where and under what conditions children are cared for in the absence of their parents. Often a grandmother or unemployable male, with little motivation and less ability to provide the kind of care so badly needed, may be left to "mind" the children. The community health nurse should attempt to set up a supportive and educational program to be sure that the child is properly protected and receiving the best care possible. Nursing plans for the substitute child care agent or agency should be as carefully and as comprehensively planned as would be the program for the natural mother.

The improvement of parental competence is certainly a powerful factor in assuring adequate protection for children, and the community health nurse is in an exceptionally favorable position to contribute to the development of this competence. Working with other groups involved with children and parents (such as Neighborhood Head Start Programs, Early Learning Centers or church-sponsored preschool programs) can extend the impact of the nurse's program in this area.

The Role of the Community Nurse in Childhood
Illness and Disability

The nature of the community health nursing required to deal with the prevention and care of illness and disability in children will depend on the causes of death and disability in one's assigned population and on the degree to which these conditions may be averted or their progress modified by community nursing action.

Some of the most important causes of death or disability may be little affected by community nursing action, or they may require nonspecific action such as improvement of the general health and health awareness of families; for other childhood illnesses, specific community nursing may be a major factor in prevention or care.

The overriding causes of death among infants are due to prenatal or natal conditions; these account for about 60 per cent of the neonatal deaths (death in the first 28 days of life). Low birth weight increases the risk enormously (nearly two-thirds of the infants who die have low birth weight). There are also striking demographic variations: the infant mortality of black babies was 92 per cent higher than that of white babies in 1976; individual states' infant mortality rates ranged from 12.7 to 25.9 in 1973; and infant mortality in large cities (population 500,000 or more) was found to be much higher than the national average.[26] Pneumonia and accidents are also among the leading causes of death in infants.

For children one to four years of age, accidents are the leading cause of death, followed by birth defects, cancer and pneumonia/influenza. Motor vehicle accidents account for the largest percentage of deaths due to accident among all children. For school children 5 to 14 years of age, accidents, cancer and birth defects head the list.[27] However, since death rates in the group aged 1 to 15 years are low, estimates of illness may be more significant as an indicator of required nursing action.

Studies on the patterns of illness in children, conducted by the National Center for Health Statistics as part of their program for a continuing national health survey, provide much information that is useful for planning community health nursing. The most striking fact to emerge from a recent study was the great frequency of illness among children.

In a survey of children and youth conducted by the National Center for Health Statistics, the most prevalent childhood infectious disease (other than the common cold) was measles, usually occuring between 4 to 6 years of age. Chicken pox and mumps were the next most commonly reported diseases.[28] The most common chronic conditions listed in the same survey were allergies and recurrent earaches (approximately 23 per cent of those examined). Lead poisoning associated with iron deficiency is another prevalent disease, especially among low-income populations living in old and poorly maintained houses. Sixty-four community-based programs estimated the prevalence rate to be 175 per 100,000 children between one and five years of age.[29]

Other chronic problems of the school age child that community health nurses will frequently deal with when helping families are included under the heading, Developmental Disabilities. This includes mild to severe mental retardation, learning disorders, and speech and vision difficulties, to name a few. An estimated 100,000 children are identified as mentally retarded each year, most cases detected during school age. In about 90 percent of cases, the retardation is mild (IQ 50 to 70), and with proper support and nurturing, these children can live and learn in the community. As many as 20 per cent of school-age children have reading or learning disabilities. These youngsters can, with appropriate medical and education attention, function well within normal range for their age. Child abuse and neglect, poor nutrition, poverty, high-risk pregnancies, and traumatic birth have all been linked to various developmental disabilities.

THE MAJOR AREAS OF COMMUNITY HEALTH NURSING EFFORT

There will be differences in the programs of community health nurses; these differences will depend on the availability of resources, the programs of related agencies, and the adequacy of each community

health nursing staff. However, certain areas may be identified as likely to engage any community health nurses' attention.
1. Preventing prematurity and caring for the premature
2. Contributing to the reduction of congenital defects and developmental disabilities
3. Preventing and caring for victims of accidents and injury
4. Recognizing and caring for illness
5. Preventing or controlling communicable disease
6. Securing early and continuing care for handicapping conditions

Prematurity Care

In 1976, 83 per cent of the live births were "low birth weight" infants, who weighed less than 2500 grams.[30] These babies operate at a handicap because they are physiologically ill-equipped to stand the rigors of adapting to extrauterine life. They are much more likely than full-term babies to suffer from congenital defects, retardation, and neurologic defects. Infants below this weight are more than twenty times as likely to die within the first year.

Many maternal factors are associated with prematurity: lack of prenatal care, poor nutrition, smoking, alcohol and drug abuse, and age (especially teenage pregnancies). Prematurity tends to occur more often among women who have had multiple pregnancies or experienced previous fetal loss or obstetric complications, suffer from chronic hypertension, or are poorly nourished. Low-income groups must be considered as at special risk. The community health nurse may provide more intensive supervision and anticipatory guidance to this high-risk group.

Although premature care in the critical early days is usually provided in the hospital, the community health nurse may do much to help the parents in caring for the baby after his return from the hospital. The mother's separation from the baby at the critical period immediately after birth may cause some estrangement, and the size and appearance of the baby may add to her uneasiness. Because she is starting her maternal responsibilities a little later than other mothers, she may need more than the usual encouragement and reassurance. In addition, the mother must take greater care in avoiding exposure of the baby to infectious disease, and she may expect more feeding problems than usual. For these reasons, families with low birth weight babies may require extra nursing effort in the period of early infancy.

Reduction of Birth Defects

Birth defects include congenital physical anomalies, mental retardation, and genetic diseases. The causes of birth defects lie in the alteration of the genes or of the chromosomal structure and in the uterine environment of the developing fetus. Preventive measures to be taken against congenital anomalies must then be directed toward genetic controls, the avoidance of conditions that might impair the uterine environment, and the use of methods for in utero detection of abnormalities of fetal growth.

For the community health nurse, this three-fold plan requires, primarily, an intensification of the maternal health supervision that is needed by all mothers. A careful history is essential and should include a record of exposure to x-rays or infectious diseases during early pregnancy; possible familial genetic defect; an estimation of the probable nutritional state of the mother; careful observations of any unexpected occurrence during pregnancy; and reported use of drugs of which the effects are not yet fully known. This approach also involves encouraging and supporting parents in securing prompt and adequate medical appraisal, ideally before conception but certainly early in pregnancy, interpreting medical findings, and helping to implement medical recommendations.

Accident Prevention

An occasional home "safety check" or discussion on street and school safety may be a good opener for the kind of instruction required to prevent accidents, but the real pay-off comes only when the family has developed ingrained habits of safe behavior. Fastening infants and children into the appropriate size car seat restraint should be automatic, even on short trips.

Dangerous household substances such as ammonia or other cleaning agents must be stored out of the reach of children. The all-adult family commonly keeps medicines, cosmetics, detergents, paints, and many other substances readily accessible. Every family member must learn new safety habits when a toddler becomes part of the family. Replacing medicines out of reach immediately after use, keeping floors and stairways free from clutter, proper storing of guns and ammunition — a general *awareness* of risks is important.

The establishment of safe play areas for children, both in and out of the home, may likewise require specific family effort. A grandmother caring for the child of a working mother may find it easier for the child to play in the street where he is certain to find playmates than to take him to the safe play area in a nearby park. It may be difficult to provide a "fenced-in" area in the home that will keep small children in sight and protected from stoves or open heaters.

The suburban father driving to the supermarket on a sunny morning when he'd rather by playing golf must be in the *habit* of checking the area behind his car and backing out slowly. Children who are cycling need to learn the habit of riding carefully and only on the proper side of the street.

The care of accidental injury must be immediate. Ideally, one member of every family should be prepared — through a Red Cross or other first-aid course — to deal with emergencies. In any event, the mother or other responsible person should be familiarized with care of common emergencies. It is wise to post directions for first-aid care of accidents or other emergencies in a conspicuous and readily available place. In many communities, there is a poison control center that operates on a round-the-clock basis. All families in which there are small children should know about this resource and have this telephone number, along with the number of the physician or other emergency medical source of care, in a prominent and convenient place near the telephone.

Every child care person, including baby-sitters and part-time care persons, should know:

1. The importance of knowing *exactly where* a small child is at all times.
2. Who and how to call for immediate help in case of accident or emergency.
3. Methods of "child proofing" a home and yard for prevention of accidents.
4. The importance of defensive action against accidents: for example, defensive driving; defensive organization of home, school, and play areas; and teaching children to handle equipment properly *before* there is an accident.
5. The importance of continuing, automatic application of the known safety rules, including the use of "reminders," such as a red "twister" on all poison containers.
6. Exactly where to find immediate instructions of what to do before the doctor can get there.

This information should be routinely included in a community health nursing service rendered to *any* growing family. One mother suggested that the nurse distribute gummed labels containing the telephone number of the doctor, poison center, fire department, and public health nurse. The nurse should also be sure her own knowledge of first-aid and emergency care is up-to-date!

Care of Acute Illnesses

For the most part, the acute illnesses of children can be cared for by some family member. Thus, in planning for community nursing care to families, it must be recognized that someone in each family should be educated as a primary care-giver. This individual is the one who will recognize any deviation from usual behavior, who will be able to take the initiative in seeking such care, who will be able to use the care wisely, and who can herself administer the simple nursing required, with or without the help of a community health nurse.

To achieve care for acute illnesses, the mother or other child care agent will need to know:
1. How to tell whether the child is ill
2. How and where to go for help if illness is present
3. How to give simple care to the sick child at home

Systematic instruction such as that provided in Red Cross or adult education classes has many advantages but does not reach all who need it. The community health nurse must find other ways of reaching individuals or small groups. Much is done in this respect when the nurse is called in to provide care to a sick child and, in the course of care, teaches the whole family. However, the number of illnesses attended by the community health nurse is known to be small, and this, too is at best a haphazard approach to meeting the need. Much ingenuity and resourcefulness are required to find alternate ways; volunteer teachers, short-trained workers, school or other agency-sponsored courses, and the everyone-teach-one approach are some of the methods that have been tried and found successful.

Control of Communicable Diseases

Although deaths from, and the incidence of, communicable diseases in children have dropped to very low levels, unless immunization measures are fully maintained there is always the threat of new outbreaks. The Center for Disease Control, USPHS recommends that children should be immunized against pertussis, diphtheria, tetanus, poliomyelitis, measles, rubella, and mumps. Each health department will have its own recommended schedule for these immunizations; and schedules may also be found in most public health or pediatric textbooks, in reports of the American Academy of Pediatrics, and in the American Public Health Association's publication, *Control of Communicable Diseases in Man.*

The Center for Disease Control recommends the schedule shown in Table 12–3. In addition, they suggest tuberculosis testing at 1 year, 2 years, 4 years, and 6 years.

Recent studies show that in some groups the proportion of children not receiving recommended immunizations is substantial. A national survey in 1976 found that children having received at least three doses of diphtheria-tetanus-pertussis vaccine had dropped to a low level (71 per cent).[31] As of 1978, 68 per cent of the children 1 to 4 years of age had at least three doses of DTP vaccine, and only 61 per cent had at least three doses of polio vaccine.[32] Even though most groups do receive the primary series of immunizations, recommended "booster" dosages are much less frequently secured.

Table 12–3   SCHEDULE FOR CHILDHOOD IMMUNIZATION

Age[1]	Diphtheria Pertussis Tetanus	Polio	Measles	Rubella	Mumps
2 months	•	•			
4 months	•	•			
6 months	•	• (optional)			
15 months[2]			•	•	•
18 months	•	•			
4–6 years	•	•			
14–16 years[3]	•				

[1] Immunizations beginning in early infancy are the recommended practice. They can be provided in later years, however, according to a schedule recommended by a family physician.

[2] Measles, rubella, and mumps vaccines can be given in a combined form, at about 15 months of age, with a single injection.

[3] Children should receive a sixth tetanus-diphtheria injection (booster) at 14–16 years, and every 10 years thereafter.

Source: *Parents' Guide to Childhood Immunization.* Washington D.C., U.S. Government Printing Office, USDHEW, Center for Disease Control, 1977.

The community health nurse should familiarize herself with the available immunization agents, with the recommendations of the local health department, and with the requirements of the board of education regarding immunization for children in school. She should work with and through school and welfare workers, school children, volunteers, and any and all channels to emphasize the importance of immunization. Her own records should contribute to knowledge of the immunization levels achieved in the community. Above all, she should locate and deal with the barriers that prevent those who need this care from actually acquiring it.

Care of Children with Birth Defects

Children with birth defects may not be readily identified. Some handicaps are discovered in the course of medical evaluation very soon after birth; but other defects, such as hearing loss and mental retardation, may not be clearly demonstrated until several years have passed. The community health nurse, therefore, has considerable responsibility both for personal observation of the family and for sharpening and interpreting the observations of family members so they can identify any deviation from normal function that might require medical investigation.

Parents may dislike and tend to avoid the fact of developmental disabilities and, as a result, may overrepresent the child's abilities or create a plausible explanation for his inabilities. This is particularly likely to happen with the mentally retarded child. Sometimes a nurse may recognize long before the parents do that the child is not developing properly. It may take persistent and careful questioning to learn all of the factors that affect the child's behavior (deafness without mental retardation, for example, may be a factor in slow development) in order to provide the physician with pertinent, complete data. Additionally, it may take skill and tact to see that the child gets care without unduly alarming the parents.

Early recognition and care of developmental disabilities are as important in treating the condition as it is in securing the necessary family adjustments to the condition. It is particularly vital to ascertain hearing loss early, since deafness brings with it a degree of sensory deprivation that may seriously affect the cognitive development of the child. For that reason, screening tests for hearing loss are usually recommended between 9 and 12 months and at least once again during the preschool period. Children at special risk should be checked more frequently. These children include those whose mothers had rubella or other viral disease during pregnancy, those with a family history of deafness, and those who suffered respiratory distress after a difficult delivery.

The community health nursing care required for developmental disabilities will vary enormously from case to case and will depend largely on the availability of nursing, social work, or educational help. In any event, the community health nurse will be one member of a group concerned with meeting the needs of the child and his family, and she will be required to plan with others to provide the care required to meet the family's total needs. The nurse will need to consider these phases of care:

1. Teaching the family how to provide required care, such as feeding, exercises, protection from injury, substitute social experiences for the child barred from usual contacts, the handling of equipment, and where to obtain special equipment (e.g., cups with big handles or easily handled spoons).

2. Reassuring the family of their adequacy in the situation, constantly pointing out their successes and special contributions, putting into perspective their lapses into irritability or despondency, and pointing out the facilities available to provide help for situations the family is unable to handle.

3. Reassuring the parent of the humanity and the likability of the extremely disabled child, that he can appeal to others as well as to his family. This reassurance is sometimes made most apparent by the nurse's own attitude in dealing with the child; she should treat him not as a sick child but as one with known limitations.

4. Providing an anchor — that is, being someone who will listen, who will understand, who can be asked questions when new problems arise, who will stand by as a family makes difficult decisions and learns new attitudes and skills.

Most communities have special programs for children with developmental diabilities. Diagnostic, evaluation, and treatment centers are usually available in urban communities. They may be located in the health department, in a special clinic system administered by a crippled children's authority, in a teaching hospital associated with a medical school, or in a voluntary agency. These centers are characterized by the availability of a multidiscipline staff that is able to make a comprehensive assessment of the child's potential for development and to institute wide-spectrum treatment.

Day care centers for the handicapped child may be available within a "normal" day care group; of, if the condition is very severe, there may be day care services especially for the handicapped. Such services provide an opportunity for socialization and also serve to relieve the mother from the sometimes exhausting and frustrating task of care. Voluntary groups, such as the National Association for Retarded Children, may sponsor mutual support or educational programs. The community health nurse should familiarize herself with the available facilities and help parents and teaching staff interpret the special problems and needs of each child.

The Malnourished Child. Some problems of children are rooted in the failure of parents or other care personnel to meet the developmental and protective needs of their charges. The malnourished child may range from minimal to extreme levels of distress. Severe protein and calorie malnutrition, found too frequently in developing countries, is fortunately rare in the United States. However, it does occur, and hospital treatment is usually required to protect the child from any possible infection or illness while nutritional balance is being re-established. More often, the nurse will encounter less dramatic forms of malnutrition: the grossly obese child, (whose gluttony may suggest either insecurity, emotional deprivation, or merely the influence of parents who feel a fat child is a well child) and the child with moderate protein deficit or anemia. These less obvious kinds of malnutrition can cause considerable developmental damage and should not be treated lightly.

Sometimes where there is no overt evidence of malnutrition and tests for nutritional adequacy are not readily available, malnutrition can be assumed on the basis of knowledge of food intake. The community health nurse may help locate these poorly fed children. If the situation warrants it and facilities are available, the child may be referred for complete nutritional study or for counseling by a nutritionist. Alternatively, the nurse may move directly to influence parents and to institute a better diet, using the help of the nutritionist if necessary. Sometimes malnutrition is due to inadequate income, and parents who are well aware of what is needed may be unable to supply the food they would like to provide for their children. In this case, conferences with welfare agencies may locate some additional funds or food supplements. The current food stamp plan enables families to purchase more food per dollar of their own expenditure. This plan is financed by federal funds and is operated by welfare agencies.

In developed countries, the problem of malnutrition is most often one of poor allocation of available money, poor habits of shopping, or food preferences rooted in cultural ethnic tradition. A child may get sweets, but not vitamins. Changing food habits is not easy, since they tend to be socially linked and rooted in cultural habits; however, an attempt to change the food intake of the children may motivate a change in the whole family pattern.

Failure to Thrive. Children that appear listless, show no anger when left by their parents, fail to gain weight, eat and sleep poorly, cry very little, or show excessive irritability or vomit without any discernible physical reason are initially lumped together as babies who are "failing to thrive." This condition is almost always associated with psychosocial, as well as physical, problems and requires the services of several agents to assess the situation and to deal with the multiple causes.

Failure to thrive is often associated with a disturbed mother-child relationship, which may result in infrequent tactile contact with the child and consequent sensory deprivation. The cause for the disturbance may be difficult to locate. The mother may have felt that this baby threatened her life or her marriage, she may not have wanted the baby, or perhaps she has been unable to respond as she felt she should to her child. As the baby shows the result of this deprivation, the mother may become more anxious and consequently even less able to establish a warm and reciprocal relationship.

Sometimes the baby's welfare assumes minor importance when other conditions are extremely threatening. The father of the family may be absent, ineffectual, or even threatening to the baby. The mother may feel socially alienated, depressed, and frustrated by conditions that she feels impotent to change and that offer no hope in the future. The baby may be in the charge of a care agent who is indifferent or insensitive to his needs or who has no interest in the child except as a source of income.

Because of her traditionally warm relationship with a family, the community health nurse is in a good position to look for early signs of failure to develop a suitable mother-child relationship and of characteristic responses of the infant who is not thriving. Using available help from other disciplines, she may be able to support the mother before the situation becomes serious. The mother may be encouraged to voice her dislike or fear of the baby, to investigate the possibility of help in preventing future unwanted pregnancies, and to express her frustrations at her living conditions, even though little can be done to improve them. As the mother's acceptance of the baby grows, her fear of him and her guilt may be reduced by specific instruction in care and by reiterated statements of confidence in her ability to be a mother.

When the family is under the care of a multidiscipline group or clinic, the community health nurse can provide information about the home and the family, help explain behavior in terms of the competing emotional demands and the stresses the mother faces, or assess the mother's strength and the capacity of her husband or other family members to support her efforts. By mobilizing the help of relatives and neighbors, the nurse may alleviate some of the sources of the mother's frustration. The provision of a homemaker or the institution of day care or early school experience for older children are other examples of the kind of help needed.

Of all problems the community health nurse faces, a child's failure to thrive is probably the one that demands the broadest spectrum of interest and action, requires the most intensive work with others, and offers the highest stakes in terms of the baby's and the mother's future.

Adolescence

Adolescence is a period of relatively good health, in spite of the turbulence caused by rapid physical, sexual, and emotional growth. This age group is characterized by frequent mood changes, unpredictable behavior, and the testing of rules and parental controls. Much is made of the negative aspects of the adolescent phase, yet very little is known about normal adolescents who develop without overt problems and are interesting energetic people full of good ideas and hope. The person who is properly prepared for the physical and emotional changes, who is secure in his feelings of self-worth, and who has some aspirations and goals for the future will be more likely to work through this developmental stage in a constructive way. Without these attributes, adolescence can be an overwhelmingly stressful time.

The special health needs of teenagers are in large part the result of society's loosely defined symbols of adulthood and the "discontinuity" individuals in this age group feel with other generations. Developmental milestones must be achieved in these areas: (1) self-image, identity, and desire for self esteem; (2) acceptance of change within themselves; (3) struggle to attain independence; (4) relationship with peers; (5) relationship with the opposite sex; (6) cognitive and vocational achievement; and (7) ability to control moods of depression and desires to act out.[33] L. Fine suggests viewing the development in this age group within stages, i.e., early, middle, and late adolescence within the family, peer groups, and the school setting.[34]

The most frequent disorders reported by adolescents are acne and obesity, problems directly related to self image. Statistics of this population have also shown accidents and emotional disorders to be of significant concern along with drug abuse, alcohol abuse, smoking, contraception, pregnancy and venereal disease.[35]

Certain orthopedic problems such as slipped epiphysis and scoliosis and other chronic conditions also appear most frequently during adolescence.

Because of the prevalence of these conditions, many school health programs now screen routinely for hypertension, sickle cell disease, scoliosis, and tuberculosis.

SPECIAL CONCERNS

Precocious Sexual Activity

Each person matures at his or her own rate, but the general trend is for girls' bodies to develop between the ages of 11 to 13 with some girls beginning to change as early as 8 or 9. The average age of menarche in the United States is 12.5 years, with full physical maturation seven years later. Boys begin to change sometime between the ages of 10 to 15.

From statistics on teenage pregnancies and sexually transmissible diseases, we know that more teenagers are sexually active at an earlier age than ever before. One fourth of American teenage girls have had at least one pregnancy before age 19. Birth rates for teenagers aged 16 to 19 are declining, but they are increasing for girls under 16.[36]

Sexual freedom has brought a greater acceptance of human sexual expression as well as greater risk of sexually transmissible diseases. Adolescents account for a large percentage of the reported cases of gonorrhea, syphilis, as well as other venereal diseases. (See Chapter 18.) Sex education and health guidance by responsible adults, including parents, teachers, church leaders, and health workers are necessary to develop a responsible attitude toward sexual behavior.

Runaways

There is increased public awareness of the growing numbers of runaway youth, the estimated number being between one to five million, and more than 50 per cent of these are girls. The average age of this population is 15 years and is frequently the result of family disruption or because of problems the youth want to keep secret, such as pregnancy or drug abuse. These youth often become involved in prostitution, drugs, and crime, and they tend to drift aimlessly from city to city.

The immediate needs of this population are for food, housing, clothing, and medical care. Shelters are being established and a National Telephone Hotline for runaway youth is in operation to assist communication between the children and parents (toll free number is 800-621-4000).[37]

The community health nurse can help organize shelters and counseling services for these youth, provide needed health services in many instances and encourage schools, churches and clubs to be aware of precipitating factors in family life.

The Adolescent with a Handicap

The problem for the adolescent with a handicap may not be from the particular limitation itself, as much as it is from the strong desire to be like and be accepted by peers. Difficulties for adolescents with some level of mental retardation can be even more upsetting for the family as well as the child. Even though functional level may be limited, the retarded youngster may desire individual achievement like others. With sexual development comes the normal desire for social interactions with the opposite sex.

The community health nurse can help parents anticipate the needs of their child, know about specialized counseling and vocational training, and assist in providing anticipatory guidance to children in the following areas: physiologic changes, emotions, and contraceptive information; awareness of self, body parts and processes; peer relationships and social interactions; and responsibility to society.[38]

Homicide, Suicide and Fatal Motor Vehicle Accidents

The death rate among Americans aged 15 to 24 is higher now than it was twenty years ago. Young men are at particular risk of violent death due to greater risk-taking and aggressive behavior. Homicides, suicides and accidents account for about three-fourths of all deaths in adolescence — approximately 48,000 deaths in 1977.[39]

Transition from childhood to adulthood can be terribly disruptive in terms of emotional stability. Although broad social issues and general social and economic stability are known to have an effect, the family has the most direct influence on adolescents during this period. Whatever the community health nurse can do to help strengthen the family, both on an individual basis and working with other concerned groups, may be the best effort in terms of adolescents developing a healthy outlook about themselves.

Case Load Management is Based on a Priority System

The almost limitless opportunities offered to the community health nurse to improve the health of the growing family make it immediately clear that it will not be possible for her to give all of the services she knows would be useful. For this reason, it is necessary to establish a priority system based on the likely impact of nursing service in a given situation and the realities of the nurse supply and demand.

In prenatal care, lifesaving and the reduction of morbidity may have highest priority, and the risk rate becomes the criterion for selection of care. The identification of high-risk mothers has been discussed previously. In some settings it is as effective to select high-risk populations as it is to identify high-risk individuals. In very low-income areas or migrant groups, for example, women at special risk will include the majority of those involved in the reproductive process. In other situations, as in a mixed income county, the selection may be on a family-by-family basis.

Patients at special risk require additional care, but the intensity and urgency of the care provided by the community health nurse is dependent not only upon the risk but also upon the help provided from other sources. Thus, a mother at high risk who is seen frequently in a clinic where there is a strong surveillance and teaching program and who has great inner strength and a supportive family may need less community health nursing than does the wife whose physical risk is less but whose husband is abroad on military duty. For this reason, it is helpful to categorize families in terms of the urgency and intensity of their need for community health nursing care in order to assure differential care.

The highest priority for community nursing support may go to unwilling or obviously inadequate parents and their children, whether they are classified as high risk or not. Here, the possibility of longterm damage due to parental deprivation may be lessened by the nurse in the community. In many cases the major effect of community health nursing will not be shown by a reduction of deaths or even by a great reduction of morbidity but rather in the improvement of the quality of childbearing and child rearing.

The community health nurse is an important member of the group concerned with well-child care and parent education. As a member of this group, she not only takes responsibility for the nursing phases of the work, but she also participates in the overall planning and evaluation of the care provided. She is as responsible as every other professional member for assuring that the total operation meets the needs of a given population efficiently and effectively.

The diverse problems families must face in raising children can often be overwhelming to the neophyte community health nurse. Her efforts, seen in isolation, cannot begin to make an impact on many of the overwhelming social problems she will face in working with families. Identifying other social and political groups in the community involved in meeting these larger social problems, using available resources from federal, state and local programs and making these resources work for families, have the potential for a larger payoff. On the other hand, the value of the community health nurse's care and concern for individual families cannot be underestimated.

REFERENCES

1. U.S. Department of Commerce: *Social Indicators*. Washington, D.C., U.S. Government Printing Office, 1977, pp. 95–96, Table 5–8.
2. Ibid., pp. 197 (Table 5–13) and 200 (Table 5–16).
3. See Gould, R.: *Transformations*. New York, Simon and Schuster, 1978; and Sheehy, G.: *Passages: Predictable Crises in Adult Life*. New York, E. P. Dutton, 1976.
4. *Information Please Almanac*. New York, Simon and Schuster, 1977, p. 721.
5. National Center for Health Statistics: *Births, Marriages, Divorces, and Deaths for 1977*. Monthly Vital Statistics Reports, Vol 26, No. 12. Hyattsville, Md., DHEW Pub. No. (PHS) 78–1120, Public Health Service, March 1978b.
6. National Center for Health Statistics: *Health-United States 1979*. Hyattsville, Md., Public Health Service, U.S. Department of Health, Education, and Welfare, Pub. No. (PHS) 80–1232, 1979, p. 142.
7. Barnard, K. E., and Douglas, H. B. (eds.): *Child Health Assessment. Part I: A Literature Review*. Washington, D.C., U.S. Government Printing Office, U.S. Department of Health, Education, and Welfare, December 1974, pp. 26–33.
8. Fogarty International Center for Advanced Study in Health Sciences, National Institutes of Health, and the American College of Preventive Medicine: *Preventive Medicine*. New York, Prodist, 1976, p. 296.
9. Klaus, M. H., and Kennell, J. H.: *Maternal-Infant Bonding*. St. Louis, Mo., C. V. Mosby Co., 1976, pp. 38–98.
10. Fogarty, International Center et al., p. 296.
11. Lubic, R. W.: Alternative patterns of nurse midwifery care. The birthing center. J. Nurse Midwif., *21*:44, 1976.
12. Hochman, G.: What happens when children have children? *Philadelphia Inquirer*, July 16, 1978, p. 1.
13. Zelnik, M., and Kantner, J.: Contraceptive patterns and premarital pregnancy among women aged 15–19 in 1976. Fam. Plan. Persp., *10*:135, 1978.
14. Hochman, p. 13.
15. Johns Hopk. Gaz., May 5, 1977, p. 1.
16. Klerman, L. V., and Jekel, J. F.: School-Age Mothers: Problems, Programs, and Policy, Hamden, Ct., The Shoe String Press, 1973, p. 44.
17. Goldstein, H., and Wallace, H.: Services for the needs of pregnant teenagers in large cities of the United States, 1976. Pub. Health Rep., *93*:46, 1978.
18. Kennell, J. H., et al.: Maternal behavior one year after early and extended post-partum contact. Dev. Med. Child Neurol., *16*:172, 1974.
19. Kennedy, J. C.: The high risk maternal-infant acquaintance process. Nurs. Clin. North Am., *8*:549, 1973.
20. Frankenburg, W. K., and North, A. F.: *A Guide to Screening for the Early and Periodic Screening, Diagnosis and Treatment Program Under Medicaid*. Washington, D.C., U.S. Department of Health, Education, and Welfare, Social and Rehabilitation Services, 1974.
21. Brazelton, T. B.: *The Neonatal Behavioral Assessment Scale*. Philadelphia, J. B. Lippincott Co., 1973.
22. Frankenburg, W. K., and Dodds, J. B.: Denver Developmental Screening Test. J. Pediatr., *71*:181, 1967.
23. Caldwell, B. M.: *Instruction Manual Inventory for Infants* (Home Observation for Measurement of the Environment). Little Rock, Ark., 1970.
24. Eiger, M., and Olds, S. W.: *The Complete Book of Breastfeeding*. New York, Bantam Books, 1972.
25. Surgeon General's Report: *Healthy People*. Washington, D.C., U.S. Government Printing Office, Department of Health, Education, and Welfare, Public Health Service, 1979, p. 93.
26. *Preventing Disease/Promoting Health–Objectives for the Nation*. (Draft) U.S. Department of Health, Education, and Welfare, August 1979, p. 17.
27. U.S. Department of Commerce, Bureau of the Census: *Characteristics of American Children and Youth, 1976*. Current Population Reports, Special Studies Series P-23, No. 66, p. 37.
28. *Examination and Health History Findings Among Children and Youths 6–17 years*. Washington, D.C., U.S. Department of Health, Education, and Welfare, U.S. National Health survey, Series 11, No. 129, 1973.
29. *Morbidity and Mortality Weekly Report, Annual Summary, 1978*. CDC, Department

of Health, Education, and Welfare, Public Health Service, Atlanta, Ga., 1979, p. 84.
30. Surgeon General's Report, p. 24.
31. *Characteristics of American Children and Youth: 1976,* p. 34.
32. *Health – United States 1979,* p. 121.
33. White, R. W.: *Growth and Organization in Personality.* New York, Holt, Rinehart, and Winston, Inc., 1972, p. 288.
34. Fine, L.: What's a normal adolescent? Clin. Pediatr., *12*:1, 1973.
35. Sternlieb, J., and Manon, L.: A survey of health problems, practices, and needs of youth. Pediatrics, *49*:177, 1972.
36. The Surgeon General's Report, p. 48.
37. Millar, H.: Approaches to Adolescent Health Care in the 1970's. Department of Health, Education, and Welfare, (HSA 76–5014), 1975, p. 21.
38. Siantz, M. L.: *The Nurse and the Developmentally Disabled Adolescent.* Baltimore, University Park Press, 1977.
39. Surgeon General's Report, p. 43.

SUGGESTED READINGS

Abernathy, V., Illegitimate conception among teenagers. Am. J. Pub. Health, *64*: 662, 1974.
Arms, S.: *Immaculate Deception.* Boston, Houghton Mifflin Co., 1975.
Babson, S.: *Primer on Prematurity and High-Risk Pregnancy.* St. Louis, Mo., C. V. Mosby Co., 1966.
Barnard, K.: Trends in the care and prevention of developmental disabilities. Am. J. Nurs., 75:1700, 1975.
Barnard, K., and Erickson, M.: *Teaching Children with Development Problems: A Family Care Approach,* 2nd ed. St. Louis, Mo., C. V. Mosby Co., 1976.
Blair, C. L., and Salerno, E. M.: *The Expanding Family: Childbearing.* Boston, Little, Brown & Co., 1976.
Boston Children's Medical Center (Richard Feinbloom): *Child Health Encyclopedia.* New York, Merlord Lawrence Book (Delta Special 1975.
Brazelton, T. B.: *Infants and Mothers – Differences in Development.* New York, Delta Book, 1969.
Caplan, F. (ed.): *The Parenting Advisor.* Garden City, N.Y., Anchor Pres/Doubleday, 1977.
Card, J. J., and Wise, L. L.: Teenage mothers and teenage fathers: The impact of early childbearing on the parents' personal and professional lives. Fam. Plan. Persp. *10*:199, 1978.
Chapman, P.: Violence and the health of American youth. *In* Task Force Reports: *Preventive Medicine USA.* New York, Prodist, 1976, pp. 119–128.
Cognitive and affective learning for self-directed health behavior. J. School Health, *46*:385, 1976.
Cohen, B., Lilienfeld, M., and Huang, P. C.: *Genetic Issues in Public Health & Medicine.* Springfield, Ill., Charles C Thomas, 1978.
Coles, R.: *Migrants, Sharecroppers, Mountaineers,* Vol. II of *Children of Crisis.* Boston, Little, Brown & Co., 1971.
Coles, R.: *The South Goes North,* Vol. III of *Children of Crisis.* Boston, Little, Brown & Co., 1971.
Consequences of Malnutrition. Hearings before the Select Committee on Nutrition and Human Needs of the U.S. Senate, 93rd Congress. Washington, D. C., U.S. Government Printing Office, (Stock No. 5270–01998).
Craven, R. F., and Sharp, B. H.: The effects of illness on family functions. NSG Forum, *71*:186, 1972.
Davidson, N. and Cameron, J.: Health services to mothers. *In* Reinhardt, A., and Quinn, M.: *Family Centered Community Nursing.* St. Louis, Mo., C. V. Mosby Co., 1973, p. 201.
Department of Health, Education, and Welfare: *Handbook of Common Poisonings in Children.* Washington, D.C., U.S. Government Printing Office, (FDA 76–7004).
Diffendal, E.: *Day Care for School Age Children.* Washington, D. C., Day Care and Child Development Council of America, 1974.

Duvall, E. M: *Marriage and Family Development,* 5th ed. Philadelphia, J. B. Lippincott Co., 1977.

11 Million Teenagers: What Can Be Done About the Epidemic of Adolescent Pregnancies in the U.S. New York, The Alan Guttmacher Institute, Planned Parenthood Federation of America, Inc., 1976.

Children's Defense Fund: *EPSDT, Does it Spell Health Care for Poor Children?* Washington, D.C., June 1977.

Epstein, J., and McCartney, M.: A home birth service that works. Birth Fam. J., 4:71, 1977.

Erickson, E.: *Childhood and Society.* New York, W. W. Norton & Co., 1963.

Erickson, M.: *Assessment and Management of Developmental Changes in Children.* St. Louis, Mo., C. V. Mosby Co., 1976.

Ferrer, T. L. (ed.): Symposium on restructuring maternity care, counseling patients with genetic abnormalities, Nurs. Clin. North Am., 10:293, 1975.

Fox, G. L.: The family's influence on adolescent sexual behavior. Child. Today, 8:21, 1979.

Fraiberg, S.: *Every Child's Birthright: In Defense of Mothering.* New York, Basic Books Inc., 1977.

Fraiberg, S.: *The Magic Years.* New York, Charles Scribner's Sons, 1959.

Freed, A.: *T. A. for Tots.* Sacramento, Jalmers Press Inc., 1974.

Fuchs, F.: Genetic amniocentesis. Sci. Amer., 242:47, 1980.

Garfinkel, J., et al.: *Infant Maternal and Childhood Mortality in the U.S., 1968–1973.* Washington, D.C., U.S. Government Printing Office, HSA 75-5013, 1975.

Gesell, A.: *Infant and Child in the Culture of Today.* New York, Harper and Row, 1974.

Gesell, A., Ilg, F. I., and Ames, L. B.: *Youth, the Years from Ten to Sixteen.* New York, Harper and Row, 1956.

Ginott, H.: *Between Parent and Child.* New York, Macmillan Co., 1965.

Gordon, T.: *P.E.T. — Parent Effectiveness Training.* New York, New American Library, 1975.

Green, M.: *A Sigh of Relief – First Aid Handbook for Childhood Emergencies.* New York, Bantam Books, 1977.

Hanlon, J.: *Public Health Administration and Practice,* 6th ed. St. Louis, Mo., C. V. Mosby Co., 1979, Chapter 17.

Harnish, Y.: *Patient Care Guides, Practical Information for Public Health Nurses.* (#21-1610), National League for Nursing, 111:1, 1976.

Haynes, U.: *A Developmental Approach to Casefinding.* Washington, D. C., U.S. Department of Health, Education and Welfare, PHS, DHEW Pub. No. (HSA) 5-5403, 1975.

Heber, R., and Garber, H.: *The Milwaukee Project: A study of the use of the family intervention to prevent cultural-family retardation. In* Friedlander, B. Z., Sterritt, G. M., and Kirk, G. E., (eds.): *Exceptional Infant,* Vol. III. New York, Brunner/Mazel, 1975.

Helfer, R. and Kemper, H.: *Child Abuse and Neglect: The Family and the Community.* Cambridge, Mass., Bellinger Pub. Co., 1976.

Ilg, F. and Ames, L.: *Child Behavior from Birth to Ten.* New York, Harper & Row, 1955.

Immunizations — (1976) Trends for Children 1–4 Years. Center for Disease Control, 4204-3.1, U.S. Immunization Survey, 1975, 1976, CDC 76–8221.

Justice, B. and Justice, R.: *The Abusing Family.* New York, Human Sciences Press, 1976.

Kadushin, A.: Child welfare services — Past and present. Child. Today, 5:16, 1976.

Kauffman, M. C., and Cunningham, A.: Epidemiologic analysis of outcomes in maternal and infant health in evaluating effectiveness of three part care teams. Am. J. Pub. Health, 60:1712, 1970.

Kempe, R. S., and Kempe, C. H.: *Child Abuse, The Developing Child Series.* Cambridge, Mass., Harvard University Press, 1978.

Kessner, D.: *Infant Death: An Analysis by Maternal Risk and Health Care.* Washington, D. C., Institute of Medicine, National Academy of Sciences, 1973.

Korones, S. B., with J. Lancaster: *High-Risk Newborn Infants; the Basis for Intensive Nursing Care,* 2nd ed. St. Louis, C. V. Mosby Co., 1976.

LeBow, M. D.: *Behavior Modification, A significant Method in Nursing Practice.* Englewood Cliffs, N.J., Princeton Hall, Inc., 1973.

Lee, F. E., and Glasser, J. H.: Role of lay midwifery in maternity care in a large metropolitan area. Pub. Health Rep., 89:537, 1974.

Legislative Base — Maternal and Child Health Programs (1975–1976). Washington, D. C., Department of Health, Education and Welfare (HSA) (77–5221).

Leonard, S. W.: How. first-time fathers feel toward their newborns. Mat. Child Nurs., *1*:361, 1976. No. 6, November/December 1976, pp. 361–365.

Lopez, R.: *Adolescent Medicine: Topics,* Vol. 1. New York, Spectrum Publications, Inc., 1976.

Lubic, R. W.: Alternative patterns of nurse-midwifery care. J. Nurse Midwifery, *21*:24, 1976.

Malter, S.: Genetic Counseling: A responsibility of health care professionals. Nurs. Forum, *16*:26, 1977.

Marquart, R.: Expectant fathers: What are their needs? Mat. Child Nurs. *1*:32, 1976.

McBride, A., B.: *The Growth and Development of Mothers.* New York, Harper & Row, 1973.

Mead, M.: The job of the children's mother's husband. *In* Goode, W. J. (ed.): *The Contemporary American Family.* Chicago, Quadrangle Books, 1971.

Meglen, M. C., and Burst, H. V.: Nurse midwives make a difference. Nurs. Outlook, *22*:386, 1974.

Meleis, A., and Swendsen, L.: Does nursing intervention make a difference? A test of role supplementation. *In* Western Interstate Commission on Higher Education: *Community Nursing Research,* Vol. 8, *Nursing Research Priorities: Choice or Chance.* Boulder, Colo., 1977, pp. 308–324.

Millar, H.: *Approaches to Adolescent Health Care in the 1970's* Washington, D.C., U.S. Government Printing Office, (HSA 75–5014), 1975.

Morris, A. G.: The use of the well baby clinic to promote early intellectual development in parent education. Am. J. Pub. Health, *66*:73–74, 1976.

Murray, R., and Zenter, J.: *Nursing Assessment and Health Promotion Through the Life Span.* 2nd ed. Englewood Cliffs, N.J. Prentice-Hall, Inc., 1979.

Parenting: An Annotated Bibliography. Children's Bureau/Administration for Children, Youth and Families, Office of Human Development Services, Department of Health, Education and Welfare, (OHDS 78–30134), 1978.

Parents' Guide to Childhood Immunization. U.S. Department of Health, Education, and Welfare, PHS (No. OS–77–50058), 1977.

Pavenstedt, E.: To help infants weather disorganized family life. *In* Reinhardt, A., and Quinn, M.: *Family-Centered Community Nursing.* St. Louis, C. V. Mosby, 1973, pp. 216–223.

Record, J. C., and Cohen, H. R.: Introduction of midwifery in a prepaid group practice. Am. J. Pub. Health, *62*:354, 1972.

Ritchie, A., and Swanson, L. A.: Childbirth outside the hospital — The resurgence of home and clinic deliveries. MCN, *1*:372, 1976.

Salk, L.: *What Every Child Would Like His Parents to Know.* New York, David McKay Co., 1972.

Schulz, D.: *The Changing Family — Its Function and Future.* Englewood Cliffs, N.J., Prentice-Hall, Inc., 1972.

Schwartz, J. L., and Schwartz, L. (ed.): *Vulnerable Infants: A Psychosocial Dilemma.* New York, McGraw-Hill Book Co., 1977.

Smoyak, S.: Symposium on parenting. Nurs. Clin. North Am., *12*:447, 1977.

Southard, S. C., et al.: A comprehensive protocol for evaluating the safety of toys for preschool children. Clin. Pediatr., *15*:107, 1976.

Steele, S. (ed.): *Nursing Care of the Child with Long-Term Illness,* 2nd ed. New York, Appleton-Century-Crofts, 1977.

Taylor, D.: A new way to teach teens about contraceptives, MCN, *1*:378, 1976.

Teenage childbearing, 1966–1975. Pub. Health Rep., *93*:96, 1978.

Tichy, A., and Malasanos, L.: The physiological role of hormones in puberty. MCN, *1*:384, 1976.

Trends in Prematurity United States: 1950–67. National Center for Health Statistics, 1972.

White, B.: *The First Three Years of Life.* Englewood Cliffs, N.J., Prentice-Hall, Inc., 1975.

World Health Organization: *Pregnancy and Abortion in Adolescence.* Report of WHO Meeting, Technical Report Series, No. 583, Geneva, 1975.

Zelnik, M., and Kantner, J.: Sexual and contraceptive experience of young unmarried women in the United States, 1976 and 1971. Fam. Plan. Prosp. *9*:55, 1977.

RESOURCES

American Academy of Pediatrics
1801 Hinman Avenue
Evanston, Illinois 60204

American Association for Gifted Children, Inc.
15 Gramercy Park
New York, N.Y. 10003

American Dental Association
211 East Chicago Avenue
Chicago, Illinois 60611

American Public Welfare Association
1660 L Street, N.W.
Suite 607
Washington, D.C. 20036

Association for Childhood Education International
3615 Wisconsin Avenue, N.W.
Washington, D.C. 20016

Child Welfare League of America
1346 Connecticut Avenue, N.W.
Washington, D.C.

Children's Defense Fund
1520 New Hampshire Avenue, N.W.
Washington, D.C. 20036

Children's Defense Fund of the Washington Research Project
1746 Cambridge St.
Cambridge, Massachusetts 02138

Children's Foundation
1038 Connecticut Avenue, N.W.
Suite 614
Washington, D.C.

Consumer Product Safety Commission
Bureau of Information and Education
Product Safety Information Division
5401 Westbard Avenue
Washington, D.C. 20207

Day Care Committee of the APHA
1015 18th St., N.W.
Washington, D.C. 20036

Epilepsy Foundation of America
1828 L Street, N.W.
Washington, D.C. 20036

Family Service Association of America
44 East 23d Street
New York, N.Y. 10010

Foundation for Child Development
345 East 46th Street
New York, N.Y. 10017

LaLeche League International, Inc.
9616 Minneapolis Avenue
Franklin Park, Illinois 60131

Maternity Center Assoc. (MCA)
48 East 92d Street
New York, N.Y. 10028

National Association for the Education of Young Children
1834 Connecticut Avenue, N.W.
Washington, D.C. 20009

National Association for Retarded Children
2709 Avenue E, East
Arlington, Texas 76011

National Easter Seal Society for Crippled Children and Adults
2023 West Ogden Avenue
Chicago, Illinois 60612

National Foundation — March of Dimes
1275 Mamaroneck Avenue
White Plains, N.Y. 10605

National Safety Council
423 N. Michigan Avenue
Chicago, Illinois 60611

SIECUS
84 Fifth Ave., Suite 407
New York, N.Y. 10011

U.S. Children's Bureau
Public Health Service
U.S. Department of Health and Human Services

Publications, U.S. Government Printing Office

"A Developmental Approach to Case Finding," (DHEW Pub. No. (HSA 79-5210) Office for Maternal and Child Health, H.S.A., D.H.H.S.

"Your Child from One to Six," (OHDS 77–30026) Office of Human Development

"Your Child from Six to Twelve," (OHD 76-30040) Office of Human Development

"Prenatal Care," (OCD 75–17), Office of Human Development

"Partners & Parents — Home Start," (OHDS 78–31106), Office of Human Development

"The Role of Parents as Teachers," (Office of Education, #107–080–01490–4)

FEDERAL PROGRAMS RELATED TO CHILD HEALTH

Appalachian Regional Development Act of 1965, as amended: Health programs and Child Development programs

Child Abuse Prevention and Treatment Act, as amended: child abuse and neglect prevention and treatment

Child Nutrition Act of 1966, as amended: Special Supplemental Food Program for Women, Infants, and Children (WIC)

Community Mental Health Centers Amendments of 1975: Comprehensive Services support and special children's services

Community Services Act of 1974: Headstart

Developmental Disabilities Services and Facilities Construction Act of 1975, as amended: Developmental Disabilities basic support

Domestic Volunteer Service Act of 1973: mini grant program

Economic Opportunity Act of 1964, as amended by Community Services Act of 1974: Community Action Programs

Education for All Handicapped Children Act: state incentive grant program

Education of the Handicapped Act, Title VI, Pt. C.: Handicapped early childhood assistance and handicapped innovative programs, deaf-blind centers

Elementary and Secondary Education Art, Titles I and III: services for disadvantaged students and educational innovation and support

Lead Based Paint Poisoning Prevention Act, as amended: childhood lead-based paint poisoning control

Military Medical Benefits Act of 1966, as amended: Civilian Health and Medical Program of the Uniformed Services (CHAMPUS) and uniformed Services Health Benefits Program

Public Health Service Act

Title III, Sec. 314(d): Comprehensive Public Health Services
Title III, Sec. 317 and 318: Immunization Grants
Title III, Sec. 319: Migrant Health Grants
Title III, Sec. 331: National Health Service Corps
        Sec. 330: Community Health Centers, including Rural and Urban Health Initiatives
Title X: Family Planning Projects
P.L. 83–568: Indian Health Serivces
Title XIII: Health Maintenance Organization Development
Titles XV and XVI: Health Planning
P.L. 95–623 Amendment of 1978: Adolescent Health Services and Pregnancy Prevention and Care

Social Security Act

Title V: Maternal and Child Health, Crippled Children Services Program of Projects
Title XI, Sec. 1110: Health to Underserved Rural Areas
Title XIX: Medicaid, including esp EPSDT, rural health clinic services, and other selected aspects of medicaid
Title XX: Social Services

CHAPTER 13

FAMILY HEALTH NURSING: THE MIDDLE YEARS

The middle years between the ages of 40 and 65 are as filled with change and stress as the years for younger age groups. The way a family functions in maintaining health and coping with illness is directly related to issues and problems adults need to confront during these years. The concepts of youth as vitality and growth and old age as vulnerable and withering, prevalent in our society, add to the burden of middle age.

There are basic biophysical, social, and emotional changes that evolve in an orderly sequence as part of the "life cycle" that Livinson describes as common to all man.[1] He and other researchers have divided the adult years into early adulthood (20–30), settling-down years (30–40), midlife transition (40–50), and the culminating years (50–60).[2, 3]

For most adults, there are periods of disequilibrium due to personalized review of where the individual is, what he has done, where he can go, and the disparity between dreams and reality.

PHYSICAL CHANGES

Persons in the 40 to 60 age group are caught between aging pains and growing pains. Their bodies may be telling them to slow down while they feel the pressure of less time. Hair begins to turn gray; skin becomes dry and wrinkled, and there may be decreased muscle tone.

Studies in biophysical changes have documented normal aging to include a progressive decrease in bone density, a 30 per cent decrease in cardiac output, a 50 per cent decrease in maximum breathing capacity, a decrease in esophageal and gastric mobility, and a 50 per cent decrease in the basal metabolic rate. There is also a decrease in deep sleep, and a gradual diminishing of sexual function, although this varies with the opportunity for regular sexual expression.[4, 5, 6]

People may become excessively involved in body monitoring, experimenting with exercise programs, jogging, and faddish diets in an effort to allay signs of aging.

Women must adjust to the physical and psychologic changes that accompany menopause. For most women, this occurs at about age 50 and continues until the ovaries stop producing estrogen and progesterone. The changing hormone level results in vasomotor instability (hot flashes), numbness in extremities, cold hands and feet, and headaches. Irregular menstrual cycles with decreased flow, spotting, and skipped periods is another sign of menopause.[7] Emotional lability — i.e., sudden changes of mood and depression — frequently accompany menopause. Family members may be confused by these changes if they are not assured that this is normal and related to hormonal imbalance.[8]

SOCIAL CHANGES

There are considerable social pressures for persons in the 40 to 65 age group that result in increased mental strain and frustration. These pressures will be discussed in terms of changing family roles, work, and civic and social responsibilities.

Changing Family Roles. This is the time when children are moving away from home and striking out to seek their own identities, leaving parents to feel rejected and confused. The "empty nest" syndrome is especially difficult for women who have not cultivated interests outside the home. For the working mother, children moving into adulthood may be a "blessed relief," allowing her more time for her own career. Launching children into integrated adult lives is difficult and frequently associated with increased economic pressure as well as emotional strain.

It is common for marital relationships to be tense during this age period. In a study by Lurie, only 42 per cent of "empty nest" women viewed their spouses positively compared to 80 per cent in other age groups.[9]

Many women in their mid-years are returning to a profession or finding their first opportunities for advancement. This, too, can be a strain on marital relationships. Divorce rates increase most rapidly for those over 30. Studies have also shown that extramarital relationships are more common in this age group.[10]

If the child rearing years have not been shared, couples may find themselves in the middle years with very little in common and, with children gone, with no real reason for maintaining a relationship.

Couples in middle years must also work through changing relationships with aging parents. Aging parents may become ill, need physical care as well as economic support from their children and, in other aspects of daily living, may be dependent on the middle aged couple.

This role reversal is made more difficult if there are "left-over" feelings of not living up to parent's expectations, anger, and guilt. Community health nurses are often confronted with what seems to be lack of concern on the part of children in caring for their older parents. The problem may not be lack of caring so much as the need for resolving old parent-child relationships.

Work and Career Roles. Men are especially tied to work and achievement of career goals, although an increasing number of women have aspirations outside the family. Studies have shown this to be a time of introspection, self-evaluation, increased reflection, and recapitulation of previous experience.[11]

A persons' feeling of self-worth and status is directly related to the work they do. Industrial workers, persons with disorderly job changes, and those with frequent unemployment records have less attachment to work as part of their self-concept.[12]

People in their middle years may feel they have reached a plateau in their careers, that opportunities for advancement are given to younger persons. It is more difficult to find work if one loses a job.

On the other hand, a study by Dennis shows the years between 40 and 60 to be the most productive in terms of creative output.[13] Persons in this age group are in control of economic life for old and young. Many feel they are at the forefront of their careers — able to use a wide array of strategies and skills, able to manipulate the environment, and, in general to excel in many directions.

Civic and Social Responsibilities. The evaluation of personal goals and values may lead to a more active role in civic and social organizations. Middle-aged people often seek posts of leadership that give vent to their need for recognition and an arena for expressing social values and expanding latent talents beyond the job and family.

EMOTIONAL CHANGES

All changes have an emotional, social, and physical component. The changing time perspective, plans for retirement and leisure, and fear of widowhood and death of friends are a few of the major emotional issues that makes a direct impact on life style for this age group.

Around age 40, one begins to count years in terms of amount of time left to live rather than time since birth. The middle-aged person begins to note that young adults look like children to them and that these children are treating them with deference. Theirs is a younger generation of which one is not a part. This change in time frame can be very upsetting to a person who still sees himself as "young."

Planning for retirement becomes a necessity instead of a far-off unrelated event. The "rite of passage" is seen by many as moving from productive maturity to non-productive old age. Men may not want to give up this important part of their self-image. The woman who has moved from school to workplace to kitchen and back to workplace may not be ready for retirement at 65. She may feel she is just beginning. Depending on an individual's resources, the economic and social consequences are also substantial.

Some corporations and employers have started special classes to help workers prepare for retirement. Information about social security benefits, second career opportunities (paid and volunteer), health maintenance, and financial planning are frequent topics discussed.

The effort of filling leisure time is difficult for some people. Without the structure of work, they find it difficult to organize their lives.

Another very real concern for people in the middle years is fear of widowhood and loss of friends. Widowed persons, usually women, were heads of households 80 per cent of the time in the 1970 census.[14] A wife may nag her husband to exercise, lose weight, and stop smoking in attempts to "keep him healthy."

There is pressure to re-examine goals and values when close friends die or become seriously ill. Reaction to usual life stresses may change and normal aches and pains become magnified due to fears of "something serious."

NURSING IMPLICATIONS

The specific knowledge based on physical changes and developmental tasks in the adult years is widening, increasing the potential impact of nursing intervention. As with other stages of family and individual development, the community health nurse is in a key position to use this knowledge in assisting families in their adjustment to change, maintenance of health, prevention of illness, and adaptation to disease.

Family function is directly related to the normal stresses of the adult years. The community health nurse can help families by explaining the stages of development during the middle years, by helping all members of the family express feelings, and by supporting work toward positive resolution of problems. When counseling adolescents in a clinic or school health program, the nurse will need to understand the reactions of middle-aged parents to their childrens' problems and intrepret these to the child. If the wage-earner develops a chronic disease requiring care by a frustrated spouse, it may be necessary to express feelings of guilt and dissatisfactions with other aspects of life before coping with the disease process can occur.

By increasing a person's self-awareness, the nurse can sometimes assist in the developmental process. Seeing stress as "usual for one's age" can make problems more possible to live with, given life a more reasonable perspective, and help in the process of acceptance of the many changes during this period.

The middle years are important in terms of preventive programs for physical and emotional diseases. A regular exercise program using daily activities to best advantage is helpful, as is a diet lower in caloric intake. Sporadic exercise and over-eating are risk factors for disease. The importance of a well-regulated exercise program and prudent diet undertaken with medical guidance cannot be over-emphasized. Regular medical exams or attendance at adult health clinics may hold the greatest benefit for this age group. Through assessment of body systems, vital signs, blood pressure, blood and urine tests, sigmoidoscopy and chest x-ray exam, the physician can proceed with early detection of common diseases for this age group. Diagnosis of adult diabetes, cancer, and cardiovascular diseases can be made with better prognosis for treatment. Self-examinations of the breast and detection of signs and symptoms of cancer of the prostate and the uterus can be taught, as can the early signs of heart disease. Persons need to be encouraged to participate in screening programs, — such as those for high blood pressure for stroke and hypertension and pap smears for cancer of the cervix — and to continue with routine maintanence for eyes, ears, and dental care. Glaucoma, hearing loss, and peridontal disease can be treated or prevented if detected early.

Fatigue and anxiety may result in depression or chronic irritability. The community health nurse must be ready to discuss and explore the reasons for these feelings and help the family see the direct effect of life style on emotional and physical health. Too much introspection and involvement in self may cause depression as well. The community health nurse, with assistance from other community resources, may be able to help individuals into useful community volunteer programs that increase self-esteem while helping others.

The increased intake of drugs, tobacco, and alcohol is a common method used in attempting to cope with the stresses of middle age. Behavior patterns are difficult to change, but the community health nurse can be alert to opportunities for reinforcing health teaching in these areas.

Acute illness during the middle years is frequently associated with stress. Coronary heart disease, ulcers, colitis and low back pain are a few common diseases with a strong emotional component. Besides assisting families in obtaining care and working out treatment routines, the community health nurse can help families focus on the problem causing the stress.

Mortality and morbidity from the major chronic diseases increase rapidly during this age period. Table 13–1 shows the death rates for selected diseases in this age group. Cardiovascular diseases and malignant neoplasm account for the greatest number of deaths in all age groups. Along with arthritis and rheumatism, they also account for a large percentage of the morbidity during the middle years.[15]

The changes in life style necessitated by the presence of one or

Table 13-1 DEATH FROM SELECTED DISEASES BY AGE IN U.S.—1977°

Disease	35 to 44 Rate	45 to 54 Rate	55 to 64 Rate
Neoplasms—All	50.9	182.5	440.5
digestive organs	8.9	36.1	105.6
respiratory system	10.6	55.1	137.3
breast	8.9	27.0	44.1
genital organs	5.0	15.0	39.7
Diabetes mellitus	3.7	9.6	27.2
Major cardiovascular disease	62.3	230.8	636.7
Ischemic heart disease	38.4	166.3	466.5
Cerebrovascular disease	10.3	28.7	79.5
Cirrhosis of liver	15.3	33.8	45.4
All accidents (other than auto)	18.9	22.6	28.9
Suicides	16.8	18.9	19.4

°Rate per 100,000 estimated population in specific group.
From National Center for Health Statistics: *Monthly Vital Statistic Report, Final Mortality Statistics*—1977. Washington, D.C., U.S. Government Printing Office, (PHS) 79–1120, May 1979.

more of these diseases can be overwhelming to a family. Family coping strengths will be diminished and rehabilitation difficult if there is too much conflict in the home from other common stresses. Perhaps that fundamental skill of "good listening," accompanied with concrete assistance in care of the sick, can help the family most in their efforts in adapting to chronic disease. The skills inherent in the nursing process must be used in helping families in this difficult adjustment.

Change is unpredictable, making the middle-aged family vulnerable to the unknown. This may be painful to some, and challenging to others. If adult years are dominated by disorganization, poverty, unemployment, and oppressive work, energies must go to surviving rather than restructuring life values. The nurse needs to be an articulate advocate for changing social and work institutions in our society, in light of known adult needs. The needs of the middle-aged family must be viewed as part of the total community system.

REFERENCES

1. Livinson, D., et al.: *The Seasons of a Man's Life.* New York, Alfred Knopf, 1978.
2. See also Neugarten, B.: *Middle Age and Aging.* Chicago, University of Chicago Press, 1968, Chapters 1 and 2.
3. Gould, R.: *Transformations.* New York, Simon and Schuster, 1978.
4. Smith, D., Bierman, E. C., and Robinson, N. M. (eds.): *Biologic Ages of Man: From Conception through Old Age,* 2nd ed. Philadelphia, W. B. Saunders Co., 1978.
5. Masters, W. H., and Johnson, V. E.: *Human Sexual Inadequacy.* Boston, Little, Brown & Co., 1970.
6. Kirkendall, L. A., and Rubin, I.: *Sexuality and the Life Cycle.* Study Guide No. 8., New York, SIECUS, 1969.

7. Cali, R. W.: Management of the climacteric and postmenopausal woman. Med. Clin. North Am., 56:789, 1972.
8. Galloway, K.: The change of life. Am. J. Nurs., 75:1006, 1975.
9. Lurie, E.: Sex and stage differences in perceptions of marital and family relationships. J. Marr. Fam., 36:260, 1974.
10. Kinsey, A. C.: *Sexual Behavior in the Human Female*. Philadelphia, W. B. Saunders Co., 1953, p. 417.
11. Neugarten, p. 139; Livinson, p. 60.
12. Wilensky: in Neugarten, p. 321.
13. Dennis, W.: in Neugarten, p. 106.
14. U.S. Bureau of the Census: *Marital Status and Living Arrangements*. Washington D.C., Current Population Reports, Series P-20, No., 242, 1972.
15. U.S. Department of Health, Education, and Welfare: *Limitation of Activity and Mobility Due to Chronic Diseases — 1972*. Washington, D.C., Vital and Health Statistics Series 10–96, 1974.

SUGGESTED READINGS

Bahnson, C. B., and Cassel, J.: Behavioral factors associated with the etiology of physical disease, Am. J. Pub. Health, 64:1033, 1974.
Diekelmann, N., et al.: The middle years — parts 1–8. Am. J. Nurs., 75:994, 1975.
Diekelmann, N.: *Primary Health Care of the Well Adult*. New York, McGraw Hill Book Co. (Blakiston), 1977.
Dresen, S.: The middle years: The sexually active middle adult. Am. J. Nurs., 75:1001, 1975.
Duvall, E.: *Family Development*, 5th ed., Philadelphia, J. B. Lippincott Co., 1977, Chapter 14.
Galton, L.: *The Silent Disease: Hypertension*. New York, Crown Publishers, 1973.
Gould, R.: *Transformations*. New York, Simon and Schuster, 1978.
Hargreaves, A. G.: Making the most of the middle years. Am. J. Nurs., 75:1761, 1975.
Livinson, D., et al.: *The Seasons of A Man's Life*. New York, Alfred Knopf, 1978.
Lowenthal, M., and Chiriboga, D.: Transition to the empty nest: Crisis, challenge, or relief? Arch. Gen. Psychiatry, 26:8, 1972.
Mead, M.: *Culture and Commitment: A Study of the Generation Gap*. New York, Natural History Press/Doubleday and Co., Inc., 1970.
Miller, Michael: Seeking advice for cancer symptoms. Am. J. Pub. Health, 63:955, 1973.
Murray, Ruth: Body image development in adulthood. Nurs. Clin. North Am., 7:622, 1972.
Neugarten, Bernice: The awareness of middle age. In Neugarten, B. (ed.), *Middle Age and Aging*, Chicago, University of Chicago Press, 1968.
Peplau, H. E.: Mid-life crises. Am. J. Nurs., 75:1761, 1975.
Smith, D., Bierman, E., and Robinson, N.: *Biologic Ages of Man: Conception Through Old Age*, 2nd ed., Philadelphia, W. B. Saunders Co., 1978.
Stevenson, Joanne S.: *Issues and Crises During Middlescence*. New York, Appleton Century Crofts, 1977.
Streib, G. F., and Schneider, C. J.: *Retirement in American Society: Impact and Process*. Ithaca, N.Y., Cornell University Press, 1971.
Wang, Mamie K.: A health maintenance service for chronically ill patients. Am. J. Pub. Health, 60:713, 1970.

RESOURCES

American Association of Retired Persons
  1225 Connecticut Avenue, N.W.
  Washington, D.C. 20036

American Heart Association
7320 Greenville Ave., Dallas, Texas 75231
(Cardiopulmonary resuscitation courses, diet counseling, smoking withdrawal programs, stroke clubs)

Local Educational Institutions
(Continuing education programs)

Local Industries and Unions
(Programs for preparing for retirement)

Metropolitan Life Insurance Co.
(Information on disease prevention)
One Madison Ave.
New York, N.Y. 10010

CHAPTER 14

FAMILY HEALTH NURSING CARE: THE AGING FAMILY

In some cultures, the aged are accorded great respect and favor. Aging is a dignified and not unwelcome prelude to a peaceful death.[1] In some technically advanced societies, however, an opposite view often prevails. "Ageism" — the unreasoning belief that people who achieve a specified age are automatically different and of less worth than their juniors — is far too prevalent. The aged are stereotyped as feeble, incapable of work, sick, asexual, childlike, and unable to make decisions for themselves. This public attitude does much to shape the nursing problems of older families.

Physical changes are, of course, expected and inevitable. But far too often they are hastened by incongruous expectations that discourage dependency-delaying tactics. The economic disadvantage among the elderly still further impedes the realization of optimum health and independence.

The reality is that people differ widely in the occurrence and pattern of aging symptoms and that most elders do not need intensive care. In 1977 only 5 per cent of those 65 or older were in nursing homes or other institutions, the remaining 95 per cent were in their own communities and, for the most part, maintaining their own households.[2, 3] While this condition may reflect inadequacy of facilities rather than the absence of need, it suggests a high level of potential demand for noninstitutional assistance. Many physical or behavioral problems are not due to the physical condition itself but to social mobility or economic conditions that are correctable.[4]

SOCIAL CONTEXT

Socioeconomic issues affect families along several fronts. These include retirement, diminished family size, transportation, general housing, and clothing.

266

Retirement. Most people stop working at or before age 65. (Recent legislation advancing the mandatory retirement age to 70 may change this.) Retirement is welcomed by some — especially for those whose work held no particular challenge or rewards and for those who have developed strong lateral interests such as gardening, volunteer work, travel, or the arts. For most, however, retirement means a loss of identity and, often, a negative self-image. It is difficult for many retirees to find essential duties to perform.[5]

Retirement almost always means a reduction in income. Annuities and social security payments are likely to be much smaller than the previous salary.[6, 7] Even with cost of living adjustments, families dependent on fixed incomes must live frugally to survive, particularly when threatened with overall inflation. Also, decreasing resources tend to make one feel weak and vulnerable.

Diminished Family Size. The death of friends and family further decrease support during critical periods. Couples become more interdependent after retirement, and the loss of a spouse is extraordinarily stressful, especially if the couple had been living in an single-family dwelling rather than a group facility. The loss of close friends who represented family can cause as much grief as the loss of a family member. Often, children or extended family members live far away, possibly because of job requirements, or because the retiree has chosen to live in a more salubrious climate. Feelings of loneliness and isolation are often expressed by the elderly.

Transportation. Nonadaptive environments also increase the problems of the elderly. Inadequate transportation, inaccessible shops, or inflexible service facilities may make life more difficult. Buses or rapid transportation systems are often designed for the young and fleet of foot, with steps too high, hand-holds unreachable, or doors that close too quickly. Shopping markets are often far away or located in centers accessible only by car. As a consequence, the elderly may become dependent on others for shopping or must buy in expensive neighborhood convenience stores.

General Housing. Housing may be similarly nonadaptive, except in segregated areas. Lack of ramps, inadequate handrails, awkward kitchen storage, and poorly secured doors in high crime areas may needlessly endanger the older resident. Neighborhoods, as well as people, change from "young married" to elderly populations; from well-off to substandard. Neighbors move away or die; churches relocate; crime increases; and "mom and pop" stores at the corner give up to the less accessible and less adaptable supermarket. The young and sociable friendly visitors of the past are now career women with little time for charitable or friendly responses to their community elderly. Visiting nurse services are increasingly expensive and unavailable to those who do not qualify for compensation services or who need intensive technical care. The community health nurse finds herself in the business of creating a community substitute. The support structure crumbles.

Things "give out" and sometimes replacements are beyond the means of the family. Lumpy mattresses, wobbly chairs, and dim lighting are hazardous to health and demeaning to the human spirit.

Clothing. This is another basic human need that may cause problems for the elderly. Because of the elderly person's limited range of motion, the way in which sleeves are put in, the location of zippers, and the basic design become very important. Selections and colors are almost always limited and costs are high. Being able to dress oneself and feel good about physical appearance are essential for a positive self-image.

It is apparent that geriatric health care must provide more than medical care. The socioeconomic and psychologic aspects of care that exert either positive or negative influences will be the decisive factors in how well the elderly cope with the aging process.

SOME COMMON PROBLEMS AND THEIR IMPLICATIONS FOR COMMUNITY HEALTH NURSING

Four areas of community health nursing concerns commonly found with elderly clientele will be discussed as typical of the myriad health problems that occur: (1) the prevention and management of illness, (2) the maintenance of general health and nutrition, (3) the prevention of accidents, and (4) combatting ageism. (See Chapter 24, Long Term Illness.)

The management of illness or disability is an almost universal problem among the aged population, especially in the later decades of senescence. Of the more than 20 million Americans over 65, 80 per cent reported one or more chronic illnesses requiring medical supervision.[8]

Within the elderly age group, the proportion of people 75 years and over is getting larger. In 1970, those 75 years and over accounted for 38 per cent of those 65 and over. By the year 2000, it is expected that about 45 per cent of the older population will be 75 years old and over.[9]

The prevalence of chronic conditions and the utilization of health services increase more rapidly after age 75. Thus, it is likely there will be an increased need for care of illness within this age group, if they are to continue to lead active lives.

The primary community approach to control disease at all ages is to prevent its occurrence whenever possible, and to minimize its affects through aversive action.

Periodic health examinations, usually annual, are important for those 65 and over. This examination may be performed by a physician or other qualified health professional and backed by laboratory support. Such an examination may reveal pre-morbid conditions, such as heightened blood pressure, or changes in cardiac rhythms that may be dealt with before disease is present.

Immunization — especially against certain influenza strains — is often recommended. The exact proposals change from time to time, the local health authority or the patient's medical advisor can advise on this. Anticipatory discussion and practice for the older person (or those caring for the elderly) may lead to faster and better response in an emergency or in early recognition of disease. "CPR" (cardio-pulmonary resuscitation) classes are available in many communities. Courses that include recognition and care of stroke and simple first aid are useful, and are often a good social experience as well.

When disease is present, it must be recognized and dealt with. There are common problems that every family faces in this process.

Acceptance and Adaptation to the Demands of Chronic Disease. There is a tendency to deny illness or to take the fatalistic attitude that since one will die anyway there is no use in fighting back. This is especially true when regimens are complex or the client doesn't believe in the effectiveness of treatment. The person with emphysema may continue to smoke, ignoring advice and disputing the basis of care. A diabetic will return repeatedly to the hospital because he or she has ignored a prescribed diet. The community health nurse can assist families by simplifying regimens as much as possible, adapting treatment to existing life styles, and teaching family members how to be helpful without being over-protective. Sometimes talking with another person who is coping with a similar problem can be helpful to patients and their families.

Assuring Adequate Health Surveillance and Continuity of Care. Surveillance systems must include periodic professional estimates of change in condition and reaction to therapy as well as continuing systematic appraisal by family or neighbors. Some regular contact is especially important for couples in which both husband and wife have impairments or for the elderly person living alone. Physical disabilities such as poor vision or hearing or lack of strength increase the problems of self-care. Fear of going outside in high crime areas also produces a need for care. Sensory deterioration may cause elderly clients to miss symptoms of impaired function such as a bruise or pain during a cardiac episode. Careful monitoring and firsthand observing by nursing personnel are essential. Nurses with extra skill in gerontology may take responsibility for health surveillance in the families' home environment. Medical supervision has traditionally meant getting the patient to the medical source — involving social services, transportation services, and an interested person serving as ombudsman and aide to see that the patient receives required care. The community health nurse can help coordinate these activities. Some agencies find patient-classification systems that document coping level and/or physical function helpful in planning and monitoring care.[11]

Monitoring Drug Usage. Most elderly clients have more than one disease and have complex medication schedules. Monitoring drug usage for medication errors, for efficacy, for toxic effects from prolonged usage, and for antagonistic effects with prescribed as well as over-the-counter drugs will always be difficult. Drugs that are well tolerated by younger persons may cause exaggerated or ineffective responses in the elderly because of slower absorbtion, slower circulation, and decreased kidney function. Confusion may be due to toxicity or electrolyte disturbance. The frequency of errors in drug taking among the elderly has been shown to be as high as 59 per cent, including errors of commission, ommission, erratic dosage, and/or overdose.[12, 13] The community health nurse must inform herself of the side effects of commonly used drugs such as Digitalis, diuretics, and sedatives and have a quick and current reference source to check others.[14]

The development of consultant back up is imperative. Drug committees made up of pharmacists and physicians may be helpful. Agency policy needs to be clear regarding discontinuation as well as administration of drugs ordered by physicians. There is a tendency, once a drug has been prescribed, to continue the prescription for life.[15]

Maintaining Family and Neighbor Support Systems. The community health nurse can supervise and supplement the personal and therapeutic care given by family members and others. An elderly man may be able to care for his bedridden spouse, but may need help with procedures to prevent bedsores, or advice on good body mechanics when moving his spouse from wheelchair to bed. Observational skills of the caring person may need to be bolstered with specific information and "how to" demonstrations. People providing care also need relief from these duties. Often the care provider is also elderly and has problems of his or her own. The community health nurse needs to be supportive of both and to keep a diligent eye on the changing capacity of care providers.

Management of Crisis. The community health nurse must check to see that the patient and support group are organized for potential emergencies. There should be a clear plan of what to do and who to call if there is a sudden change in condition — the physician, a neighbor, or an agency center. This alert system needs to be reviewed periodically.

Financing of Health Care. Families may need help in understanding the benefits and limitations of their insurance programs, whether Medicare, Medicaid, or one of a variety of private insurance services. The community health nurse should be sure her own information is current with respect to community resources. Other possible sources of help are the local welfare agencies, health department, and senior citizen centers or special interest groups such as AARP (American Association of Retired Persons).

The community health nurse who is directly or partially responsible for personal care services should keep in particularly close contact with the local social security office personnel, in order to assist families and also to enlist the aid of the social security personnel in explaining the benefits to which the client is entitled.

THE MAINTENANCE OF GENERAL
HEALTH AND NUTRITION

Most elderly persons in our society are amazingly adept at managing the changes of physical functioning that occur with aging, and continue to lead a normal life, often with zest and energy. For many, it is the renaissance of heightened awareness, when a person can reflect on what has been and use this information for continued development and planning for the future. The important element seems to be the balance between physical activity, social activities, rest, and stress. Exercise, passive or active, is important for health maintenance. A recent Health, Education, and Welfare pamphlet outlines various methods of exercising for older individuals.[16] The community health nurse can assist clients in selecting activities suitable for them, encouraging continued walks and the learning of new activities.

Regular contact with family and friends helps people to feel a part of society. Maintaining interest in people outside the family, such as participants in political, social, or civic concerns, affords new interests as well as refining old ones and helps to achieve new goals and values. Active listening, supporting the investigation of new ideas, and obtaining books from the library (in large print if possible) may be all that is needed on the part of the nurse. Nurses may also help elderly clients by being aware of the normality of sexual drives among the elderly and providing for discussion of physiological and emotional constraints. Discussion of possible modification of sexual techniques to adapt to physiologic change or impairments can provide practical support. Referring to resources may be helpful in developing appropriate sexual skills.[17]

The advent of "Social Security Sin" — cohabitation among elderly social security beneficiaries, since marriage would result in a decrease in benefits — was a response to insensitivity of administrators of the sexual needs of the elderly. (This problem has since been corrected.)

Patterns of rest and stress have a large impact on overall health. The community health nurse can assist clients in planning the day around resting needs, using times of peak energy to their best advantage, and making sure rest times are not disturbed. Eliminating stress is more difficult. If stress is environmental (sound, light, color, and crowding), the nurse may help to secure change. Other sources of stress and frustration caused by living style or physical and mental impairment are more difficult to control, but helping the person recognize and understand stressful situations clearly can be helpful.

Maintenance of adequate nutritional practices is frequently beyond the capability of the aging family. Difficulties in shopping may limit the types and quantity of food available. Many stores do not package meats and vegetables in small enough quantity for one or two people. Lack of

272 / FAMILY HEALTH NURSING CARE: THE AGING FAMILY

sufficient income all too often leads to poor food choices — paying the rent may take precedence over buying nutritious, fresh foods. Inadequate storage and cooking equipment can also be a problem, especially for those living in rented rooms, in single occupancy dwellings, in deteriorated hotels, and in delapidated housing they cannot afford to leave or repair. The skyrocketing cost of electricity and gas may force some families to use makeshift heating and cooking sources that may be unsafe or grossly inadequate. Hot lunches provided by the community may supplement home-cooked foods. Poor housekeeping practices, either habitual or a recent sign of depleted energy, may lead to food spoilage. There may be a general loss of appetite due to poorly fitted dentures, restricted activity, constipation, and restrictive (low salt) diets.

Nursing intervention may be helpful in locating ways to shop and extend available food, in changing consumer behavior, in recruiting shopping and housekeeping assistance, and in using community resources such as Meals on Wheels and supplemental food programs such as the National Food Stamp program.

Watching the "reduced for quick sale" merchandise, using day old bread, and taking advantage of specials can help stretch the food budget. Support in taking an assertive stand with supermarkets — either individually or as an organized group — is often helpful in obtaining smaller quantity packaging. Store managers can suggest a time for shopping that will suit the special needs of the elderly. Community agencies may provide bus services to larger stores. The recruitment of shoppers or household aides will differ in every community. There may be organized home health aide programs operating within the agency in which the nurse is working or under other auspices. Informal sources or methods may also help. "Adopt a grandparent" programs provide an opportunity for a continuing relation between visitors and families who benefit from the human contact as well as the specific services provided. Church groups and schools may be interested in helping young people to learn more about their communities and to deal with intergeneration relationships. Informal connections often develop and can be encouraged. For example, one man of 80 shopped twice a week for "his three ladies" who were unable to shop for themselves.

Nurses can help locate sources for repairing dentures and for routine dental work. Sometimes the local dental auxilliary can be of assistance. Using dental school clinics may also provide less expensive care.

Increasing fluid intake and selecting fresh fruits and vegetables can help alleviate constipation. Appetite can be stimulated and balanced diets promoted by using attractive presentation of food, variety, different spices and by adapting special diets to personal and cultural tastes.[18, 19]

Prevention of Accidents

The prevention of accidents involves both the management of the environment so as to minimize the risk, and development of behavior patterns that are conducive to safety. In both instances, developing a "safe" environment or habits for the elderly may require methods different from those for younger groups, to compensate for sensory loss and slowed or unsteady reactions to danger.

In the home, falls and burns are major hazards for the elderly. Problems may be identified by analysis of every day activities and the equipment used for each activity in relation to the surrounding in which the activity takes place. Bathrooms should be considered risk areas for those with motor difficulties, susceptibility to giddiness, or low levels of energy. In general, hot tub baths should be avoided and baths should be scheduled so someone is within call in case of trouble. Walk-in showers are easier to use, provided the heat of the water supply is steady. The local gas and electric company can be helpful in checking stoves, heaters, and the dependability of pilot lights. With outdoor activities such as gardening or mowing the lawn, the safety of equipment should also be considered as well as the energy it requires for operation.

Frequently encountered hazards are: torn or worn carpets, especially on landings, inadequate hall lighting, lack of secure hand rails on stairs and hand grips in bath tubs, and poorly secured doors and windows in high crime areas. All small equipment such as toasters, irons, and lamps should be checked for faulty wiring.

Even when the environment is as safe as possible, careless behavior may create hazards. Storing utensils or food in areas that require reaching across a stove, climbing a wobbly stool, or wearing unsuitable clothing can cause accidents. Being too impatient and trying to work too fast can easily lead to disaster.

Street accidents present much the same combination of environmental and behavioral factors. If traffic lights change too quickly, it may be impossible for an elderly person to cross a busy street safely. Littered streets or alleys may cause stumbling. If crime rates are high, the safest daylight hours should be chosen, known trouble spots avoided, and walking confined to the curb side of the sidewalk. The community health nurse can help by documenting trouble spots and bringing this information to the appropriate public persons or agencies, either by representing the individual(s) or organizing ad hoc groups of individuals to present his/her own case for needed action.

Many elderly people continue to drive until very late in life, especially in rural communities. Limiting driving to daylight and non-rush hour traffic times should be encouraged. The community health nurse may alert individuals to available alternatives when weather is foul and encourage the use of streets with less traffic and with traffic control lights. Loss of driving privileges is a bleak reminder of approaching dependency, and the nurse may need to provide sympathetic support for elder citizens who can no longer drive safely.

COMBATING AGEISM

The community health nurse can be a significant contributor to understanding the needs of the elderly and combating ageism. In working with families and other helping agencies, the community health nurse can alert others to the negative affect of treating older people as though they were children, over-protecting the handicapped individual, or assuming that all people over 65 will act alike.

The nurse may involve different age groups in working with the elderly, in both service and educational settings. Nursery schools may spend time and share activities with a nursing home population. Community organizations or school groups may be interested in direct service projects with the elderly. Skills and knowledge of elderly persons may be tapped for the needs of the younger generation. For instance, in the *Foxfire* projects, a group of young people visited elderly citizens and collected historical information about the way mountain people lived and worked, adding to living history while learning to appreciate the contributions of the elderly.[20]

RESOURCES FOR CARE

The paucity of resources for care of the aging is striking. Too few professional personnel are alert to the needs of elderly families. Public health agencies need to be more rigorous in case finding, especially for adults over 75 years of age, women, and those confined to their homes.[21] The community health nurse could work cooperatively with physicians in providing care, health teaching, and continuing observation of the chronically ill. The nurse may participate in the establishment of well-adult clinics for health screening and teaching, and help organize older citizen groups for purposes of teaching, sharing, and counseling.[22]

Day-care centers for the aging are increasing in number. Some of these are essentially therapeutic — individuals come to the center for necessary treatments, but live at home. These centers are usually controlled and staffed by a hospital or similar facility. Another type of day-care facility is directed primarily toward meeting the social needs of the older group. These facilities may provide health advice, low-cost hot meals, work on handicraft skills, and social and recreational activities for their patrons. These centers are usually community-based and linked with other programs (such as general health surveillance or case finding measures). The staff is likely to be largely volunteer.

The community health nurse may help in stating the needs for such facilities when they are not available; to advise with hospital-linked staff or volunteers on available resources for referral, to develop screening measures to reach this group regularly, and to offer more intensive nursing care as needed. When there is no such facility, the community health nurse may document the need for action and refer local leaders to appropriate action channels. The proliferation of residential facilities for older families from the single condominium to the large self-contained community for the elderly creates a new opportunity for community health participation in preventive and curative care. The more traditional foster home or boarding home also invites nursing participation in the support of patients and their caretakers. The community health nurse may be asked to support the patient or caretaker by demonstration and advice, to assume responsibility when more sophisticated care is required, and to interpret regulations or standards of care.

Legislators are reluctant to move decisively to improve care for the elderly because of the high costs of care and the relatively low impact of programs on the general health.[23] The community health nurse may provide essential planning data and document unmet needs, evaluate outcome of public and voluntary programs, and communicate this information to key individuals and groups. The U.S. Senate Special Committee on Aging has served as a focus for gathering information, documenting, and developing legislation for national action. The political clout of senior citizens themselves has grown as their numbers have increased, and period of activity is extended. Organizations such as the National Association of Retired Persons and the National Council of Senior Citizens have active legislative programs as well as local service activities.

Citizen groups such as Common Cause and Public Citizens, Inc., have lent support and expertise in the areas of political action, consumer protection, and legal services. There is a need for consumer protection with regard to all products, but especially in the areas of health insurance, auto insurance, unsafe drugs, questionable therapeutic devices, and unscrupulous door-to-door salesmen. There is a growing awareness of the need for legal services for the elderly to protect individuals from fraud and violence, infringement of civil liberties due to impairments (especially when an individual is unable to manage his own affairs), and the right to die naturally and with dignity.

The variety of issues, complexities of needs, and the constraints of time and money mean that the community health nurse must summon all her skills and imagination in working with the "golden years" population.

REFERENCES

1. de Beauvoir, S.: *The Coming of Age*. New York, Warner Books, Inc., 1973.
2. National Center for Health Statistics: *Health in the Later Years of Life*. Washington, D.C., U.S. Government Printing Office, Pub. No. 1722–0178, October 1971.
3. National Center for Health Statistics: *National Nursing Home Survey 1977*. Washington, D.C., U.S. Department of Health, Education, and Welfare, 1979.
4. Comfort, A.: *A Good Age*. New York, Crown, 1976.
5. Carp, F. M. (ed.): *Retirement*. New York, Behavioral Publications, Inc., 1972.
6. Social Security Administration: *Planning for the Later Years*. Washington, D.C., U.S. Government Printing Office, Pub. No. 3000 8–67.
7. Social Security Administration: *Your Social Security*. Washington, D.C., U.S. Government Printing Office, Department of Health, Education, and Welfare, Pub. No. SS1–35, 1970.
8. Committee on Nursing Care: *Nursing and Long-Term Care: Toward Quality Care of Aging*. St. Louis, Mo., American Nurses' Association, 1975, p. 19.
9. Bureau of the Census: *Projections of the Population of the U.S., 1977–2050*. Washington, D.C., U.S. Government Printing Office, Current Population Reports, Series P–25, Pub. No. 704, July 1977.
10. Caring for the Aged: An AJN Feature. Am. J. Nurs., 73:2049, 1973.
11. Katz, S., et al.: Studies in illness in the aged — the index of ADL, A standardized measure of biological and physiological function. J.A.M.A., 185:914, 1963.
12. Kayne, R. C.: Drugs and the aged. *In* Burnside, I. M.: *Nursing the Aged*. New York, McGraw-Hill Book Co., 1976.
13. Schwartz, D., et al.: Medication errors made by the elderly, chronically ill patients. Am. J. Pub. Health, 52:2018, 1962.
14. Roberts, J., et al.: *Pharmacological Intervention in the Aging Process*. New York, Plenum Press, 1978.
15. Judge, T. G., and Caird, F. I.: *Drug Treatment of the Elderly Patient*. Kent, Eng., Pitman Medical, 1978.
16. U.S. Department of Health, Education, and Welfare, National Institutes of Health, Office of Human Development: *The Fitness Challenge*. Washington, D.C., U.S. Government Printing Office, Pub. No. OHD 75–20802, 1975.
17. Butler, R.: *Sex Over 60*. New York, Harper and Row, 1976.
18. Schroeder, H. A.: Nutrition. *In* Cowdy, E. V., and Franz, U.S.: *Care of the Geriatric Patient*. St. Louis, Mo., C.V. Mosby Co., 1971.
19. U.S. Department of Agriculture: *Food Guide for Older Folks*. Washington, D.C., U.S. Government Printing Office, 1975.
20. Eliot, E.; *The Foxfire Book*, Vols. I–V. Garden City, NY, Doubleday and Co., 1972.
21. Managan, D., et al.: Older adults: A community survey of health needs. Nurs. Res., 23:426, 1974.
22. Anderson, E. G.: Senior citizens' health conferences. Nurs. Outlook, 21:580, 1973.
23. Trager, B.: Home health services and health insurance. Med. Care, 9:89, 1971.

SUGGESTED READINGS

Aiken, L.: *Later Life*, Philadelphia, W.B. Saunders Co., 1978.
Alfano, G.: There are no routine patients. Am. J. Nurs., 75:1804, 1975.
Atchley, R. C.: *The Social Forces in Later Life*, 2nd ed. Belmont, Ca., Wadsworth, 1977.
Binstock, R. H., and Shanos, E. (eds.): *Handbook of Aging and the Social Sciences*. New York, Van Nostrand Reinhold Co., 1977.
Burnside, I. M. (ed.): *Working With the Elderly: Group Process and Techniques*. North Scituate, Mass., Duxbury Press, 1978.
Butler, R. N., and Lewis, N. E.: *Aging and Mental Health*, 2nd ed. St. Louis, Mosby, 1977.
Costello, M.: Sex, intimacy, and aging. Am. J. Nurs. 75:1330, 1975.
Davies, L.: Attitudes toward old age and aging as shown by humor. The Gerontologist, 17:220, 1977.
Duvall, E.: *Family Development*, 5th ed. Philadelphia, J. B. Lippincott Co., 1977.

Eliopoulos, C.: *Gerontological Nursing.* New York, Harper & Row, 1979.

Eliopoulos, C.: Assessment and action in gerontological nursing. Fam. Comm. Health, *1*:81, 1978.

Hayflick, L.: The cell biology of human aging. New Engl. J. Med., *295*:1302, 1976.

Hess, P., and Day, C.: *Understanding the Aging Patient.* The Robert J. Brody Co. (Prentice Hall), Bowie, Md., 1977.

International Federation on Aging: *Home Help Services for the Aging Around the World.* Washington, D.C., International Federation on Aging, 1975.

Keith, P.: A preliminary investigation of the role of public health nurses in evaluation of services for the aged. Am. J. Pub. Health, 66:379, 1976.

Kubler-Ross, E.: *Death: The Final Stage of Growth.* Englewood Cliffs, N.J., Prentice Hall, 1975.

Managan, D., et al.: Older adults: A community survey of health needs. Nurs. Res., *23*:5, 1974.

Miller, M. A.: Remotivation therapy: A way to reach the confused elderly patient. J. Gerontol. Nurs., *1*:28, 1975.

Moss, F. E., and Halamandaris, V. J.: *Too Old, Too Sick, Too Bad.* Germantown, Md., Aspen Systems Corp., 1977.

Murray, R. B., and Zentner, J. P.: *Nursing Assessment and Health Promotion Through the Life Span,* 2nd ed. Englewood Cliffs, N.J., Prentice Hall, 1979, Chapters 9 and 10.

Neugarten, B. L., and Havighurst, R. J.: *Social Policy, Social Ethics and The Aging Society,* National Science Foundation (No. NSD/RA-760247), Washington, D.C., U.S. Government Printing Office, 1976.

Nodell, W., et al., Symposium on use of drugs in the elderly patient. Med. Clin. North Am. 29:6, 1974.

Ostfeld, A., and Gibson, D. (eds.): *Epidemiology of Aging.* Summary Report and Selected Papers, Bethesda, Md., U.S. Dept. of HEW (NIH 75-711), June, 1972.

Roberts, J., et al.: *Pharmacological Intervention in the Aging Process.* New York, Plenum Press, 1978.

Robinson, C., and Lawler, M.: *Normal and Therapeutic Nutrition,* 15th ed. New York, Macmillan, 1977.

Schwartz, D.: Safe self-medication for elderly outpatients. Am. J. Nurs., 75:1808, 1975.

Schwartz, D.: Aging and the field of nursing. *In* Riley, M. W., et al. (eds.): *Aging and Society,* Vol. 2. New York, Russell Sage Foundation, 1969.

Shanas, Ethel: Health status of older people. Am. J. Pub. Health, *64*:261, 1974.

Silverstone, B., and Hyman, H. K.: *You and Your Aging Parent.* New York, Pantheon Books (Random House), 1976.

Sorenson, A. W., and Lyon, J. L.: Nutritional epidemiology: A research approach. Fam. Comm. Health, *1*:69, 1979.

Tedrow, Jack L.: Emotional, physical and legal aspects of aging. *In* Reinhardt, A., and Quinn, M. (eds.): *Current Practice in Family Centered Community Care,* St. Louis, C.V. Mosby, 1977, pp. 261–282.

Trager, B.: Home health services and health insurance. Med. Care, 9:89, 1971.

United Nations: *International Directory of Organizations Concerned with the Aged.* New York, Department of Economic and Social Affairs, 1977.

U.S. Department of Agriculture: Food Guide for Older Folks. Washington, D.C., U.S. Government Printing Office, 1976.

U.S. Senate Special Committee on Aging: *Home Health Service in the U.S.,* by Brahma Trager, Home Health Consultant, Washington, D.C., U.S. Government Printing Office, 1972.

The White House Conference on Aging, 1971: "Toward a National Policy on Aging: Final Report," Vols. 1–2, 1973.

RESOURCES

Informal resources, such as neighbors, family members, church acquaintances or service groups, local hospital personnel, the family physician and his staff, and the school child needing participation to expand his understanding of older people, are the mainstay of the helping programs for the aging family. In addition, the organizations listed below have programs relevant to the elderly.

American Association of Homes for the Aging
   529 14th Street, N.W.
   Washington, D.C. 20004

American Association of Retired Persons
   1225 Connecticut Avenue, N.W.
   Washington, D.C. 20036

The American Geriatrics Society
   10 Columbus Circle
   New York, N.Y. 10019

American Red Cross
   17th Street between D and E, N.W.
   Washington, D.C. 20006

Center for Law and Social Policy
   1751 W Street, N.W.
   Washington, D.C. 20006

Common Cause
   2020 M Street, N.W.
   Washington, D.C. 20006

The Gerontological Society
   1 Dupont Circle
   Washington, D.C. 20036

Gray Panthers
   6342 Greene Street
   Philadelphia, Pa. 19144

International Senior Citizens Association
   11753 Wilshire Blvd.
   Los Angeles, Ca. 90025

National Committee Against Discrimination in Housing
   1425 H Street, N.W.
   Washington, D.C. 20005

National Council for Homemaker, Home Health Aide Services Inc.
   1790 Broadway
   New York, N.Y. 10019

National Council of Health Care Services
1200 First Street, N.W.
Washington, D.C. 20005

National Council of Senior Citizens
1911 K Street, N.W.
Washington, D.C. 20005

National Council on the Aging
1828 L Street, N.W.
Washington, D.C. 20036

Public Citizens, Inc.
1346 Connecticut Avenue, N.W.
Washington, D.C. 20006

U.S. Department of Health and Human Services
Government Printing Office
Washington, D.C.

Publications: *Older Americans Act of 1965 and Related Acts*
Social Security Handbook, 1974
Your Medicare Handbook, 1977
National Clearing House on Aging, *Inventory of Federal Statistical Programs*

CHAPTER 15

HEALTHY SEXUALITY: A COMPONENT OF FAMILY HEALTH

Recent emphasis on sexuality as an important dimension in health is a natural outgrowth of social and technologic change. Throughout history, attitudes toward sex have ranged from the public orgies of Imperial Rome to the starchy morals of the buttoned-up Victorians (when sex was the manly obligation of the husband and the womanly duty of the wife, pleasure was never admitted, and clear distinctions were made between legitimate and illegitimate unions). In our own century, we have gone from the titillations of the Edwardians, to the energetic promiscuity of the flapper era, to the rigid social code of the fifties, and on into the "swinging seventies." These reversals have never been absolute, however, and fortunately there have always been writers and commentators like Chaucer, Rabelais, and James Thurber to remind us that sex is still good for an occasional laugh.

At the moment, we are in the midst of a reaction to conservative ideals. Not everyone is happy about it, particularly about the more extreme manifestations, such as highly visible hard-core pornography and openly tolerated sex among teenagers. But the beneficial effects of this relaxed attitude are considerable — if only because, for the first time, some of the darker and sadder aspects of sex are being brought out into the open. The community health nurse should include good sexual adjustment as one of the criteria for total family health.

Nurses themselves will vary in the degree to which they are comfortable discussing sexual matters. Nevertheless, the development of a healthy sexuality is important, and community health nurses must be cognizant of it and, when necessary either directly or through referral, institute action to improve sexual attitudes and behavior.

SEXUAL COUNSELING

The actual program of sexual counseling will be shared with counselors who are specialists in the field, teachers, clergy, and social workers. There are four main goals in such counseling:

1. To maximize the sexual adjustment of bonded couples — married or cohabiting, homosexual or heterosexual.
2. To help those engaged in casual or exploratory sexual behavior to use this experience constructively for themselves and their partners.
3 To promote socially and personally *responsible* behavior in matters relating to sex.
4. To encourage social and legislative measures to reduce discrimination against atypical minorities such as homosexuals and to assure fairness in dealing with prostitutes and sexual offenders.

Sexual Adjustment Among Established Couples

There is ample evidence that many couples, especially those well into their married years, fail to realize the potential of healthy sexuality for enriching their relationship to each other or to the general quality of their lives. The sexual experience can provide comfort, reassurance, relaxation, and pleasure to an extraordinary degree.

Yet, all too often, couples fall into dull sex patterns characterized by routine performance, unequal enjoyment, sometimes even outright displeasure or hostility. These patterns *can* be changed, but adaptation of sex behavior cannot be achieved by the application of a few technical innovations. It requires a real willingness on the part of both partners to work at it, to open their minds to exploration of new approaches, to take time to communicate fully with each other, and to recognize the egalitarian "giving" quality of effective sexual activity.

Because of the complexity and privacy of this relationship and because of the existence of many residual taboos, many couples will need professional help to accomplish desired changes.

Exploratory Sexual Experiences

For many (if not most) young people, there is a period of sexual activity that is essentially exploratory, temporary, and definitely not expected to lead to marriage. This can take many forms and be of varying duration: overt cohabitation; regular dating, including sex; combined drug and group sex episodes; or brief overnight flings with casual acquaintance (e.g., a pick-up encountered in a bar). None of this is new, although it may now be more frequent and more open.

Such experimentation may provide experience in close and sometimes demanding or complicated relationships; this is a part of growing up. The usefulness of exploratory sex will depend upon the degree to which these experiences are constructive. There are obvious dangers in the drug- and bar-associated activities that make them unlikely to lead to more lasting unions.

The Promotion of Socially and Personally Responsible Behavior

Sexual liasons (permanent, semipermanent, or transitory) must be approached *responsibly*. Both partners should accept their commitment to prevent and deal with unexpected and undesirable eventualities, such as venereal disease or unwanted pregnancy, with each partner recognizing the value of the other and striving for mutuality rather than dominance or exploitation.

Adolescents faced with strong sex urges, but not yet ready for marriage, may need help. Fortunately, teen-age marriages, which are so prone to heartbreak and disillusionment, appear to be on the decline. Frequently, these marriages are the result of sexual experimentation that inadvertently or sometimes purposely led to pregnancy. It would be helpful if the economic and managerial realities of marriage could be taught in school — not as special "sex education" lecture but as a course on the finite nature of money, the truth about genitally transmitted diseases, the obligations of parenthood, and the disadvantages of bonds that are forged too early. In this way the school and, to a lesser extent, the community agency offer a setting in which young people can discuss their particular problems and decide for themselves what is meant by words such as, responsibility, commitment, respect, and honor. This new morality, which purports to be so carefree, has in fact plunged young people into a world full of demands and responsibilities, which their parents never had to face at so early an age.

There is a danger, too, that current standards are creating a new kind of competitiveness regarding sex. The message we get from many books, films, magazines is that strenuous, prolonged, and flamboyant sexual activity is the goal to strive for: every red-blooded American boy and girl "wants it all the time." Actually, sex is a matter of taste; people will differ as to how much they want and how often. Nurses, parents, practicing professionals, and friends also have a responsibility to protect and minister to the desires of those who choose abstinence.

Social and Legislative Measures Are Needed

Despite the new sexual freedom, much of our thinking about sex is still dominated by the social beliefs and constraints of the Victorian era. In the area of general sex behavior, it is important to develop the social sanctions to assure equal rights and opportunities for all. Considerable leadership is being provided by SIECUS (Sex Information and Education Council of the United States), a sex and marriage counseling service established for the purpose of educating professionals in all the helping disciplines to recognize that sexuality is a valid component of being human at all ages.

But leadership is needed at every level. In schools, churches, service agencies, and informal groups, community health nurses can play an important part by fostering discussion and explaining or interpreting different points of view. Among young people in particular, there is a wealth of knowledge that could be shared with receptive elders.

Society still apparently feels threatened by homosexuals and prostitutes, seeing in their activities only the corrupting and unhealthy aspects of sex. Emotions are very strong on this subject, probably because such groups represent the *non*-procreative side of sex; therefore, they can, by older standards, be equated with unholy lust and lewdness.

Following in the wake of the Black Power and Women's Liberation movements, the gay population and prostitutes are now organizing to secure their own legal rights and establish their claims to social acceptance and dignity. Until they have attained these goals, the community health nurse should encourage appropriate legislative action and humanitarian activities within the community, and show by her own example that she endorses the right of fair treatment for *all* people.

Sex offenders *do* represent a threat to the community. The community health nurse must be alert to detect potential offenders and be prepared to take positive action with actual offenders; but she should also treat the offender and his family with compassion and understanding. She should be aware of laws and statues relating to this problem, and of sources of legal and psychiatric help to which she can turn for assistance.

Legislation relating to rape is important, but even more important is the way in which such legislation is implemented. All too often since the burden of proof rests on the victim, it is unclear whether it is the offender or the victim who is on trial. (See Chapter 20.)

NEW ATTITUDES AND SEXUAL ADJUSTMENT

The community as well as the individual and family has a stake in the development of healthy sexuality. Poor sexual adjustment may produce physical symptoms such as fatigue and neurosis as well as social maladjustments growing from frustration. Open and permissive premarital or extramarital sex may increase exposure to genitally transmitted disease. Different standards of behavior may create tensions between the generations. At the same time, the newer relaxed attitudes may make those who are actually or potentially endangered by disease or stress seek needed diagnosis and care, and take the responsibility of securing care for others.

Today, the availability of measures for birth control makes sex for the purpose of procreation only a small part of sexual expression. At one time, particularly in agrarian societies, large families were considered essential to provide the needed manpower to work the land. A man needed legitimate heirs to inherit his property or his wealth. Sex for its own sake was wicked, a decadent indulgence. Now, fears of overpopulation and a new awareness of the finite quality of natural resources have made the small family desirable and voluntary childlessness respectable. Sex *can* be enjoyed for its own sake, and treated as an enriching dimension to life. It is not, however, a commodity to be treated lightly. Sexual experience can have many faces — serious, romantic, entertaining, passionate, and soothing. Sometimes it can be brutal and terrifying. Good sexual adjustment is a worthwhile and important goal for family health.

Attitudes toward sex are by far the most important factor in achieving successful sexual adjustment. The following suggest a set of desirable sexual assumptions:

1. Sex is an important, legitimate, and powerful dimension of human behavior.
2. Enjoyment of sex is a natural and desirable thing.
3. Sex is an egalitarian activity in which neither partner controls, coerces, or exploits the other and in which either partner may take the initiative.
4. Sexual satisfaction is cumulative; good experiences of the past make future success likely. Sexual expression can extend to later years, even into the eighth decade of life.

Many people already share these assumptions, especially if they comply with the early examples set by parents in the home. For others it may mean a sharp reversal of present beliefs, practices, and ideals.

The roots of sexual behavior lie in early experiences. Parental or school guidance can assure that little girls and little boys learn to expect quality of opportunity, yet feel comfortable being a girl or a boy. Prohibitions regarding discussion or exhibition of sexual organs, or flippant falsehoods about intercourse, pregnancy, or birth can have serious repercussions. On the other hand, honest accurate information provided when it is requested or indicated by developmental stages, health education that includes references to human reproduction and sexuality, and many other specific incidental activities will put sex in perspective and may prevent future misconceptions and frustrations.

Even more important are the role models set by parents. Children are observant, and they absorb atmospheres. Denigration, discontent, and emotional dishonesty spread from one generation to another. Remarks such as "Father is late *again*, and I worked so hard on the dinner," or "We won't tell him how much we paid for this, he'd have a fit," as well as spiteful concentration on cooking or household chores as soon as a tired husband returns from work are imprinted on the young mind and create an image of the role of wife as someone who can be neglectful, complaining, and deceitful. Spontaneous expressions of affection, hugs, and non-routine kisses, a compliment — even a good fight if it clears the air — communicate an environment of trust and security. Parental responsibility for making a marriage work is a lesson of great importance.

Attitudes about women have been modified and are changing dramatically. In sexual matters, the double standard prevailed until very recently. By this warped standard, men were allowed and even expected to exercise complete sexual freedom without strings or conditions. It was the responsibility of the woman to demonstrate control and defend her virtue. If a woman became pregnant out of wedlock or if a wife succumbed to seduction, she was stigmatized as a tramp or a trollop, while the man remained blameless. Modern mores are more equitable.

Legislation has also improved attitudes to women. It is harder to exploit a woman who is guaranteed the right to vote and equal job opportunities and equal pay for equal work than one who is totally dependent upon her husband.

Underlying Problems

Problems such as lack of communication, endangered or lowered self-esteem, differences in sex drive, or competing demands for energy may interfere with sexual fulfillment. Couples who have always covered up basic disagreement or discontent, who habitually deny or avoid problems rather than talk them out, will have difficulty in communicating their needs and desires regarding sex.

Partners may differ in the intensity of their sex drive, and this will require understanding, patience, and openness, and sometimes considerable change in the patterns of sexual expression. There may be differences, too, in the energy demands placed upon one or both partners. The young mother with active preschool children, or the wife who is combining a job and homemaking, may find little energy left for sexual activity. The suburban husband, tired from the demands of his career, commuting, and wearying weekend domestic chores, may likewise have less energy and subtlety to bring to the marital bed.

The relation between sexual performance and self-esteem needs to be emphasized, and especially at points when self-esteem is threatened — a fortieth birthday or at retirement, or when long-term illness has been discovered, for example. These critical points deserve special efforts at maintaining a viable sexual relationship. When there is disability due to age, illness, or points of stress such as menopause, adaptations may be necessary to permit continuance of sexual expression at a time when reassurance of one's manhood or womanhood is urgently needed.[1]

In each of these cases, facing the problem is essential. Encouraging open expression of all these problems is important. Group discussions on sexual adjustment, simulation conversations with the nurse as a preparation for talking with spouse or children may be helpful in bringing out the reluctant partner or partners.

SEXUAL ALTERNATIVES

Same sex sexuality is increasingly acknowledged as a legitimate option for a minority of the population. Despite tremendous advances in recognition and acceptance of the "gay" sexual orientation, assimilation is far from complete or general. Negative attitudes, especially when held by close family members or friends, place an additional strain on lesbian and male homosexual couples. They may feel that it is necessary to conceal their relationship, or they may be persuaded that their association is indeed undesirable or abnormal.

Single sex couples have the same needs for communication and continuity and the commitment of deep sexual attachments, and face essentially the same problems as do heterosexual couples. They may require more support because of excessive social pressures.

Group sex represents another option. In this situation, a varying number of couples or individuals engage in free and open sex relationships at the same time. For some this is a temporary experience, usually at the point of high sexual drive, that is later discarded in favor of a single couple relationship; for others it may be continuing. In communes, the sexual mode may be group sex or it may be a "bonded pair" relationship, in which a couple is either married or recognized by the group as being temporarily or for an extended period committed to one another.

"Swinging couples" are commited to sex without continuing involvement. In most cases, the basic bond between couples is expected to hold fast, while shared sex with other couples is transitory and variable.

THE ROLE OF THE COMMUNITY HEALTH NURSE

The preceding discussion focuses on the totality of the concerns regarding healthy sexuality, and requires the participation of many individuals and groups. Just what one particular community health nurse will do will be conditioned by what others are doing. Most important is the mode of behavior adopted by parents or by families as a whole, and in a more general way by the community. Additionally, action will be taken by general service agencies, welfare organizations, schools, occupational health services, and health maintenance organizations, to mention a few. Lastly, there will be active contributions from specialized agencies such as SIECUS, and by organizations such as the American Psychiatric Association and the National Organization of Women.

The community health nurse will need to have a concept of the total effort to promote healthy sexuality, and the programs undertaken in a formal way by other groups. In family care, she should estimate the general pattern of sexuality and assess the quality of information transmitted to children in any particular family. Regardless of how much is done by others, the community health nurse should try to estimate how far the family's needs are being met, and what is still lacking.

Whatever the scope and character of her role in promoting sexual health, the community health nurse will need to develop an adequate body of specific knowledge regarding sexual behavior and legislation pertaining to sexual offenders. In addition, she should clarify and, if necessary, obtain help with any ambiguities she herself may feel regarding the subject of sex so she can participate and contribute within the community to her fullest capacity.

REFERENCE

1. Dresden, S. E.: The middle years: the sexually active middle adults. Am. J. Nurs. 75:1001, 1975.

SUGGESTED READINGS

Abernethy, V.: *Population Pressure and Cultural Adjustment*. New York, Human Sciences Press, 1979.

Baizerman, M., Thompson, J., and Stafford-White, K.: Adolescent prostitution. Child. Today, 8:20, 1979.

Barrett, J. E.: Family life education-parental involvement. J. School Health, 49:15, 1979.

Beis, R. H.: Sex: Purpose and natural law. Humanist, 39:31, 1979.

Broderick, C.: Normal sociosexual development. *In* Broderick, C., and Bernard, J. (eds.): *The Individual, Sex, and Society*. Baltimore, Johns Hopkins Press, 1969.

Cohen, T. B.: Observations on school children in the People's Republic of China. J. Am. Acad. Child Psych., 16:165, 1977.

Evans, R. B.: Homosexuality and the role of the family physician. Med. Aspects of Human Sex., 13:10, 1979.

Franzblau, S., Sprafkin, J. N., and Rubinstein, E. A.: Sex on T.V.: A content analysis. J. Commun., 27:164, 1977.

Friedeman, J. S.: Development of a sexual knowledge inventory for elderly persons. Nurs. Res., 28:372, 1979.

Gruis, M. L., and Wagner, A.: Sexuality during the climacteric. Postgrad. Med., 65:197, 1979.

Harrison, B.: Toward a just social order. J. Curr. Soc. Issues, 15:63, 1978.

James, J., and Meyerding, J.: Early sexual experience and prostitution. Am. J. Psych., *134*:1381, 1977.

Krueger, J. C., et al.: Relationship between nurse counseling and sexual adjustment after hysterectomy. Nurs. Res., *28*:145, 1979.

Lief, N., and Payne, T.: Sexuality knowledge and attitudes. Am. J. Nurs., *75*:2026, 1975.

Luria, Z., and Rose, M. D.: *Psychology of Human Sexuality.* New York, John Wiley and Sons, 1979.

Masters, W. H., and Johnson, V. E.: *Homosexuality in Perspective.* Boston, Little, Brown and Co., 1979.

Masters, W. H., and Johnson, V. E.: *Human Sexual Inadequacy.* Boston, Little, Brown and Co., 1970.

Masters, W. H., and Johnson, V. E.: *Human Sexual Response.* Boston, Little, Brown and Co., 1966.

McKinnon, I.: Child pornography. FBI Law Enforcement Bulletin. *48*:18, 1979.

Morin, S. F., Schultz, S. J.: The gay movement and the rights of children. J Soc. Issues, *37*:137, 1978.

Payne, T.: Sexuality of nurses: Correlation of knowledge, attitudes and behavior. Nurs. Res., *25*:286, 1976.

Sexuality and patient care. Communicating Nurs. Res., *11*:77, 1978.

Shirreffs, J. H., et al.: Adolescent perceptions of sex education needs. J. School Health, *49*:343, 1979.

Surawiez, F., and Winick, C.: Debate: Should prostitution be legalized? Med. Aspects Human Sex., *13*:120, 1979.

"The New Morality: An Exclusive Poll on What Americans Really Think About Sex," *Time*, November 21: 111, 1977.

Whitley, M. P., and Willingham, D.: Adding a sexual assessment to the health interview. J. Psych. Nurs. Mental Health Serv., *16*:17, 1978.

Wolf, W., and Fligstein, N.: Sex and authority in the workplace. Am. Sociol. Rev., *44*:235, 1979.

Woods, N. F.: Human sexuality and the family. Current Pract. Obstet. Gynecol. Nurs., *2*:199, 1978.

Woodward, C. A.: Understanding pornography consumption. J. Psych. Nurs. Mental Health Serv., *16*:36, 1978.

Chapter 16

THE COMMUNITY:
THE COMMITMENT

While the major contribution of the community health nurse is undeniably the improvement of family health and well-being, it is the community as a whole that represents the final commitment. Both the American Nurses' Association and the World Health Organization have emphasized this commitment in statements on community nursing practice.[1, 2]

This emphasis arises from increasing acceptance of the principle, equal access to available health care is a universal right. If everyone is entitled to equal access in accordance to their needs, then the whole population unit becomes the "patient." It is no longer considered moral to provide exquisite care for a few, while many go without care or are eligible for only a few benefits. While at the present time distribution of health care services is far from equitable, public pressure for increased care to the economically disadvantaged, the elderly, and the handicapped plus others underserved is growing, making change highly probable.

Another force for community focus is the increasing understanding of the interdependence of man and his complex social and physical environment. The crime-ridden community, the geographic "pockets" of high-infant mortality, and the mining community are environments that work with the specific agent or risk factor contributing to disease in populations. It becomes increasingly clear that many health problems can be resolved only by the concerted action of the community as a whole. Rat control, water quality, lead poisoning in children, smoking and substance abuse, highway accidents, are all examples of problems needing total community action.

The community — all of the people within given boundaries — are, in the final analysis, the true nursing load; for community health nursing is, by definition, concerned with all people. While higher priorities for care may be allocated to specially vulnerable families or groups within the community, those admitted for care do not represent the total group

289

with which the nurse is involved. Awareness of the needs of those *not* under continuing nursing supervision as well as the needs of those receiving care, is essential to understanding of the community health.

The community health nurse, as one of the links in human services, operates in the context of the functioning community, sharing the responsibility for building community capability to deal with its health problems effectively.

"COMMUNITY" MAY MEAN MANY THINGS

The sociologist, psychologist, demographer, architect or industrialist will each have his own way of looking at the community. And so will the community health nurse. The World Health Organization's Expert Committee report on community health nursing contains a simple, and useful definition:

A community is a social group determined by geographic boundaries and/or common values and interests. Its members know and interact with one another. It functions within a particular social structure and exhibits and creates norms, values and social institutions.[3]

The people living in a community may range, in terms of homogeneity, from a group that shares a common cultural background and a well-defined value system to a collection of many individuals thrown together by chance without any recognized common interests.

The community may be a neighborhood or cluster of families, an ethnic group, an industry or place of work, or a school. Sometimes the community is no more than a meeting place (such as a shopping mall or street corner), where adolescents meet on a regular basis — "hanging around" in fellowship and identification with one another.

Some communities are stereotyped — e.g., the ghetto, the rural community, septic tank suburbia, or the hippie community. Such labeling is dangerous, as wide differences do exist within each group.[4]

The community also represents an environment that may have a positive or negative impact on health. The rate and direction of economic growth, the decision to build a large residential facility or nuclear power plant, or the development of a vermiculite mine will all change the physical and social environment in a variety of ways. These changes could bring needed economic growth to a community; or they could threaten the usual ways of doing things, dislocate large numbers of families, or pollute the air.

The community may also be looked upon as a support system. It is a tremendous, though often ignored, manpower reservoir. The innate or easily taught skills that would enable people to watch their own health and maintain surveillance over their communities could be exploited. The opportunities for care exchange and use of existing groups in the community for health purposes are untapped resources. The people, the managers, and the institutions must identify with each other, and recognize their interdependence. A cluster of families may keep an eye on one another's children, check on an elderly neighbor, or watch each other's homes when one family is away. The nurse needs to use these informal understandings as well as the formal ones in the community, as an extender of available nursing care.

The community serves as a channel for political action on behalf of its members. Efforts to personalize civic programs, secure greater consumer participation on organization's boards, and develop local health planning groups are part of the potential political action. Such groups can lobby for better services for the elderly, document the need for a child guidance center, or influence health policies in prisons and schools. Groups like these may be useful in evaluating the nursing program in relationship to the perceived needs of the community and recommending different service modalities. According to Borgese, "The primary reason for the existence of a political community — or of any other community — is that in it and through it, individuals do what they cannot do by themselves. The community thus enhances the individual more than it limits him."[5]

A COMMUNITY FOCUS MAY REQUIRE
SOME PROFESSIONAL REORIENTATION

Nurses, like most members of the helping professions, tend to focus on individuals and families rather than on what they may see as the less personal population-in-environment unit of care. Although well sensitized to the physical and interpersonal indices of human disorder, nurses may be less attuned to the statistical cry for help that is the community's symptom of illness. A community focus places as much emphasis on the proportion of pregnant women receiving adequate nursing support as on the quality of nursing service provided to an individual family. It offers the same sensitivity to the mood and self-respect of a neighborhood — as reflected in the appearance of streets and alleys and in the condition of its schools — as it does to the mood and self-respect of the family. It offers responsiveness to the need for concerted neighborhood action to change the dangerous play habits of children, as well as responsiveness to individual needs.

This focus requires a nursing approach different from the one-by-one approach of family care. For example, the identification and neutralization of the hostile individual or family who is not receiving care may be necessary to avoid building distrust of helping agencies among other potential recipients of care. Enlisting the help of those who exert influence in the community may require changing social patterns that are deeply ingrained.

For most nurses, "thinking community" takes some readjustment and conscious effort, for without this point of view, it is impossible to realize fully the benefits nurses can provide to the community.

THE COMMUNITY NURSE'S SHARE IN COMMUNITY PLANNING VARIES

The pattern of assignment influences the planning procedures. If the community health nurse is the sole professional nurse representative or the nursing group leader for a community, she will obviously carry the major responsibility for adapting the general program to local needs. If she is a member of a nursing group or of a multidiscipline group planning for the health care of a community, her responsibility may be smaller in scope, but she will still be expected to contribute to program planning through the evaluation of new methods and suggestions for change.

Agency tolerance for difference and experimentation affects the scope of planning responsibility. In some agencies, there is a greater tolerance for innovation; other agencies may tend toward greater central-ization of decision and methodology. However, it is safe to say that in most instances, nurses in the field underestimate rather than overesti-mate the degree of freedom they have. Usually the attitude of the central office is far less rigid than that which is perceived by the nurse.

The strength and influence of community groups concerned with nursing affect the demand for change and individualized planning. For the most part, community action and planning groups are geared to changing and to increasing the relevance and impact of human services. They expect to be heard, to influence decision making, and, above all, to get more of the good things of life for the community they represent. When such groups are numerous and active, they will expect the community health nurse to find some way of responding to their demands for increased or improved service; this would, in turn, demand adaptations to the existing nursing program.

The pattern for the delivery of nursing services requires varying degrees of "merge" in planning the nursing program. When there are several agencies providing nursing care in an area, the planning task becomes more complex, since the nursing program in any one agency must be related to that program in other agencies in order to assure the best possible coverage. Even when there is only one designated commu-nity health nurse in a community or neighborhood, other health groups (such as hospital outpatient nursing services, personnel employed by the family physician, or "good neighbors" who help out in an emergency) may participate in the work of community nursing.

THE PROCESS OF DEVELOPING THE LOCAL COMMUNITY NURSING PROGRAM

Careful planning at the local community level helps to assure that the nursing services will be accessible, acceptable, and pertinent. Even when they are in close proximity, localities are likely to differ consider-ably not only in the health conditions they experience but also in the degree of family independence, patterns of use of health services, and the sources of influence in health matters.

Planning guides the choices that have to be made. Rarely is the nurse in a situation where the demands for nursing do not outrun the available nursing time. Pressures for more nursing care or for nursing care of a specific kind come from many sources and differ from one locality to another. Each newly developed health program is "crucial"; each newly elected government official has promises to keep; and each nurse is pushed by her professional training, her professional affiliations, and her professional conscience to extend and improve the services she can offer. Emphasis on participation and building the decision-making capacity of the communities has brought about an opportunity for a new kind of nursing care. The public, too, has increased its appetite for health care (especially among the low-income groups) and is increasingly aware of its right to decide what care is required and what they are entitled to. Thus the nurse or nursing group must constantly choose among various priorities or courses of action, basing the choice on conditions specific to the neighborhood.

Planning makes performance evaluation meaningful. What is "good" community health nursing in one area may be inadequate or inappropriate in another setting, even though on the surface the communities and the services afforded seem very similar. Local community-focused planning helps to clarify the specific outcomes that may be used as criteria for success.

Realistic planning is an antidote to frustration. Faced with both internal and external pressures and demands, the community health nurse serving a specified neighborhood may become frustrated or dissipate her nursing energy in scattered or low-impact activities. Planning helps to identify the things that will *not* be done as well as those that will be done, to indicate limits as well as hopes for nursing achievement. Defining the necessary accommodation by means of a rational process helps to relieve the nurse of unnecessary anxiety or guilt about the things that cannot be done and provides for the collection of evidence of tangible accomplishments.

In developing the nursing program, the community health nurse will use the general processes of assessing, planning, implementing, and evaluating, which have previously been discussed. She will use many of the approaches involved in community health diagnosis and, also, those which are generic to nursing. However, as she draws upon these general concepts and skills and relates them to the special social and environmental conditions and her own professional style, she will fashion a program that is highly singular.

Get the "Feel" of the Community

Nurses newly assigned to a setting may have a strong compulsion to act. Because there are so many problems to be dealt with and so much that could be done, there is a tendency to wade right in with advice and change. This desire to help immediately is satisfying to both the provider and the recipient of service, but it is important that the nurse not commit herself prematurely to a course of action that may later prove untenable. Precipitate action may lead to serious errors of judgment in terms of the need for and acceptability of the proposed changes.

During the first days in a new neighborhood, it is better for the community health nurse to act like a sponge — absorbing all the sights and sounds and smells without making any effort to systematize or even to understand them. The tone of voice used in neighbor-to-neighbor conversation, the effort to beautify the surroundings, the way in which workers in the hospital or welfare office refer to their clients ("those people" as contrasted to "such a good mother even though she has never learned to keep house"), the ways in which people congregate on the street or in other gathering places, or the attitudes of the landlords toward children are examples of observations that may provide valuable clues to community dynamics. The nurse visiting families of a different race, nationality, or social background from her own can learn much about intergroup relationships from the way in which she herself is received into a family or from the family's casual references to school or job situations.

Such reactions as these between the people or between the people and their environment have a bearing on the choice of nursing strategies, but the meaning of any single aspect of this relationship must be seen in the context of the whole. If made too soon, a systematic assessment of these factors may bias observation and obscure these interrelationships.

First impressions provide a basis for action pending more definitive study. Obviously, the community nurse is not going to postpone all action until it is possible to construct a detailed plan. During the early period in a new setting it is possible to size up what seem to be the overriding problems, to get an idea of what health matters are most urgent to the people of the community, and to make a rough estimate of the ability of the population as individuals and as a community to care for its health needs. These impressions will provide a basis for immediate action and will allow the nurse to be visible and helping while taking a systematic look at nursing-action needs and alternatives.

Develop and Use a Community Data Bank

Good program development depends upon good data, and every community health nurse must allocate some time to the collection and analysis of pertinent facts about the setting in which she works. One useful way of going about this is to develop a "data bank," a place where pertinent information about the community is gathered together for ready reference.

A community-oriented health record form — encompassing a data base for community assessment, stated community problems, and specified goals and objectives with plans for nursing intervention and evaluation — was developed at the University of Texas School of Public Health.[6] With use of this tool, nurses are able to systematically collect and update the community data base, plan more carefully, and monitor and reflect the efforts of nursing intervention on a community's health.

Population Characteristics

The bank should include data about both the general and the health characteristics of the population. The general characteristics of the population are important to program planning. Trends in the size of the population, age and sex distribution, family size, occupations, educational attainment, or racial or national origins influence the demands for nursing care.

Health characteristics — including trends in mortality and morbidity, illnesses causing absence from school, or health conditions for which people have been referred for nursing service — are of obvious importance. Utilization patterns — usual sources of primary medical care or the nature of the attendance group at screening services — are also clues to problems requiring nursing intervention. Patterns of family health maintenance, such as child rearing, family management, and eating habits, constitute another important area of planning data.

Environment Characteristics

Data about the environment should also be considered. Significant information about the physical environment might include the nature of traffic patterns (e.g., the safety of crossings or high-speed freeways), general conditions of housing, the safety and adequacy of school buildings and school grounds, natural hazards, and pesticides in common use in rural areas.

Data about the social environment may include the general level of interchange among subgroups in the community, habits of recreation (whether family-focused, individual, "home grown," or commercial), or intergenerational relationships.

Formal and Informal Community Resources

Information about available resources for medical or health care and the conditions of their use may be supplemented by information about non-health groups or individuals that are available to give help. For example, it is necessary to know which persons are eligible to use a particular clinic, when they may attend, what the charges are likely to be, and what person should inquiries be addressed to. It may also be important to know whether the city or state health department has a consultant in tuberculosis care who can be asked for advice, whether a local industry employs a nurse who will inform workers of special health programs, or whether a retired librarian may be called upon to secure books for shut-ins.

Trends in Service Activities

It is not safe to assume that what has been done through community nursing service accurately reflects the current nursing needs of the population, but past activity records do reflect the expectations that have been engendered in the public with respect to nursing service. Any contemplated substantive program change must be seen in the context of these expectations and habits of use.

Information about service inputs (that is, the time spent in nursing and the activities that have been undertaken) and service outputs (such as the number of cases brought to medical treatment or that show improvement) are obviously important to planning.

Systematic collection and organization of data maximize its usefulness. It is obvious that in planning for a small population unit such as a neighborhood, information must be gathered in bits and pieces; some of the data will be specific for the neighborhood, such as that for a census tract, and some data will be extrapolated from that relating to larger population groups.

The community health nurse must see data collection as a continuing task; she must add to the available facts such new data as are uncovered and constantly update existing community information.

Depending on the nature of the data, it may be useful to tabulate it in order to provide for quick comparison (as with trends in utilization of particular services), to establish separate files (such as a resource file), or simply to file the various compilations and reports together in a readily accessible spot. The important thing is to make it easy to see the inter-relatedness of these various units of information as they affect the provision of care. For example, it is important to see the changing service input trends as they relate to changes in the nature of the population or to the introduction of new sources of health care in the community. When the method of collecting and storing these data is already established, the community health nurse may need only to learn how to maintain them and to use them in a synthesized way.

Relating Nursing Efforts to Those of Other Groups

Information from the data bank will need to be supplemented with further information secured through conferences with other groups that are responsible for nursing or related programs. For instance, it is important to know if the local hospital is planning any change in program or organization that would affect the community nursing support. The nurse should inquire if the medical director in the neighborhood health unit is making plans that might require a change in the nursing support program: A special immunization campaign or potential new mental health facilities must be taken into account in the development of the community nursing program.

ENGAGE NEIGHBORHOOD RESIDENTS IN NURSING

Engaging neighborhood residents in nursing is a problem of philosophy and method. Hans Spiegel said, "Probably no other issue is as vital to the success of solving America's urban crisis than the viable participation of urban residents in planning the neighborhoods and cities in which they live and the social programs that directly affect them."[7] This belief has been reiterated by many leaders in social planning and action and has been applied to rural as well as urban settings. Although the concept of citizen participation appears to have wide acceptance, there is little agreement on the scope of such participation or on the methods by which it might be best achieved.

Community health nursing, or public health nursing, has traditionally adhered to the philosophy that the individuals and communities served should share in the decisions made about care. There is a long history of the involvement of the public in boards, committees, and other community action groups as well as that of individuals, groups of patients, and families in their own nursing care. However, many nurses feel that this philosophy has not been implemented as fully as possible and that low-income groups in particular have not been adequately represented in community planning and action for nursing care. Recent trends in social planning suggest that much more frequent and forceful citizen involvement is likely to develop. This development offers both a challenge and an opportunity for community health nursing.

Citizen Participation Serves Practical Purposes

Participation Clarifies the Needs that Nursing Should Meet. The perception of need will obviously vary between the health professional and the local community representative, since these perceptions are based on different experiences, training, and values. The professional must avoid falling into the trap of feeling that what the professional wants to do represents the "true need" and what the public wants the professional to do is the "demand." What hurts is the problem, and what hurts — whether the real or fancied condescension of the nurse, the absence of a night consultation service, the failure of the nurse to intercede with another agency for the family, or frank illness — is best known by those who feel the hurt. In the give and take between community representatives and the nurse or nursing group, each can put forth their facts, ideas, and feelings and, hopefully, arrive at a decision as to the nursing action that should be taken.

Participation Validates the Goals that Are Established for the Nursing Service. Community residents are apt to make a pretty good guess as to whether or not nursing might help a situation and as to how far the residents of the community can go in coping with a problem on their own.

Participation Brings New Skills and Knowledge into Service. In the course of dealing with the day-in and day-out problems of living in a low-income neighborhood, in an isolated rural area, or on a military post, residents learn ways of coping with the special problems they face. They know the problems of managing food stamps, of finding ways for the overworked farm boy to help at home and still join the school band, and of managing an alcoholic member of the family. Those with experience as welfare recipients know the pros and cons of the young mother's difficult decision whether to remain on welfare or to leave her child in the care of others and become self-supporting. Only the residents of a Hutterite community can appreciate fully the pressure to maintain traditional patterns of child rearing and the problems of adapting to the world outside.

Participation Has Value in Itself. For those who are unaccustomed to having much control over the important things in their lives, participation offers an opportunity to take some definitive action, to feel less impotent, and to exercise their right to choose. Even when the participation is limited to criticizing the shortcomings of the present program, system, or personnel, at least it is positive action on the part of the consumer. For others, more accustomed to having a voice in their own affairs, participation offers an opportunity to contribute in a meaningful way to an important service and often leads to greater health knowledge and to a greater commitment to the cause of improving the health of the public.

Community Leaders

The community health nurse hopes that every community resident who has any contact with nursing will participate in some way in the nursing-care program. In addition, some residents may be expected to exert unusual influence over the actions of their neighbors or to engage actively in the process of social change in the community. Sanders points out that these leaders may come in many styles, including the "top leadership" group, which has general influence in many areas; those whose leadership is exerted primarily in one system of the community, such as the health system; and those who hold elective offices or jobs that provide them with channels for influence, such as committee members or physicians, or who are recognized as spokesmen for specific groups.[8]

It is important to remember that it is not easy to separate the true from the apparent sources of leadership. The most vocal and frequently elected committee member may have status; but when decisions are made, others may play the key role. Elected committees may or may not be considered by the community as truly representing them. Also, leadership capability in many cases, especially in urban populations, may be latent. For example, in a public housing unit, the community health nurse may come upon a resident who has never been active (in the organized sense) in influencing his neighbors but, when asked to help in a discussion group, shows great ability at analyzing problems, seeing alternative solutions, and motivating others toward a new way of thinking.

Leadership capacity rests partly on personal endowment, on the ability and the desire to understand others, and on the capacity to "get through" to the strength of their impulse to act rather than withdraw in the face of a problem. The quality of the leadership will also be affected by the nature of the problems, by the leaders' knowledge of the problems, and by the ways in which their actions will affect others involved in the decision.

It is important to know to what extent those representative of or speaking for the community have had experience in problem definition and independent decision and to what extent they have — either from their general background knowledge or from materials provided them — the facts upon which a decision should rest. The neighborhood council may be working from an entirely inadequate knowledge of the financial situation of the larger community or of the long-range effects of certain actions that may be proposed. If they have lived largely in a setting in which the options for action are sharply limited, they may not be experienced in weighing alternative actions. (The community health nurse may appreciate this as she herself struggles with decisions about alternative courses of nursing action!) The nurse's persistent search for indigenous leadership must be accompanied by definite planning to develop and use the leadership available.

Training in collaborative decision making is important not only for community residents but also for professional and other service personnel who are responsible for providing the required care. The community representative needs to be provided with information and explanation about the conditions that set restraints within which decisions must be made. He must learn that any suggestion made will receive full and careful consideration, and he must distinguish between those things about which his group can make the final decision and those that must be left to the professional or paid worker. For example, no one would suppose that a neighborhood committee could decide what medication should be ordered for a specific condition or whether or not certain technical nursing procedures could be entrusted to one with less than professional preparation.

On the other hand, professional workers must also be trained in the art of collaborative decision making and action. It is sometimes difficult for the professional worker who lacks many of the experiences of his clients to realize that the expertise of the community resident may far exceed his own in matters related to the scheduling of services or to the interpersonal relationships in the service setting.

To assure some continuity in citizen participation, the community health nurse or nursing group may want to establish a citizens' advisory or action committee for nursing. This may be a separate committee that is elected or appointed by the neighborhood group, or it may be a subcommittee of the community health committee. In either case, the charge to the committee should be clearly stated. There should be provision for rotation of membership in order to increase the opportunities for participation. Regular meetings should be held, and records should be kept of the committee's actions and recommendations.

NURSING GOALS AND PRIORITIES GROW OUT OF THE COMMUNITIES NEEDS

The observant nurse will soon learn that the things she sees as nursing needs do not always coincide with what the community residents and their organizations see as nursing needs. In establishing goals and priorities as a base for program development, the nurse must take time to broaden her outlook, so that she can see needs in a very relative sense. The object is to achieve a synthesis of her own concept of what sort of nursing care should be provided in these particular families and institutional groups with the ideas of those responsible for the overall health program development, and with the consumers' concepts of nursing care (either as they are formally expressed in committee reports or as they are deduced from nursing encounters with individuals and families).

The achievement of this synthesized view of community nursing needs requires a great deal of discussion with the relevant individuals and groups: physicians, health-care facilities personnel, welfare groups, and formal or informal action groups. It also requires that the nurse have a clear image of community health nursing practice in the conceptual sense: For instance, she should react almost automatically to the word *need* as representing a relationship between the demands set by a health condition, the ability of the family to cope with that demand, and the likelihood that nursing will affect the condition in some favorable way; she should also realize that what constitutes a "here-and-now" need may be totally different at another time or another place; and she should recognize the validity of the perceived need and the legitimacy of her concern with the needs of the non-served, as well as the served, population. Each step used in defining need should be checked out against the basic concepts that underlie nursing practice.

Goals

On the basis of the explorations and decisions made in the course of involving institutional and citizen representatives in the nursing problem and using her own assessment of the situation, the community health nurse can develop a clearly stated set of goals and also a set of specific outcomes, *indicators*, that can be used to determine whether or not these goals have been realized.

Thus, the nurse planning for the maternity phases of the community health program might set (among others) two primary goals:

Goal I: Expectant mothers will receive comprehensive prenatal care in the first trimester.

Goal II: The family environment, animate and inanimate, will provide age-appropriate stimulation for the child or children.

She can then set forth the specific outcomes toward which effort might be directed and by which progress should be measured. For example:

Indicators for Goal I

1. An increase in the proportion of those registering for care within the first trimester from the present 49 per cent to 75 per cent (as indicated by the total number of births recorded in the community).
2. Specified tests and services for at least 85 per cent of those under nursing supervison (as indicated on the family record).

Indicators for Goal II

1. Parents and responsible caretakers are aware of normal growth and development (as indicated by interview on home visit), or parents' initial and later responses to hypothetical child rearing problems (as recorded on special survey forms show an increment in the proportion of positive responses in the course of care over the first year of life).
2. The home situation includes a variety of objects and activities for children to explore and manipulate as measured by the Caldwell Home Inventory.[9]

Priority should be given to areas that represent a significant health threat or that represent a major concern of the community residents. For instance, emphasis may be placed on the care of unmarried adolescent pregnant girls, or on the improvement of the food intake of expectant and nursing mothers, or on interceding with community care agencies for more personalized care.

These goals and priorities should be written down and kept on file. They should be agreed upon by the nurse, her agency administrative personnel (which may mean her supervisor or the nursing consultant standing in for the administration), and those representatives of the community who are working with the nurse on program development.

THE ACTION AGENDA DIRECTS EFFORT

Once the community health nurse has established the goals and priorities of her local community's program, there is need for an action agenda that will give some order to the implementation phase of the program. The action agenda is usually set up for a minimum of one year (sometimes two, if the agency is on a biennial plan and budget) with supplementary planning within shorter time units such as a month or week or, when necessary, at even more frequent intervals. Specific schedules and plans may be drawn up on a quarterly, monthly, or weekly basis, depending on the nature of the nursing work to be done.

If the nurse is working in a large agency, there may be action agenda plans already developed within which her planning will occur. She may also find that there are general priorities or commitments and that her plan is essentially an adaptation of the larger one. The action agenda should show:

1. The general distribution of nursing time and effort, as related to program and supportive responsibilities.
2. The implementation modalities that are to be used.
3. The timetable, including progress checkpoints.

The Distribution of Nursing Time

The distribution of nursing time and effort involves both fixed commitments and choices. *Fixed commitments* may be formally or informally derived. The nurse working in a community setting is almost always either one of a group of workers serving a special group or part of an organization serving the larger community. The obligations or commitments made by the larger organization will be binding upon her. Some nursing activities may be required by law — certain school examination procedures, for example. Other commitments may grow from contracts or less formal agreements. There may be a contract wth an industry to provide certain home-care servies to their beneficiaries; an agreement with a hospital to provide nursing support to a satellite clinic operating in the neighborhood; or an informal understanding with a neighborhood action group that specified services will be available in the evening as well as during the day.

The community health nurse should familiarize herself with the terms of these fixed commitments, known what nursing obligations are implied, and to what degree the programs may be altered within the agreements made. Time can then be allocated for these activities.

The nurse has a greater opportunity to make *choices* in the optional or flexible portion of the program; for example, the selection of expectant parents for community health nursing supervision, the intensity of care provided these families, the scheduling of services, and the choice of methods for reaching these families may be subject to the choice of the community health nurse.

Within these optional service areas, there will be some programs or aspects of programs that have a higher value than others, either intrinsically, or for the present time, or for the particular place. There will be population groups or mini-neighborhoods that seem to have a greater need than groups living elsewhere. Programming is easier if there is a classification system for identifying high-priority families and populations. For example, each family or neighborhood cluster may be rated A, B, or C, depending on the intensity of their nursing need. Some agencies have established classification schemes but, for the most part, these are not fully developed. Again, the community health nurse has a great opportunity to influence community health nursing practice by her own efforts in this direction. In determining the value level of a particular element of service, consideration should be given to:

1. *The urgency of the situation.* For example, the urgency of providing nutritional advice or supplementation to the low-income expectant mother is exceedingly high — the effects of neglect are probably great — and timing is of prime importance. Suspected but still undiagnosed tuberculosis or venereal disease would fall into the same category of urgency.

2. *The likely impact of nursing intervention.* For example, it is less likely that nursing intervention will change the situation of a chronic alcoholic than it will affect the use of available preventive health measures.

3. *The social or medical importance of the changes* that might be secured through nursing intervention. For example, the nurse may be able to persuade an elderly patient with tuberculosis, who is being cared for reasonably well by an equally elderly spouse, to seek hospital care and more definitive treatment. However, the social benefit of this nursing intervention may be little compared to other possible uses of the nurse's time — for example, improving family functioning in a three-generation family faced with catastrophic illness.

It must be reiterated that the judgment of those receiving service as well as that of health professionals is important in making these determinations.

A realistic estimate of available time is the first step in time allocation. The general distribution of time and effort must take account of supportive as well as direct service activities: time must be allowed for educational or supervisory work with auxiliaries or students, for program review and evaluation, and for writing reports. Non-service time — travel time, sick time, and holiday time — must also be reckoned with.

Thus, a nurse working in a relatively settled suburb and responsible for a population of approximately 3,000 might find her time divided something like this:

Total working hours... 1,920 (240 days)
Off-the-job hours
    Holidays: 40 hours (5 days)
    Sick leave average: 48 (6 days)
    Total   88 (11 days)
Total on-the-job hours.. 1,832 (229 days)
Nonservice hours
    Travel, estimated on experience: 420 hours
    Total   420
Total "available" on-the-job hours 1,412
    Time required for supportive activities — program
    planning, reports, giving or receiving supervision —
    based on past experience.
        Average of 1.5 hours per working day: 344 hours.
        Total   344
Time available for direct care activities .... 1,068 hours

IMPLEMENTATION MODALITIES

Modes of implementating care will vary in time cost and impact value from one community to another. For example, there may be a choice between the use of a group approach and the use of an individual approach to counseling families in home care of the chronically ill. Some of the questions that might be raised include:

1. Is group contact the method of choice because it offers an opportunity to promote participation of community residents in their own care?
2. Are the people in this community likely to attend such group activities? Will this program reach those who need it most?
3. Are there ready-made groups — organized church groups, for instance — in the community that might be used?
4. Does the group approach lend itself to the use of supplementary volunteer or paid services that might conserve nursing time? For example, does the adult education department of the public school system or the local chapter of the American Red Cross have facilities for offering these courses, thus conserving the time of the community health nurse?
5. Are the problems of the groups sufficiently similar, so that group work will have a general appeal?

6. If the community health nurse is to undertake this program herself, will it save or cost time ? If the group approach is more expensive than the individual approach, is the likely impact sufficiently greater to compensate for the difference in cost? On the basis of these two factors is the group approach a "good buy"?

These kinds of questions will help each nurse to evaluate the relative merit of a number of possible channels for service. Some general considerations about various implementation modalities are listed in Table 16–1.

TIMETABLE AND CHECKPOINTS

The community health nurse's calendar is usually a two-part affair: a tentative effort schedule that extends over the year and a current schedule that may be compiled for a period of a month or so. A timetable or calendar helps to keep the nursing effort on course.

All fixed commitments, such as visits to schools, clinics, and staff meetings, should be scheduled first. Plans for group instruction or group problem solving that require a longterm commitment should also be blocked out early in the planning period. More flexibly timed events, such as home visiting and other types of family-nurse conference, may then be planned around this base.

The calendar should specifically indicate "checkpoints," when time is allowed for a review of progress and for documenting and evaluating the services afforded. The frequency of such checkpoints will depend on the nature of the case load. In generalized programs in which there is considerable group work and numerous fixed commitments, a quarterly review may be adequate; in other settings, such as home-care agencies, a more frequent review may be required. The important thing is to provide for reviews in advance.

The nurse's schedule should be duplicated, so that it can be made available to recipient groups (such as the community nursing committee or the school) and also to the administrative or supervisory personnel with whom the nurse is working.

COORDINATION — ANSWER TO FRAGMENTATION?

As the number of agencies and the types of service personnel continue to expand, it becomes increasingly important to assure that the various programs and services mesh in such a way that all of the resources are used efficiently to the benefit of the public. The community health nurse has a particular responsibility for the promotion of measures that will help coordinate and rationalize these many services.

Table 16–1 GENERAL CONSIDERATIONS OF VARIOUS IMPLEMENTATION MODALITIES

Implementation Modality	Advantages	Disadvantages	Constraints or Problems
1. Home visits by nurse or nursing group member.	Highly individualized care. Direct observation of family functioning. Immediate adaptation to home facilities Access to family members other than patient.	Costly in time, especially if distance is great. Indigenous non-nurse resources may not be used fully in solution of problems.	Securing adequate coverage of the population.
2. Nursing or nursing group contact in clinic, office, place of work, center, etc.	Conserves nursing time, since patient does the traveling. Easy use of other service personnel such as social worker or dentist. Use of special demonstration or teaching materials not readily transported to the home. Helps to establish family-agency ties.	Does not provide first-hand observation of family functioning. Seems less personal to the recipient of care. Works a hardship on family if carfare, baby tending, etc. are required. Does not "reach out" to those reluctant to secure care.	"Institutional flavor"; proper setting for care may be hard to achieve.
3. "Do it yourself" visits' to homes by neighborhood volunteers or paid workers.	Expresses a neighborhood commitment. Easy communication, since visitor and visitee have similar backgrounds and problems. Ego-building value by providing a "giving" rather than "receiving" experience for the volunteer and a job for the paid worker. Inexpensive way to reach previously unreached groups.	Input is hard to control; the indigenous worker may communicate very well, but what is communicated may be inaccurate or harmful. Neighborhood residents may not want their neighbors to "know too much" about them. Important problems may be missed because of lack of training of visitor.	Selecting visitors trusted by the population and responsible in carrying out tasks. Professional staff must learn to accept and work with this group of workers.

4. Relay service: training others to do tasks now done by nursing, as for instance training community volunteers or civic groups to do screening measures, to teach home care of the sick, etc.	Multiplier effect: allows extremely rapid dissemination of information or simple services.	May miss health problems in families. What can be taught must usually be limited to well-defined areas because judgment in health matters may be limited.	Requires nursing time for development, teaching, and supervision.
5. Group instruction.	Use of demonstration equipment. Economy in use of ready-made groups. Mutual stimulation among class members.	Interests and present knowledge may vary so widely that general content is not suitable.	Availability of transportation, meeting places, and teaching equipment.
6. Group problem solving.	Inculcates a problem-solving approach that should carry over to new problems. Builds self-confidence of participants in health matters. Assures relevance of content.	Problems of a few may dominate all. Costly in time and may require additional preparation of nurse.	Nurse must be sufficiently competent in the content. Nurse must be willing to accept validity of problems identified by group, even if they seem tangential to her.
7. "Kitchen-party," "teach-ins," or discussions: a small number of neighbors meeting in one of the participants' homes.	Commitment of groups. Lessens travel time for participants. Saves nurse's time if common problems exist. Organization and set-up time is absorbed by recipients of care.	Social, rather than learning, aspects may predominate. May lead to too great expenditure of time or money on part of hostess.	Members must be used to or able to meet comfortably under such circumstances. There must be common problems in which all share an interest.
8. Calculated lack of nursing action when community interest or potential impact seems low or when family can and should take responsibility.	Conserves time for accepted perceived needs. Builds family independence and self-confidence. Avoids negative recipient response if they see the service as unnecessary.	May produce an unbalanced program.	Cannot be used if the activity is in a fixed commitment class or has a high safety value. Difficult to evaluate long-term effects on nursing impact, and misjudgment may result.

Coordination of nursing effort takes place in the context of agreements and policies that are developed at broader responsibility levels: the geneal policy of the *whole community* with respect to the development of resources and programs and commitments to program elements; the policies and contracts of the *community agency* of which the community health nurse is a part, and the *local community level*, where those directly responsible for providing care plan together for a mutual effort. It is at this last level that the community health nurse is most frequently directly involved, although she may suggest or help evaluate the operation of the larger system.

The barriers to interagency coordination must be identified. These barriers may include lack of any systematic means of communication, conflicting interests and goals of various autonomous agencies providing care, or pressures upon local units from national or regional units of their organization. For example, a psychiatric hospital, under great pressure, is convinced of the need for minimizing hospital stay and looks to possible home-care programs; whereas a community health nursing service may want to protect and preserve family functioning, which may be threatened by the hospital's effort for home care.

The importance of *maximal coordination* cannot be overemphasized. *Maximal coordination* of nursing services means much more than providing for an adequate referral system. Lack of coordination wastes scarce nursing resources, decreases the likelihood that nursing services will reach all who need them, neutralizes benefits by poor follow-through, and subjects the public to the frustration and the time costs of making their way through a labyrinth of service institutions or of waiting many hours only to find they are at the wrong facility.

Criteria for Evaluating Coordination

1. Whenever possible, one agency should take primary responsibility for the nursing care of a particular family or population group and for knowing the nature and extent of the nursing services given.
2. Each agency should be apprised of nursing services provided by other agencies to clients under their care.
3. The referral system should assure that complete and specific information is transmitted to the referral agency often enough to avoid any discontinuity in care.
4. The referred family or group should be involved in the referral process, including the initial decision to refer.
5. The referral system should be as economical as possible in the professional time that it requires.
6. The right of individuals and groups to protection of privacy should be scrupulously observed in planning and referral processes.
7. The agencies involved should clarify the philosophy upon which

they provide care and the nature of each agency's commitment to the community.

8. The coordinating system should be reviewed periodically to be certain that it is functioning effectively.

Coordination Methods

One of the most commonly used methods of coordination of care facilities, and one which is useful in small communities with few resources or where long-standing and satisfactory working relationships have been developed, is *frequent face-to-face conversation and interchange*. Thus, the nurse in a rural county may "visit with" the family physician or the hospital nursing department in her area at periodic intervals, during which they discuss mutual problems with respect to referral and to coordinating their efforts. The nurse, the welfare worker, and the teacher may get together occasionally at lunch to review situations or programs in which all three have some stake. Even when more sophisticated methods are in use, this simple verbal interchange continues to play a part in the overall coordination of the program.

In the sophisticated and resource-rich community, more systematic measures may be required. These methods may include:

1. The development of a *coordinating committee*, consisting of representatives from each of the agencies providing nursing care to a population group. This committee may meet regularly to agree upon procedures, records, forms, and techniques of family information and to discuss problems in the coordination process. Such a committee may also develop a community-wide referral system to which all agencies would adhere.

2. The appointment of a *liaison nurse* who functions on an interagency basis. Most often, this worker is found in the hospital serving the local community; she is either employed by the hospital or, in some instances, by a health department or other community agency and assigned to work with the hospital. Sometimes one liaison nurse is assigned to a community agency and visits all of the hospitals used by residents of that area, or community health nurses may be assigned in rotation to this service.

The primary function of the liaison nurse is to provide a link between the hospital and the other agencies of the community. The liaison nurse (usually with a background in public health) works with the nursing, social service, and medical staffs of the hospital as they plan patient care; makes round; suggests points at which the community agency might be called upon to support the family during the patient's hospitalization; and reassures the patient that someone is looking after the family in his absence. She helps the community health nurse to assess the suitability of the home for the patient's return, and she encourages the staff and patient to make full use of available community services. It is her responsibility to make certain that the referrals provide complete and specific information about the care needed. She helps develop and maintain procedures for interagency communication by contributing to the development of referral forms, initiating referral, conferring as necessary with other agencies, and helping with referral to resources other than nursing. She also interprets the programs and goals of one agency to other agencies.

3. Regularly scheduled *interagency case conferences* may also provide a channel for implementing and improving the coordination effort. Thus, the experience of each agency with a particular family can be shared, and common problems or service gaps can be identified. When the "patient" is a population group, a similar mechanism may be used in which agencies meet regularly to discuss their work with respect to a particular problem. For example, one conference might be on the care of the adolescent unmarried mother or on the care of the discharged mental hospital patient.

Whatever method or methods are used to assure coordination of services, it is important to check the effectiveness of the system periodically. It is good to know whether or not the users of the system are happy with it; but it is even more important to see how well the system is guiding care. The records of representative families, population groups, or recipients of a given type of service might be reviewed to establish the degree to which practice is consistent with the established criteria. What is the time lag between the identification of need for home care and the receipt of the request for such care by the community agency? How well were the identified needs of the family or group met through the combined agency effort?

The effectiveness and efficiency of the community nursing program will be largely determined by the quality of the planning that goes into its development. It is well worth the time invested to make this development as orderly and as thoughtful as possible.

REFERENCES

1. American Nurses' Association: *A Conceptual Model of Community Health Nursing.* Kansas City, Mo., American Nurses' Association, 1980.
2. World Health Organization: *Community Health Nursing: Report of an Expert Committee.* Geneva, World Health Organization, Technical Report Series No. 558, 1974.
3. World Health Organization, p. 7.
4. Berger, B.: Myths of American suburbia; Vef, H.: Soulside, Black ghetto culture and the community. *In* Bell, C., and Newby, H.: *A Sociology of Community: A Selection of Readings.* Portland, Ore., Frank Cass and Co., Ltd., 1974.
5. Borgese, E. M.: Last days of the superpowers. Center Mag., 3:2, 1970.
6. Anderson, E. G., et al.: *The Development and Implementation of a Curriculum Model for Community Nurse Practitioners.* Washington, D. C., U.S. Government Printing Office, DHEW Pub. No. HRA77-24, August 1977, pp. 53–70.
7. Spiegle, H. (ed.): *Citizen Participtation in Urban Development,* Vol. I. Washington, D.C., National Training Laboratory Institute for Applied Behavioral Science (associated with the National Education Association), 1968, p. iii.

8. Sanders, I.: *In* Freeman, H., Levine, S. and Reeder, L.: *Handbook of Medical Sociology.* Englewood Cliffs, N. J., Prentice-Hall, Inc., 1979, pp. 420–424.
9. Erickson, M. L.: *Assessment and Management of Developmental Changes in Children.* St. Louis, Mo., C. V. Mosby Co., 1976, pp. 120–127.

SUGGESTED READINGS

Abrams, H. K.: A community perspective on health care, Nurs. Outlook, *19*:82, 1971.
Archer, S. E., and Fleshman, R.: *Community Health Nursing.* North Scituate, Mass., Duxbury Press, 1979, pp. 21–53.
Associated Hospital Service of New York, Home Care Department: *A Proposal: Shared Coordinated Home Care Service.* New York, Associated Hospital Service, 1973.
Barron, E.: Hospital, hotel, agencies coordinate care for the aged. Hospitals, *49*:44, 1977.
Barry, M., and Sheps, C.: A new model for health planning. Am. J. Pub. Health, *59*:226, 1969.
Bell, C., and Newby, H. (eds.): *A Sociology of Community: A Selection of Readings.* Portland, Ore., Frank Cass & Co., Ltd., 1974.
Biddle, W. W., and Biddle, L. J.: *The Community Development Process: The Rediscovery of Local Initiative.* New York, Holt, Reinhart, and Winston, Inc., 1965.
Blackford, J. S.: The professional and the contemporary youth scene. Nurs. Clin. North Am., *5*:261, 1970.
Blythe, R.: *Akenfield: Portrait of an English Village.* New York, Bell, 1969.
Brickner, P., and Sharer, L.: Hospital provides home care for elderly at one-half nursing home costs. Forum, *6*:7, 1977.
Brinton, D.: Value differences between nurses and low income families. Nurs. Res., *21*:46, 1972.
Bristow, O., Stickney, C., and Thompson, S.: *Discharge Planning for Continuity of Care.* New York, National League for Nursing, Pub. No. 21-1604, 1967.
Bruhn, J.: Planning for social change: Dilemmas for health planning. Am. J. Pub. Health, *63*:602, 1973.
Cahn, E. S., and Passett, B.: *Citizen Participation: Effecting Community Change.* New York, Praeger Publishers, Inc., 1971.
Chermayeff, S., and Tzonis, A., *Shape of Community: Realization of Human Potential.* Baltimore, Penguin Books, 1971.
Cobey, J. H.: The supervisor as motivator. Nurs. Outlook. *19*:801, 1971.
Connely, P. B.: The hidden enemies of health and the APHA. Am. J. Pub. Health, *61*:7, 1971.
Cox, F. M. (ed.): *Strategies of Community Organization,* 2nd ed. Itasca, Ill., F. E. Peacock, Inc., 1973.
Daniels, R. S.: Governance and administration of human services in urban low income communities. Am. J. Pub. Health, *63*:715, 1973.
Decker, F., et al.: Using patient outcomes to evaluate community health nursing. Nurs. Outlook, *27*:278, 1979.
Densen, P. M.: *Patient Classification for Long-Term Care: User's Manual.* Washington, D.C., U.S. Government Printing Office, DHEW Pub. No. (HRA) 74-3107, 1973.
Fifer, E. Z.: Hangups in health planning. Am. J. Pub. Health, *59*:765, 1969.
Hall, J. E., and Weaver, B. R.: *Distributive Nursing Practice: A Systems Approach to Community Health.* Philadelphia, J. B. Lippincott Co., 1977, Chapter 10.
Heley, R. W.: Continuity of care. Nurs. Times, *72*:955, 1976.
Home Health Care: *A Discussion Paper, Intra-departmental HHC Policy Working Group:* U.S. Department of Health, Education and Welfare, League Exchange, (113) 111-ix, 1–54, 1977.
Jones, Y. W., and Partridge, K. B.: Community nurses' perceptions: An aid to the administrator. J. Nurs. Admin. *2*:22, 1972.
Kane, R., and Kane, R.: *Long-Term Care in Six Countries: Implications for the United States.* Washington, D.C., U.S. Government Printing Office, 1976.
Katz, A., and Felton, J. S.: *Health and Community.* New York, Free Press, 1965, pp. 838–851.

Katz, H. P., et al.: Quality assessment of a telephone care system utilizing non-physician personnel. Am. J. Pub. Health, 68:31, 1978.

Kincaid, K.: *A Walden Two Experiment: The First Five Years of Twin Oaks Community.* NewYork, Morrow, 1972.

Klein, D. L.: *Community Dynamics and Mental Health.* New York, John Wiley & Sons, 1968.

Kramer, M.: Consumer's influence on health care. Nurs. Outlook, 20:574, 1972.

Kramer, R. M., and Specht, H.: *Readings in Community Organization Practice.* Englewood Cliffs, N. J., Prentice-Hall, Inc., 1975.

Lassey, W. R. (ed.): *Leadership and Social Change.* Iowa City, University Assoc., 1971.

Lavor, J., and Collender, M.: Home health cost effectiveness: What are we measuring? Med. Care, 14:866, 1976.

Lebon, J.: Consumer assessments of the quality of medical care. Med. Care, 12:328, 1974.

Lind, A.: The future of citizen involvement. Futurist, 9:316, 1975

Mayers, M.: Home visit — Ritual or therapy? Nurs. Outlook. 21:328, 1973.

McNeil, H. V., and Holland, S. S.: A comparative study of public health nurse teaching in groups and in home visits. Am. J. Pub. Health, 62:1629, 1972.

McNeil, J., and Bergner, L.: Use of mobile unit to provide health care for preschoolers in rural King County, Washington. Pub. Health Rep., 90:344, 1975.

Mickey, J. E.: Findings of study of extra hospital nursing needs. Am. J. Pub. Health, 53:1047, 1963.

Milio, N.: *The Care of Health in Communities: Access for Outcasts.* New York, Macmillan Co., 1975.

Moreland, H. and Schmidt, V.: Making referrals is everybody's business. Am. J. Nurs., 74:96, 1974.

Morris, R., and Harris, E.: Home health services in Massachusetts, 1971: Their role in care of the long-term sick. Am. J. Pub. Health, 62:1088, 1972.

Mustard, S., and Stebbins, S. L. (eds.): *Introduction to Public Health,* 4th ed. New York, Macmillan Co., 1968, chapter 2.

Novello, D. J.: *The Consumer's Role in Health Care.* New York, National League for Nursing, NLN Pub (52-1727), 1978.

Nuchalls, K. B.: Who decides what the nurse can do? Nurs. Outlook, 22:676, 1974.

O'Donnell, E. J.: The neighborhood service center. *Welfare in Rio,* 6:11, 1968.

Osborne, O. H.: Issues in achieving effective professional alliances. Nurs. Digest, 4:56, 1976.

Robinson, P.: Community nursing in a changing climate. Nurs. Outlook, 19:410, 1971.

Rosen, H. M., Metsch, J. M., and Levey, S. (eds.) *The Consumer and the Health Care System: Social and Managerial Prospectives,* New York, Spectrum Pub. Inc., 1977.

Ross, M. G., and Lappin, W.: *Community Organization Theory and Principles.* New York, Harper and Row, 1967.

Ruth, M. V., and Partridge, K. B.: Differences in perception of education and practice. Nurs. Outlook, 26:622, 1978.

Sanders, I.: In Freeman, H., et al. (eds.): *Handbook of Medical Sociology.* 3rd ed. Englewood Cliffs, N.J., Prentice-Hall, Inc., 1979, pp. 412–433.

Scott, Clarissa S.: Health and healing practices among five ethnic groups in Miami, Florida. PH Rep. 89, Nov./Dec., 1974, pp. 524–532.

Shortell, Stephen M.: Continuity of medical care: Conceptualization and measurement. Medical Care, 14:377, 1976.

Tinkham, C., and Voorhies, E.: *Community Health Nursing. Evolution and Process,* 2nd ed. Ch. 10. The Community as the Patient. New York, Appleton-Century-Crofts, 1977.

Tolkoff-Rubin, N. E.: Coordinated home care: The Massachusetts General Hospital experience. Medical Care, 16:453, 1978.

Tuckett, D., and Kaufert, J. (eds.): *Basic Readings in Medical Sociology,* London, Tavistock Pub. Limited, 1978.

U.S. Public Health Service: The Effects of Continued Care, a Study of Chronic Illness in the Home. DHEW Pub. No. (HSM) 73–3010, Washington, D.C., U.S. Government Printing Office, 1973.

WHO Technical Report Series #558: Community Health Nursing: Report of a WHO Expert Committee, Geneva (Switzerland) WHO, 1974.

WHO: The Community — New Focus for Nursing. WHO Chronicle, 29, 1975, pp. 91–96.

Widmer, G., Brill, R., and Schlosser, A.: Home health care: Services and cost. Nurs. Outlook, *26*:488, 1978.

Will, M. B.: Referral: A process not a forum. Nursing, 7:44, 1977.

Williams, C. A.: Community health nursing — What is it? Nurs. Outlook, *25*:250, 1977.

World Health Organization: Statistical Indices of Family Health, Report of WHO Study Group, Geneva, 1976.

Zbrowski, M., and Herzog, E.: *Life Is with People,* New York, Schocken Books, 1972.

Zimmer, James G.: Length of stay and hospital bed misutilization. Med. Care, *12*:May, 1974.

CHAPTER 17

COMMUNITY DIAGNOSIS: KEYSTONE OF PUBLIC HEALTH PRACTICE

The basis of community health action must be an accurate assessment of the state of health of the community as a whole. For this reason, community health diagnosis is the keystone of community health practice.

In the past, estimation of the health of a population was often equated with death rates and the prevalence, incidence, and distribution of disease and disability. However, as health goals extend to encompass the improvement of the quality of health as well as the prevention and treatment of disease, and as the impact of ecologic and psychologic forces on health and health care are more clearly understood, the concept of community health diagnosis becomes more complex.

AN ECOLOGIC APPROACH IS ESSENTIAL

Basic to community health diagnosis today is the acceptance of the validity of the ecologic approach. The science of ecology concerns the interaction of man and his natural or manmade environment. Payne attributes much of the failure to solve the health problems of the world's peoples to the lack of this ecologic approach:

We have tended to regard man simply as a biological animal with biological needs, which can be satisfied by the expenditure of enough dollars and the provision of a few relatively simple physical necessities. We have largely ignored the fact that he is a social animal and that it may be at least as important

314

to his health to satisfy his social needs and behavioral urges as his purely biological ones.[1]

Thus, community health diagnosis reflects not only the cumulative record of health conditions and threats in a population group but also (1) an evaluation of the dynamic situation in which that group is experiencing, adapting to, and modifying all of the biological, physical, and social forces that have a bearing on community health and (2) the relationship and interaction of these forces.

MULTIDISCIPLINARY SKILLS ARE REQUIRED

Community health diagnosis may take place at all levels — from the judgment supported by information collected from neighborhood residents by a single neighborhood worker to a full-scale report on health and health care for a nation based on information gathered by highly specialized and sophisticated techniques.

The development of a full-scale appraisal of community health involves the collection and analysis of many kinds of data and the combined judgment of several health and health-related disciplines. It will include the whole complex of public, voluntary, and private health institutions. Some of the required expertise will come from professionals in the traditional public health disciplines — the community health physician, nurse, engineer, social worker, and biostatistician. Some help will come from more specialized workers — the anthropologist, economist, behavioral scientist, sociologist, and planning specialist. Also, it is increasingly apparent that community health assessment should involve the recipient of the health care service.

Such full-scale diagnosis for planning by community health councils has become an ongoing effort of many local and state governments. Aided by federal legislation, the National Health Planning and Resources Development Act (PL 93-641), these groups have developed complex methodologies dependent upon a variety of skills for assessing community need. (See National Health Planning Information Center [NHPIC], p. 335.)

There continues to be a need for "hands-on" community assessment. The community health nurse will be involved in assessment primarily as a reporter of conditions in the area in which she works or as one who weighs the conclusions of the investigators against her own experience in the field. When a community health assessment is available, it should be studied by each community nurse as the perspective from which her own responsibility can be viewed.

In many situations, the need is for a relatively simple assessment in which health workers estimate the health of the neighborhood, county, or village in which they work. There may be data available that, when combined with judgments based on observation and inquiry, provide a satisfactory basis on which to plan health programs. It is in these situations that the community health nurse is most likely to be involved in planning and carrying out an assessment of community health.

THREE CONSIDERATIONS OF COMMUNITY HEALTH DIAGNOSIS

The community nurse should be aware of the process by which a community health diagnosis is made, for the steps will be the same at all levels even though there will be differences in the scope and sophistication of methods. Community health diagnosis is based on three interdependent, interacting, and constantly changing conditions:
1. The health status of the community, including the population's level of vulnerability.
2. Community health capability, or the ability of the community to deal with its health problems.
3. Community action potentials, or the ways and directions in which the community is likely to work on its health problems.

Any theoretical statement of the nature of the assessment will involve readily available and precise data as well as data that are elusive and iffy in character — that is, areas in which a rigorous examination of the situation is possible as opposed to areas in which educated guesses may be the best available method of investigation. Most community health leaders would agree that no need is more pressing than the one for research into the assessment of community health in order to provide not only a guide for action but also a much needed base for the evaluation of health care.

THE HEALTH STATUS OF THE COMMUNITY

The health status of the population involves people in their environment. Consequently, the estimate of the health status of the community includes two inter-related factors: people factors and environmental factors.

People Factors

People factors include the following:
1. *The characteristics and the growth trends of the population as a whole.*
   This includes the relationships between birth and death rates and immigration and emigration rates; changes in the age, sex, or racial

characteristics of the population; educational achievement levels; residence characteristics; and mobility.

2. *Trends in the death experience of the community, with special attention directed to untimely death.*

The quality of the death experience is not necessarily shown in the death rate alone; the medical cause of death may also be a valuable indicator. For example, a high infant mortality rate or a high tuberculosis rate is generally considered to be evidence of inadequate preventive health services. Along with deaths from accidental causes, deaths from diseases such as measles, poliomyelitis, or diphtheria — for which preventive measures are available — are a sharp reminder of human waste. A rate used especially in developing countries as an index of untimely death is the "proportional mortality rate," developed by Swaroop.[2] This rate compares the number of deaths occurring in individuals 50 years old or older to the total number of deaths in the community. Its validity rests on the assumption that deaths in the younger age group have a higher preventability.

The medical cause of death may, however, be inadequate as a single measure of the quality of the community's death experience. If one accepts the theory of multiple causation and believes that the necessary and sufficient causes of disease may include personal-behavioral and social conditions as well as biologic or pathologic conditions, it is important to know the conditions (other than disease itself) that are associated with a particular category of deaths.[3] Examples of this type of association are found in the relationship between poverty and certain disease entities such as tuberculosis, mental illness, and infant mortality and the relationship between cigarette smoking and death from lung cancer. Effects of occupation and life style — especially as related to the amount of exposure and response to stress — and those of climate, culture, and degree of social integration, are other areas that may affect the incidence of untimely death in a community. For this reason, it is important to know in which subgroups of the population deaths occur and the characteristics of the health behavior that may have a bearing on the prevention of untimely death. Such as analysis provides a base for remedial action.

3. *The prevalence of presymptomatic illness.*

There are more and more data on the existence of presymptomatic illness in population groups. Indices such as rising blood pressure, an increase in the cholesterol volume of blood, or small increases in blood sugar levels are examples of presymptomatic illness. These estimates may be made on the basis of special surveys or as part of a screening program.

4. *The number and location of vulnerable or special risk groups in the community.*

Special-risk groups are not characterized by a disease or other condition requiring medical care but by a personal or social condition that makes them unusually susceptible to illness or lowers their capacity to deal with disease or disability. Communities characterized by extensive poverty clearly present a higher degree of vulnerability to health impairment, as do those in which there is a high proportion of mothers with obstetric complications or a great number of unmarried teenage mothers. Relatives of diabetic patients, or of those patients who are markedly overweight or underweight, or those with an inappropriate food intake also fall into the increased risk group. Multiproblem families — those receiving care for a number of health or social conditions — are also considered to be a high risk group.

Vulnerability is also characterized by inappropriate or risky health behavior. Thus, in judging the quality of health in the population, it is helpful to know to what degree cigarette smoking, drug addiction, or excessive use of alcohol are prevalent. Careless habits with motor vehicles may be characteristic of communities or groups; the farm area where young children are permitted to drive tractors or operate other large equipment or the high school group that takes pride in reckless driving are examples. Patterns of utilization of the available health services also reflect vulnerability levels. The extensive use of folk medicines and treatments; "shopping about" for medical care, so that continuing care is made impossible; and delay in seeking care may constitute a distinct threat to health. Habits like these increase the vulnerability of the population.

5. *The number and characteristics of those functioning below their potential health level.*

Even though this is not always an easy determination to make, the community health nurse frequently encounters individuals or groups who are obviously functioning at a level far below that which they could achieve. The chronically fatigued worker who has poor sleep habits and is unwilling to work within his physical limits, the mildly depressed housewife who sees life as an endless battle to catch up with her ironing, and the irritable, dyspeptic executive goaded to compete beyond reasonable limits are examples of functional underachievement. It is at this point that one moves from the concept of health as an avoidance of disease, disability, and death to the concept of health as a positive force for improving the quality of life.

The implication of this list of human factors is that the difficulties of community health assessment are increasing. This increase may be partly due to a past preoccupation with illness and death as the principal indicators of health status and a resultant failure to move toward more precise methods for the diagnosis of the less obvious indicators of health status. However, the promotion of preventive and maintenance health care rests largely in the recognition of these less obvious deviations from health and in the development of measures to deal with them. The young worker who is helped to see the futility of accepting his chronic fatigue as inevitable may never become the tuberculosis patient who has to be identified, diagnosed, and treated. In affluent countries where disease-control measures are well developed, it seems logical that these qualitative aspects of an individual's health will receive increasing attention.

Environmental Factors

Environmental factors include the following:
1. The physical environment, such as the purity of the air and water, the adequacy of housing, and the quality of the work and home environment.
2. The social environment, including the "metabolism" of institutions within the community, the stability of the population, the quality of social planning that attempts to prevent alienation of subgroups in the community, the effectiveness and acceptability of communication networks that provide for group identification, and the provision made for recreation.

Some environmental problems — e.g., the industrial air pollution and the quality of the community water supply — are amenable only to large-scale action. Others are matters that can be dealt with by individuals or families: air can be polluted with excessive smoke from burning leaves or with incautiously used insecticides; the quality of housing can be seriously impaired by poor maintenance. Rats, stairways without handrails, unvented gas heaters, and a school without proper handwashing equipment are examples of the kinds of environmental control problems with which the community health nurse will be concerned.

In the past the major focus has been on the physical aspects of the environment, but the importance of the social environment and of the interdependence of physical and social aspects is increasingly clear. For example, it has been noted that although resettled slum dwellers are in technically improved physical surroundings, they may be less happy than they were in their old environment where the social ties were different. Conversely, some who transfer from drab city slums to areas where the individuality of their dwelling is emphasized (e.g., where there are separate yards for play), have improved the quality of housekeeping to a degree not seen when the move is only to another city apartment. Many housing experts now take into account the establishment of socializing centers that will take the place of the neighborhood store or the front stoop of the tenement. They recognize the need of elderly people to see green grass from their windows and the importance of finding ways to involve people with the management of their environment. Welfare officials are finding that a modicum of beauty in the surroundings, in addition to the essentials for life, may be a powerful stimulus to self-respect.

THE HEALTH CAPABILITY OF THE COMMUNITY

Health capability of a community is represented by the degree to which it is able to cope with its health problems and needs — to what extent its economic, institutional, and human resources are able to assure the well-being of its people.

The general economy is an obvious and powerful factor in this respect. An affluent country or community almost always has greater potential for health action than does the community in which income levels are low. For health planning, it is also important to know how the wealth of the community is distributed. If the country is characterized as wealthy, but the wealth is concentrated in a small privileged group, there may be large segments of the population whose situation does not reflect the general economic condition. On the other hand, a depressed economy may be reflected in general conditions of living that have a negative influence on health capability: a low level of educational achievement associated with inadequate school resources will slow down health education efforts and reduce the available pool of secondary school graduates from which the health professions recruit; poor roads or lack of public transportation may make health facilities inaccessible even when they do exist in adequate quantity and quality; inadequate nutrition may sap the energies of the people, so that they become indifferent to all but the most crisis-oriented health services.

Institutional Resources

Institutional resources, such as hospitals, nursing homes, and other community health facilities (health departments, visiting nurse associations) are apt to vary widely in quantity and quality from community to community. In addition to the actual number of facilities (or the ratio of beds or services to the population), it is important to know to what degree these facilities are inadequately equipped, how geographically and financially accessible they are to the people they serve, and how well or how poorly they are staffed to suit their functions. For example, a community may have what appears to be a good supply of nursing homes. However, if these institutions charge more than most of the people in the community can afford to pay; if they are located at great distances from the users of care; and if they are staffed with virtually no professional nursing supervision, the community is not capable of handling its problem of nursing-home care.

The ways in which resources are organized and used may be as critical as their availability. For example, if health agencies have the equipment and the know-how to provide preventive as well as curative services but programs are administered so that care is limited to those who are already ill or if the facilities are utilized by only a few of the population, the resources are still inadequate in relation to the needs of the population. If hospital beds are available for immediate care of cancer patients but admission policies are so rigid that they cause undue delay, the end result may still be insufficient. The adequacy of facilities may not be apparent when there is lack of coordination, gaps and overlapping of services, or institutional isolation. For example, if a hospital has not developed adequate measures for referral, the posthospital cardiac patient may lose much of the benefit of his hospital stay, or he may have to utilize hospital services to a higher degree than should be necessary. If every institution relies only on its own information about a patient instead of using the information available from other groups, its effectiveness, as well as that of other groups, is reduced, and the institution is able to provide less care than one might expect from the ratio of the facilities to the population. Good community-wide planning maximizes the care provided.

Human Resources

In health care, two kinds of human resources must be considered: the professional resources of the community itself (such as nurses and physicians) and the informal resources found in the general population.

Formal Human Resources. The availability and quality of health manpower will vary widely. The nature of the medical supply in the large city may be such that there is a great complement of specialists, but very few general practitioners; ample facilities for hospital care, but virtually no home visiting by the physician; and excellent care for crises, but little continuing health surveillance. In the rural area, there may be a general practitioner available who represents a first-line health resource, but specialization backup may be at some distance. Manpower in community agencies may also vary; there may be a good supply of professional nurses but a small group from which to draw nurses' aides or other auxiliaries, a situation that might be reversed in another community. In some communities, there is a strong complement of specialized workers on the health teams in hospitals and in other community health agencies, whereas in other areas there may be essentially the old "three-part team" in public health — the physician, nurse, and sanitarian — with specialists available at intervals or through referral to another community.

With respect to health manpower, it is important to reemphasize that the organization and coordination of manpower resources are as important as the numbers and types of personnel available. If, for example, the physical therapist is available in the hospital but does not participate in the training of nurses who must provide post-hospital care, there is a lack of manpower from the standpoint of the community health agency — even though the number of physical therapists is judged to be adequate for the community as a whole. If short-trained workers receive inadequate, on-the-spot guidance, they may be available in adequate quantity but not in quality.

Informal Human Resources. The importance of informal health resources is equal to if not greater than that of professional institutional resources for health care. For example, the self-reliance and general responsibility of a community provides a valuable resource for health care. In a rural community where there is little affluence but also little poverty, individuals, families, and small neighborhood groups may have developed great abilities to care for their own health; older and wiser women in the community can be a natural resource to the young wife and mother, church groups may provide home care for families when the mother is ill or otherwise unable to care for her family; and home nursing and transportation to health facilities may be undertaken by neighbors. On the other hand, in the very low income neighborhood in a large city — where educational achievement is low, dependency is high, and instability in family structure is common — the immediately available resources for self-help are more limited, and health professionals may have to provide many of the services that, in other settings, would be provided by the individuals themselves.

Human resources may also vary between communities made up largely of retired persons and suburban areas populated by young families. The variance grows out of the particular abilities of different age groups with respect to their own care and to their ability to help with the care of others. Again, in communities where most people work outside the home, less dependence on self and neighbors for health advice can be expected than in areas where most of the married women do not work.

The Health Action Potentials of the Community

Community action patterns affect health planning. Each community will differ in its patterns of health action — depending on the value people assign to health as compared to their other life needs, their characteristic way of taking action, the political system by which they govern themselves, and the habits they have developed regarding social action. These characteristic ways of thinking and acting apply to individuals as well as to the institutions within the community. They are of great importance in health diagnosis since they determine the ways in which the community as a whole will respond to its health needs and the measures for improving the health situation that are likely to prove relevant, acceptable, and effective.

Consider the following analogy: the doctor needs to know not only the nature and severity of his patient's infection but also the efficacy and ways in which this individual moves to deal with the assaults to his life. Does he tend to give up in despair and turn to someone else to make his decisions? Does he delay as long as possible in taking a required action? Does he deal with any impairment with aggressive determination? In many instances, the medical-care treatment must be as dependent upon this knowledge of the patient's ability to deal with problems as upon the accuracy of the diagnosis and the propriety of the treatment.

The assessment of the action patterns of a community involves an estimate of the basic values and beliefs about health that provide the impetus for action, the institutional system that supports the action, and the habits the community has developed for dealing with common problems.

Characteristic Beliefs and Behaviors

Within a community, there may be identifiable subgroups that have developed their own ways of life and of working on their common problems. The "town-and-gown" schism of college towns is one example of this — an example that most colleges and universities are trying to eliminate. "Little Italy" or "west of the railroad tracks" or "the hollow" may be recognized by those who dwell there to have an individual identity and to merit care and social action consistent with their special values, life ways, and problems. It is important to know not only the kinds of subgroups that exist but also the degree to which they share in and differ from the values of the larger community, for from community values spring the community health goals — those things the community considers "good" in health care. (For further discussion of special communities, see Chapter 26.)

In some communities, traditional ways of behavior will be strictly followed, with many of the details of daily living subject to elaborate rituals and rules. In others, individuality may be stressed; or there may even be great rigidity in the need to be different. In one neighborhood, kinship bonds may be exceedingly strong; in times of trouble, help is usually sought from a mother, an aunt or other relative, or a wise neighbor. Other communities seen to follow the "I-don't-bother-my-neighbors-and-they-don't-bother-me" rule, and each family deals only with its own problems.

The value assigned to health care as compared with other life needs is often frequently culturally determined. In some communities, health will be high in the hierarchy of life values, and health information and care will be sought and welcomed. In other areas, competing values may take precedence — "getting ahead" may seem more important to the business executive than does developing a way of life that will reduce stress. The struggle for sheer survival of those in pioneer or poverty situations may put all but the most immediate and urgent health needs low on the priority scale. In some communities, the decisions of a prestigious leader (such as a village priest or mayor) may influence the behavior of the whole group. In other areas, the sources of influence are much more diffused — a situation prevalent in large urban areas where people tend to associate with a particular group of people at work, another at church, and a third at home.

These characteristic ways of behavior are exceedingly important to the health planner. For example, if one of the health goals is to have women within certain age groups examine their breasts periodically as a means of early detection of abnormality, the education might be planned on a one-by-one basis — with the health worker talking with individuals (in their homes or at a clinic) about the reason for the procedure, the technique used, and the steps to take if anything unusual is found. If neighborhood ties are strong, the instruction might be given in neighborhood groups; in this situation, the educator has the advantage of reaching larger numbers and the opportunity of using the group members themselves for mutual aid. If the strong-leader pattern prevails, attention should be placed on reaching and convincing the leaders before any attempt is made to contact the target population.

The Community's Political System

The inter-relationship between the political and government structure and the people it serves is an important factor in predicting the means by which the population will move to meet its health needs. Although *politics* is often used as a derogatory term — synonymous with lack of integrity and commitment to the public — the political system does represent the way in which a population group has organized in order to facilitate collective action and exert some control over its collective behavior. The stability and responsiveness of the political structure have considerable effect upon the ability of the community to develop continuing and stable health programs. The way in which the several groups of people within the community sees "the government" also affects their expectations concerning government health action, their willingness to support and participate in government-sponsored health activities, and, often, the way in which they relate to the health department, the school nurse, or other government workers.

The relationship between the political system and government units also has an effect on the way in which the community's health tasks will be accomplished. The degree to which health personnel are subject to political appointment has an effect on long-term planning, since (1) political control tends to produce less continuous staffing than does the merit system and (2) political control may attract job applicants whose talents adhere more to party loyalty than to professional expertise. In general, it is considered desirable in a democracy that those positions which are essentially policy making in nature should be tied to the political system, since elected officials — especially those at higher levels of responsibility — are usually committed to some kind of change and can accomplish this best if the policy-making staff is similarly minded. On the other hand, positions that are primarily of an administrating and implementing nature may lose much by a political appointment, since the continuity of program implementation is determined at this level — thus, stability in the work force is beneficial. It is important to know to what extent health personnel are subject to political appointment; also important is the degree to which the political establishment concerns itself with health programs. Do they "leave it to the experts," giving little attention or support to the programs as they develop? Or do they take an active part in representing the public's needs and in striving for effective and efficient health-care systems?

The Community's Habits of Action

Both the report of the National Commission on Community Health Services and the Comprehensive Health Planning Act use the phrase *partnership for health* to describe the relationship that should exist between health efforts of government at all levels and private and voluntary health services. In the United States and Canada — as in many industrialized countries of the world where private and government health-care systems are well developed — the relationship between the two is of major significance to the health of the community. This relationship may be hostile, with each party feeling that the other is failing to act in the true interests of the community. It may be based on a scrupulous observance of declared spheres of influence, with neither party trespassing into areas that are considered within the other's province. It may be a true partnership, with government agencies and voluntary agencies, private medical and health practitioners and government health employees, and hospitals and other community agencies combining their efforts to define and correct the health problems of the community. Obviously, the last pattern is the most desirable; however, all too often, the relationship that exists lies somewhere between the first and third patterns of cooperation.

To understand the health action patterns of a community, it is important to know in what ways the different levels of government interact — the flow of money, advice, and support from national, to state, to local agencies and from the community agency to the various smaller geographic or cultural units within the community. It is important to know how the government agency interacts with the private physician. Does it move to his support, provide him with consultation and patient-care services that will strengthen his work, and share responsibility with him on a planned basis? Or are both groups acting as isolated entities? It is also important to know how government agencies interact with voluntary agencies. Does the local health officer welcome the help of the people from the local tuberculosis association and keep them informed of the health department's plans? Or does he secretly wish they would disappear and let him get on with the job? Does the government agency work with the local nurses' association on salary problems? Or does it get involved only when involvement cannot be avoided?

"Who Does What" Is an Important Question. Within each community, there is apt to be a relatively small group of individuals (or institutions) that exert considerable influence on the decisions of others in the community and so become in effect the decision makers in many matters of public concern. Such a power structure has engaged the interest of sociologists for many years and has engendered some controversy over the means by which such individuals can be recognized. Studies indicate that power tends to be a specialized rather than a generalized attribute; the person or group exerting the influence may vary in different subgroups or in different problem areas: the individual who is in a strong position of power with respect to health decisions may not be the same one who initiates a program for city beautification. Furthermore, the person who is most vocal and visible as a committee member may not be the one who is exerting the pressure; a behind-the-scenes leader may, in fact, have greater control. Thus, in seeking out the leadership group in a community, it is important to distinguish the figurehead from the individual who truly exerts an influence on the decisions made.

Of considerable interest in recent years is the emergence of increased power among both the organized poor and students. These two groups have exerted considerable influence on local and national decisions — the exact antithesis of their former power stance. With respect to leadership power among the poor, the change undoubtedly represents both a shift in the nature of the problems engaging the social planners and a defined public commitment to the development of leadership in this group. The result is that, in many communities, there is a new type of leader whose influence derives from his sharing in and knowledge of the problems of extreme poverty and whose natural capacity for leadership has been carefully fostered as a matter of social policy.

"Who Talks to Whom" Provides Action Clues. The network of communication that is built up within families and groups has an important part to play in the development of community health plans and therefore is logically included in the community assessment process. Informal influence, such as that found within the family or work unit, has been recognized as a powerful factor in securing health action; and the degree to which such informal influence is favorable to good health practice is a matter of concern to health officials.

The patterns and the force of influence within a family differ greatly. When kinship ties are strong and communication among family members is extensive, the opinions and judgments of even the remote relative may exert considerable influence on family health decisions and attitudes. In some families, relatives are the first-line help sought in emergencies of all types, and family response to the needs of its members may be prompt and generous. In other instances, family ties are weak, and the first source of help or advice may be a community agency or professional worker.

Informal influence may also be exerted through friendship and organizational affiliations. Studies have shown that most people develop friendships of a continuing type. Bell and Boat[4] found that only a small proportion of the groups they studied could not identify "best friends."

In addition to individual and family communication networks, the number and types of groups with which community members are affiliated may have a strong influence on the way they perceive and act in health matters. The stand taken by an individual's church may influence his or her attitude concerning contraception; the official position taken by a labor union may influence its members' judgments about the best methods for delivery of health care services; social affiliations may affect one's perception of the value of health care. Freeman and Lambert have found that most community groups influenced health behavior to some degree in both a positive and a negative way.[5] Thus, it is important to know insofar as possible the channels of communication and the network of social relationships that exist in a group as a basis for understanding the ways in which they might be expected to take health action.

Communities Have Their Own Styles of Response. Communities develop their own style of responding to health problems in the way they organize to take action as well as in the characteristic course of action followed.

Some communities tend to organize for health care on a community-wide basis, with plans and action designed for the city or county or state as a whole. In other areas, action may be developed within a loose structure of community-wide planning, with considerable diversity in the programs of smaller groups within the community. In still other communities, each small group appears to go its own way with little relationship to the plans or actions of other groups.

Some communities tend to organize for health care under well-defined goals. Others move within a vague general commitment to health care "rocking along" with current programs or leaving the decision to the health administrator. When the goal-oriented approach is used, the goals may be set by the health professionals, representatives of the community, a political body, or some combination of these groups. These goals may be minimal — to have safe streets and to protect the population from dangerously ill people and epidemics — or the more inclusive and operatively stated — to give the old people the medical and nursing care they need or to give mentally retarded children educational and health opportunities to maximize their skills. Sometimes these goals are consciously arrived at, explicitly stated, and deliberately pursued. More often, what the community wants and is willing to support in health care is not formalized but is nevertheless expressed in health behavior such as their patterns of utilization of available services, legislative action, or response to the care provided. Local and regional health planning agencies developed under the Comprehensive Health Planning Act have afforded a formalized mechanism for such community effort.

Families or subgroups within the community also organize for their own health care in different ways. They may plan on an expedient crisis basis, using the emergency room of the local hospital as their primary source of care; they may take a more prudent approach through prepaid insurance and a wider use of preventive care; they may rely entirely on the medical center specialist group for medical care or on the general practitioner for first-line care of illness, using the medical center only for serious problems.

THE NURSE'S SOURCES OF COMMUNITY HEALTH DATA

The community health nurse must investigate the many sources of information that will shed light on the health situation of a community. Official agency records, state or local published reports of vital statistics and services provided, formal and informal conferences with community leaders will all yield many facts and opinions that together produce a picture of the situation.

Official Vital Statistics Provide a Useful Base

The decennial census of the United States provides basic information about numbers of people, much of which is detailed for states or for local communities, such as counties and municipalities. The census tract data are available in all counties included in metropolitan areas (average 3,000–4,000 population). The infrequency of the count, however, means that there will be times when the data for the local area are incomplete or inaccurate — for instance, when a recent major extension of housing increases the population within a matter of months. However, the census is a valuable source of data that shows trends over time and provides the national picture as a backdrop against which the local situation may be viewed in perspective.

Local vital records or reports, generally available through the local or state health department, may prove more immediately useful. Reports of birth and deaths frequently include more information than the mere fact of birth or death. A birth certificate, for instance, may include such information as whether or not the mother received prenatal care, and it may give facts about the delivery as well.

Surveys or Survey Reports Supplement Official Records

The purpose of the United States Center for Health Statistics is the continuing assembly and interpretation of health data for the population as a whole. In addition to the usual information about births, deaths, and reportable diseases, there is provision for a continuous survey of the population based on probability sampling techniques that yield data regarding the prevalence (i.e., the number of individuals suffering from a particular condition at a given point in time) and incidence (i.e., the number of new cases over a specified period, usually one year) or illness or disability. Programs of the center have broadened to include data from the health examination survey, nutrition examination survey, health resources utilization, health resources, and family growth, as well as the traditional health interview survey.[6] Content of each may be modified from time to time to secure data of particular interest. Special surveys may be undertaken for disease-related occurrences, such as the incidence of smoking or the blood cholesterol levels of given age groups. Some of the studies combine household survey procedures and medical examination procedures. The various reports of the center are published by the Government Printing Office and are available in most health libraries and in many public libraries. Such survey data represent one of the valuable tools for public health practice.[7]

Some local communities, states and regions, and health services research centers carry on household surveys and epidemiologic studies of current problems affecting the total population in a specified area. Local surveys are organized to provide data not otherwise available or to answer specific questions. For example, a household survey might be planned to find out what differences exist in the utilization of local health resources. Surveys may be oriented to epidemiologic, behavioral, or biologic data and will vary widely in methodology. However, their two primary characteristics are that they are based on a sample that is sufficiently representative of the population being studied to render the findings predictive for the whole group and that the methodology is such that it minimizes the likelihood of unreliable findings.

Central Registries on Specified Conditions

Central registries may be maintained for specified conditions, such as crippling, handicap, cancer, tuberculosis, or mental illness. The purpose of such a registry is to make available at all times a count of those reported as suffering from particular diseases or impairments and the status of each case with respect to disease state and treatment. Such accounting makes it easy to plan for shifts in program as the size of the register grows or shrinks and as the characteristics of those persons listed in the register change.

Agency Records Provide Current Data

Records of hospital admissions and discharges, health department reports or case records, and insurance groups records may provide data about health in the community and the services that the people are receiving. Records of illness, physical examination reports, and records of absence in schools and industries are sources of information of illness in special age or vocational groups. However, agency records that are not directly concerned with illness and its treatment are often considered unreliable sources. For example, nursing records are probably a poor source to use for determining to what extent patient teaching programs are being implemented.

Another source of useful information is reports of screening experience — both special screening efforts and the ongoing screening that may be done in schools, industries, or in the health center for the general public.

Systematic Observation and Inquiry

Systematic observation and inquiry are good sources of community health data. For example, systematically querying prenatal patients on their reasons for seeking medical care may produce information on attitudes toward prenatal care. Visits to nursing home administrators, groups concerned with helping the elderly obtain needed care and services, professionals trying to implement legislation and regulations for care of the elderly — as well as talking with and observing older families coping in their own environment — will help to identify problems and vulnerable groups in this age population. This type of inquiry can be escalated to full-scale research when the occasion warrants. Sometimes it is possible to engage in this kind of research as part of an ongoing job, or with assistance from others in the agency, or in cooperation with a university that may conduct the study.

Current journals, such as the nursing and public health journals, often provide information about other communities, information that may be valid in one's own setting. More specialized journals may report on community studies, such as reports of adherence to regimen among tuberculosis patients; again, these reports might have significance for one's own community.

There is a great wealth of sources. The individual involved has the responsibility of seeking out those that provide suitable data on which to base an estimate of the health of the community.

ANALYSIS OF HEALTH DATA

The assembly of available factual data, observations, and judgments about the health conditions and the health functioning of the community is only the first step in diagnosis. The rest of the process involves the ordering and synthesis of these bits and pieces of information (which are likely to vary greatly in their quality: that is, in their reliability and applicability) into some kind of whole that permits drawing inferences that will serve as the basis for program planning. This means that the data must be studied and related in an orderly way.

Data Must Be Seen in Perspective

Current information about health conditions and health behavior represents just one point in a long process. First, it is important to see present conditions in the perspective of time; in other words, one must recognize trends. For example, current deaths from accidental causes need to be seen in terms of the type and the number of such deaths in the past. Is the overall rate climbing or falling? Are rates for certain types of accidents changing? If the data are seen in the perspective of time, their meaning is amplified.

Second, it is important to see statistics in the perspective of the larger environmental forces that might have significance: the greater likelihood of accidental death due to an increased number of motor vehicles; improved housing that lessens the number of home accidents; shifts in parent-youth or youth-society relationships that are conducive to aberrant behavior on the part of young people. Is the increasing venereal disease rate largely accounted for by small population clusters, or is it distributed throughout the community? Is good utilization of facilities associated with their location, with the participation of the consumers in the management of the facility, or with the kind of personnel employed in the facility? The search is for those things in the environment that could be associated with an observed change, whether that change is favorable or unfavorable.

Quantitative and Qualitative Facets of the Data Must Be Balanced

The number of cases of dental caries represents a tremendous problem in terms of size. However, in terms of impact on total health, this number may be less important than the one indicating a rising venereal disease rate. In terms of avoidability — another quality criterion — it would perhaps add up to a lesser level of importance than, say, the number of cases of measles among children. Nutritional deficiencies carry a different qualitative value in an affluent country than they would in a country where frank underfeeding is associated with economic inability to secure adequate food supplies. Therefore, unless qualitative criteria are applied, the statistical magnitude of a problem may dangerously distort its real importance.

INFERENCES PROVIDE A BASE FOR ACTION

Once relationships become clear, it is possible to move toward inference: the general conclusions that may be made on the basis of the data. For example, it may be apparent that a particular community will not respond well at a particular time to a crash program for tuberculosis control. This may be because they accept the disease as inevitable and because transportation and manpower deficits make it difficult to get the required medication or to provide the necessary supportive care to direct people in taking the medication. Furthermore, folk medicine may be a powerful deterrent, and the relationship between the indigenous practitioners and the organized health unit are characterized by a lack of understanding and trust. The first thrust might thus be toward caring for individuals and postponing the mass action.

In another instance the conclusion might be that it is essential to move quickly into a measles vaccination program, even though it will be difficult to get supplies and to work out satisfactory arrangements with private physicians. The public is impatient; they are used to having new discoveries placed into the program early; the product is safe; the physicians for the most part are likely to "go along" with a crash program if it is properly presented; other urgent programs will be disarranged but not seriously impeded by the requirements of this one; and a group of volunteer workers in low-income areas are anxious to have a specific program to work on. In this situation, the forces for quick action outweigh the forces for a more deliberative approach.

In other instances, inferences may be made about the possible outcomes of the program. The combination of multiple and serious health impairment, low income, negative attitudes toward authority, and a great need for identity in a low-income urban group might lead one to infer that goals should be set at a more moderate level. At the same time, service requirements may need to be built beyond the point that the health conditions themselves warrant in order to establish a level of direct help that would obviously demonstrate an honest and sustained effort to help.

The inference stage is the transition between diagnosis and program planning. It defines and sets the limitations, the imperatives, and the maximizing opportunities that appear to exist, and it indicates the kinds of approaches that might be expected to be useful. Thus armed, the health worker is in a position to move to specific program planning and implementation.

The simplicity or complexity of community health diagnosis depends on the situation and on the preparation and availability of the professional worker. Some appreciation of the community in these broad terms is an essential background for the nurse as she plans for the nursing care of population groups, however large or small these groups may be. As she studies the needs for nursing care within the population for which she is responsible, she will use to some extent the observations and the processes required for more elaborate community health diagnosis.

REFERENCES

1. Payne, A. M. M.: The environment in human ecology: General considerations. *In* Pan American Health Organization: *Environmental Determinants of Community Well-Being.* Washington, D.C., 1965, p. 3.
2. Swaroop, S.: *Introduction to Health Statistics.* Baltimore, Williams and Wilkins Co., 1960, p. 182.
3. See for example Bahnson, C. B.: Behavioral factors associated with the etiology of physical disease. Am. J. Pub. Health, *64*:1033, 1974.
4. Bell, W., and Boat, M.: Urban neighborhoods and informal sociological relationships. Am. J. Sociol., *62*:391, 1957.
5. Freeman, H. E., and Lambert, C.: The influence of community groups on health matters. Human Organiz., *24*:353, 1966.
6. Copies of all reports listed here, as well as catalogues, can be obtained free of charge by calling (301) 436-"NCHS" (24-hour publications "hotline") or writing to:
National Center for Health Statistics
Scientific and Technical Information Branch
3700 East-West Highway, Room I-57
Hyattsville, MD 20782
7. For a current listing of topics, see National Center for Health Statistics: *Current Listing and Topical Index to the Vital and Health Statistics Series.* DHEW Pub. No. (PHS) 79-1301.

SUGGESTED READINGS

Bayer, M.: Community diagnosis — Through sense, sight, and sound. Nurs. Outlook, *21*:712, 1973.
Bellow, T. A.: Community health nurses and community organization. *In* Archer, S. E., and Fleshman, R.: *Community Health Nursing.* North Scituate, Mass. Duxbury Press, 1975.
Bennis, W., et al.: *The Planning of Change,* 3rd ed. New York, Holt, Rinehart and Winston, 1976.
Berger, D. G., and Gardner, E. A: Use of community surveys in mental health planning. Am. J. Publ. Health, *61*:110, 1971.
Blum, H. L.: *Planning for Health: Development and Application of Social Change Theory.* New York, Human Sciences Press, 1974.
Bock, W.: Field techniques in delineating the structure of community leadership. Human Organiz., *24*:358, 1965.
Bowman, R. A., and Culpepper, R. C.: Power: Rx for change. Am. J. Nurs., *74*:1053, 1974.
Boyer, J. S., Reinhardt, A., and Quinn, M. (eds.): in *Community Assessment in Family-Centered Community Nursing.* St. Louis, C. V. Mosby Co., 1973.
Cox, F. M. (ed.): *Strategies of Community Organization,* Itasca, Ill., F. E. Peacock, Inc., 1973.
Davies, M. (ed.): *Use of Epidemiology in Planning Health Services.* Proceedings of International Epidemiological Association; Belgrade, Yugoslavia, January 1973.
Dodge, W. F., et al.: Patterns of maternal desires for child health care. Am. J. Pub. Health, *60*:1421, 1970.
Florida State Board of Health: *A Study of Extra-Hospital Nursing Needs in a Retirement Area.* Final Report of St. Petersburg, Florida, 1964.
Freeman, H. E., Levine, S., and Reeder, L. P. (eds.): *Handbook of Medical Sociology,* 3rd ed. Englewood Cliffs, N.J., Prentice-Hall, Inc., 1979.

Fuchs, V. R.: *Who Shall Live? Health, Economics and Social Change.* New York, Basic Books, Inc., 1975.

Hanchett, E. S.: Community Health Assessment: A Conceptual Tool Kit. New York, John Wiley, 1979.

Hanlon, J. J.: *Public Health Administration and Practice,* 6th ed. St. Louis, Mo., C. V. Mosby Co., 1974, Chapter 39.

Isaacs, G.: Frontier nursing service: Family nursing in rural areas. Clin. Obstet. Gynecol., *15*:394, 1972.

Linder, F.: The health of the American people. Sci. Am., *214*:21, 1966.

Logan, R. F. L.: Assessment of sickness and health in a community. Med. Care, 2:173, 1964.

MacMahon, B., and Pugh, T.: *Epidemiology: Principles and Methods.* Boston, Little, Brown and Co., 1970.

Magalhaes, M., and Albold, M.: Teaching public health nursing by the city block. Am. J. Nurs., *62*:82, 1962.

Mechanic, D.: *Politics, Medicine and Social Science.* New York, Wiley Interscience, 1974.

Moe, E.: Nature of today's community; Reinhardt, A. M., and Chatlin, E. D.: Assessment of health needs in a community: The basis for program planning. *In* Reinhardt, A., and Quinn, M. (eds.): *Current Practice in Family-Centered Community Nursing.* St. Louis, Mo., C. V. Mosby Co., 1977.

Morris, J. N.: *Uses of epidemiology,* 3rd ed. Baltimore, Williams and Wilkins Co., 1976.

Mullane, M. K.: Nursing care and political arena. Nurs. Outlook, *23*:699, 1975.

Novello, D. J.: The National Health Planning and Resources Development Act. Nurs. Outlook, *24*:354, 1976.

Oglesby, M., and Carl, M. K.: The development and evaluation of a health care system: A heuristic model. Nurs. Res., *23*:334, 1974.

Palmiere, D.: Types of planning in the health care system. Am. J. Pub. Health, *62*:1112, 1972.

Partridge, K. B.: Community and professional participation in decision making at a health center. Health Serv. Rep., *88*:527, 1973.

Regester, D. C.: Community mental health — For whose community? Am. J. Pub. Health, *64*:886, 1974.

Reinke, W. A.: *Health Planning: Qualitative Aspects and Quantitative Techniques.* Baltimore, Johns Hopkins University Press, 1972.

Roghmann, K. J., and Haggerty, R. J.: The diary as a research instrument in the study of health and illness behavior. Med. Care, *10*:143, 1972.

Rothman, J.: *Planning and Organizing for Social Change.* New York, Columbia University Press, 1974.

Ruybal, S. E., Bauwens, E., and Fosla, M. J.: Community assessment: An epidemiological approach. Nurs. Outlook, *23*:365, 1975.

Schwenger, C. W., and Sayers, L. A.: A Canadian survey by public health nurses of the health and living conditions of the aged. Am. J. Pub. Health, *61*:1189, 1971.

Scott, J. M.: The changing health care environment: Its implications for nursing. Am. J. Pub. Health, *64*:364, 1974.

Shiloh, A., and Selavan, I. (eds.): *Ethnic Groups of America: Their Morbidity, Mortality and Behavior Disorders.* Vols. I and II. Springfield, Ill., Charles C Thomas, Publisher, 1973 (Vol. I) and 1974 (Vol. II).

Silver, G.: Community participation and health resource allocation. Int. J. Health Sci., 3:117, 1973.

Somers, A.: Who's in charge here — or Alice searches for a king in Mediland. New Engl. J. Med., *287*:849, 1972.

Spector, R.: *Cultural Diversity in Health and Illness.* New York, Appleton-Century-Crofts, 1979.

Stensland, P. G.: Old professional in a new world. Adult Leader., April 1973. Reprinted from Nurs. Dig., *1*:76, 1973.

Susser, M.: *Causal Thinking in the Health Sciences: Concepts and Strategies of Epidemiology.* New York, Oxford University Press, 1973.

U.S. Public Health Service: *The Cooperative Federal-State-Local Health Statistics System.* Pub. HSM 72-1209, Rockville, Maryland.

U.S. Public Health Service: *Facts at Your Fingertips, A Guide to Sources of Statistical*

Information on Major Health Topics, 3rd ed., Department of Health, Education and Welfare (PHS) 79-1246, National Center for Health Statistics, 1978.

Wilkins, R.: Data collection and classification in services for the mentally retarded. W. H. O. Chron., 27:194, 1973.

World Health Organization: *Community Health Nursing, Technical Report Series 558.* Report of a WHO Expert Committee. Geneva, 1974, pp. 7–10.

World Health Organization: *Measurement of Levels of Health. Technical Report Series No. 137.* Geneva, 1957.

World Health Organization: *Statistical Indices of Family Health.* Report of WHO Study Group, Geneva, 1976.

RESOURCES

National Health Planning Information Center
  (NHPIC)
Bureau of Health Planning and Resources
  Development
HRA, DHHS
P.O. Box 1600
Prince Georges Plaza Branch
Hyattsville, Maryland 20788

National Center for Health Statistics
Scientific and Technical Information Branch
3700 East-West Highway, Room 1-57
Hyattsville, Maryland 20782
Phone 301/436-NCHS (24-hour publications hotline)

CHAPTER 18

THE COMMUNITY HEALTH NURSE IN THE EARLY DETECTION AND CONTROL OF DISEASE

The control of disease is a central concern of community health agencies. Public health agencies, originally concerned primarily with the control of communicable diseases, have broadened their concern to include the control of many other diseases and, in particular, of the control of chronic illness.

The incidence of acute communicable diseases has been dramatically reduced as sanitary measures and new immunizing agents have become available. Smallpox is considered to be eradicated; diphtheria and poliomyelitis have been brought to very low levels in developed countries; measles and rubella are becoming equally rare. However, occasional outbreaks do occur, and vigilance is still necessary until these diseases are completely eradicated. Venereal disease, hepatitis, and tuberculosis continue to present problems.

The control of noncommunicable disease is a much more complex problem than the control of communicable disease. For many diseases, knowledge about causation is scanty, and the roles of the multiple contributing factors are not clear. Furthermore, much of the required care is provided by private physicians, and their aid must be enlisted if control is to be achieved.

METHODS OF DISEASE CONTROL

The control of disease is a dynamic process; it is a problem in which the pieces of the puzzle are constantly being rearranged. The distribu-
336

tion of disease may change as social and economic conditions change. New methods of prevention and cure continue to be discovered at a rapid pace, and incidence rates may fall precipitously over a very short period (as was true after the introduction of penicillin). Acceptance of the concept of multiple causation of disease opens an almost inexhaustible source of intriguing lines of inquiry in which it sometimes appears that nonmedical factors outweigh the medical in effecting change. Thus, the control of disease in populations must be a constant process of study, action, and restudy. Control programs enhance efforts to define the nature and distribution of disease in the population, to institute the preventive measures that are available, and to secure prompt and adequate curative and rehabilitative care.

Epidemiology — The Basis for Action

Epidemiology is the study of the distribution and determinants of disease in populations. Infectious diseases, chronic diseases, and social systems have been studied using this approach. The distinctive characteristic of epidemiology is its focus on health in populations as distinct from the health of individuals. Current definitions also stress the concept of excessive prevalence of a condition, based on comparisons of one population group to another.[1]

Define the Nature, Extent, and Distribution of Disease

Obviously, it is vital to know the incidence and prevalence of specific diseases in the population in order to judge the size of the problem with which the health system must deal. A knowledge of trends concerning incidence and prevalence is essential in order to plan control programs for the future.

Knowledge of the distribution of the disease among various segments of the population is essential for developing more precise measures for control and gaining increased insight into the nature of the disease process. Knowledge of the age, socioeconomic, and occupational groups that are particularly affected provides valuable clues to causative or influential factors of the disease; these data also provide a basis for case selection and program direction.

Define the Determinants and Consequences of Disease

A knowledge of the determinants and consequences of a disease is essential to its control. The search for the determinants of disease has moved from a narrow focus on the specific causative organisms or event without which the disease or condition *cannot* occur, to a wide-angle view of the multiple factors that determine whether or not the disease actually *will* occur. For example, infection with the tubercle bacillus is *necessary* for tuberculosis to develop in an individual, but it may not be *sufficient* to cause the disease. Stress, poor nutrition, crowding, or inadequate health practices and facilities for health care may be just as important in explaining why — given the same degree of exposure to the causative organism — some people contract the disease while others do not.

Thus it may be important to know not only the disease state of the population but also the pattern of pre-disease states or disease-associated conditions. For example, it may be useful to estimate the nutritonal levels, immunization status, birth weights, or smoking habits of the population; these indices help to elucidate the nature of the disease experience and suggest the relative vulnerability of specified populations.

Knowledge of the health or social consequences of disease is also an essential for control of disease, since it provides an index for evaluating the urgency for the control measures and a means of determining the value of the program to the community.

Primary and Secondary Preventive Measures

Preventive measures may be primary or secondary, with varying levels of specificity. Some measures, such as measles immunization or abstinence from smoking, are expected to prevent the occurrence of the disease. Other measures, such as early detection of disease or programs of rehabilitation that maximize functioning of the disabled, are expected to minimize the effects of the disease once it occurs.

Commonly used preventive measures vary widely in the degree to which their utility has been validated. For example, smoking is almost certainly implicated in the development of certain respiratory diseases, and "tender loving care" by parent or parent surrogate is quite clearly associated with an infant's ability to thrive. Other preventive measures — e.g., health education measures as a means of reducing the incidence of venereal disease or counseling services as a measure for reducing emotional stress among college students — are more speculative.

When the means of prevention are not known, reliance must be placed on secondary preventive measures and the alleviation of the effects of the disease. When the causes of a disease are multiple (as is the case with tuberculosis), and there is a lack of precise information about the reinforcing effect of contributing conditions that exist concurrently, prevention may involve many components.

Thus, in some instances, "instituting preventive measures" may indeed represent a clear-cut, obvious program — for example, the current efforts to immunize children against rubella in order to protect their mothers from infection that may endanger future offspring. In other instances, however, "instituting preventive measures" may imply a concerted attack that includes efforts to reduce the stress factors in the physical or social environment — e.g., to provide nutritional guidance to increase the hemoglobin level, to institute welfare services to support a more adequate level of living, and to refer to a marriage counselor to reduce stress arising from domestic difficulties.

Prompt and Adequate Care

Prompt and adequate care means more than the provision of care facilities. Prompt and adequate care requires that the condition be put under care as soon as the need arises and that the care encompass secondary prevention and rehabilitation, as well as curative content. It implies that the recipients are willing to accept the care provided and that the professionals providing the care are adequate in number and competency. It also implies that the facilities are adequate enough to permit the professionals to work efficiently as well as being accessible and acceptable to the users. Thus, "prompt and adequate care" is as much a responsibility and function of the individual who is ill as it is of the community that is obligated to see that the necessary care is available. It is as much a function of the consumer — whether patient or taxpayer — as it is of the health professional.

The provision of direct therapeutic intervention must be combined with measures designed to produce an informed and highly motivated population, an adequate supply of professional personnel of appropriate levels of preparation, and an action program that develops the facilities and the procedures necessary to reach those who require care.

Prompt and adequate care in the present-day context must also encompass provisions for social and environmental, as well as medical, action.

THE ROLE OF THE COMMUNITY HEALTH NURSE IN DISEASE CONTROL

Control Through Ongoing Activity

The community health nurse has many opportunities for disease control action in the course of her daily work. The alert community health nurse discovers many disease problems other than those conditions for which service was initiated. The visit to a preschool child may lead to the discovery of an older family member whose fatigue, cough, and listlessness indicate possible disease. The routine visit to a school may turn up information about an increase in the number of sore throats or gastrointestinal upsets among the pupils and teachers, indicating the need for an epidemiologic investigation. For patients who have a long-term illness and who are being cared for at home, the community health nurse may be a major observer of changes that suggest intervention to prevent secondary complications.

The ongoing educational activities of the nurse also do much to further the disease-control program. These activities may range from general public education, which is designed to alert the public or a large segment of the population to a particular problem, to the type of intensive family teaching that occurs in the home care of the stroke patient. Education may be directed toward others in the professional community (such as nurses working in physician's offices or in industry) in order to increase their contribution to disease-control efforts. It may be directed to those who have, or are at special risk of having, a specific disease, such as inactive tuberculosis patients or families in which diabetes has appeared. Education may be directed toward the "deciders" in a particular community (such as elected officials, labor leaders, or clergymen). These leaders may sanction or encourage a particular course of action, thus building community commitment to the program.

The ongoing health promotional activities of the nurse contribute to the improvement of the general condition of the population and to increasing its resistance to disease or to improving its capacity to cope with disease, physically and emotionally, when it occurs. For example, the child who has learned the value of handwashing in school may be less likely to pick up infections transmitted hand-to-mouth; the well-nourished expectant mother may be at less risk during pregnancy; the person who has learned to deal realistically with life problems and who has established an "emotional reserve" may be better equipped to handle catastrophic illness, should it occur. Although not all "good" health behavior can be shown as directly influencing disease occurrence or severity, the assumption of such a relationship is usually made as a working hypothesis on which to base the planning of control programs. Much further research is needed to document or disprove these hypotheses.

Anticipatory Guidance and Supportive Measures

A second large contribution that is made in the course of the nurse's daily work is the anticipatory guidance that is provided when the risk is known to be high. Lewis Thomas calls this the ". . . nontechnology, impossible to measure in terms of its capacity to alter either the natural cause of disease or its eventual outcome."[2] Much time and effort are spent in listening, encouraging, and reinforcing family strengths during periods of stress. When a member of a family is known to have diabetes or tuberculosis, a special anticipatory guidance effort will alert the family to the early symptoms of trouble and to the value of periodic screening for the disease. The high-strung mother may receive specific knowledge about symptoms of illness in order to reduce her undue stress due to the imagined ills of her child as well as the consequent stress build-up of the family as a whole. In areas where the teenage pregnancy rate is high, the school nurse would most likely be particularly alert to signs of pregnancy among the group she services. She might also encourage referral by others in teaching and counseling positions, and arrange with teachers to include information in the general health instruction program on the signs of pregnancy, the dangers of nonmedical abortion, and the sources of help for expectant mothers. If it is consistent with school and community policy, information on the availability of contraceptive advice and the conditions under which this advice can be obtained may also be included. All of these measures can help in securing early and adequate care. They are not special activities of community health nursing; rather, they are just the application of good nursing practice.

Epidemiologic Investigations

Epidemiologic investigations may be *descriptive:* they may deal with the occurrence and distribution of disease or health states of different segments of the population, of different communities or settings, or of trends over time; also, they may describe observable phenomena, such as the clustering of cases or the patterns of epidemics. Other forms of epidemiologic investigation are *analytic,* seeking out statistical associations that help to explain the occurrence and pattern of disease, and *experimental,* testing a hypothesis by rigorous research techniques. Thus, epidemiologic investigation may take many forms, involve many methodologies, and engage many different types of practitioners.

The community health nurse, working with the epidemiologist and the biostatistician, may participate in epidemiologic investigation through the following activities:

1. She may serve as an advance intelligence officer regarding conditions that merit epidemiologic study. The community health nurse may notice that within a low-income area, a particular neighborhood or cultural cluster tends to seek care and to adhere to recommended medical procedures, whereas other groups, subject to the same economic pressures, fail to do so. A study of the characteristics of this phenomenon may lead to a better understanding of the factors associated with compliance and may cause the modification of certain care practices.

2. She may collect data essential to epidemiologic analysis. This may be done as part of an organized study in which an epidemiologist or research officer has designed a study or developed formal interview schedules or report-forms for securing and transmitting required data. The fact-finding interview described in the preceding chapter is a major tool in this effort. On other occasions, the community health nurse may be on her own, collecting data to be submitted to the epidemiologist for use in a decision on the best way to evaluate the situation. Here, the nurse's knowledge of disease and disease processes is vitally important, since the need is not for information *per se* but for information relevant to the particular disease or situation.

3. She may participate in the design of epidemiologic investigation by identifying relevant areas of information not already included or by indicating possible nonmedical factors that might be significant in the analysis of data. For example, the nurse might point out that patterns of absence in industry appear to be related not only to the worker's characteristics but also to the supervisory style of the worker's immediate superiors.

4. She may motivate and assist the subjects of epidemiologic investigations in cooperating in disease investigation and control. The person with tuberculosis may find it difficult (and sometimes impossible) to identify the probable source of his infection or to admit that he did not take the prescribed medications. The willingness of each patient to try to provide required information and to "level" with the study personnel will influence the amount of knowledge that can be accumulated about the disease and its treatment. The busy mother of a small infant may find it difficult to set aside a period time to talk with a household interviewer about her childbearing experience and her feelings about the professional care she received unless she can see the ultimate benefits of the study. The nurse's own conviction of the importance of learning more about disease and disease-related conditions and her understanding of the importance to the study of the cooperation of those being studied will undoubtedly influence the quality of data secured. There is an increasing use of long-term prospective studies of factors associated with disease or health behavior, often involving the use of study cohorts that are followed over many years. In this case, maintaining the integrity of the study is extremely important. Keeping families "in the study" — returning for periodic tests or interviews, reporting frequently, or maintaining specified dietary records or practices — may be of major concern to the investigator. This may become a nursing assignment in itself, with the nurse assigned to the project to maintain contact with the family and to encourage and assist family members in their part of the study. In some instances, investigators have offered comprehensive nursing care as a bonus for participation. Thus, a community health nurse assigned to a long-term follow-up project for brain-damaged children might provide general nursing support to the family. Establishing such a service-oriented and close

relationship may lead to the family's identification with the purpose of the project and may increase each member's willingness to participate fully over an extended period of time.

5. She may use the results of epidemiologic investigation as a springboard for the improvement of community health nursing practice. The findings of epidemiologic studies may help to pinpoint the nursing needs of the population groups, to identify the crucial components of the care required, or to suggest areas of investigation in nursing practice.

The Nurse May Implement Regulations for Control

The community health nurse may be involved in the implementation of regulations for the control of disease. The nurse may support the efforts of the disease-control program to secure adequate reporting of disease as well as facilitate the reporting made by private physicians or by others required to report. She may be called upon to report breaches in the observation of required practices of individuals who are afflicted with a communicable disease or to explain and interpret the nature of the constraints imposed upon the patient by the regulations that do exist. Thus the school health nurse must be prepared to interpret and to follow regulations regarding exclusion from school for medical reasons, and to support compulsory immunization programs for children.

The nurse will want to have readily available the regulations regarding the reporting of disease and the public safety practices required of the family and of others associated with the patient. The community agency usually provides the nurse with such guides. If the agency cannot provide the guides, the nurse may need to secure the information from the local or state health department.

EARLY DETECTION OF DISEASE

The early detection of disease has assumed increasing importance both in private medical practice and in community health programs; it has, in fact, become a basic health service. This undoubtedly reflects the more hopeful and aggressive approach to preventing or moderating the effect of illness, especially long-term illness.

Major Approaches to Detection

Screening

Screening was defined by the Commission on Chronic Illness in 1951 as the following:

The presumptive identification of unrecognized disease or defect by the application of tests, examinations, or other procedures which can be applied rapidly.

Screening sorts out apparently well persons who probably do have disease from those who probably do not.[3]

It should be noted that screening does not include diagnosis; rather, screening identifies those who need more definitive study.

Screening is a valuable measure in that it can reach large numbers of people at a low cost and, for the most part, does not demand the services of the physician. The patient may be responsible for securing necessary specimens and for submitting these for analysis.

Screening measures may be directed toward a single disease or health condition, such as tuberculosis or food intake; or it may be *multiphasic* — that is, directed toward several diseases or health conditions. The Early and Periodic Screening, Diagnosis and Treatment (EPSDT) programs, designed for children eligible for medical assistance, include screening for hearing, vision, growth and nutrition, developmental problems, tuberculin sensitivity, bacteriuria, anemia, sickle cell disease trait, and increased lead absorption.[4]

Screening measures should not be undertaken for conditions with a negligible prevalence in a given community. For example, screening for parasites would be appropriate only where there was a known problem. The following is a list of criteria for selecting conditions for screening measures:

1. The condition sought should be an important problem.
2. There should be an accepted treatment for patients with recognized disease.
3. Facilities for diagnosis and treatment should be available.
4. There should be a recognized latent or early symptomatic stage.
5. There should be a suitable test or examination.
6. The test or examination should be acceptable to the population.
7. The natural history of the condition, including its development from latent to declared disease, should be adequately understood.
8. There should be an agreed policy on whom to treat as patients.
9. The cost of case finding (including diagnosis and subsequent treatment of patients) should be economically balanced in relation to the possible expenditure on medical care as a whole.
10. Case finding should be a continuing process and not a "once for all" project.[5]

Screening measures may be directed toward the population as a whole (mass screening), or they may be aimed at selected groups within the population. Tuberculosis screening, for example, may be primarily directed toward low-income groups or other groups at special risk in large cities; screening for cervical cancer is directed toward women in the age group 25 years and over; and vision and auditory screening may be directed at preschool and school-age children.

Physical Assessment

The physical assessment is usually accompanied by laboratory or other technical diagnostic procedures and, increasingly, is given along with health counseling by the physician, or nurse (or by another designated associate, such as a social worker or nutritionist). This procedure offers a more comprehensive health assessment than does screening. The examination may be undertaken by the family physician, by an organized clinic group or research team, or by a practitioner in a particular setting (e.g., the industry or school). In 1947, the American Medical Association established standards for the physicians' examination and suggested a schedule for such examinations throughout life:

Prenatal ....monthly to biweekly examinations
First 6 months..biweekly examinations
Second 6 months ....monthly examinations
1 to 2 years..quarterly examinations
2 to 5 years..semiannual examinations
5 to 15 years ....examination every 2 to 3 years
15 to 35 years...examination every 2 years
35 to 60 years...annual examinations
60+ years ....semiannual examinations

Since 1947, a great variety of schedules have been proposed for school-age children, for industrial populations, and for the general public. For the most part, subsequent recommendations proposed wider spacing of examinations. However, the changes appear to have been based upon feasibility rather than on need factors. Breslow and Somers recommend a life-time health monitoring program designed to incorporate cost-effective and health-effective prevention measures into ongoing health services. They define health goals and services based on clinical and epidemiologic criteria specific to 10 different age groups ranging from infancy to 75 and over. For example, in the age group 40 to 59, tests for hypertension and for cervical, mammary, and gastrointestinal cancer would be conducted along with interviews on smoking, drinking, and dietary intake.[7]

Regular medical examinations may be provided on a "selected population" basis for those with hazardous industrial jobs, for vulnerable families, for low-income populations, or for others at special risk. In the detection of handicapping conditions in children, a "risk register" or a "special service register" may be used. Under this system, factors associated with high risk are identified; then, for each family, designated health workers record the presence or absence of these risk factors. The names of the individuals exposed to risk factors are entered into the special register; these people are seen more frequently than are the others in that age group. A World Health Organization working paper estimated that about 20 per cent of the children born might be expected to fall into the risk-associated group and that within this 20 per cent, about 80 per cent of children with disabilities would be found.[8] The trend is definitely toward a broad-spectrum health examination with high reliance on laboratory tests and on the observations of the physician and of other professional personnel.

Interview or Questionnaire Survey

Individual or household interviews or questionnaires may also be used as a measure of securing data on the probable presence of illness, presymptomatic disorders, or prejudicial health conditions or behavior (such as smoking). These interviews are, for the most part, "structured" — that is, designed to cover specific content in a uniform way.

Self-administered health questionnaires are sometimes used either as a self-screening device or as an adjunct to physical examination. Follow-up counseling is provided to those whose questionnaire returns indicate problems; referral to medical care is made when indicated.

In addition to their use as a measure for individual health assessment, such interviews may be administered to a probability-sample in the population at large or to special groups, such as a school population, in order to establish the prevalence of specified conditions.

Continuing Surveillance

Continuing observation by physician, teacher, nurse, or other professional worker or by others sensitized to make pertinent observations is also an effectvie disease-detection measure. For example, observation of the young child, undertaken by the parent and monitored by the nurse, may reveal symptoms of impaired hearing: e.g., difficulty in waking or a lack of response to speech or a ringing telephone. The teacher's observation of a child who appears to block out the outside world and to retreat to nonresponsive indifference may lead to early recognition of a psychiatric disorder.

EARLY DETECTION OF ABNORMALITY

Discovery of unrecognized disease is a focal concern of early detection measures, but it is not the only purpose served. The uncovering of developmental irregularities, predisease conditions, and poor health practices, although less dramatic, may provide equally important findings. In particular, many health workers feel that the discovery of a slight elevation of blood pressure, a heightened cholesterol level, or obesity may indicate a higher than normal risk of specific disease — thus leading to treatment that may lessen the risk. Overcompetitive work habits or a beginning dependence on alcohol may be as important to executive health as is diabetes; the overanxious parent may be as much a danger to her child as is the mother who has tuberculosis.

Early detection measures may also yield important data regarding prevalence and incidence of specific health conditions. Perhaps the most notable development of such data is the continuing household interview and health examination program of the National Health Survey. Through the use of representative sampling units of the population, the survey provides data that make possible an estimation of characteristic health patterns and trends for the population of the country as a whole.

Since early detection measures start with presumably well populations, they contribute to the accumulation of data that are necessary to define more clearly what is "health" and what is "normal." At present, there are large areas of borderline illness — i.e., conditions that do not warrant a diagnosis of disease but are of sufficient impact to reduce one's effectiveness in meeting family or work responsibilities or to suggest a threat of illness.

Lastly, early detection measures may serve an important health education or health promotion end. Inquiry about smoking or inadequate sleep may lead to changed behavior.

Inquiries and tests for specific diseases may lead to a greater awareness of the symptoms of these diseases, to more prompt self-disclosure should these symptoms occur, or to the institution of regular self-inspection (such as regular self-examination of the breast).

THE OUTCOMES OF DETECTION PROGRAMS VARY

The outcome of a specific program will vary with the program's purpose, specific goals, and the population served. Glaucoma screening for those over 35 years of age is likely to yield a high number of new cases, since the incidence of glaucoma is great and since the onset of chronic glaucoma (which constitutes about 85 per cent of the total cases) is insidious and not easily recognized.

Screening for cervical cancer, if persistently undertaken, can enable the health professional to discover the disease at the preinvasive (and hence, more treatable) period. Even when the number of new cases uncovered is small (as in phenylketonuria (PKU) testing of infants), if the possiblity of treatment is bright, the savings to the individual and to the community may be great.

Screening measures, however, are not always indicated. For example, nutritional suveys might be expected to be quite effective in identifying previously unknown nutritional deficit in low-income communities, but this detection measure is too expensive for the high-income community, where a smaller yield is likely.

Yankauer and his associates have shown that school health examinations uncover few cases of previously unrecognized disease. He points out, however, that other purposes of the examination, such as education in and motivation toward the use of preventive health care, may make the procedure worthwhile.[9]

It is important for the nurse as a participant in or supporter of early disease detection programs to know what outcomes the sponsors of the program expect.

THE ROLE OF THE COMMUNITY HEALTH NURSE IN DETECTION PROGRAMS

The community health nurse, directly or indirectly, does much to support and implement programs for early detection of disease and abnormalities.

Motivation of Participants

The community health nurse motivates families and groups to use available resources. A persistent and troublesome problem in using early detection methods as a measure of health improvement is assuring that those who should receive the benefits of screening or other measures actually do receive them. In settings such as school and industry, utilization of preventive care facilities is encouraged by the organization's sponsorship and by the pressures to conform to the behavior of the majority. In some instances, these procedures may be required as a condition of admission to school or the retainment of a job. Community-sponsored programs, on the other hand, tend to be unevenly utilized.

Motivation may be a very individual thing, and the community health nurse's role may be to help the susceptible group to recognize and deal with the barriers to seeking such care. Steps that appear useful are:

1. Use all channels to inform families, groups, sources of referral (doctors, schools), and the community as a whole of the opportunity provided and of the advantages of participation.

2. Make special efforts to reach the most vulnerable groups with the message; inform and enlist local leaders, and "reach out" to families most in need through special home visiting and group discussions in the school or the community.

3. Try to anticipate and deal with "hang-ups," such as fears of finding out about disease or a dislike of using public health care facilities.

4. Make participation easy or, at least, possible by making provisions for such needs as child care or transportation.

5. Offer help to private physicians in the required, more definitive follow-up care for his patients.

6. Identify those who do *not* participate and try to uncover the reasons for their nonparticipation. This information will be most helpful in the preparation of future programs.

The Nurse May Be the Screener

Nurses are expanding their role in patient care with startling speed; and, in many instances, this role expansion involves taking on certain screening responsibilities. Nurses in schools and in industry have traditionally provided considerable screening service, aided by teachers and other health personnel. For many years, nurses in rural or inaccessible areas have served as screening agents. In some localities, nursing clinics to which patients come for a variety of tests, as well as for nurse counseling, have functioned for several years. In the past, these responsibilities were usually undertaken because no other professional worker was available. At present, however, there is considerable pressure for nurses in urban areas to take on expanded screening functions. Even though physicians are available, there is a feeling that the community health nurse is, by training and temperament, well adapted to the provision of such screening; it is also felt that it may be easier for the family to deal with the nurse, especially if the nurse-family relationship has been a close one. The problem of follow-up care is simplified when the nurse, backed by laboratory services, takes a central role in the actual screening.

In most instances where the nurse's role in screening is to be enlarged, the agency will make the decision as to which procedures can be safely delegated and will arrange for any additional training that the nurse may need to absorb this responsibility. If the nurse is working in a setting where such administrative support is not available (for example, if she is the only nurse in an independent project), she must take on the responsibility that any professional worker would in the control of his or her own practice. The community health nurse must be sure that she is not assuming responsibilities that either contravene medical or nursing practice acts or require a level of skill or judgment beyond her professional training. If she is unsure of herself or if she does not know sources for special training, the nurse may want to seek the help of the city or state nursing consultant, the local nurses' association, or the nursing administrator in a larger agency in the community.

Recruitment and Training of Screeners

Screening may be done by the nurse herself or by trained, paid or volunteer workers. Whether screening is continuing (as in self-examination of the breast or in a teacher's observations of school children) or only periodic (as in school or industrial health examinations), the community health nurse may be expected to recruit some or all of the members of the screening team — or, in the case of individual self-screening, to enlist the individual in this effort — and to provide for any needed training.

The *recruitment* of screening agents must be directed toward those individuals who have sufficient commitment to follow through with the task once it is undertaken and who can appreciate the necessity for accuracy and consistency in following the recommended procedures. It is advisable to recruit a few stand-by helpers to fill in if someone else must be absent. Consideration should also be given to enlisting the help of the consumer group as a measure of increasing interest and commitment to the project. Sometimes ready-made groups may be used, such as members of the parent-teacher association or graduates of a Red Cross home nursing class.

Timing of the screening service and of the training sessions should be consistent with the other demands made upon the screening team. If, for example, teachers are to help with screening procedures, the times should be worked out with the responsible administrator in order to interfere as little as possible with regular teaching duties. If parents are the screeners, schedules should be arranged so as not to conflict with home responsibilities.

A *review of content and procedure* may be necessary. The nurse should allow herself enough time to be sure her own knowledge of the screening program is up-to-date and accurate. The content and procedures of the program should be checked with a nurse consultant or with current nursing literature. When the screening involves the use of equipment, manufacturers may be able to provide assistance.

A *training program*, with a mini-curriculum, will have to be developed; this program should allow for:

1. Definition and interpretation of the purpose of the screening effort.

2. Presentation and discussion of the basic principles or concepts involved.

3. Explanation of the procedures involved.

4. Demonstration and practice of the procedures.

A *plan for supervision* of trainees must also be developed. This may involve observation of the screeners at work and review conferences with individuals or groups. In most instances, questionable or negative findings are checked by another screener who has had more experience.

The plan for recording, reporting, and follow-up care should be built into the training program.

Sometimes the community health nurse arranges only for screening personnel who have already been fully trained either by a voluntary association (such as the Society for the Prevention of Blindness) or by the agency. If this is the case, the nurse's reponsibility for teaching and supervision will be limited.

The Nurse May Be the Interviewer

When interview data are the basis of a survey or study, the community health nurse may be the interviewer. In this case, the primary purpose is not to secure change but rather to secure information.

Sometimes the interview is focused on a single individual who can provide information about his own symptoms, experience, plans, or feelings. He may be the "index case" (that is, the person first reported for care); he may be someone who is closely associated with the patient (a contact) and who may also have the disease; or he may be a parent. Sometimes the focus of the fact finding is the household, and data are secured regarding all members residing in the household.

In the nurse's handling of this responsibility, as in the whole fabric of nursing practice in any setting, the general skills of interviewing are exceedingly important. The purpose of the fact-finding interview may be to describe events, behavior, values, perceptions, or feelings. There are three types of fact-finding interviews with which the community health nurse may be involved:

1. *The epidemiologic investigation,* in which the purpose is to assemble relevant information about the onset and course of the disease, the possible sources of the disease, the other individuals who might be affected, and the presence or absence of factors that may be associated with the occurrence of disease.

2. *The individual or household survey interview,* which is designed to secure data on the incidence and prevalence of health or health-related conditions and to gather information of a behavioral, demographic, or personal nature that may be related to the occurrence of these conditions.

3. *The in-depth interview,* which is designed to describe, in detail an occurrence or a situation from several viewpoints.

The purposes of the interview will determine the type of interview and the methods that are used.

The fact-finding interview may be integral to nursing care or may be separate from it. In some cases, the fact-finding interview is undertaken in the course of providing care to the family and may be used not only as a means of securing information but also as a vehicle for explaining or teaching (as is often the case in caring for communicable diseases or screening for developmental disabilities).

In other instances, the fact-finding interview may be purposely divorced from care. This is important when the interview is part of a study, and it is essential that the responses be obtained under uniform conditions. The interjection of service, advice, or comment may in itself influence the nature of the responses. To provide even incidental assistance might make the findings unreliable.

The Interview May Be Structured or Unstructured

The Structured, Standardized Interview. The purpose of the structured, standardized interview is to collect data under uniform circumstances in order to minimize the differences in response that might be caused by the bias or the manner of the interviewer or by the way in which the question was asked. Thus, the structured interview attempts to subject each respondent to precisely the same stimulus. An interview schedule is developed and tested; each question is spelled out in detail, and even the introduction of the interviewer is prescribed. It is extremely important that the questions asked are in exactly the same words and order in which they appear on the schedule, since the timing of "sensitive" or of "recall" questions may affect the answer. If there is no response to a question, the interviewer should not offer an explanation or probe for an answer unless the directions specifically permit this; and the interviewer should respect any limitations that might be set with respect to "probe" questions. Care must be taken not to suggest a "correct" answer by tone of voice or by expression.

Questions unrelated to the interview should not be answered until after the interview has been completed. If a request for advice or service is made, the request should be noted and another time set for such care, since the interposition of service may affect the answers supplied.

The Unstructured, Unstandardized Interview. The unstructured, unstandardized interview is generally used when the nurse's goal is not to compare responses but to use the responses as a means of understanding or explaining a situation. This type of interview is more exploratory, and the quality of the results depends on the skill of the nurse — her ability to ask questions that encourage adequate responses and to recognize certain verbal and nonverbal clues, which may indicate that a different line of questioning might produce useful information. The content of the questions, the method of the questioning, and the timing and arrangement of various facets of the inquiry are matters left to the interviewer. This kind of interview allows for great flexibility in adapting to differences among individuals.

The nurse's general interviewing skill will come into play in the unstructured, unstandardized interview. The intuitive response to observations of subtle changes in the appearance or manner of the interviewee — the delayed response, the "closed-down" expression, or the flicker of interest and response that signals an interpersonal breakthrough — are important elements in fact gathering. The technique and skill of the nurse in the timing and wording of sensitive questions — the matter of fact tone of voice or the prior sanction of a negative response ("Do you find it hard to remember to take all of your pills?") — will influence the quality of response.

The Epidemiologic Interview

The epidemiologic interview usually combines both structured and unstructured approaches. Usually, there is a form that indicates the kind of information the epidemiologist will need in order to assess the situation. Since these forms may be rather general, the nurse may want to supplement them with information related to the particular disease being investigated. In any event, she should refresh her memory of the nature of the disease and its transmission before proceeding to the interview.

There is more freedom in the way the questions are asked than there is in the structured interview, and probing is not only permissible but also highly desirable when information is not forthcoming. For example, if a patient with salmonella infection cannot recall eating food other than that which was eaten by other (and unaffected) members of her family, the nurse may raise questions about lunch with the neighbors, or an overlooked between-meal snack, or "just a taste" of something. If the unanswered or incompletely answered question is a sensitive one (as when the inquiry concerns an issue such as sexual contact), the nurse may choose to rephrase the question and ask it later on in the interview when a greater degree of trust has been developed. When the reply involves recall of something that happened some time ago, there may be a need for a "check" question. For example, if the mother reports the onset of disease in a child as occurring on Tuesday, the nurse might check by asking later, "Did Johnnie go to school on Monday?"

Subjective observations or comments may be a helpful supplement to the interview data, if this practice is consistent with the study design. For example, even in the structured interview, the nurse interviewer might express some doubt about the validity or completeness of responses by means of a recorded comment such as "the respondent appeared overanxious to give the right answers and reiterated several times that she was doing exactly what the clinic told her to do," or "the respondent appeared reluctant to answer the question, although she did not refuse to do so," or "the respondent was preoccupied and anxious about a son who has just been hospitalized following an automobile accident."

The Surveys

A survey is as good as its sample. Most interview surveys are based on information secured from a sample that is representative of the whole population. Interviewees are carefully selected to assure this representativeness. However, if a substantial number of the sample group is not located, refuses to participate, or provides only partial or obviously unreliable answers, the findings will be much less useful. The nurse interviewer can make a valuable contribution to the study by locating all members of the sample group and encouraging them to participate in the study.

The Nurse May Be the Organizer

Sometimes the community health nurse is responsible for arranging for the screening or examination activity. When this is the case, a manual or a set of directions will probably be available, indicating the necessary steps and governing regulations. In general, it is important for the nurse to do the following:

1. Notify the eligible population (or, in the case of minors, their parents).

2. Interpret the purpose and limitations of the procedure to the eligible population and, when indicated, to other community sources of care such as family physicians.

3. Secure the necessary authorization. This includes getting parental permission for the examination or procedure and clearing the general plan and schedule with appropriate authorities (e.g., school personnel or the medical director of health).

4. Recruit and train volunteer assistants.

5. Schedule the activities and post and announce the schedule well in advance of the date.

6. Arrange for anticipated follow-up activities.

The Nurse Is Involved in Follow-Up Care

The community health nurse is inevitably involved in follow-up activities such as the following:

1. Providing post-survey health counseling, including interpreting the meaning of the screening or the examination to the public.

2. Making referrals to sources of further study or care.

3. Reporting on follow-up outcomes and other data useful in evaluation of the screening activity.

Post-Survey Health Counseling

Provision for post-survey health counseling requires that the nurse must be thoroughly acquainted with the survey or screening procedure that has been used and with the meaning of the findings. In particular, the nurse should be able to answer the following questions:

1. How *sensitive* and how *specific* were the tests used? In other words, what is the likelihood that those persons having the disease or abnormal condition would be identified by the test used? If, for example, a test has a large number of false negative results, it is important that the family continues to be alert to any sign of possible disease. On the other hand, if the test is likely to yield a large number of false positive results, the family should be informed of this and not worry unduly. Above all, the community health nurse should emphasize that no screening system is fool-proof and that continuous observation and reporting of any unusual development is necessary.

2. What are the criteria for referral for care? In screening or survey procedures, there are usually a significant number of instances in which no disease is found but predisposing conditions — such as obesity, high cholesterol level, marginal hearing, or vision disabilities — are seen. The responsible screening or survey team will decide the level at which referral will be made and to what extent those with predisease condi-

tions will be encouraged to seek further diagnostic work-up or anticipatory care.

3. What can be done to deal with the disease or predisease condition discovered? There will be some instances in which nurse counseling may be indicated — for instance, in mild obesity or poor habits of daily hygiene. There may be community resources available for anticipatory or definitive care. Unfortunately, there will be some conditions for which little can be done to improve the situation or for which community resources have not been developed. In these instances, general supportive measures may be all that can be given.

Referrals

In making referrals to other sources of care, the community health nurse may need to locate new resources or to strengthen ties with sources of help not frequently used. Local chapters of voluntary health agencies, such as the American Heart Association or the National Tuberculosis and Respiratory Disease Association, may be helpful in locating resources for care. When making a referral to the family physician, the community health nurse may need to acquaint him with the survey or screening procedure that was used. She also may need to offer her own help in follow-up care either by working directly with the patients and their families or, if there is a nurse employed in the physician's office, by providing her with information and materials.

Evaluation of the Detection Effort

The community health nurse's accurate and prompt reporting of the action taken by those referred for further study is important to assure adequate care for each participant; it is also a means of evaluating the screening effort. In the long run, it is the number of persons who receive care, not the number of persons discovered to have disease or abnormality, that tests the usefulness of the screening measure.

Response to the screening program and the degree of effort required to implement the recommendations for postscreening care are useful in evaluating the methodology used. The nurse's observations or judgments concerning the families' reasons on whether or not to use the screening opportunity can be a valuable contribution to the evaluation of the acceptability of the methods used and to the improved development for future programs.

It is obvious that follow-up activities for screening programs will require substantial nursing time. This time requirement must be taken into account when planning the screening program.

There seems to be every indication that organized early–disease-detection methods will continue to expand and that methodologies will be further refined. The community health nurse will inevitably be involved with these activities; through her involvement, she can increase her ability to contribute to preventive health care.

SPECIAL PROBLEMS IN THE CONTROL OF COMMUNICABLE DISEASE

As has already been noted, the impact of communicable disease on the health of the public has been sharply reduced; nevertheless, the problem of communicable disease control still persists, although to a lesser degree than existed previously. The problem may be the more harassing to the community health professional because it is so often preventable.

Goals Change with Changing Technology and Resources

Payne states that the goal of communicable disease control is "to reduce the incidence of the disease to a tolerable level as quickly as possible within the resources available."[9a] The "tolerable level" depends on the degree to which the disease can be prevented or ameliorated and on the community's ability to take the required action. For some diseases (polio, malaria, and syphilis, for example), it is felt by many that complete eradication, as in the case of smallpox, is a feasible goal. In other instances where the determinants are complex and the treatment is less well defined, the goal of eradication may be an unrealistic one. In the case of gonorrhea, for instance, the determinants and limitations of present diagnostic methods are such that control is difficult; and, thus, eradication is probably not possible, even though treatment methods are well advanced. Furthermore, diseases wax and wane in occurrence and virulence. As some diseases are brought under control, other diseases (such as hepatitis, influenza, and the newly emerging viral diseases) continue to baffle and challenge the health professional. From time to time, there are epidemics of previously unrecognized disease, as occurred in the case of Lassa fever in Nigeria and Legionnaires' Disease in Philadelphia. Gregg expresses the problems in these terms: "Infectious disease is the final expression of interaction between a progressively changing and aging host population, an endlessly adaptable parasite, and a constant pressure from a man-made environment."[10]

THE ROLE OF THE COMMUNITY HEALTH NURSE IN COMMUNICABLE DISEASE CONTROL

The community health nurse has a dual role of care and control. The nursing care of a patient with communicable disease is no less important than it is for any type of illness. The emphasis here will be upon the control measures, but this should in no way be considered as minimizing the focal role of personal care.

Disease control measures have special emphasis when the disease is communicable. The general methods of disease control apply, of course, to infectious as well as noninfectious diseases. However, certain aspects of the control procedure should be emphasized.

Reporting Disease

Reporting is of prime importance in establishing the prevalence and incidence of disease. All states and most local communities have regulations requiring the reporting of communicable diseases not only by the physician responsible for the diagnosis but also, in many instances, by householders or anyone else having knowledge of, or reason to suspect, the existence of a communicable disease. Reporting is carried out at all levels of government in order to maintain an epidemiologic intelligence system that facilitates control. Local intelligence is relayed to states; states give the information to the appropriate national agency; and the national agency informs the World Health Organization. The specific diseases to be reported are established by each government unit, but all listings include the diseases designated by the World Health Organization as those reportable internationally.

The community health nurse may be involved in several ways in insuring adequate reporting. First, she may educate the public concerning the importance of securing care for what may be a communicable disease. If parents feel a disease is a natural occurrence in childhood and fail to seek medical assistance, the disease is not diagnosed and is not reported. The nurse may assist the family physician in reporting by seeing that he has the necessary regulations and forms and by reminding him of the need to report. She may report any suspicious symptoms she herself observes, such as an increased number of reported gastrointestinal upsets; and she may request a visit by the epidemiologist if her observations suggest that further disease investigation is required.

Maintaining a Safe Level of Immunization

The community health nurse contributes to the achievement of a safe level of immunization in the population. The need to intensify the immunization effort has been recognized nationally. The impetus for the extension and improvement of immunization for preschool children was provided by the passage of the Vaccination Assistance Act of 1962 and the 1965 amendments to this act (Public Law 89–109). Essentially, this legislation provides assistance in planning for and organizing immunization programs, purchasing immunization materials, and developing studies to determine needs. Immunization needs are not limited to children. Protection against diseases such as influenza, tetanus, or cholera may be recommended under certain circumstances for adults:

travelers, employees with high exposure to disease, elderly people, pregnant women, or those living in groups (such as nursing home residents).

The nurse should familiarize herself with the immunization measures that are available in her locality — the people for whom these measures are recommended, the ages or intervals of administration, the conditions and cost of implementation. Textbook information in this area must be supplemented by more current sources because of the rapid development of new immunizing agents and methods.

The nurse may be called upon to give immunizations, to interpret the need for them to potential users, and to inform others who may influence potential users. She may be called upon to organize special immunization clinics or special programs for immunizing special groups.

The community health nurse should get whatever information is available on the immunization level of her community and determine how close this level comes to the "epidemic safe" 85 per cent level for the more important diseases. This information may be available from the local health department, or it may be estimated on the basis of records of children entering school, of industrial populations, or of clinic groups.

The sharp decline in diseases for which specific immunizing agents are available may lead to complacency about the immunization status of the population. Surveys all too often indicate that the level of immunization among some segments of the population is far below a satisfactory level. In the 1976 U. S. Immunization Survey it was found that, of the population 1 to 4 years of age, only 61.6 per cent had 3+ doses of polio vaccine, 71.4 per cent had 3+ doses of DTP vaccine, and 65.9 per cent had measles vaccine.[11] These rates are below levels considered medically necessary to protect the population from epidemics.

The percentage of the population receiving such protective care varies greatly with socioeconomic status, even when immunization is available without charge. The community health nurse can do much to even out these differences.

Controlling the Spread of Infection

The community health nurse contributes to the control of the spread of infection by the following three measures:

1. Monitoring the care provided for those who suffer from an infectious disease and who are being cared for in a nonhospital setting.

2. Securing compliance with regulations affecting those with communicable disease or those who have been exposed to communicable disease. Regulations may include exclusion from school or from specified occupations and the observance of reasonable precautions in protecting others from infection.

3. Inculcating personal health behavior that prevents the spread of communicable disease.

Home care of communicable disease is for the most part limited to minor communicable diseases or to longterm illnesses that are considered under reasonable control. The major effort, of course, is to assure the safety and the comfort of the patient. Whether the nurse is providing a major part of the care or whether the family is providing care under the general direction of the nurse, provision should be made for adequate daily care, for the maintenance of nutrition, and for the relief of the patient's boredom and stress. In particular, efforts should be made to make the patient feel a part of the family despite his isolation and the avoidance of close contact.

Isolation measures become much less restrictive as more is known about the spread of infection and as treatment becomes more effective in controlling infectivity. For example, the effectiveness of chemotherapy in producing a negative sputum and the knowledge of the great importance of the airborne droplets in the transmission of infection has made it possible to dispense with much of the strict isolation and cautionary procedures — the boiling of dishes and the burning of materials handled by the patient — in favor of simple separation of the patient from the stream of family traffic and from very close contact with others.

It is the nurse's responsibility to know the methods by which the disease is spread and the measures that must be taken to prevent the transmission of the disease. She must be satisfied that the person who gives care in her absence thoroughly understands the principles on which these measures are based. The procedures should be as simple as possible, since the home situation is much different from that of the hospital. The nurse's skill in estimating the family's capability for care is an important element in determining the way in which this information will be transmitted.

The nurse should also be aware of groups that might be particularly susceptible to infection and that, consequently, require special protection (such as the very young child or the elderly person).

In most instances, the agency will provide a quick reference guide to communicable diseases. The guide would indicate the symptoms, incubation period, method of transmission, and principal control measures in regard to a specific disease. If a guide of this type is not available, the nurse should be sure to secure a source for such information that can be kept for ready reference.[12]

Exclusion of the diseased individual from certain types of occupation or from school may be necessary to protect other vulnerable groups. The nurse can do much to encourage patients not only to follow the required exclusion regulations but also to act in advance of the need. For instance, mothers may be encouraged to keep small children home from school when they have symptoms of an upper respiratory infection. The nurse should be familiar with the regulations and should be prepared to explain the reason for their existence.

The inculcation of health habits that prevent transmission of disease plays an important part in disease control. The school nurse, the visiting nurse, and the nurse in the clinic setting can incorporate such teaching into her ongoing services to patients in many ways.

In the area of disease control, as in all other areas of the health program, the nurse has an important function. Perhaps her most important contribution is that of "just good nursing" to those she serves.

SYPHILIS AND GONORRHEA: PERSISTENT PROBLEMS

It is believed that syphilis can be eradicated. Yet in 1978, 20,362 cases of primary or secondary syphilis were reported. (See *Center for Disease Control Monthly Report* for latest figures.) Information from the most recent Joint Statement of the Center for Disease Control and the American Social Health Association suggests the number of reported cases understates the problem due to inaccurate reporting, their estimates being closer to 80,000 new cases annually.[13] Although the reported rate is declining somewhat, there is still concern because of the possible long-term and costly effects of the disease.

Gonorrhea continues to be the most frequently reported communicable disease with 1,000,177 cases reported in 1978, a rate of 465.9/100,000 population.[14]

In part, changes in reported cases reflect increased case-finding activities, particularly in females, but they also reflect real changes in disease incidence.

The reasons given for increases in venereal disease (VD) are many — greater sexual freedom, ease of cure, and the occurrence of "silent" disease or asymptomatic gonorrhea in both men and women. Incidence varies greatly by geographic locality, by age group (teenagers and young adults comprise the majority of those affected), and by frequency of contact with multiple partners (homosexual males accounted for over half the incidence of gonorrhea in one large metropolitan area).[15] For example, the overall rate for gonorrhea in 1977 was 465.9 cases per 100,000 population. The rate for those in the age group 15 to 19 was 1212.4 per 100,000 population.

Gonorrhea is a serious disease with complications such as pelvic inflammatory disease, sterility, urethritis, and acute arthritis in young adults.

Although very different in manifestation and occurrence, syphilis and gonorrhea have certain characteristics in common that influence the kind of action required for their control:

1. Both diseases are endemic in the population; incidence is a worldwide problem. Aside from influenza and measles, VD is the most frequently transmitted disease in epidemic form.

2. The roots of the problem are social-behavioral rather than biologic, and they are difficult to control.

3. Reported incidence does not tell the whole story. Many cases are cared for by private physicians and clinics and a large number go unreported.

4. Venereal disease, especially gonorrhea, is a disease of youth. Rates vary from 1 in 87 teenagers to 1 in 33 in some areas.

General Approach to the Control of VD

The basis for any VD control program is the interruption of transmission from infected host to susceptible person. This assumes knowledge of characteristics of agent and host, host-agent interactions as reflected by natural history of the disease, and environmental factors. For the community health nurse, this will include responsibilities for primary prevention (prevention of infection), for secondary prevention (prevention of disability or death in those infected), and tertiary (rehabilitation) care.

Nursing Efforts Directed Toward Primary Prevention of VD

The community health nurse contributes to the primary prevention of venereal disease through her educational and motivational efforts provided in ongoing activities with families and the public and through special educational programs aimed at populations at risk. Working with existing community groups (such as a school, clinic, or PTA,) and industries, she may develop or assist others in developing programs with information about promiscuity, individual responsibility for knowing signs and symptoms of disease and seeking diagnosis and treatment, and resources for treatment. The use of peer group motivation toward responsible behavior may be a powerful influence, and group work with open and frank discussion can be an effective method. In the Joint Statement survey, health officers were asked to describe the effectiveness of health education on teenage VD rates in their area. Most felt there was an increase in numbers of teenagers reporting to clinics. One-to-one contact in high incidence areas, using trained aids to provide information, was found to be a successful method.[16]

The nurse may need to encourage families to discuss sexuality more openly and with specific information. One study showed that mothers rarely talked about sex with their daughters, assuming that they had received the necessary information elsewhere.[17] Adolescents need to understand early signs of disease and the kind of sexual behavior that increases risk.

The nurse may be involved in research efforts in demonstrating and evaluating new approaches to control programs, developing and testing interviewing methodologies, or in research programs that test host susceptibility to immunization. Ethical issues involved in this type of research need to be well thought out and all future implications defined, as recent controversy over the Tuskegee Study of Untreated Syphilis has shown.[18]

Nursing Efforts Directed Toward Secondary Prevention of VD

The community health nurse contributes to the secondary prevention of VD through case finding, through case management, and through assisting others in the control team.

Case Finding

The nurse contributes to case finding in three ways:
1. By contact tracing and cluster identification.
2. By direct or delegated general case finding measures in vulnerable populations.
3. By participating in mass or crash programs or screening measures.

Contact Tracing. The highest new-case yield comes from the investigation of those who have been exposed to the infection by a known case, and the backbone of the case finding program must be contact tracing. The success of such a venture must, in the long run, rest with the index case's willingness to divulge the names of those individuals who might be contacts. Experienced investigators indicate that patients rarely provide a complete list of contacts during the first interview and that, in most instances, a follow-up interview is essential in order to complete the list. Contact interviewing must be of a high quality in order to motivate the individual not only to get treatment himself but also to encourage others to seek care as well. Sensitivity and timing are of the utmost importance in achieving this end.

Cluster Identification. Recently, emphasis has been placed on cluster approaches — that is, bringing in for interview and diagnosis those people with whom the patient is closely associated but who are not necessarily named as contacts. If the patient is fully convinced of the need for his own care, he may be persuaded of the importance of naming those among his acquaintance that might have been exposed and enable them to secure prompt treatment. In some instances, prophylactic treatment may be prescribed for contacts who do not show clinical or serologic symptoms in order to abort the disease if it is incubating.

General Case Finding. General case finding measures include incorporation of venereal disease content into all services provided to groups that are particularly vulnerable and maintaining a high alert to the possibility of venereal infection. It must be remembered that venereal disease is not limited to a particular social class; outbreaks have occurred frequently in "good" schools and in "highly respectable" families. However, the incidence does tend to be greater among mobile groups in the population, such as agricultural migrant workers; among those with inadequate family life or other problems of social adjustment; and among those living in areas with poor homes and few recreational facilities.

Case Management

The nurse contributes to venereal disease case management in several ways. She may, of course, provide therapeutic care in treatment centers. She may use therapeutic and counseling interviews with patients and their contacts to increase their understanding of the disease and its treatment and to promote their active participation in caring for themselves and in safeguarding others. The person who has a venereal disease is in many instances upset about it: he may feel embarrassed or stigmatized or that he has been wronged by the source of his infection. His feelings of self-respect and personal worth may be damaged, and an already poor self-image may be even more depressed. Properly used, this experience may be constructive and may increase the individual's responsibility and self-respect rather than diminish them.

In the case of minors, it is possible in most states to treat the child without parental consent or knowledge. It may be possible for the professional worker to notify the contact of the possible infection without involving or naming the patient who identified the contact. This may be the easy way to accomplish the job; it is not easy for a teenager to face his family with the fact of his infection or for a young person to tell another. However, when it is possible for the patient himself to explain his plight or to bring in a friend for treatment, he is being given an opportunity for responsible behavior that may accomplish much more than case finding per se.

In her contacts with patients, it is especially important that the nurse must come to terms with her own feelings about venereal disease and sexual behavior and realize how her own feelings may influence her ability to help. Sometimes it is not possible for a nurse to get through to a particular patient. When this is the case, the nurse may want to seek help from a more experienced interviewer; and if she still finds difficulty, she may suggest that someone else try. There is clear evidence that both the quality of the service and the attitudes with which it is delivered are important factors in the utilization of VD clinics.

In all work with venereal disease, it is, of course, especially important not to violate a confidence. All information should be kept in locked files, and all personnel working with this patient group should be fully briefed on the confidentiality of all record or interview content.

Interviewing has been used intensively and extensively with the patient who has syphilis. It has been much less frequently used for those with gonorrhea. This may change, and contact investigation applied to encourage patients to refer their sexual partners for examination. The question could be raised as to whether or not the failure to use this powerful tool is hampering the control effort.

Assisting Others in the Control Team

The community health nurse may support others in their care of patients with venereal disease. She may work with a venereal disease investigator, a disease control officer, or a nonmedical epidemiologist, all of whom may also function in this program. These workers may have backgrounds that range from on-the-job training to master's degrees in public health. All will have had some training in interviewing and epidemiologic investigation. They may participate in field investigations, in contact tracing, and in other case-finding measures and may also carry treatment responsibilities. When there is such a member in the service group, it is obvious that there will be much sharing of responsibility between him and the nurse. Each can do much to support the other's activities; however, frequent exchange of information is vital to effective activity.

The community health nurse can be of particular help to the family physician or specialist providing care for venereal disease. In most instances he will be dealing with a relatively small number of cases of this type and will welcome the assistance of the nurse. The community health nurse might provide him or his office nurse or receptionist with materials or information, or she might work directly with his patients and their contacts. The health department will usually provide for epidemiologic follow-up for all reported cases, but the nurse can offer more patient-focused care in addition to this. The nurse may also reassure the physician, as well as the patient, that the patient's right to privacy will be respected.

The Importance of Funding

Figure 18–1 traces the levels of federal appropriations for VD control from 1947 to 1979. There seems to be a trend in disease rate with the rise and fall of public support. Overconfidence in drug therapy and decreased vilgilance in control programs is a possible explanation for the shift in funding during the mid-1950's. Serious interest in control of all forms of VD must be engendered in the public. Programs now frequently screen for approximately 20 different sexually transmitted diseases. Sufficient resources are directly related to how extensive and aggressive the VD control program can be.

Whether in the field of cancer, heart disease, hepatitis, or venereal infection, the disease control program represents an engrossing area of the nurse's work. Disease control requires the full use of every facet of

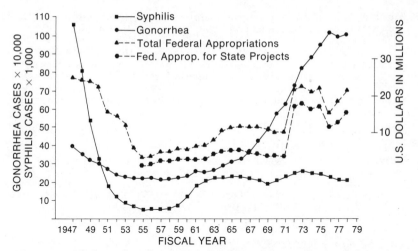

Figure 18-1 Reported civilian cases of primary and secondary syphilis and gonor-rhea, (United States), fiscal years 1947–1978; total federal appropriations, fiscal years 1947–1978; and for state projects, fiscal years 1955–1978, expressed as constant dollars (base fiscal year 1967 = 1.00) (Developed by John C. Hume, M.D., Dr. P.H., Johns Hopkins School of Hygiene and Public Health, 1979.)

nursing practice, and the results are likely to be commensurate with the energy expended and the satisfactions are deep.

REFERENCES

1. MacMahon, B., and Pugh, T.: *Epidemiology and Methods.* Boston, Little, Brown & Co., 1970, pp. 1–5 and Maxcy-Rosenau, in Sartwell, P. E. (ed.): *Preventive Medicine and Public Health,* 10th ed. New York, Appleton-Century-Crofts, 1977, pp. 1–4.
2. Thomas, L.: *The Lives of a Cell.* New York, Bantam Books, Inc., 1974, p. 36.
3. Commission on Chronic Illness: *Chronic Illness in the United States, Vol. I — Prevention of Chronic Illness.* Cambridge, Mass., Harvard University Press, 1957, p. 45.
4. *A Guide to Screening-EPSDT-Medicaid, SRS/HEW.* In cooperation with the American Academy of Pediatrics (P.O. Box 1034, Evanston, Ill., 60204), 1974.
5. Hart, C.R. (ed.): *Screening in General Practice.* New York, Churchill-Livingstone, 1975, pp. 12–13.
6. *Periodic Health Examination: A Manual for Physicians.* Chicago, American Medical Association, 1947.
7. Breslow, L., and Somers, A.: The lifetime health-monitoring program. New Eng J. Med., 296:601, 1977.
8. World Health Organization: *Early detection of handicaps in children.* WHO Chron., 22:16, 1968.
9. Yankauer, A., et al.: A study of case finding methods in elementary school: Methodology and initial results. Am. J. Pub. Health, 52:656, 1962.
9a. Payne, A.M.M.: Approaches to communicable disease control. WHO Chronicle, 22:3, Jan, 1968.
10. Gregg, M. R.: Communicable disease trends in the United States. Am. J. Nurs., 68:88, 1968.
11. Center for Disease Control, Immunization Division: *Summary of Immunization Status for Polio, DTP, Measles, Rubella, and Mumps.* Atlanta, Ga., Department of Health, Education, and Welfare, 1976.

12. For example, see Benenson, A. (ed.): *Control of Communicable Diseases in Man*, 12th ed. Washington, D.C. American Public Health Association, 1975.
13. Center for Disease Control and the American Social Health Association: *The 1975 Joint Statement — Today's VD Control Problem. The American Social Health Association, the American Public Health Association, the American Venereal Disease Association, and the Association of State and Territorial Health Officers*, p. 13.
14. Center for Disease Control: Monthly Morbidity and Mortality Report, P.H.S., D.H.E.W., Atlanta, Ga.
15. Dritz, S. K., et al.: Patterns of sexually transmitted enteric diseases in a city. Lancet, 2:3, 1977.
16. Ibid., Today's VD control problem, pp. 39–40.
17. Block, D.: Sex education practices of mothers. J. Sex. Educ. Ther., 4:7, 1978.
18. See for example Brandt, A. M.: *Racism and Research, the Case of the Tuskegee Syphilis Study, The Experiment and HEW's Ethical Review*, Hastings Center Report, December 1978; and Kampmeier, R. H.: The Tuskegee Study of untreated syphilis. S. Med. J., 65:1247, 1972.

SUGGESTED READINGS

Baker, S. P.: Injury control. *In* Sartwell, P. E. (ed.): *Preventive Medicine and Public Health*, 10th ed. New York, Appleton-Century-Crofts, 1973.

Blank, F. L.: Infectious diseases in primitive societies. Science, 187:515, 1975.

Bloch, D.: Sex education practices of mothers. J. Sex Educ. Ther., 4:7, 1978.

Bonser, R. S. A., Knight, B. H., and West, R. R.: Sudden infant death syndrome in Cardiff. Association with epidemic influenza and with temperature, 1955–1974. Int. J. Epidemiol., 7:335, 1978.

Breslow, L.: Early case findings, treatment, and mortality from cervix and breast cancer. Prev. Med., 1:141, 1972.

Burnet, F., and White, D.: *The Natural History of Infectious Disease*, 4th ed. Cambridge University Press, 1972.

Dershewitz, R. A., and Williamson, J. W.: Prevention of childhood household injuries. A controlled clinical trial. Am. J. Pub. Health, 67:1148, 1977.

Dritz, S. K., et al.: Patterns of sexually transmitted diseases in a city. Lancet, 2:3, 1977.

Early detection of handicaps in children. WHO Chronicle, 22:16, 1968.

Ennals, D.: Complacency can kill. Nurs. Mirror, 145:9, 1977.

Erhardt, C. L., and Berlin, J. (eds.): *Mortality and Morbidity in the United States*. Cambridge, Mass., Harvard University Press, 1974.

Fleming, W. L.: Syphilis through the ages. Med. Clin. North Am., 48:587, 1964.

Foster, S.: Participation of the public in global smallpox eradication. Publ. Health Rep., Vol. 93:142, 1978.

Frame, P. S., and Carlson, S. J.: A critical review of periodic health screening using specific screening criteria. J. Fam. Pract., 2:29, 1975.

Fraser, D. W., et al.: Legionnaire's disease: Description of an epidemic of pneumonia. New Engl. J. Med., 297:1189, 1977.

Fraser, D., and McDade, J.: Legionellosis. Sci. Am., 241:82, 1979.

Gillum, R., et al.: Community surveillance for cerebrovascular disease: The Framingham cardiovascular disease survey. Pub. Health Rep., 93:438, 1978.

A Guide to Screening — EPSDT — Medicaid, SRS/HEW. In cooperation with the American Academy of Pediatrics, P.O. Box 1034, Evanston, Illinois 60204, 1974.

Haddon, W.: On the escape of tigers: An ecologic note. Tech. Rev. (MIT), 72:44, 1970.

Harmison, L. T.: Toxic substances and health. Publ. Health Rep., 93:3, 1978.

Harnish, Y.: *Patient Care Guides — Practical Information for Public Health Nurses*. New York, National League for Nursing, Pub. No. 21–1610, 1976.

Harnish, Y.: *Patient Care in Tuberculosis*. New York, National League for Nursing, Pub. No. 45–1414, 1973.

Hingson, R.: Obtaining optimal attendance at mass immunization programs. Health Serv. Rep., 89:53, 1974.

Holland, W. W.: Screening for disease: Taking stock. Lancet 2:1494, 1974.

Hume, J. C.: Trichomoniasis — Eight reasons why you should take it seriously. Med. Times, Vol. 106:59, 1978.

Hyde, M.: *VD: The Silent Epidemic*. New York, McGraw-Hill Book Co., 1973, p. 64.

Infection Control. New York, National League for Nursing, Pub. No. 20–1582, 1975.

Judson, F., and Wolfe, F.: Tracing and treating contacts of gonorrhea patients in a clinic for sexually transmitted diseases. Pub. Health Rep., 93:460, 1978.

Kessler, I., and Levin, M.: *The Community as an Epidemiologic Laboratory, A Casebook of Community Studies*. Baltimore, The Johns Hopkins Press, 1970. See Chapter 6, The Framingham study 20 years later.

Kessner, D.: Screening high-risk populations: A challenge to primary medical care, J. Commun. Health, 1:216, 1976.

Khoury, S.: Screening for hypertension in Washington, D.C. 1971, Health Ser. Rep., 88:824, 1973.

Kleinman, G., and Cant, S.: Occupational disease surveillance in Washington. J. Occup. Med. 10: 750, 1978.

Kork, S.: *Epidemiology and Community Medicine*, New York, Appleton-Century-Crofts, 1974.

Leavell, H. R., and Clark, E. G.: *Textbook of Preventive Medicine*, New York, McGraw-Hill Book Co., 1953.

Lilienfeld, A.: *Foundations of Epidemiology*, New York, Oxford University Press, 1976.

Maxcy-Rosenau, and Last, V. M. (eds.): *Public Health and Preventive Medicine*, 11th ed. New York, Appleton-Century-Crofts, 1980.

McCormack, W. M.: Treatment of gonorrhea — Is penicillin passé? New Engl. J. Med., 296:934, 1977.

McGrath, P., and LaLiberte, E. B.: Level of basic venereal disease knowledge among Jr. and Sr. high school nurses in Massachusetts. Nurs. Res., 23:31, 1974.

McInnis, J. K.: Do patients take antituberculosis drugs? Am. J. Nurs., 70:10, 1970.

McNeil, W. H.: *Plagues and Peoples*. New York, Anchor/Doubleday, 1976.

Morrison, S. F., and Arnold, C. R.: Pts. of common communicable disease. Nurs. Clin. North Am., 5:143, 1976.

Mortimer, E. A.: Immunization against infectious disease. Science, 200:902, 1978.

Morton, B. M.: *VD, A Guide for Nurses and Counselors*. Boston, Little, Brown and Co., 1976.

Nahmias, A., and Roizman, B.: Infection with herpes simplex viruses 1 and 2. New Eng. J. Med. 289:781, 1973.

Olsen, D., Kane, R., and Proctor, P.: A controlled trial of multiphasic screening. New Eng. J. Med., 294:925, 1976.

Pellegrino, E. D.: Preventive health care and the allied health professions. *In* Hamburg, J. (ed.): *Review of Allied Health Education*. Lexington, Ky., University Press of Kentucky, 1974, pp. 1–18.

Pisa, Z., and Strasser, T.: *Community Cardiovascular Disease Control Programmes*. Geneva, World Health Organization, 1976.

Preventive Medicine USA: Theory, Practice and Application of Prevention in Personal Health Services. Quality Control and Evaluation of Preventive Health Services. New York, Prodist, 1976.

Prothero, R. M.: Disease and Mobility: A neglected factor in epidemiology. Int. J. Epidemiol., 6:259, 1977.

Reid, D. D.: *Epidemiological Methods in the Study of Mental Disorders*. Geneva, World Health Organization, 1960.

Rice, M. J., and Kaplon, E. L.: Rheumatic fever in Minnesota: II, Evaluation of hospitalized patients and utilization of a state rheumatic fever registry. Am. J. Pub. Health, 69:767, 1979.

Roberts, E., Kline, D., and Gagnon, J.: *Family Life and Sexual Learning: A Study of the Role of Parents in the Sexual Learning of Children*. Cambridge, Mass., The Project on Human Sexual Development of Population, Education, Inc., 1978.

Robertson, L. S., and Zador, P. L.: Driver education and fatal crash involvement of teenaged drivers. Am. J. Pub. Health, 68:959, 1978.

Rosebury, T.: *Microbes and Morals*. New York, Viking Press, 1971.

Rosen, G.: *Preventive Medicine in the United States*, 1900–1975, 1st ed. New York, Science History Publications, 1975.

Ruccione, K.: Variations on a theme; The role of a cancer nurse epidemiologist. Oncol. Nurs. For., 4:8, 1977.

Schneiderman, G., et al.: Tay-Sachs disease and cancer screening programs: Psychosocial aspects. Prog. Clin. Biol. Res., 18:395, 1977.

Shamansky, S. L., and Clausen, C. L.: Levels of prevention: Examination of the concept. Nurs. Outlook, 28:104, 1980.

Skinner, F. A., et al.: *Gonorrhea: Epidemiology and Pathogenesis.* New York, Academic Press, 1977.

Sparling, F.: *Dx & Rx* of syphilis. New Engl. J. Med., 284:642, 1971.

Stewart, P. L., et al.: The nurse's role in the swine influenza immunization program. Nurs. For., 16:128, 1977.

Syphilotherapy, 1976. J. Am. V. D. Assoc., 3:98, 1976.

Terris, M.: Breaking the barriers to prevention: Legislative approaches. Bull. N.Y. Acad. Med., 51:242, 1975.

Terris, M.: The epidemiologic tradition. Pub. Health Rep. 94:203, 1979.

Thorner, R. M., and Remlin, Q. R.: *Principles and Procedures in the Evaluation of Screening for Disease.* Washington, D.C., (Reprint of Public Health Monograph No. 67), U.S. Government Printing Office, May 1967 (National Center for Health Services Research, DHEW).

Today's VD Control Problem 1975. American Social Health Association with APHA, American Venereal Disease Association, and Association of State and Territorial Health Officers.

Toman, K.: *Tuberculosis Case-Finding and Chemotherapy, Questions and Answers.* WHO, Geneva, World Health Organization, 1979.

White, K., and Henderson, M.: *Epidemiology as a Fundamental Science, Its Uses in Health Services Planning, Administration and Evaluation.* New York, Oxford University Press, 1976.

Witte, J.: Recent advances in public health: Immunization. Am. J. Publ. Health, 64:934, 1974.

World Health Organization: *Second Report of Expert Committee on Smallpox Eradication.* Geneva, WHO Technical Report Series No. 493, 1972.

Yankauer, A., Frantz, R., Drislane, A., and Katz, S.: A study of case finding methods in elementary school: Methodology and initial results. Am. J. Pub. Health, 52:656, 1962.

Zapka, J., and Averill, B.: Self care for colds: A cost-effective alternative to upper respiratory infection management. Am. J. Pub. Health. 69:814, 1979.

Zweighaft, R. M., et al.: Lassa fever: Response to an imported case. New Engl. J. Med., 297:803, 1977.

RESOURCES

American Academy of Pediatrics: *Report of the Committee on Infectious Disease* (Red Book)
P.O. Box 1034
Evanston, Illinois 60204

American Association of Poison Control Centers
c/o Academy of Medicine of Cleveland
Poison Information Center
10525 Carnegie Avenue
Cleveland, Ohio 44106

American Cancer Society
777 3rd Avenue
New York, N.Y. 10017

See also local chapters.

American Heart Association
7320 Greenville Avenue
Dallas, Texas 75231

Programs: diet counseling, smoking withdrawal,
    stroke clubs, prevention
    and control of rheumatic fever, and
    many publications.

American Public Health Association
1015 Eighteenth Street, N.W.
Washington, D.C. 20036

British Journal of Venereal Disease
British Medical Association

The International Bank for Reconstruction
    and Development/The World Bank
19th St. and I, N.W.
Washington, D.C. 20006

National Safety Council
444 N. Michigan Avenue
Chicago, Illinois 60611

Programs: defensive driving, biking,
    educational materials.

Sexually Transmitted Disease:
Journal of the American Venereal Disease Association

Sexually Transmitted Disease (STD)
Fact Sheet, 34th ed.,
Center for Disease Control
Atlanta, Georgia

Technical Information Center for Smoking and
    Health (DHHS)
Office on Smoking and Health
Rockville, Md. 20857

U.S. Consumer Product Safety Commission
Hazard Identification and Analysis
National Injury Information Clearinghouse
Washington, D.C. 20207
Telephone: (301) 492-6424

U.S. Department of Health and
  Human Services, Public Health Service
Center for Disease Control
Atlanta, Georgia 30333
Telephone: (404) 329-3534

Recent statistics on reportable diseases,
  recommended treatment schedules, public
  education information.

Weekly Morbidity and Mortality Report
U.S. Public Health Service
Center for Disease Control
Atlanta, Georgia

Includes new information and recommendations
  regarding immunizations

World Health Organization (WHO)
Geneva, Switzerland

CHAPTER 19

MENTAL HEALTH AND MENTAL DISORDER

Mental health and mental illness are perhaps the most tantalizing of the problems faced in community health practice. Mental illness is a worldwide problem of staggering proportions and a major cause of disability. It is a field in which the "unknowns" in causation and treatment greatly outnumber the "knowns." Mental health concerns spill over into every health problem and into every health discipline. Furthermore, the conditions associated with mental illness do not always fall solely within the range of health efforts; equally these conditions may be a concern of education, welfare, or environment. The challenge for community health is to devise strategies to prevent, contain, or alleviate the effects of mental disorder while recognizing the legitimate concern of other human services as well as providing the leadership required to coordinate the contributions of related groups. The nature of the problem provides an unusual opportunity for the community health nurse, since she can mobilize multiple sources of care and form a bridge between the family and its socioeconomic-cultural milieu.

Current Concepts of Mental Health and Mental Illness Are Diffuse and At Variance

There is currently no universally accepted definition of mental health.[1] This creates obvious difficulties in program planning and in comparative research, since there may be little consistency in diagnosis or problem definition. Estimates of prevalence or incidence will be affected by the current or local definition of mental health and mental illness. Program evaluation will vary depending upon the desired outcome, which will also vary with definition.

371

"Mental health" may be seen by some as the absence of mental illness or mental disorder sufficiently serious to interfere with one's usual occupation. At the other end of the semantic scale, some might define mental health in terms of Maslow's concept of "creative self-hood," which is characterized by such attributes as superior perception of reality, problem centering, freshness of perception, and richness of emotional reaction.[2] Goerke and Stebbins suggest that good mental health might be characterized by normal behavior, absence of mental disease, adjustment to environment, perception of reality, and personality integration.[3] Carstairs suggests that two models may be identified — an illness model and a positive health model — and that programs will vary depending on whatever model (or mixture of the two models) is adopted.[4] In the illness model, emphasis would be placed on the prevention, diagnosis, treatment, and rehabilitation of those afflicted with mental disorders. Mental disorder usually refers to the organic and functional psychoses, neuroses, personality disorders, alcoholism, drug dependence, and behavioral disorders.[5] The International Classification of Diseases Nomenclature (ICDA) also includes mental retardation under this category. In the positive health model, which is more sociologically oriented, emphasis would be placed on maladaptive behavior and general problems of growth and development, environmental change, and realization of genetic potential.

Some attempts at definition are based on the establishment of norms for psychologic functioning — e.g., self-awareness, self-acceptance, undistorted perception of reality, and a sense of identity or of environmental mastery; however, such norms are, for the most part, societally determined and require constant revision. For example, norms of sexual behavior, of rebellion (at community conditions), and of familial roles are undergoing intense change. Divorce — once considered evidence of "social pathology" — might be seen today as a practical assessment of reality or as creative coping.

What does seem clear is that mental health is a sociomedical-educational phenomenon, manifested in a variety of ways, and interwoven with and dependent upon general health, social, educational, and environmental conditions. In the broadest interpretation of mental health, the implication is that everyone in the population would be involved.

The Dimensions of the Mental Health and Mental Disorder Problem Are Only Loosely Defined, But

us discussion, it is obvious that estimates of the size ental health problem in a given population will vary s may also vary with the availability of diagnostic and treatment facilities and with the level of the general health care structure. A major problem for epidemiologists centers on the disagreement about criteria for diagnosing mental disorders and the difficulty in case identification when surveys are conducted in untreated communities. The current estimate of the prevalence of mental disorders in the United States is that at least 10 per cent of the population is affected at any given point in a year. When newer and more precise methods are used for large population studies, prevalence rates are expected to be between 15 to 20 per cent of the population.[6]

On a worldwide basis, it has been estimated that severe mental illness affects 1 to 2 per cent of the population, and that this rate would be much higher if milder cases of mental illness were also included.[7]

Mental health treatment, once considered only long-term in nature, relied heavily on institutional settings for care. Today, care is predominantly acute, with a shifting locus of care to outpatient settings. Between 1971 and 1975, the number of days of care in mental health inpatient settings decreased by 32 per cent. These changes were particularly striking for state mental hospitals with the advent of deinstitutionalization.[8] In 1975, the specialty mental health sector — i.e., mental health clinics or community mental health centers — provided services for an estimated 15 per cent of the U.S. population. About 22 per cent, or 7 million people, were not treated or seen by either sector.[9]

Admissions to care facilities for mental disorders have concentrated heavily in the middle age groups, with 40 per cent between the ages of 25 and 44 years. Compared with their distribution in the population at large, minority races were overrepresented in admissions to mental health facilities, with an excess of at least 20 per cent for each age group.[10] The most frequent disorders seen among all 1975 admissions were depression (accounting for 17 per cent of the total admitted), and schizophrenia (accounting for 16 per cent).

Patterns of occurrence of specific conditions change with age, sociocultural, and economic conditions. For example, schizophrenia occurs more often in low-income families; suicide occurs most often in young adults and increases at times of political upheaval. Depression is prevalent among the elderly, while manic-depressive states and alcoholism hit hardest at those in their middle years.[11] For males, alcohol disorder and schizophrenia (with 18 per cent and 17 per cent, respectively) were the leading diagnoses at admission. For females, depressive disorder accounted for 23 per cent of the total admitted.[12]

The cost of mental illness and mental disorders is staggering. One estimate, based on loss of earnings as well as direct-care costs, was set at 21 billion dollars (for 1971) and another at 26.2 billion dollars annually.[13, 14] These figures would be even higher today.

Despite restriction in benefits for mental and nervous conditions, in 1973 these conditions accounted for 7.3 per cent, or 61.6 million dollars, of the total benefits disbursed by Blue Cross and Blue Shield, compared to 3.9 per cent of the total disbursements in the period of 1960 to 1965. It is estimated that Medicare and Medicaid benefits for psychiatric care amount to over 400 million dollars every year.[15]

Numbers of patients and costs of care represent only part of the total impact of mental disorder. For example, the human costs of alcoholism may have the most impact on the patient's family — the distraught wife and embarrassed children who go through their own special hells. The parents of a severely brain-damaged child, faced with the stress of a complex and rending set of decisions, may be as much at risk as the afflicted child. The children of a mentally disordered elderly parent face adjustments and decisions that may strain family finances and energy and threaten long-standing values or self-concepts.

New Knowledge Is Expanding the Treatment Potential

Recent biologic, psychiatric, and sociocultural research has already influenced patterns of care, and promises even greater change. The giant steps made in the development of psychoanalytic theory and techniques; of electroconvulsive therapy; and of specific drug therapies for schizophrenia, depression, manic-depressive states, and hyperactivity have already resulted in significant expansion of the opportunities for care. Advances in biologic knowledge are expected to have as much of an impact on care as those in the psychiatric field, if not more so. One important breakthrough has been the discovery that information is transmitted through the brain and nervous system by the release of biochemicals called *neurotransmitters*, which bridge the gap between cells. One such neurotransmitter, norepinephrine, has been shown to be affected by drugs used in the treatment of depressive or affective disorders.[16] This is expected to lead to new understanding and extension of drug therapies. Although much is still unknown about the interaction of these substances, the pace of discovery is a rapid one.

There is increasing evidence that heredity plays a role in mental illness. Apparently, heredity strongly influences susceptibility to schizophrenia and manic depression, although the genetic factor by itself does not cause disease.

Discovery of the relationship between *biologic rhythms* and human behavior has great importance for preventive and curative efforts in mental disorder. Susceptibility to psychic assault, openness to treatment measures, and general coping levels probably vary widely in accordance with the highly individual biologic time clock of each person.

Epidemiologic data about mental disorder and mental health continue to accumulate, but at a slower pace — hampered by the absence, in many instances, of any single *obligatory* factor in the development of mental disorder. It has been shown, however, that schizophrenia is a familial condition, more frequent among low-income groups, and that life styles characterized by pressure and stress increase the risk of breakdown.

Advances in learning theory offer new opportunities for treatment. A recent report states the following:

> The development and application of learning theory rank with the discovery of neurotransmitters and of drugs to treat schizophrenia and depression as one of the greatest advances in the mental health field in recent times.[17]

The process of behavior modification through *operant conditioning* has been developed and incorporated into psychiatric care.[18] Although based on classical conditioning theory, it differs in that it is concerned with voluntary behavior, and substitutes rewards and punishments as a stimulus for desired behavior. Reinforcement measures are meticulously developed to accommodate the individual's concept of a desirable response. For example, the restraint shown by a child in dealing with a toppling tower of blocks may be reinforced by sympathetic and approving parental comment; an adolescent who has conquered alcohol addiction may be further strengthened by being asked to help others who wish to be cured. Sometimes just recording progress is enough (e.g., a successful dieter's weight loss chart).

A greater understanding has developed concerning motivation, and it is now known to be a far more complex phenomenon than had previously been supposed. The dramatic potential of *biofeedback,* and the possibility of voluntary control of bodily responses formerly thought to be outside the control of the individual, is remarkable.

A new appreciation of the importance of individual *membership in and interaction with significant social groups* in molding personality, in encouraging socially relevant behavior, and in improving the physical and social environment has also made a vital contribution to mental health care.

There is mounting evidence of the relationship between mental health problems and situational or social factors. The *sense of community* — the belonging, sharing, and commitment to a family, group, or neighborhood — is highly important to most people in providing support and direction. In the past, such identity was almost inescapable; however, the increase in family mobility, the size and impersonal attitude of government and industry, and the relinquishment of helping services to the professionals has eroded these natural affiliations. Nevertheless, people continue to seek community in whatever form they find to be available and satisfying. Many of these "communities," however, are nontraditional and transient.[19]

In the midst of these widespread developments, *traditional treatment measures continue to be useful.* Psychoanalytic therapy, group therapy (and its more recent relative, family therapy), electroconvulsive therapy, client-centered therapy, transactional therapy, and milieu therapy all continue to hold an important place in mental health care; in addition, the possibilities of psychopharmaceutical intervention continue to expand.

The current situation is one offering an incredible array of thera-peutic measures drawn from many fields of knowledge. Even more choices are likely to be offered in the near future, since much research in mental health is at the breakthrough point. Despite these advances, much is still unknown. The agent in causation seems clearly multiple rather than single, and it is likely that many reinforcing factors are involved in producing mental disorder.

Many of the new treatment opportunities require skills that already exist (or exist in part) in community health nursing practice. These include the concepts of mobilizing families and groups to act on their own behalf in terms of health care, of offering support as integral to professional practice, and of changing health behavior. Community mental health, however, is an area in which "back-up" sources are of great importance, since the pace of discovery and change is so fast. The community mental health or psychiatric nurse specialist in a health care agency and the worker in a diagnostic and treatment center — along with other, similar sources of information — are crucial to community health practice in this fascinating field.

New Insights Alter Pattern of Care

There are several broad changes in the patterns of care that can be identified.

1. *There is a shift away from the traditional Freudian concentra-tion on the individual and his unconscious motivational conflicts.* Greater emphasis is being placed on social-interpersonal– and situational-oriented care. Group, community, and family therapies are being increasingly used. Symptomatic treatment, which is based primar-ily upon pharmaceutical intervention, offers the opportunity for provid-ing short-term and less expensive care as well as for reaching a larger proportion of those needing care.

Family therapy is of particular interest to community health nurses, and they frequently play a supporting role in such care. Family therapy acknowledges the profound reciprocal influence of the family and its members, and the therapeutic power that may be engendered as a result; the therapy process engages the family in the recognition and sub-sequent alteration of destructive behavior. The family as a whole may have problems of communication with each other and with the world outside. Zuk sees the professional worker in family mental health as a go-between for the family.[20] The desired outcomes of family therapy are to mobilize and support the family in dealing with mental disorder and to promote the development of family functioning as a favorable milieu in which all family members can develop their own potential and support each other.

Community mental health therapy is directed toward identifying and dealing with mental health or mental disorder as it exists in the population as a whole and toward increasing the effectiveness of the community in caring for its members. This involves not only the provision of care for individuals and families but also the development of policies and programs that enable the community to become a favorable milieu for the mental health of the total population. Thus, the community itself, as well as the sick or threatened person or family, becomes the care unit. The objectives for the community as a whole are as follows: to provide an ambiance that is conducive to mental health and capable of securing appropriate care for the mentally disordered; to foster communication and mutual effort between the community and its mental health care system as well as between the community and its agencies and the people; and to broaden public understanding and support concerning mental health problems. To achieve these objectives, the efforts of many institutions and groups will have to be coordinated — e.g., inpatient facilities, community mental health centers, clinics, health maintenance organizations with mental health facilities, teaching hospitals, private physicians, informal groups, patients, and their families.

As in any community service, and traditionally in public health efforts, the *community*—i.e., the structural and interpersonal entity which represents the totality of the human habitat — is the basic service unit.[21]

2. *There is a strong shift away from extended hospital care in favor of environments such as the home, boarding home, or foster home.* New therapeutic procedures lend themselves well to such care, and the costs are well below those required for institutional care. This change was undoubtedly influenced by many factors, such as the following: increased availability and use of outpatient and after care facilities; development and use of psychoactive drug treatment; greater use of community mental health centers and their affiliation with state mental hospitals; development of effective screening procedures to prevent inappropriate admissions; changes in state legislation regarding commitment and retention in facilities; and deliberate administrative efforts to reduce the inpatient population.

3. *Comprehensive Mental Health Centers*, a major provision of the 1963 legislation, offer a focus of leadership as well as additional care facilities. In order to qualify for Federal assistance, each center must provide at least five basic services: (1) in-patient care; (2) out-patient care; (3) partial hospitalization (day, night, hospital care); (4) emergency services 24 hours a day; and (5) consultative and educational services.

The center is also required to plan for care in conjunction with other resources; this places the center in the over-all planning stream of the community. The law provides for "catchment areas," ranging in size from 75,000 to 200,000 people, that serve as a population planning base. Unfortunately, the fact that these catchment areas do not always coincide with other health service areas creates some problems. In 1977 there were 649 federally funded community Mental Health Centers.[22]

It is expected that the psychiatric hospital, freed from the excessive burden of being the major source of care, will develop more specialized and intensive treatment programs.

4. *The care team is changing.* The traditional care team of psychiatrist, psychologist, social worker, and nurse has changed beyond recognition. The pressure to expand services so as to reach those in need of care was one factor in the development of new types of personnel. Another factor was the increasing acceptance of the importance of sociocultural elements in the treatment of mental disorder along with the realization that indigenous or "like-experience" personnel might be more effective than professional workers in certain aspects of care. Professions not previously used for direct care now seem indispensable—the neighborhood organizer, the planner, the educator, and the lawyer. The place of the family is central, and family members function as regular members of the care team.

The following types of workers may be included in the team, although the configuration will differ widely:

a. Members of health and health-related professions with special training in mental health — psychiatrist, clinical psychologist, psychiatric nurse specialist or practitioner, and psychiatric social worker.

b. Members of health and health-related disciplines without special preparation in mental health — registered nurses, family physicians, health educators, and community health nurses.

c. Members of professions supportive to the health profession but not of it — educators, community planners, and data specialists.

d. Mid-level practitioners prepared either in basic health and health-related areas or in mental health — practical nurses, mental health associates, or social work associates. The mental health associate is an intriguing newcomer; trained usually at the associate degree level, he is equipped to provide a variety of direct care functions.

e. Short-trained paid and volunteer workers equipped to provide intensive care within a limited range — such as crisis care, hot-line service for suicide or drug counseling, and service as a patient advocate.

f. Informal participants, usually providing care to a restricted clientele, such as a friend or relative of the patient. A typical example of this category might be a community-oriented resident in a housing complex for the elderly who maintains an alert among fellow residents, and reports their needs for attention. Another particularly strong member of this group is the person with "like experience" — e.g., the ex-hospital client or the spouse of an alcoholic.

The nursing care component is of particular concern to the community health nurse, as a source of referral, patient care information, joint care planning, and consultation. A survey in 1975 indicated that 39,228 registered nurses were employed in mental health facilities. About 48 per cent of these were working in hospitals; 13 per cent were working in outpatient facilities; and 10.6 per cent were working in community mental health centers.[23] In community health nursing, most mental health activity is incorporated into the work of generalized nursing. However, the recent increase of autonomous mental health facilities in communities has been reflected in the assignment of nurses to special programs in mental health.

The number of psychiatric nurse specialists and practitioners is growing rapidly, and constitutes a valuable source of care for families who need more than can be provided by a generalized community health nurse. They are also an important and easily reached source of consultation about an immediate problem of care or assistance.

Role Change and Role Diffusion Are Common and Sometimes Sweeping

The rapid proliferation of categories of personnel has required compensatory shifts of role among all workers. Furthermore, the concepts of hierarchical control and rigidly prescribed duties simply do not work when applied to mental health care, in which interpersonal skills and specialized knowledge or experience play such a large part. In crisis care, the choice of therapist may be less a factor of depth and sophistication of training than of the likelihood that a particular worker can establish contact quickly with a particular client. In short-term care, it may be desirable to prevent attachment of the client to a single worker; thus, several workers may share responsibility for care. Expertise is not distributed hierarchically: the short-trained aide who is an ex-addict may be more adept at dealing with a client who is "tripping"—i.e., experiencing drug-induced hallucinations—than is the professional worker without such experience. (Conversely, an ex-addict who believes that he achieved his cure by will power alone and that anyone could emulate him if they just tried may be a very poor therapist.)

This blurring of roles, while deplored by some, does seem to be well adapted to the special problems of mental health and mental disorder. DeYoung describes in detail the diffusion of roles, with attendant benefits and constraints, in a family crisis situation.[24] Meldman gives a pertinent description of role-sharing between psychiatrist and nurse-practitioner in a private practice setting.[25] Role diffusion, in effect, pools the skills of the entire staff and permits more precise matching between the training of the worker and the problems of the client. It may also allow for more rapid response to client needs, since any of several types of worker may be able to handle a particular problem.

The merging of roles, however, does place a premium on case management and joint planning of care. The indigenous worker may be well received by the suicide-prone client and his family; however, if the counseling provided is inappropriate, the effort can be totally wasted or even counterproductive. Communication and informal interchange must be free and frequent to avoid confusion and to assure a forward-moving treatment program that is both relevant and coordinated.

Community Health Nursing Intervention Is Fluid, Multifaceted, Basic, and Opportunistic

Mental health care has long held a high priority in community nursing practice. The staff mental health consultant was a familiar figure in public health services as early as the twenties. As schools of nursing intensified their concern with mental health and mental illness, and as graduates became more aware of mental health problems, the consultant services were reduced but emphasis on the mental health component in all care remained high. In the fifties—when new treatment possibilities made shorter hospital stays possible and more home care feasible— psychiatric consultants began to appear in community agencies in increasing numbers. Case finding, referral, care of the mentally ill at home, and supportive services to families expanded.

The *goals of community health nursing intervention* provide a basis for planning the mental health effort. Inevitably, these goals will coincide at some points with the aims of other community health and mental health groups. The goals should provide a guide in the development of nursing measures to achieve community mental health, such as:

1. To help prevent the occurrence of mental disorder or of conditions conducive to mental disorder by strengthening individual, family, and group support systems and by diminishing illness-inducing behavior and adverse environmental conditions.

2. To contribute to the early discovery of mental disorder by identifying vulnerable individuals, families, and groups and by providing surveillance of such groups with prompt referral for specific diagnosis and care.

3. To increase the feasibility of out-patient care of the mentally ill by the provision of such therapeutic care as is compatible with the situation and by the supervision of such care provided by family members or workers in foster or boarding homes.

4. To strengthen the linkage among clients, the agencies that serve them, and the general community through interpretation and support.

5. To contribute to the rehabilitation of those with mental illness through direct nursing support and through referral to rehabilitation facilities.

6. To help improve the available care force through participation in the recruitment, training, supervision, and evaluation of employed personnel, students, family members, and volunteers.

7. To participate in the management of mental health care by systematically searching out, documenting, and reporting conditions and supplying information that might contribute to the understanding or treatment of mental health problems.

Obviously, the community health nurse cannot be solely responsible for reaching these goals, but nursing *concern* must embrace each one. The level and nature of responsibility assumed and the patterns of sharing with other agents will vary widely. Boundaries and limits of service may be set by interagency understandings or formal agreements, or there may be an informal sharing agreement worked out on a one-to-one basis by those providing the care. For instance, in an urban setting with a community mental health center, crisis or immediate care as well as much of the continuing care of those with mental health problems may be the responsibility of the psychiatric team of the center, with the community health nurse contributing largely through case-finding referral, and general support (such as strengthening the family).

In other settings where specialized services are not immediately available, the community health nurse may be the primary care agent, providing not only crisis care but also referral, follow-up for diagnosis and prescription of therapy, post-hospital care, and over-all care management.

The exact pattern of intervention is often a matter of individual judgment on whether to initiate simple supportive measures or to refer the individual for skilled psychiatric care at a mental health clinic or center — for example, whether to provide advice to an obese client with symptoms of insecurity or to seek psychiatric back-up and guidance for a patient referral.

Good General Community Nursing Care Offers a Valuable Means of Reducing Risk

"Mental health" elements pervade every area of community health nursing commitment: e.g., strengthening the family's ability to cope with health problems (which is the most basic commitment in community health nursing); increasing parenting skills; assisting families to meet the stress of long-term illness, disability, and death; helping adolescents to confront problems with drugs or with sexually transmitted disease; assuring good maternity care that minimizes the danger of brain damage to the fetus; and improving the human environment in schools and in industry through guidance in accident prevention, analysis of performance problems, and so forth. Through concurrent or anticipatory support and counseling, the community health nurse may increase the family's ability to cope on its own.

By anticipating the expected points of stress — adolescence, retirement, menopause, or adjustment (to a new community or to catastrophic illness) — it is possible for the family to examine its own strengths and weaknesses, and to develop and evaluate alternative actions in advance.

The reinforcement of problem-solving skills, basic to all community health practice, is crucial in the management of stress.

Unexpected stress brought about by sudden illness, unemployment (resulting in a drastic change of life style), or severe injury with disability may strain the family beyond its bearable limits. The immediate availability of someone to talk to, as well as the opportunity for more intensive crisis care, may bolster the family's capability. Ideal conditions exist when there is a nurse available who knows the family and who is able to have a continuing association with the family. Such affiliation makes it easier to identify the potentials of the family's own support system and to gauge more quickly what kinds of help or information the family most needs.

The *achievement of identity* is vitally important to every individual. The need for identity as a person, unique and in charge of one's own destiny, is compelling; if this need is denied, the individual may be driven to inappropriate or even disastrous behavior. Parents must understand the travail of the young child or adolescent as he confronts the world and discovers his own place in it. Husbands and wives need to comprehend the frustration of feeling that their identities are being swallowed up in the demands of work, homemaking and parenting. Community health nurses often see evidence of such frustration, and can do much to help both individuals and families through discussion or through referral to a mental health facility. Most often, detection of a problem comes in the course of providing services for another. For instance, the teacher-nurse health conference may include discussion of an obstreperous underachiever and truant pupil, or a visit to monitor blood pressure may reveal conflicts traceable to an identity problem. No nursing situation is ever like a neat little box, tidily waiting to be tagged and shelved: surprises and challenges are always "popping up."

A sense of *ethnic or neighborhood identity* may also influence behavior. Keyes observes that, while the need for identification with a community is a strong one, such identification is difficult to achieve because of mobility, urbanization, and the depersonalization of traditional assistance agencies.[26] Beyond the usual affiliations with clubs, unions, and military or veterans' organizations, according to Keyes, there are certain lengths to which people will go to establish overt identity with a group — they will cling to the society in local hangouts or the latest "in" places, make extraordinary efforts to be recognized in public places, join communes exhibiting glaringly "alternative" life styles, and indulge in showy pseudo-neighborliness without any commitment to friendship. These temporary and often shallow links are no substitute for community identification in the deeper sense. Keyes further suggests that changes in service or in political jurisdictions, which would create a smaller communal unity, might be useful in developing greater community identity. Much of what has been accomplished in community action groups under the Office of Economic Opportunity offers this kind of possibility. Some communities have organized neighborhood councils, legally recognized, that serve in an advisory relationship to the governmental structure as well as operating independently.

Psychiatrists, sociologists, city planners, and a host of other action groups are searching for a substitute for the "home town" of the past — a place where acceptance is warm and assured, where mutual assistance and consideration are taken for granted, and where one can feel a sense of commitment to the group. While the search continues, there is much that the community health nurse can do through basic practice — e.g., by encouraging neighborly exchange and joint effort or by mobilizing groups to deal with specific health problems, such as policing school crossings or providing transportation for elderly clients. A particularly useful measure is the promoting of responsible participation by the young in problems of the health of their families and their communities.

Freedom to grow is an essential ingredient of mental health, though many factors militate against it. Differences in values or behavioral norms between generations may interfere with family support of young people intent on achieving a healthy sexuality. An emphasis on conformity in the community may make it difficult for the "different" individual to express his interests. Stereotyped family roles may set unreasonable limits on development: for example, an able business woman might be unable to take advantage of opportunities for promotion because she is seen by her family as responsible solely for housekeeping.

Through listening, counseling, encouraging, and referring, the community health nurse can do much to reverse negative attitudes and patterns of behavior and to increase the inducements to healthy and satisfying growth.

Strengthening family and community support systems — a constant concern in family health nursing — has many implications for building resistance to mental illness.[27] Loneliness, which sometimes leads to despair among the elderly, is less likely to occur if the family and the community have been coached in supportive measures such as visiting, chauffeuring, and involving the individual in activities or in holiday celebrations. In the absence of kinship family, the community (concerned neighbors, church members, and high school service clubs) may act as surrogate family members to provide care and affection. These one-to-one measures may be supplemented by community-organized helping structures, such as Meals On Wheels, hot lunch programs, or recreational and day-care centers.

Helping others is good therapy, and sometimes one good idea can produce two good deeds. The young suburban mother may be less likely to turn to alcohol out of boredom or loneliness if she becomes involved in activities such as *delivering* meals to the elderly or helping at a day-care center. Husbands, too often preoccupied with their careers, should be made aware of the loneliness and isolation of suburban wives and encouraged to find ways to involve their spouses in more stimulating activities. Where there is a potential extended-family linkage, this should be encouraged as a resource for further support.

The Community Health Nurse Plays an Important Role in Preventing and Identifying Conditions Known or Suspected to Cause or Predispose to Mental Illness

The best avenue of prevention is good generic nursing in all areas of care. Thorough family care throughout the maternity cycle, besides providing surveillence for physical health problems, can assist parents in preparing to fill their familial roles as competently as possible, in controlling family size to fit family needs, and in coping with changing emotional needs of all family members. Nursing care for venereal disease will help prevent neglect of syphilis—which, if left untreated, may result in mental disorders. Effective nursing in school and industry settings will help make these environments positive values in mental health.

More specific information on predisposing factors to mental illness will also assist the nurse in defining populations at risk. For example, adolescent suicide is escalating and is currently the second leading cause of death for the group aged 12 to 24 in the United States. Several studies described by Prophit suggest a typical pattern of life events, critical periods of stress, and a characteristic biography of the adolescent who reaches such despair.[28]

The community health nurse must attempt to provide knowledge of symptoms indicating a need for care, since anyone in touch with the public is a potential case finder. It is hoped that the parent, teacher, industrial foreman, high school youth, or anyone else who is likely to have effective access to people should have basic knowledge about mental health problems such as suicide, hallucinations, delusions, and confused behavior and should know how to reach someone who can provide immediate help.

Secondary Prevention Deals with Early Recognition and Care

The purpose of secondary prevention is to minimize the effects of mental illness through early recognition and the prompt provision of adequate care. The community health nurse participates in this effort through:

1. Identifying families or groups which are especially vulnerable to mental illness.

2. Providing nursing surveillance when indicated to these families or groups.

3. Identifying probable mental disorder through observation and evaluation of behavioral clues.

4. Referring those with possible mental disease or disorder to appropriate resources for definitive diagnosis and treatment.

The *identification of vulnerable families* is based upon epidemiologic information and upon knowledge of the individual family's usual behavior. Vulnerability, in the epidemiologic sense, is the relative risk of mental illness among individuals with certain predisposing characteristics: those in susceptible age groups (adolescence, menopause), those with special attributes (such as an aggressive drive for success), those exposed to particular environmental conditions (such as industrial settings that utilize lead), or those in high-crime poverty-stricken areas.

In dealing with a specific individual or family, one must consider both the relative strength of the predisposition or threat and the countervailing forces operating within the family. For instance, risk of schizophrenia is high among adolescents, disabled elderly, and people in the midst of political upheaval. The elderly disabled person, however, may have a high resistance to emotional disorder if she believes she is safely in God's hands, and that He will not send more than she can bear.

An adolescent may have a family history of schizophrenia (already a potential problem) and be a member of a noncommunicative and emotionally cold family, which further increases the risk. Adolescents are highly susceptible to suicide; however, a particular adolescent may be less likely to take this course if he is a member of a warm and communicating family, or has firm relationships with a circle of stable and reliable friends.

Families who find it difficult to manage the problems of daily life are more likely to produce children showing maladaptive behavior than are families who cope efficiently. However, not *all* children respond by copying adult behavior. Some children develop strong resistance to emotional disruption and establish compensating patterns of behavior to meet their own needs and often to help meet the needs of other members. Children of alcoholic parents, for example, frequently develop such compensating behavior. Merrill has pointed out the ability of many families to adapt to the absence of a schizophrenic mother.[29]

Individuals or families at special risk, then, may be identified as:

1. Individuals or families sustaining *a sharp change in life style*, environment, economic condition (newly widowed women, divorcees, those having abortions, families transferring to new communities).

2. Families or individuals who *cannot cope* or manage.

3. Families with *a history of mental disorder*, especially suicide or schizophrenia.

4. Families or individuals *facing a highly disagreeable reality*: arrest or confinement, academic failure, removal to a nursing home.

5. Families with an *adverse genetic pattern*.

6. Families with *inadequate affectional networks*: lacking in warmth toward or concern for one another, "loners," isolated elderly, families engaged in a running power play — particularly when one member is most often the loser.

Vulnerable Populations May Need Intensified Care

Populations, as well as individuals and families, vary in their susceptibility to mental illness.

1. *Low income groups* are highly vulnerable. Lemkau states, "Almost all mental disorders appear to occur more frequently in the socioeconomically deprived segments of the population."[30]

2. *Prison inmates* and offenders frequently suffer from mental disorder.

3. Those living and working in *high-stress environments* — for example, working in exceptionally complex jobs or in jobs subject to frequent obsolescence of skills; living in communities suffering from racial tension and disorder; or administrating in extremely competitive fields — are more subject to mental illness.

4. *Physically and socially isolated populations* — including mobile populations living in temporary communities; rootless groups without internal identification; pockets of elderly persons stranded in a changing neighborhood — are considered vulnerable.

5. Those living in *adverse environments* (such as slums, drug cultures, high-crime districts) or, at the other end of the scale, areas stressing overconsumption (such as a social milieu where everyone strives to have more of everything than his neighbors — and much more than is needed).

Obviously, these families and communities are not the only ones that will encounter mental health problems and require some professional intervention; however, they represent a high-priority group and should be given more than the usual surveillance and assessment.

The Expansion of Out-Of-Hospital Care and Shortened Hospital Stay Increases the Responsibility of the Community Health Nurse

The community health nurse will be involved with many aspects of care of the mentally ill, including:

1. Crisis care for the sick and their families.

2. Pre-hospital, intra-hospital, and post-hospital care for the client and family.

3. Therapeutic nursing care for the mentally ill or threatened at home.

4. Interaction and involvement with other sources of care.

5. Preventive and supportive measures for families, friends, and other significant individuals or groups within the client's orbit.

Crisis Care

The general aspects of crisis care have been described elsewhere in the text.[31] The community health nurse may perform crisis care as a regular part of nursing care in all fields, including that of mental health; or she may be assigned as a full- or part-time member of a crisis team in a mental health center or Health Maintenance Organization; or she may serve primarily as a back-up for the crisis team. Crisis care is not designed to effect deep psychosocial change or to provide long-term care; rather, its purpose is to furnish symptomatic relief and support so as to enable the client to maintain his usual roles. The crisis team includes workers with diverse talents (professional, midlevel, and short-trained contributors), all of whom are engaged in the therapy effort. Resource or back-up personnel outside the team may include family members, teachers, clergy, friends, and often the community health nurse. In the selection of a tearm to work with a specific person, the ability to empathize — that is, individuals who understand alternative life styles, particular ethnic groups, adolescent behavior, or whatever is required — should be emphasized.

Typically, crisis care employs a variety of therapies, such as family, group, or couple. The community health nurse may do much to interpret and encourage use of these resources and to help communities to develop resources where none exist. She may be called upon to provide continuing supportive care when the need for crisis care has subsided.

Crisis centers supply excellent service at a relatively low cost, and they may avert lengthy hospital stays or damaging delays in securing care. One would expect, therefore, to see such services continue and expand.

Hospitalization

Hospitalization constitutes a family crisis that both threatens and relieves the family. For some patients, hospital care is the preferred plan of treatment. Sometimes hospitalization may be of short duration in order to study the condition and to establish a therapeutic plan. In other instances, it will be long — a substitute for home care when the problem is too great to be handled by the family or foster home. Both initiation of hospital care and the later re-entry of the individual into the family and community place great strain on the family.

Pre-Hospital Care May Help the Family to Adjust More Easily to Changes

While emergency hospitalization is sometimes required, there is frequently time between the decision to hospitalize and the actual transfer. This waiting time is a period of stress for all concerned; however, it offers a rich opportunity for supportive nursing action. The patient may need time to talk about his anxieties and fears about the hospital; the family may need time to clarify their own perceptions of what hospitalization means. Is it shameful, or just another medical recommendation? Is it a signal of abandoning rather than helping the sick individual?

Time is also needed to reallocate the roles of the hospitalized member. He knows his departure will alter the balance within the family, and he needs reassurance that his role will be restored to him when he returns. Often this is not a new experience for the family. As Merrill points out, frequently the family has already absorbed the roles of the sick person, since his inability to cope probably preceded the decision to seek care.[32] If hospitalization is prolonged, considerable readjustment may be needed: the mother must go to work, or the father may have to secure baby-sitting and household help. On the other hand, the need for mobilization of the family to meet this crisis may have a strengthening effect rather than a debilitating one — children may take pride in their new skills, and the father may feel that he is fulfilling his household tasks well.

The patient must also understand his part in the healing process. He may need to be prepared for the different routine and pace of life of the hospital, and its often perplexing size. The family needs to prepare itself for its supportive task — avoiding estrangement with the patient and reassuring him of his continued place in the family. They must be prepared for possibly unusual, even bizarre, behavior.

During the Period of Hospitalization, the Family May Need Continuing Support

Extra duties, taken on at the point of crisis, may grow onerous over a period of time; and optimism may be replaced by discouragement. Children may find themselves unable to cope with the absence of a parent or sibling and unable to explain the absence to their friends. Perhaps the most helpful service the community health nurse can provide is support — by visiting, by phoning, and by being available to be called upon. Sometimes hospitalized patients reject their families or become unresponsive, and the family may need help in maintaining contact with the hospitalized member. Often already overburdened by new responsibilities, the family needs a vast amount of understanding to help them as they in turn support the patient.

The Immediate Post-Hospital Period Is One of Stress for Both the Patient and the Family

The trend toward shortened hospital stay has placed burdens of adjustment and involvement in therapy on the family for which it may be ill-prepared. For example, a patient released from hospital care after several years may be suddenly thrust upon his family, who have established patterns of living adapted to his absence. They are accustomed to leaving care to the hospital and are often frightened at their new responsibility. Because of his experiences, the patient seems to be a different person on his return, almost a stranger. The family is worried about internal relationships, about the neighbors, about displays of outlandish or excessive behavior.

The patient may have acquired new ways of behaving — expressing rather than suppressing anger, talking out rather than repressing hostility. This can be good for the patient, but trying for the family.

There may be other difficult adjustments. The wife turned bread-winner may not want to relinquish her job, or the children may not want to upset the patterns of decision and action obtained while the father was away. Sometimes the patient can resume his role only gradually, so that there is some confusion in the minds of the children as to hierarchy. All may feel a degree of estrangement, and some wariness in re-establishing customary family relationships.

During this time after hospitalization, the community health nurse will interpret the family's role in therapy and provide a source of information and support. When the family has continued under community health nursing surveillance throughout the hospital experience, there will have been some preparation and training of the family for this return — discussion, clarification, coaching, and rehearsal — all of which can encourage confidence for the readjustment period. When the community health nurse is called only after the fact, it is important that she do everything possible to secure prompt referral: the first days and weeks at home are crucial, and a later referral may only compound the problems.

The plan for post-hospital care is usually developed jointly by the responsible treatment team in the hospital and the family; in this case, the community health nurse will provide follow-up professional supervision. Sometimes this is not practicable, and the community health nurse will develop a plan with the family after consultation with the medical advisers to be certain that the plans so made are consistent with over-all treatment. Institutions will vary in the specificity with which they describe (or prescribe) the contribution they expect from community nursing. In any event, the community health nurse should inform herself of the general nature of the treatment plan and the antecedent care. When the responsibility of the community health nurse is heavy, she would be wise to engage the aid of some specialist (psychiatric nursing consultant, local psychiatrist, psychiatric nurse practitioner) who is willing to be available to help with problems that do not justify a full conference with the family's medical treatment group but rather some shoring up of the nurse's own knowledge.

The provision of continuing care may involve monitoring drug regimes, counseling, family therapy, or supervising operant conditioning programs. It also involves directing the family to available community agencies and professional groups. There may also be a need to manipulate the social environment — as, for instance, working with a teacher to prepare students for the return of a classmate from a mental institution. The breadth of possible action sometimes overwhelms the nurse with little experience in this field. But with close coordination with primary treatment sources, the good offices of the public or heatlh agency librarian, and the back-up personnel mentioned above, these uncertainties can be met.

Rehabilitation Is an Essential Component of Care in Mental Illness

Mental illness, often requiring separation from one's family for extended periods of hospitalization, or resulting in social isolation, produces particularly acute demands for rehabilitative care. As hospital stay shortens, and as the concept of the family as therapist broadens, more and more of this rehabilitative effort is likely to fall upon the community or family health nurse.

The object of rehabilitation is to restore the individual to his usual social role as promptly and fully as possible. The rehabilitation effort is directed toward preserving the individual's own assets and bolstering his coping capabilities. For the adult of working age, return to work is especially important.

The return to "normal" may, in many cases, be incomplete or conditional. For example, "return to work" can mean returning to work in a protected environment or in a low-stress occupation. Ability to function within the family may depend on adherence to a drug regimen, and ability to maintain identity with and participation in social groups might be contingent upon readily available support figures. The client must set realistic goals to avoid discouragement or failure.

Rehabilitation is by nature a multidiscipline, multiagency task. Each situation may call upon a different combination of professional workers: vocational counselors, educationists, social workers, or a different agency involvement and different levels and kinds of family therapeutic effort. Planning conferences, usually sponsored by the major care facility and involving several agencies as well as the family, help establish practical goals and programs. The community health nurse is an important contributor to such conferences because of her knowledge of the family and its patterns of decison making and action and because of her ability to anticipate community responses when the time comes to reintegrate the individual into his social milieu.

Many Interventions and Problems of Care of Mental Illness Are Common to Other Nursing Services

Problems of supervising drug regimens, for example, are much the same as those presented when the illness is diabetes or tuberculosis. The patient and the family must in all cases understand what part the drug plays in the total therapy and what the drug can and cannot do. They need to know what degree of tolerance is safe in terms of exactness of dosage, missed dosages, or timing of dosage. They need to know the symptoms of drug-related side effects, and the urgency of reporting these to the medical advisor.

Family therapy is closely related to the community health nursing concept of involving the family in its own care, and recognizing the autonomy of the family in health decisions. Group work with expectant parents has much in common with group therapy, and modification of the environment, both physical and social, is basic to many situations in family health.

Moving from general approaches to specific therapy in cases of mental disorder demands familiarity with new information and refinement of skills. In turn, proficiency gained in working with the mentally ill and their families can be very useful in helping parents to develop child-rearing skills or in encouraging neighborhood committees to overcome argumentative barriers when trying to reach decisions.

When the home of the mentally ill patient is a boarding home or a foster home, the problems are similar to those dealt with in the family home. There is the same need to involve the staff or owner of the boarding or foster home as there is to involve the family in supporting the therapeutic process and in establishing and carrying out a plan of care.

Strong Linkage of the Family and Its Support Systems Maximizes the Benefits of Care and Promotes Economical Use of Available Resources

Good referral practices (preparing the family and the support source for their encounter, selecting among possible sources those most adapted to the specific situation, balancing formal and informal sources of help) are essential. The family may need help in feeling comfortable in their use of helping services. They may worry lest people know of attendance at Alcoholics Anonymous sessions, or friends may gossip about use of family counseling services. They may delay in seeking hospital care because they have heard horror stories about conditions in such hospitals. The family and the individual may need time to bring their reservations and fears into the open. A trusting relationship between nurse and client is sometimes slow in developing, and the family will often test her in many ways.

If the community health nurse (or health nurse-cum-psychiatric practitioner) is the principal referrant for the family, it is important that she and they be in touch with other sources of care and information that might at some time be involved. Community health nursing for the family does not end when the individual client is referred to specialized mental health services.

Association with informal sources of help is an important factor in prevention and care of mental illness or disorder. A good friend, loving and caring; a respected elder brother; and a grandmother or uncle may provide sources for listening and reassurance. The young person who has overcome former suicidal tendencies or who has understanding and warmth may help peers who feel suicidal or who have made suicide attempts.[33] The alcoholic may find calm sanctuary with a sympathetic, nonalcoholic married brother or sister.

The family is, of course, the most important of these support sources. Some families are unable to give support because of social pathology or personality deficiencies, but for most the ability to help a disturbed member can be strengthened if they understand the nature of the needed support and specific ways in which it can be tendered. For example, there are parents who have a very great concern and affection for their children but who cannot communicate that concern. There will be a need to discuss explicit steps that could be taken and some of the reasons why young people feel the need to resist, either as a measure of independence or as a test of the real commitment of the parents. Couples may find that simple fatigue causes rifts in understanding — for instance, making an effort to help may look like an attempt at domination. If both giver and recipient of support understand these and similar mechanisms that can get in the way of truly supportive relationships, they can improve their support potential.

The limits as well as the power of family support must be recognized: the extremely aggressive or abusive person may need professional help immediately, for example. It is necessary to establish a balance between the professional and family contributions to care — though both are indispensable. A continuing search for new formal and informal resources will increase the options available to families.

Improvement of the physical and social environment may decrease pressure or contribute to changing attitudes and concepts. The child growing up in a deteriorated, rat-infested, poorly maintained home in a neighborhood where the alleys are strewn with rubbish and garbage, with harsh and often drunken parents, is unfortunately not a rarity. Such children might be expected to have trouble in developing a sense of personal worth or easy relationships with classmates, and even more in finding a sense of community. All too often, these conditions engender sentiments such as "Why bother?" or "Let the government do it," or "Nobody's going to help you, so take what you can." It is easy to understand why such young people retreat to the self-defeating world of alcohol and drugs. Yet improvement is *not* impossible. Simply sprucing up the appearance of the local environment can add to self-esteem. Vigorous, dependable, and continuing neighborhood support will contribute to the development of healthy mental and emotional behavior.

Sometimes the focus is on the mini-environment — the small cluster of close neighbors, or the residents of a single block. The community health nurse can be a leader in pulling this small group together — encouraging, for example, a discussion on the hazards of selecting babysitters too casually, the danger of leaving older children unsupervised in empty homes, and the poor example set to children when adults drink to excess or take drugs.

Above all, joint efforts by neighbors or small groups of families in a community can demonstrate that, by working together, at least some of the problems can be solved. You don't need to hire a sanitarian to sweep the sidewalk in front of your house! Furthermore, a neighborhood organization may bring problems to the attention of civic authorities, forcing them to take remedial action.

Mental health nursing efforts may help to define the problems of mental illness in the community and, in some cases, document the outcomes of specific treatments. The community health nurse can also assist by locating mental health personnel and can promote improved mental health through liaison with a variety of treatment facilities.

The community health nurse can use available epidemiologic information to search out the most vulnerable populations. In the course of her usual services, she may identify both individuals and groups in need of mental health assistance. She can document the need for new facilities or for programmatic changes within existing ones. She can evaluate new approaches and therapies, based on observation of clients in their natural habitat, and note the effect of the intervention upon not only the individual but also others within his orbit.

Another contribution the community health nurse can make in the area of community practice is fusing together the different health and health-related services to families. In a publication of the American Public Health Association, it is stated, "An area in which the need for intelligent planning is urgent. . . is the linking or fusing of the delivery of mental health services with other health-related and social service systems."[34] The family/community perspective of community health nursing has provided most nurses with considerable experience in fusing their efforts with those of schools, industries, poverty programs, prison welfare associations, welfare agencies, and the many health agencies. This experience should be useful as well to other planners. Directly or indirectly (through providing back-up support to citizen or other action groups), the community health nurse can bring to the attention of community officials or voluntary organizations the need for specific services.

Mental health and mental illness impinge on virtually every community health nursing effort. The challenge is so broad that only through knowledgeable alertness, effective teamwork, and great precision in the selection of the appropriate nursing response can it be met.

Threats to the Nurse's Mental Health

Caring for the mentally disordered is a task that may occasion some uncertainty and frustration within the nurse. She may herself be fearful of mental illness and virtually immobilized when called upon to help another in mental distress. She may feel that much of the care required is not nursing, that it takes too much time, that it interferes with the accomplishment of "real" nursing tasks, or that it demands skills and knowledge beyond that expected of a nurse. She may find it hard to muster the necessary permissiveness and warmth in the face of slow progress or overt hostility, or she may feel that she cannot accept the concept of community mental health when she sees nursing as primarily a one-to-one nurse-patient interaction. She may find it hard to accept the ambiguity of her role — that some who receive care will, nevertheless, continue to do poorly and that some must do without care.

It is easy to become discouraged with the slow progress of families in changing health behaviors and of community resources in adapting to meet very obvious needs in all aspects of community nursing. The community health nurse may find herself overwhelmed with the larger social issues of poverty, crime, or inadequate social functioning of families, to name only a few, that she may have contact with on a daily basis. Depending on the community setting, she may have realistic fears for her own safety, especially if she is working in or near a high crime area or an area where there is known drug traffic and abandoned buildings.

The nurse may be hampered by a lack of knowledge and skill in certain areas, whether it is new psychiatric treatment methods or assessment of the newborn. This feeling of inadequacy may be strengthened when families and medical personnel are not accustomed to referring to the community health nurse as a source of help in this particular field. She may not be certain about how much she should do. There are several steps she may take to remedy such conditions. She may:

1. Read about developments in psychiatric practice, or attend continuing education courses in areas she is weak in, to increase her background knowledge.

2. Locate, with the help of her supervisor, consultant resources either in the agency or in the community.

3. Suggest inservice education topics or develop ready reference material in areas where she feels insecure. Chances are that others working in the area need more information as well.

4. Talk out her own feelings with the nursing supervisor or other appropriate professional person, such as a consulting psychiatrist or mental health nurse specialist.

5. Know the community, both broadly and intimately. Individual health problems are usually a part of the larger societal problems. Combining forces with other groups in the community can often make an impact when the one-on-one encounter may not. For example, the nurse may find that by working with others involved in child abuse or by involving the family in a self-help group, she may effect change faster than by working alone with the family. Knowing dangerous neigh-

borhoods or blocks or patterns of activity and alerting "regulars" to her plans and whereabouts can reduce risk of personal injury.

6. Tie community health nursing to the power structure of the community. This may mean learning how to work through the legislative process, working with planning bodies, or identifying community leaders and establishing reciprocal relationships that benefit the community as well as the nurses sense of relevance.

The mental health aspects of community health care are so interwoven with the individual nurse and with every other service activity that competence in this area is a crucial issue in general nursing effectiveness.

Activities that are specifically labeled "mental health" represent a claim on community health nursing time as well as an opportunity to gain insights and skills that will carry over to many other phases of the nurse's work and personal growth. Concern for improving community mental health will lead not only to seeking out those who need psychiatric help but also to modifying the community environment to make it more conducive to mental health. Here, too, the potential benefits go far beyond the immediate situation. Dealing with the ego-damaging effects of the low-income neighborhood may contribute to improvement of the health of a designated group of patients. It may also contribute to the realignment of relationships and attitudes so essential for social action and social justice. Thus, the community health nurse can wisely spend much thought and care on the development of her skills in this area of professional practice.

REFERENCES

1. Sartorius, N., and Shapiro, R. W.: A common language. World Health Chron., 27:30, 1973.
2. Maslow, A.: Cited in Teeran, R. C., and Birney, R. C.: *Theories of Motivation in Personality and Social Psychology.* Princeton, N.J., D. Van Nostrand Co., Inc., 1964, p. 118.
3. Goerke, L. S., and Stebbins, E. L.: *Mustard's Introduction to Public Health,* 5th ed. New York, Macmillan Co., 1968, p. 168.
4. Carstairs, G. M.: Mental health, what is it? World Health Chron., 27:4, 1973.
5. Public Health Service, U.S. Department of Health, Education, and Welfare: *Health: United States, 1978.* Washington, D.C., U.S. Government Printing Office, Pub. No. (PHS) 78–1232, December 1978, p. 69.
6. *Health: U.S., 1978,* p. 70.
7. Editorial. World Health Chron., 27:3, 1973.
8. *Health: U.S., 1978,* p. 71.
9. Ibid.
10. Ibid., p. 72.
11. Hanlon, J.: *Public Health Administration and Practice.* St. Louis, Mo., C. V. Mosby Co., 1974, pp. 438–446.
12. *Health: U.S., 1978,* p. 72.
13. National Institute of Mental Health, U.S. Department of Health, Education, and Welfare: *Research in the Service of Mental Health.* Washington, D.C., U.S. Government Printing Office, Pub. No. 75-37, 1975.
14. American Public Health Association: *Mental Health: The Public Health Challenge.* Washington, D.C., 1975, p. 86.

15. Ibid., pp. 91 and 97.
16. *Research in the Service of Mental Health,* pp. 8–9.
17. Ibid., p. 14.
18. See Chapter 5, Family Goals and Strategies, for further discussion of this topic.
19. Keyes, R.: *We the Lonely People: Search for Community.* New York, Harper and Row, 1973.
20. Zuk, G.: *Family Therapy: a Triadic Appraoch,* New York, Behavioral Publications, 1972.
21. See Chapter 16, The Community: The Commitment, for further discussion.
22. *Health: U.S., 1978,* p. 78
23. U.S. National Institute of Mental Health: Biometry Branch Survey and Reports Section, 1975.
24. DeYoung, C.: Nursing contribution to family crisis treatment. Nurs. Outlook, *16*:60, 1968.
25. Meldman, M. V., et al.: Public health response to nurse psychotherapists. Am. J. Nurs., *71*:1150, 1971.
26. Keyes: *We, the Lonely People: Search for Community.*
27. See Chapter 4, The Family as the Unit of Care.
28. Prophit, S. P.: The Enigma of Adolescent Suicide. *In* Mercer, R. T. (ed.): *Perspectives on Adolescent Health Care.* Philadelphia, J.B. Lippincott Co., 1979, Chapter 10.
29. Merrill, G.: How fathers manage when wives are hospitalized for schizophrenia, Soc. Psych., *4*:26, 1969.
30. Lemkau, P.: *In* American Public Health Association: *Mental Health, The Public Health Challenge,* p. 41.
31. See Chapter 26, Special Communities.
32. Merrill, How fathers manage. . . . , p. 26.
33. See for example American Association of Suicidology: *Suicide in Young People.* Houston, Texas, Dept of Psychiatry, Baylor Medical College (undated pamphlet).
34. *Mental Health, The Public Health Challenge,* p. xv.

SUGGESTED READINGS

Bassuk, E. L., and Gerson, S. Deinstitutionalization and mental health services. Sci. Am., *238*:46, 1978.
Broskowski, A., and Baker, F.: Professional, organizational and social barriers to primary prevention. Am. J. Orthopsych., *44*:707, 1974.
Brown, B. (ed.): Politics and power. Nurs. Admin. Qtly., 2:17, 1978.
Bush, M. T., Ullom, J. A., and Osborne, D. H.: The meaning of mental health: A report of two ethnoscientific studies. Nurs. Res., *24*:130, 1975.
Cronin-Stubbs, D.: Family crisis intervention: A study. J. Psych. Nurs., *16*:36, 1978.
Cuejic, H., et al.: The evolution of a school-based mental health program using a nurse as a mental health consultant. J. School Health, *49*:36, 79.
Davis, M., Kramer, M., and Strauss, A.: *Nurses in Practice: A Perspective on Work Environment.* St. Louis, Mo., C. V. Mosby Co., 1975.
Deinstitutionalization: the evolution and evaluation of health care policy in the United States and Great Britain. Milbank Mem. Fund Quart., *4*:429, 1979.
Doll, W.: Family coping with the mentally ill: An unanticipated problem of deinstitutionalization. Hosp. Com. Psych., *27*:183, 1976.
Fitzpatrick, M. L.: Safety and the community nursing experience. Nurs. Outlook, *19*:527, 1971.
Hollingshead, A. B., and Redlich, F. C.: *Social Class and Mental Illness.* New York, John Wiley & Sons, Inc., 1958.
Jones, F. H. A 4-year follow-up of vulnerable adolescents: The prediction of outcomes in early adulthood from measures of social competency, coping style, and overall level of psychopathology. J. Nerv. Mental Dis., *159*:20, 1974.
Kalish, B. V.: The promise of power. Nurs. Outlook, *26*:42, 1978.
Kramer, M., and Schmalenberg, C. (eds.): Bicultural training and new graduate role transformation. Nurs. Digest, 5: 1978.
Krauss, J. B.: The chronic psychiatric patient in the community — a model of care. Nurs. Outlook, *28*:308, 1980.

Lyon, G. G., et al.: Ways of intervening with the psychotic individual in the community. Am. J. Nurs., 79:490, 1979.

Mechanic, D.: Social structure and personal adaptation: Some neglected dimensions. *In* Coelho, G. V., Hamburg, D. A., and Adams, J. E., (eds.): *Coping and Adaptation.* New York, Basic Books, Inc., Pubs., 1974, pp. 32–44.

Mercer, R. T.: *Perspectives on Adolescent Health Care.* Philadelphia, J. B. Lippincott Co., 1979, Chapters 9 and 10.

Moos, R. H. (ed.): *Human Adaptation: Coping with Life Crises.* Lexington, Mass., Health Sciences Pub. Corp., 1976.

Naparstek, A. J., and Haskell, C. D.: Neighborhood approaches to mental health services. *In* Macht, L. B., et al. (eds.): *Neighborhood Psychiatry.* Lexington, Mass., Lexington Books, 1977.

Palermo, E.: Mental health consultation in a home care agency. J. Psych. Nurs. Mental Health Ser., 16:21, 1978.

Pasamanick, B. (ed.): *Epidemiology of Mental Disorder.* Washington, D.C., American Association for the Advancement of Science, 1959.

Pasnau, R. O.: *Consultation-Liaison Psychiatry.* New York, Grune and Stratton, 1975.

Psychology Problem Classification for Children and Youth. Washington, D.C., U.S. Government Printing Office, DHEW, PHS, Pub. No. (HSA) 77-5203, 1977.

Regier, D. A., Goldberg, I. D., and Taube, C. A.: The de facto U.S. mental health services system. Arch. Gen. Psych., 35:685, 1978.

Riedel, D. C., Tischler, G. L., and Myers, J. K. (eds.) *Patient Care Evaluation in Mental Health Programs.* Cambridge, Mass., Ballinger Pub. Co., 1974, Ch. 4.

Sartorius, N.: Epidemiology of depression. WHO Chron., 29:423, 1975.

Sheehy, G.: *Passages: Predictable Crises of Adult Life.* New York, E. P. Dutton & Co., Inc., 1976.

Stricklin, M. L.: Mental health patient assessment record: Interobserver reliability. Nurs. Res., 28:11, 1979.

U.S. President's Commission on Mental Health: *Report to the President: Vol. 2.* Washington, D.C., U.S. Government Printing Office, Task Panel Reports, 1978, pp. 1–138.

Vaughn, C. E., and Leff, J. P.: The influence of family and social factors on the course of psychiatric illness: A comparison of schizophrenic and depressed neurotic patients. Br. J. Psych., 129:125, 1976.

Waskow, I. E., and Parloff, M. B. (eds.): *Psychotherapy Change Measures.* Washington, D.C., U.S. Government Printing Office (DHEW Pub. No. ADM 74-120), 1975.

CHAPTER 20

FORCIBLE RAPE: A GROWING THREAT

Forcible rape usually refers to carnal knowledge of a woman by a man carried out against her will, without her consent, or by force.[1] There are other categories of rape; however, the discussion here will be restricted to the kinds of situations most likely to be encountered by a community health nurse. As was previously mentioned in Chapter 1, the incidence of forcible rape has been increasing — in 1978, rape affected 30.8 of every 100,000 inhabitants in the United States.[2]

The incidence of rape varies sharply with income: higher rates of rape and of attempted rape victimization were found among women whose major activities took them away from the home and those with lower family incomes than among women who spent most of their time at home and those with higher family incomes. Similar differences existed between white and non-white populations — rape among white female populations was estimated at 67 per 100,000, compared to 115 per 100,000 among non-white females.[3] More rapes occurred in the evening and nighttime hours than during the day, and more took place in an open public area such as a street or park than in any other location.[4]

While no age group is invulnerable, the majority of victims were between the ages of 16 and 24 years. The incidence in this age group in 1979 was 243 per 100,000, and 224 per 100,000 in females 12 years of age or older.[5]

Most offenders were unmarried, working as unskilled labor, or unemployed.[6] Thus, while rape is not limited to any particular age, economic, or racial group, it is a far greater problem for women under 30 in low income populations, especially in non-white groups.

The motivation to rape is not fully understood. It appears to stem from a variety of causes: sexual insecurity or the need to establish sexual identity, an unusually strong sex urge, the need to vent hostility or frustration toward society, or the need to prove manhood with a peer group. Sometimes rape is almost casual — the opportunity arises, and the offender seizes the advantage. Contrary to popular opinion, the relationship to alcohol is not clear. Research has revealed no common discernible behavior pattern or personality type as typical of the rapist. What seems apparent is that the motivation is complex and individualized, so that each situation must be seen in its own context.

There are no predictable conditions under which rape may occur. In some instances, rape is a matter of chance, perhaps touched off by the mere presence of a potential victim in conjunction with a robbery or other felony. In other instances, especially in cases of group rape, the victim may be selected in advance and the operation carefully planned.

Rape often involves physical violence beyond that associated with intercourse itself — beatings and other forms of abuse are common. Frequently there is extreme humiliation of the victim — e.g., repeated intercourse with observers present, forced engagement in cunnilingus or fellatio, and extreme verbal humiliation.

Group rape is especially ugly. Generally it has been planned; the intent is to inflict both pain and shame. The reinforcing effect of the leader on the members, and of one member on another, is such as to trigger higher levels of violence and degradation than might occur in an encounter with a single assailant.

COMMUNITY HEALTH NURSING IN A PROGRAM OF PREVENTION

Ultimately, of course, the goal is total eradication not only of forcible rape but also of all other forms of social violence. That hope, however, represents more than any one individual can realistically accomplish. The community health nurse must concentrate on what is possible and must direct her particular skills and persuasive powers where they will be most effective. She can promote development of healthy sexual attitudes through her contacts in schools with young people and their parents and with teachers and guidance counselors. She can encourage open discussion of sexuality and sexual problems, promote sex education, and be alert to early signs of possible offenders. By herself or through others (such as civic groups, police, churches, parent-teacher organizations), she can enlist the public in a safety program, with special efforts to reach those in the most vulnerable age group (16 to 24 years).

Traditionally, it has been a woman's responsibility to avoid being raped, by circumscribing her behavior. The stigma of rape was on the victim, as if her behavior or clothing provoked the attack. This attitude is totally rejected by many women today, who are working to eradicate it from our courts and from the public mind. Today women insist on the right to use public transportation, to be employed outside the home, to use recreation facilities — to go about life freely — without the fear of rape. Unfortunately, our society has to undergo many changes before freedom from fear can be a reality. Girls and women of all ages must still think in terms of *preventive action*. The following are among the many possible precautions to take and to teach:

In the Home. Women in the same neighborhood or apartment building can get together, keep an eye out for each other, and help each other avoid situations where rapes might occur — for instance, plan to go together to an isolated laundry room in a large apartment building. Install dead-bolt locks on all outside doors. Insist on adequate locks on apartment doors. Demand to see identification of anyone claiming to be a utility repairman, *before* opening the door. Instruct young girls to report to parents or teachers any one who is bothering them — sometimes young girls are afraid to say anything, because the man is a friend of the family or a relative. Baby-sitting jobs should be accepted only if a parent will take the sitter home; baby sitters should be prepared to recognize and deal with over-friendly fathers.

On the Streets. We need to pay attention to the surroundings, look alert, and pay attention to the people around us and not ignore threatening or odd behavior. Women are socialized to be polite and not draw attention to themselves. In a moment of danger, they may hesitate to scream, to run, or to throw things. An attitude of mental and physical preparedness can help. Knowing ways to fight or scream, talking with other women about their experiences and getting together to practice what you might do may be useful. Women who work late shifts can ask police for special patrols during change-of-shift times.

In Traveling. It is best to travel with others, and always a good idea to keep car doors locked while driving and to be alert when returning to a parked car at night. When using public transportation, wait in well-lighted areas; walk an extra block to use a busy stop, rather than an isolated one. Avoid hitchhiking or picking up hitchhikers, since the risks are so great. Think ahead; don't run out of gas when driving.

THE COMMUNITY HEALTH NURSE AND CARE OF THE RAPE VICTIM

Several factors combine to determine care of the rape victim. First, there is the effect of the legal situation on the attitudes of victims, offenders, and law enforcement personnel. Because rape involves a heavy jail sentence, care must be taken to protect the suspect from unfounded accusation. This requires positive determination of the occurrence of the sexual act and of the circumstances under which the act took place — whether it was by force or against the will of the victim. The victim will then be required to testify as to what happened — usually at a time when she is in all likelihood shaken, hurt, and bewildered. When the victim is known to have been promiscuous or "loose," the questioning may be particularly intensive. All too often, the implication is that it is the victim rather than the assailant who is at fault.

Indeed, probably because of deeply rooted social conventions, the victim herself may feel guilty — as though she had in some way allowed the situation to occur.

Immediately following a rape, the victim needs several different kinds of care. There is need for immediate medical attention to prevent pregnancy or genital infection. This can be not only a physical but also an emotional ordeal for a young person who is unaccustomed to gynecologic examinations and, in many instances, is suffering from shock due to the rape itself and attendant beatings or other violence. The police are working under other pressures and cannot always take time to consider the emotional state of the victim: she will need additional comforting and assistance in facing the brusqueness of the police or other officials.

Later, the victim must go to court and present her case, encountering strange procedures, a hostile defense lawyer, and a cruel sense of being exposed.

During all of this, the victim must also somehow move toward integrating this terrifying experience into her life as a whole, and re-establishing her own emotional balance.

Depending on the facilities available and to some degree on agency policy, the community health nurse may take action herself, refer elsewhere for action, or call to the attention of other treatment facilities the type of care that is required and that should be provided after the discovery of the rape.

The *rape center* is an increasingly available facility, especially in large urban centers. These are usually small privately run clinics or offices, manned largely by volunteers concerned with the prompt care and protection of the victims of rape. They try to work closely with law enforcement agencies in order to provide assistance to victims as soon as is feasible, and to follow up each case straight through to the courtroom. In some instances, the rape center provides total service — medical, professional social work, and nursing personnel, and psychiatric counseling. In others, the main role is that of referral for necessary medical care. A central modality of these centers is the use of "like-experience" personnel, usually serving on a volunteer basis. Thus the rape victim can talk to someone who has herself been raped, who comprehends the ordeal, and who can provide guidance in the practical aspects of reporting and testifying. Mostly, the victim needs someone to talk to so as to verbalize her feelings of degradation and shock, and often of betrayal. Referral to other sources provides for specialized care, but the center itself offers a "safe haven" and continuing support.

Immediate support and reassurance may be provided by an "on call" community health nurse or by a nurse functioning in a rape center. One recommendation suggested that a nurse or social worker accompany the police on rape investigations so as to provide prompt and sympathetic support to the victim.[7]

In most cases, emotional support will be needed for a fairly long time. There are predictable phases of response on the part of the victim, not dissimilar from those anticipated in other crisis situations.[8] These usually begin with acute reactions of anger, bewilderment, despair, and hysteria. Next, the victim will display evidence of outward calm and apparent adjustment; she will resume her normal routine and claim to others that she has completely recovered from the ordeal. This stage can be deceptive: the victim may in fact still be in emotional torment, but unable or unwilling to express it. Eventually, and with help, the victim will be able to integrate and resolve the experience.

The experience of either overt or submerged reaction to such trauma is understandable. Rape can leave devastating mental scars, and the need for immediate help must not be underestimated. Frigidity, unnatural fears of sex, even catatonia can be the result of neglect or inattention.

Throughout this cycle of readjustment, there will be a need for specific information — where to find free legal service, where to go for initial medical appraisal and help, what is involved in the gynecological examination, what drugs have been prescribed, and the importance of following instructions regarding them. Above all, sympathy and reassurance must be provided: The expression, "It could have happened to anyone," may need to be said over and over to relieve a sense of guilt or degradation.

The client also needs assistance in recognizing the symptoms and the general nature of the adjustment period — the recurring memory of the event, the depression, and the strained relationship with others. At this point, she may well need further support from professional or "like-experience" workers, so that she may free herself to think through her own reactions. She will also need help in recognizing that the phase of apparent outward adjustment is likely to be only one step toward final resolution.

The family as well as the patient will need help throughout this entire experience. Parents or husbands may feel that their daughter or wife has disgraced or humiliated them or that she invited or permitted the sexual activity; they can, in effect, isolate her from her usual sources of family support. They may themselves take on the guilt, feeling somehow that it was their responsibility to prevent the attack. Or they may just need help in understanding unusual behavior on the part of the victim — moodiness, or a lack of interest in family affairs.

The provision of care and emotional support at all these levels may be shared by community health nurse, social worker, and volunteer. The nurse's role will include seeing the total need, estimating the adequacy of the community response to this need, and being prepared to accept primary responsibility for care if necessary. She may share responsibility with a team operating under her direction, or participate in a team under other direction; conversely, she may refer all or part of the care to other sources.

The sex offender as well as his victim will also need help. However, the range or degree of abnormal behavior is very broad here — from the "accidental" or one-time offender to compulsive rapist or child molester — and is for the most part beyond the scope of the community health nurse. Problems of sweeping proportions, requiring massive remedial action, cannot be dealt with practically through local health care mechanisms. The energies of the community health nurse are better directed toward aiding the family and friends of the offender.

PREVENTIVE AND SUPPORTIVE ACTION WITHIN THE COMMUNITY

· There are many ways in which the community health nurse may become involved in a community's efforts to prevent potential rape. An awareness of lifestyles and living patterns of the community is an important beginning. For example, the community health nurse may draw attention to the time school children spend unsupervised at home between their return from school and their parents' return from work. When individual families cannot provide alternatives, she may encourage institution of after-school activities, or ask church groups to provide facilities, or urge children to stay with relatives or neighbors until the parents return. The simple expedient of carefully briefing children may in itself help reduce the risks. Citizens' alert groups often work with the police when incidents appear to be on the rise. The community health nurse can be of assistance by taking opportunities to share her knowledge of the community with new policemen in the area.

There are several things a community health nurse can do in order to be prepared when rapes do occur. She can work to establish a rape center in her community; she can also develop a resource list of previous rape victims who are willing to assist others, of legal aid personnel, and of strong motherly surrogates who can provide reassurance and support, especially to the truly abandoned or severely underprivileged victim.

Problems of violence are not easily analyzed, understood, or treated. It is difficult to know whether any of the interventions we know about will indeed affect the incidence or outcome of episodes of rape. However, one must assume that support and understanding can mitigate to some degree the effects of this particularly dehumanizing experience.

REFERENCES

1. Amir, M.: *Patterns of Forcible Rape*, Chicago, University of Chicago Press, 1971, p. 60.
2. U.S. Bureau of the Census, *Statistical Abstract of the U.S.: 1979*, 100th ed. Washington, D.C., 1979, p. 177.

3. McDermott, M. J.: Applications of The National Crime Survey Victimization and Attitude Data, Analytic Report SD-VAD-6, U.S. Dept. of Justice, Washington, D.C., U.S. Government Printing Office, 1979, p. 6.
4. Ibid., p. xi.
5. Ibid., p. 5.
6. Amir, *Patterns of Forcible Rape*, Chapter 12.
7. Weiss, E. H., Taub, N., and Rosenthal, J.: The Mental Health Committee: Report of the Subcommittee on the Problem of Rape in the District of Columbia. Med. Ann. D. C., *41*:703, 1972.
8. Fox, S. S., and Scherl, D. J.: Crisis intervention with victims of rape. Soc. Work, *17*:37, 1972.

SUGGESTED READINGS

Amir, M.: *Patterns of Forcible Rape*. Chicago, University of Chicago Press, 1971.

Brownmiller, S.: *Against Our Will: Men, Women, and Rape*. New York, Simon and Schuster, 1975.

Burgess, A.: The rape victim: Nursing implications. J. Prac. Nurs., *28*:14, 1978.

Burgess, A. W., and Holmstrom, L. L.: *Rape: Crisis and Recovery*. Bowie, Md., Robert J. Brady Co. — A Prentice-Hall Co., 1979.

Colderon, V. R.: Continuing education promotes social change. J. Con. Educ. Nurs., *10*:8, 1979.

Crimwell, P. E. (ed.): *Women and Mental Health: A Bibliography*. Washington, D.C., Department of Health, Education, and Welfare (Pub. No. 75-142), 1974.

Donadio, B., and White, M. A.: Seven who were raped. Nurs. Outlook, *22*: 245, 1974.

Fox, S. S., and Scherl, D. J.: Crisis intervention with victims of rape. *Soc. Work, 17*:37, 1972.

Gorline, L. L., et al.: Examining and caring for the child who has been sexually assaulted. MCN, *4*:110, 1979.

Gottesman, S. T.: Police attitudes toward rape before and after a training program. J. Psych. Nurs., *15*:14, 1977.

Hiberman, E.: *The Rape Victim*. Washington, D.C., American Psychiatric Association, 1976.

Ipema, D. K.: Rape: The process of recovery. Nurs. Res., *28*:272, 1979.

Lee, B.: Interview: Precautions against rape. Sex. Behav., *2*:33, 1972.

Weiss, E. H., Taub, N., and Rosenthal, J.: The mental health committee: Report of the Subcommittee on the Problem of Rape in the District of Columbia. Med. Ann. D. C., *41*:703, 1972.

Rape crisis intervention in Boston's Beth Israel Hospital — A model program. J. Prac. Nurs., *28*:17, 1978.

CHAPTER 21

ABUSIVE BEHAVIOR IN THE FAMILY

In recent years, the battered child has been the focus of an aroused social concern. These children are the victims of abusive parents or other care agents; they usually suffer serious physical or psychologic injury, sometimes death. Abusive behavior is a result of uncontrolled rage, unbearable frustration, or mental disorder. No particular age group is singled out, infants only weeks or months old are abused as brutally as toddlers or teenagers. Nor is any single form of abuse predominant—the victim may be beaten, kicked, drowned, sexually molested, cut, choked, or burned; some are neglected to the point of unspeakable filth or starvation.

A related problem is wife beating — a long-standing situation that is just now coming into the open. This may or may not be associated with alcoholism. Abusive behavior involves two clients: the victim, who needs protection, and the abusor, who is often desperately seeking help and who is as much a patient as the sufferer.

Neglect and abuse of the elderly is also of concern and ranges from inattention to physical battering. Financial pressures, family conflict, and degree of care needed by the elderly are associated with abuse of this age group.

Abusive behavior in the family is no respecter of class or education — it occurs in a city slum or in a penthouse, in suburbs or in rural areas, and in the wealthy or in the impoverished (and all economic levels inbetween).

Child protection is primarily a function of the states, and many have enacted legislation requiring the reporting of child abuse and ensuring protection from reprisal for those who report and testify. An important stimulus to public action was the passage of the Child Abuse Prevention and Training Act of 1974 (PL 93-247). This act directed the creation of a National Center for Child Abuse and Neglect within the Department of Health, Education, and Welfare, which provides a clearinghouse for information and resource materials and supports research and training in this field.

Although wife beating is illegal, legal authority is more diffuse and society has been less outraged. Local authorities often see wife beating as "normal" or a "familial affair," and are reluctant to intercede.

Concerns regarding domestic violence have assumed national proportions, and efforts to develop legislation that would provide shelters and educate people regarding the problem continue.

Detection Is Difficult

The abuse problem is truly of unknown proportions. One estimate is that 1 out of every 100 children is physically or sexually abused or severely neglected.[1] Domestic violence is estimated to affect one in six couples per year. Many injuries inflicted through abuse go unreported, or their true origin is concealed. Parents will bring a battered child to a clinic with plausible explanations for contusion or burns, and the child is often too young or too frightened to describe what actually happened. In "good," high-income, or in apparently happy families in particular, professional workers may find it hard to credit what they observe when the child is brought in for care. Also, if abusive behavior is not suspected, internal injuries may be missed.

Parents or other abusers are generally remorseful and contrite once the initial seizure of passion or anger has passed. They rarely mean to do as much harm as they do, and the abused person (or the rest of the family) knows it. This can result in a kind of conspiracy of silence. Families that are happy in other respects are unwilling to expose this aberrant behavior on the part of one member. The problem, especially abuse of spouses, may not be admitted until something really drastic happens — divorce proceedings, extreme bodily injury, or death.

Less dramatic, non-physical abuse is much more elusive to detect, but equally damaging to the victim. Physical abuse can be the result of sudden fury or uncontrolled impulses; often the victim (e.g., wife or child) is not the cause of the attack; he or she just happens to be handy at the time. Psychologic abuse requires some forethought; it is more subtle and insidious, and much more difficult to prove.

Recently, there has been more willingness on the part of both affected persons and the public to discuss problems of this nature. People openly admit situations that even a few years ago were considered shameful or taboo, such as homosexuality, marital discord, and abusive proclivities or experiences. Airing these problems will open the door for increased understanding and improved treatment.

ABUSIVE BEHAVIOR IS A
MULTIDISCIPLINE PROBLEM

The problems of abusive action almost always require multidisciplinary care. In this field, special importance is attached to the use of lay therapists, in addition to the usual team members. These are usually warm, outgoing, and stable individuals who have undergone a short training course. They may be nursing aides, social service aides, or simply interested citizens with no professional medical or social work background; many are volunteers. They provide a releasing presence for those who have the potential to demonstrate or have already demonstrated abusive behavior. The procedure followed by these lay therapists is uncomplicated and direct: they visit the family, show interest, listen, reassure, and refer. They work in close association with a professional team member who provides insight and overall care management.

Self-help groups are of great importance. Sometimes these are organized in national associations such as Parents Anonymous or Alcoholics Anonymous (a very helpful group when alcoholism is part of the problem). Sometimes they consist of informal interchanges among like-experience individuals or families in a clinic, or discussions between parents and personnel in a child protection service. Such affinity groups make it possible for abusers to verbalize their experiences, their sense of guilt, and, most important, the "triggering" conditions that lead to abuse behavior. If they genuinely want rehabilitation, abusers can gain understanding and practical help from one another.

Traditional psychiatric group or family therapy conducted by professional or lay leaders, emergency help by hot line, emergency house or clinic visits, foster home or day-care placement — these are all possible strategies. Their goal is to reduce the stresses leading to abusive behavior and to protect the abused or threatened person. Although sometimes necessary, criminal prosecution is rarely effective in protecting the abused; it may indeed only intensify the dangers. This is a situation in which the rapidly vanishing, extended family can be a potent resource — serving as a sanctuary and source of comfort and providing reassurance of continued family concern.

Many different groups can be involved: law enforcement agencies, legal aid, medical care facilities, schools, and churches. If it becomes necessary to remove a child from an immediately dangerous situation, the removal must be carried out by the police or other legal enforcement agency. When there is a designated center for care of abused children and adults, this special center may serve as the coordinator of efforts on behalf of the family. In the absence of such a center, local custom will determine the patterns of responsibility.

Care that is preventive in nature — e.g., offering supportive efforts to vulnerable families or individuals who are not yet abusers or documenting cases of borderline neglect or incipient non-physical abuse — may or may not be a concern of the local treatment center. It is in this area that the community health nurse may find herself most deeply engaged.

The Community Health Nurse Can Play an Important Role

Within the team as it exists on the local level, the community health nurse may serve as case-finder, reporter, and care agent, fitting her activities to those of others in the group.

1. *Identification of those most vulnerable* to abusive action, and intensification of support through direct action or referral, may prevent trouble in some instances or bring victims into protective custody more promptly.

The nurse should "have her antennae out" regarding conditions that are common breeding grounds for violence, such as the following: parents whose own childhood was characterized by brutal treatment and who show persistent immaturity and poor impulse control (low anger threshold, "hot" temper); single parents or parents of unwanted children (i.e., one who has been denied a requested abortion); little parental concern shown in a family with a large number of closely spaced children; familial history of alcoholism, drugs, or delinquency; evidence of poor marital adjustment (nagging, scolding, excessive repression of one partner or, conversely, docile and uncomplaining acceptance of intolerable conditions); and a severely handicapped child with whom parents cannot or will not cope.

2. If the danger can be brought into the open, *aversive action* may be possible. For example, the non-abusive parent with a potential abusive spouse may identify available sanctuaries such as grandparents, a kindly neighbor, or a community child protection center, and be encouraged to take children there during drinking bouts or periods of incipient rage. The person who lashes out uncontrollably under pressure should be urged to talk out the trouble and express himself with a lay therapist or other receptive person in order to deter actual abuse. When available, a hot line can provide emergency help; sometimes, all that is needed is someone to listen. Parents who cannot manage an afflicted child or who feel burdened with too many children, or who live in deep poverty may be helped to greater proficiency or, if possible, referred to facilities for relief or release time through agents such as paid or volunteer household helpers, day care, or family assistance.

3. *Early recognition and care* of abusive behavior may offer hope of minimizing the danger. Suspiciously frequent accidents that produce fractures, bruises or cuts should be carefully investigated. Often abusive parents will go to a different hospital or clinic after each incident of maltreatment; they hope to avoid accumulating a record of their actions.

Sharing of information between medical facilities would be very fruitful. The nurse should be alert for evidence of parental rejection or neglect which may not yet be technically abusive; this could include parents who refer to an infant as "it," children who are poorly diapered or underfed, or severe punishment meted out for minor insignificant offenses.

The National Center on Child Abuse and Neglect suggests the following outline for observations of abuse and neglect:

I. Signs of abuse in children needing immediate action.
   A. Any injury in an infant under 12 months of age.
   B. Gross or multiple injuries in a child of any age.
   C. Repeated injuries. Fractures in various stages of healing.
   D. Intracranial injuries.
   E. Unexplained weight loss.
   F. Severe malnutrition or failure to thrive, especially in very young children.
   G. Dehydration under unusual circumstances.
   H. Venereal disease or signs of genital trauma in children unable to understand the nature of the sex act.
II. Signs of Abuse in caregiver.
   A. Current behavior in relation to the child's condition:
      1. inappropriate affect;
      2. inadequate or conflicting history of the injury;
      3. failure to seek medical care promptly.
   B. Observations of interaction with the child:
      1. inappropriate demands and expectations of a child;
      2. unreasonable and inappropriate discipline;
      3. angry, impulsive behavior.
   C. Current living situation:
      1. stress;
      2. isolation;
      3. inadequate support.
   D. Care of other children.
   E. Childhood history of caregiver.
   F. Relationships with other agencies.[2]

Detection of wife beating is difficult. The woman can generate a variety of excuses for bruises, cuts, or fractures. Women who are abused frequently have a low self-esteem and appear helpless. They continue to accept abuse because they are convinced that their spouse will reform, because of economic hardship and need for child support, or because they are afraid they cannot make it on their own. The sense of helplessness and the lateness in obtaining needed medical services are common symptoms to look for.

ASPECTS OF COMMUNITY CONTROL

Reporting is essential in community involvement with abusive behavior. Most states make it mandatory to report suspected child abuse, and the legislation will contain conditions that pertain to reporting abuse. One definition of child abuse *for reporting purposes* is:

A child, under the age of 18, who is suffering from physical injury inflicted upon him by other than accidental means, or sexual abuse, or malnutrition, or suffering physical or emotional harm, or substantial risk thereof by reason of neglect. Reporting of neglect shall take into account the accepted child rearing practices of the cultures of which he or she is part.[3]

This definition obviously excludes many families who *need help* with problems of child abuse, either for preventing or correcting antecedent habits of harsh punishment that may lead to frank abuse. For example, a child who is physically untouched but subjected to emotional harrassment, verbal abuse, extended isolation, or who is consistently made a scapegoat within the family is at grave risk. Though the situation may not conform to the definition just quoted, nevertheless, the warning signals are clear.

It is believed that there is a large group of offenders who could avoid future abusive behavior with the aid of minimal therapy or very simple preventive measures. A few hours with a lay therapist — someone to listen — may be all that is needed to clear the air and relieve pressures. Securing daytime care for children to allow a mother some restorative quiet privacy may also be helpful. For the most part, however, preventive measures should be left to skilled professionals who are trained in this area of work.

Helping families identify stress — whether it involves the work place or life's unfulfilled expectations — can also be helpful. Identifying problems and airing these can often help bring a family toward resolution and different approaches to management of conflict and stress.

There will be times when the community health nurse may be required to testify; and, in this case, the employing agency will provide appropriate assistance. At the point of reporting and testifying, the nurse should try to deal sympathetically with the abuser and the family as well as the victim. If the abuser can face the problem squarely, knowing that support will not be withdrawn, there is a greater likelihood of rehabilitation. Many abusers want desperately to be helped, but do not know how to ask for aid.

In contacts with the public, the community health nurse can encourage candor in discussing the problem and can stress the urgency of reporting suspected abuse. A receptive attitude toward the plight of the abuser on the part of the public may encourage individuals who could gain from treatment to make the effort to seek it out.

One frequent dilemma for abused children is repeated placement and replacement in different foster homes. This is primarily a protective device, but it can lead to very real problems — a lack of family identity and a deep sense of insecurity.

Another problem that is beginning to surface is abuse of parents, especially the elderly, by their families. The problem is neither defined nor well documented, but cases of abuse have been reported.[4] Stress, history of aggressive behavior, and economic hardship seem to be important factors. To the extent that the nurse can assist families in identifying the real problems, alternative solutions can be sought that are beneficial to everyone.

The community health nurse may contribute to community control of abusive behavior by documenting the need for more care or additional facilities, not only for those already in the abuser-abusee category but also for those in the category of latent abusive behavior. For example, a community in which most wives work outside the home may be relying on unsuitable or even dangerous baby sitters with consequent direct risk to the children. Community day care or after-school recreational facilities may be badly needed. Day care centers for the elderly or supplemental help in the home may be needed.

Special care centers may be urgently required in areas where actual abusive behavior frequently surfaces and where potential or hidden abusive behavior is suspected. With her knowledge of the community, her awareness of individuals who have the potential for abusive behavior, and her familiarity with the review of case histories of those whose steps to abuse have been sequential, the nurse may help to identify groups for intensive preventive measures.

Abusive behavior is a challenging and elusive problem. By observing, documenting, counseling, and fostering interagency cooperation, the community health nurse may contribute substantially to a better understanding and wider treatment for this critical phenomenon.

REFERENCES

1. Light, R.: Abused and neglected children in America: A study of alternative policies. Harvard Educ. Rev., 43:556, 1973.
2. Public Health Service, Department of Health, Education, and Welfare: *Child Abuse/Neglect, A Guide for Detection, Prevention, and Treatment.* Washington, D.C., U.S. Government Printing Office, Pub. No. (HSA) 77-5220, 1979, pp. 5–6.
3. Department of Health, Education, and Welfare Publication: *National Conference on Child Abuse: A Summary Report, 1973.* Washington, D.C.: ADM 74–117, GAO, 1974, p. 16.
4. Battered families: A growing nightmare. U.S. News World Rep., 89:60, 1979.

SUGGESTED READINGS

Bavolek, S. J., et al.: Primary prevention of child abuse and neglect: Identification of high-risk adolescents. Child Abuse Neglect, 3:1071, 1979.
Bell, J. N.: Rescuing the battered wife. *Hum. Behav.,* 6:16, 1977.
Block, M. R., and Sinnott, J. D. (eds.): The Battered Elder Syndrome: An Exploratory Study. College Park, Md., Center on Aging, University of Maryland, 1979.
Broadhurst, D. D.: Update: What schools are doing about child abuse and neglect. Child. Today, 7:22, 1978.
Charnley, L., and Myre, G.: Parent-infant education. Child. Today, 6:18, 1977.
Densen-Gerber, J., and Hutchinson, S. F.: Sexual and commercial exploitation of children: Legislative responses and treatment challenges. Child Abuse Neglect, 3:61, 1979.
Fontana, V., et al.: The abused child, the abusing adult: Both are victims, both need your help. J. Prac. Nurs., 28:24, 1978.
Friedman, K.: The image of battered women. Am. J. Pub. Health, 67:722, 1977.

Frommer, E. A.: Predictive preventive work in vulnerable families of young children. Child Abuse Neglect, 3:777, 1979.

Gelles, R. J.: Power, sex and violence: The case of marital rape. Fam. Coord., 26:339, 1977.

Gelles, R. H., and Straus, M. A.: Violence in the American family. J. Soc. Iss., 35:15, 1979.

Giarretto, H.: Humanistic treatment of father-daughter incest. Child Abuse Neglect, 1:411, 1977.

Gordon, J. S.: Alternative human services in crisis intervention. Victimology, 2:22, 1977.

Gordon, J. S.: The runaway center as community mental health center. Am. J. Psych., 135:932, 1978.

Hall, N. M.: Group treatment for sexually abused children. Nurs. Clin. North Am., 13:701, 1978.

Harbin, H. T., and Madden, D. J.: Battered parents: A new syndrome. Am. J. Psych., 136:1288, 1979.

Helfer, R. E., and Kempe, C. N. (eds.): *Child Abuse and Neglect: The Family and the Community.* Cambridge, Mass., Ballinger Pub. Co., 1976.

Hurwitz, A.: Child abuse: A program for intervention, Nurs. Outlook, 25:575, 1977.

Jacobson, B.: Battered women: The fight to end wife beating. Civ. Rights Dig., 9:2, 1977.

Johnson, D. G.: Abuse and neglect — Not for children only! J. Gerontol. Nurs., 5:11, 1979.

Johnston, M. S. K.: Practical advice for beginning a therapeutic group for abusive parents. Child Abuse Neglect, 2:223, 1978.

Justice, B., and Duncan, D. F.: How do job-related problems contribute to child abuse. Occup. Health Safety, 47:42, 1978.

Lau, E., and Kosberg, J.: Abuse of the elderly by informal care providers. Aging, Nos. 299–300:11, Human Development Series, Department of Health, Education, and Welfare, 1979.

Lebowitz, B. D.: *Crimes Against the Elderly.* Statement before the Joint Hearings of the Subcommittee on Domestic and International Scientific Planning, Analysis and Cooperation, Committee on Science and Technology, and the Subcommittee on Housing and Consumer Interests, Select Committee on Aging, House of Representatives (96th Congress, 1st session), January 31, 1978.

McKeel, N. L.: Child abuse can be prevented. Am. J. Nurs., 78:1478, 1978.

Novak, D. B. and Meismer, D. T.: A plea for help: One community's response. Victimology. Int. J., 2:647, 1978.

Ottenberg, P.: Violence in the family: Abused wives and children. Bull. Am. Acad. Psych. Law, 5:380, 1977.

Petro, J. A., Quann, P. L., and Graham W. P.: Wife abuse: The diagnosis and its implications. J. Am. Med. Assoc., 240:240, 1978.

Straus, M. A., Gelles, R. J., and Steinmetz, S. K.: *Behind Closed Doors: Violence in the American Family.* Garden City, N.Y., Anchor Press/Doubleday, 1980.

Tilelli, J. A.: Sexual abuse of children: Clinical findings and implications for management. New Eng. J. Med., 302:319, 1980.

U.S. Department of Health, Education, and Welfare, Public Health Service: *Child Abuse/Neglect; A Guide for Detection, Prevention, and Treatment.* Washington, D.C., U.S. Government Printing Office, Pub No. (HSA) 77-5220, 1979.

RESOURCES

National Center on Child Abuse and Neglect (NCCAN), Children's Bureau, Administration for Children, Youth and Families, Offices of Human Development Services, P.O. Box 1182, Washington, D.C. 20013.

The American Humane Association, Children's Division, 5351 S. Roslyn Street, Englewood, Colorado 80110.

National Center for the Prevention and Treatment of Child Abuse and Neglect, University of Colorado Medical Center, 1205 Oneida Street, Denver, Colorado 80220.

Parents Anonymous, 22330 Hawthorne Blvd., Torrance, California 90505, Telephone (213) 371–3501.

CHAPTER 22

DEVELOPMENTAL DISABILITIES

Health care for those with developmental disabilities offers a special challenge to community health nursing. The term covers a broad spectrum of mental and physical concerns that arise as a result of congenital or acquired difficulties and that affect an age group ranging from newborn to 21 years. These problems may include neurodevelopmental difficulties, cerebral palsy, epilepsy, sensory deficits, emotional disturbances, metabolic and/or genetic disturbances and central nervous system trauma. Since all but a few children with these problems live with their families and need to adapt to community living, it becomes mandatory that the needs presented by those with developmental disabilities be viewed in the context of both the family and the community.

As defined by recent legislation, developmental disability means "a severe, chronic disability of a person" that

a. is attributable to a mental or physical impairment or combination of impairments;
b. is manifested before the person attains age 22;
c. is likely to continue indefinitely;
d. results in substantial functional limitations in three or more of the following areas of major activity: (1) self-care; (2) receptive and expressive language; (3) learning; (4) mobility, (5) self-direction; (6) capacity of independent living; and (7) economic self-sufficiency; and
e. reflects the person's need for a combination and sequence of special, interdisciplinary, or generic care, treatment or other services which are of life long or extended duration and are individually planned and coordinated.[1]

This definition excludes those of borderline intelligence or those classified as mentally retarded solely on the basis of IQ scores. The focus is upon ability to *function socially* rather than upon intelligence per se.

The problem is impressive in size and impact. Under the revised definition, developmental disabilities are estimated to effect 331,000 (3 per cent) children from infancy to two years of age, 1,053,000 (1.87 per cent) children from 3 to 17 years, and 1,858,000 (1.49 per cent) young adults and adults from 18 to 64 years.[2] An estimated six million Americans suffer from mild to severe mental retardation, and each year approximately 100,000 children are identified as mentally retarded. In about 90 per cent of cases, the retardation is defined as mild (IQ 50 to 70) and diagnosis is made at school age.[3]

The impact of developmental disabilities is profound. The condition is permanent, producing severe impairment in a large proportion of those affected; and intensive and expensive care is required to minimize disability or to provide humane institutional treatment for those who are critically impaired. This financial burden affects both family and community alike.

Recent emphasis has been on providing services within the community to assist disabled individuals to operate within the "mainstream" of normal society. For example, Congress passed the Education of Handicapped Children Act (PL 94-142) seeking to guarantee the availability of free, appropriate public education for all handicapped students in the least restrictive environment. There has been an overall trend to deinstitutionalize persons with mental retardation and provide for smaller units within the community. A certain danger is inherent in this movement — i.e., safety and adequate care of those with severe problems — but the experience so far seems to be a positive although difficult one.

The etiology of developmental disabilities is not always clear. Developmental disabilities, and specifically mental retardation, may be caused by multiple biological, psychologic, and sociocultural factors. Some of these factors are well documented; others are suspected. *Genetic factors* (inborn metabolic errors) may result in Down's syndrome, (mongolism), cretinism, phenylketonuria, incompatible Rh factor, Tay-Sachs disease (defective metabolism in early infancy), and other less common disorders. *Perinatal factors* — such as infection in the mother transmitted to the fetus, (e.g., rubella), tumors, malnutrition, and drugs — also effect developmental disabilities. Congenital rubella syndrome is a prominent threat; 20 to 25 per cent of infants born to mothers who contracted rubella in the first trimester of pregnancy develop this syndrome, which includes deafness, microcephaly, mental retardation, and bone defects.[4]

Injuries, accidents, and *childhood disease, including birth injuries,* are known to be factors in developmental disabilities. Poisoning, particularly lead poisoning, can cause mental dysfunction. Malnutrition, although difficult to isolate as a single cause, is known to affect learning potential and behavior; and difficult labors or complications of labor may be associated with lower IQ scores and cerebral palsy. Meningitis and other diseases affecting the central nervous system may also affect later development.

Environmental factors, though thought to influence growth and development, are the least documented as contributors to developmental disabilities. Available evidence suggests that the following environmental factors are important: (a) amount of inanimate stimulation; (b) amount of animate stimulation; (c) the manner in which animate stimulation is provided; (d) the teaching style used by significant adults; (e) the mother's perception of the child; (f) the amount of stress in the family; (g) general emotional stability of parents; and (h) the presence of a father or male figure.[5]

PATTERNS OF CARE HAVE CHANGED

The essential change in care for children with developmental disabilities is the adoption of a much more aggressive attack on early screening and detection as well as the pulling together of many disciplines to work with these children and their families. The goal of care is early initiation of treatment and "normalization" for both individual and the family, so that the disabled person can find a place in society; maximize what he or she can do; and, if rehabilitation is not possible, establish an environment that provides his or her life needs and self-respect. The overall strategy is a broad approach, based upon synchronized action by many different agencies, groups, and individuals.

The Developmental Disabilities Assistance and Bill of Rights Act of 1978 — which provides for university-affiliated facilities for developmental disabilities, state allotments, and special project grants — has provided strong incentives for the development of diagnostic, treatment, and rehabilitation centers. Aid for research on different care patterns has also been supported by federal, state, and voluntary programs. The result appears to be not only an increase in facilities but also a strong reorientation by the professionals and the public toward responsibility for providing for maximum growth potential.

The current community action to combat developmental disabilities centers on the following strategies:

1. A distinction between those who need therapeutic or educational care and those with simple learning difficulties who are reasonably well adjusted to their society, concentrating on those who need care.

2. A vigorous drive toward more accurate diagnosis and development of more adequate processes and programs for care.

3. A strong effort to avoid institutional care for those who can be cared for in the home, foster home, or other noninstitutional setting. This is beneficial in two ways: it provides an economic approach to care, and it serves to keep the disabled in the mainstream of society.

4. Special education facilities for children with developmental disabilities within the general education system and intensive efforts toward vocational training for those able to work, plus education and involvement of potential employers to encourage hiring of disabled persons.

5. A strengthening of general programs where neglect may lead to problems. These include maternity care (especially neonatal and intranatal care), and control of syphilis and diabetes, protection from rubella, and the prompt care of toxemia.

6. A "human rights" emphasis in relating developmental disabilities to society. These new strategies have produced a widespread effort toward guarantees of human rights for the disabled in terms of the following: their right to appropriate treatment; their right to decent living conditions in institutions; their right to affection and esteem; and (though this is a delicate issue, with no simple solutions) their right to marry and procreate or to make their own decisions concerning sterilization.

These strategies are directed toward three objectives: (1) helping the family to utilize all available preventive measures; (2) mobilizing the support systems within the family and the community; and (3) guiding the developmentally disabled to reach his highest potential while at the same time encouraging the system to realize its greatest potential for help. Many of these activities will be woven into other services — maternal and child health care, school and occupational health consultation, or family health surveillance.

THE COMMUNITY HEALTH NURSE PLAYS
A SIGNIFICANT ROLE IN CARE

The community health nurse contributes to the prevention, control, and amelioration of handicapping developmental disabilities largely through its integration into all facets of service.

1. The nurse can help families to secure *early and competent care* throughout the maternity cycle. This includes making sure that prospective mothers and adolescents presumed to be capable of becoming pregnant are all inoculated against rubella. The nurse may also be called upon to supervise and coordinate the activities of subprofessional workers who are involved in the medical system.

Families known to be at special risk (such as those with a history of mental retardation) should be referred for genetic advice or counseling. Early warning and education can prevent birth injuries or unnecessary exposure of the fetus to maternal infection, and can lead to early identification of other potential problems.

2. The nurse can maintain an *"epi-alert" for precursors of developmental disabilities* and special surveillance of those in jeopardy; for example, pregnant women 38 years old or older (in offspring of this age group, Down's syndrome is much more prevalent); those exposed to lead poisoning; or cases of blood incompatibilities between parents. This mandates at least a minimal genetic pedigree as part of any family history where the parents are of child bearing age.

3. The nurse should provide for *developmental surveillance* direct-

ly or by referral, or through support of others who can recognize and appraise deviant developmental patterns. This is desirable for all families, but essential for those vulnerable to developmental problems. For example, slowness in crawling, walking, talking, unusual difficulty in weaning, poor schoolwork or excessively sluggish behavior, and other physical or behavioral signs help identify potential problems. There are a variety of tools for assessing the development of children, neonate through older age groups.[6] The community health nurse working with families will find these screening tools very helpful in gathering specific information and observations about the family and the child with special problems. This kind of surveillance is conducted in conjunction with other professionals (teachers, social workers, psychiatrists, physicians) who can advise and alert the nurse or, in turn, be advised or alerted by her.

4. The nurse should *provide appropriate information or referral* services to other professional personnel for *parents who risk producing children with developmental disabilities*, so that they can make early and enlightened decisions regarding childbearing.

When preconceptual care is possible, the potential parents will need help in considering the alternatives. They should be advised on available contraceptive measures, abortion, or the means of securing voluntary sterilization; they must be informed of the likelihood of producing an impaired child if they proceed. Once the decision has been made — whatever it is — prompt referral is vital.

In some instances, the diagnosis of mental retardation may be made in utero early enough to allow parents to decide whether or not to allow the pregnancy to continue. Amniocentesis is considered safe for the mother and poses very little risk to the fetus. However, parents often need reassurance that the tests are reliable; and, if the outcome is positive, they may need extensive support in deciding whether or not to continue the pregnancy.

5. The community health nurse can *identify conditions* that might be confused with mental retardation and, thus, lead to a false diagnosis. As soon as possible, children should have tests at a very early age to identify any losses in hearing or vision that could interfere with normal learning. This should be part of a comprehensive preschool physical examination. By the time the child reaches school, it may be too late to reverse the effect on learning abilities. Severe infection or illness at any age may also produce slowed responses.

Poor school achievers should receive an intensive medical appraisal to rule out special learning disabilities or neurological disorders such as dyslexia which might lead to a false diagnosis and thus waste time in securing the necessary treatment.

6. The nurse should *sustain the family* in their support of the child with a developmental disability. The family will need reinforcement during periods of crisis, and perhaps even more during the chronic

problem of continued care. This will become increasingly important as more and more mentally retarded and developmentally disabled individuals are being cared for in the home.

There are three points that can create great stress within a family: (1) the point of initial diagnosis; (2) the point of institutionalization for those severely handicapped; (3) and the point at which the child achieves sexual maturity, when questions of reproduction and/or limitations thereof may be raised. The nursing support provided at these points will be the same as that for all crisis care.

The diagnosis of mental retardation is often not a surprising one to the family, but most parents hope that their worst fears will not be realized. Some will reject the diagnosis, going from one authority to another for further consultation, and usually magnifying the significance of every tiny gain by the child. Their reactions are often the result of simple fright; they are frightened of the exorbitant amount of care which will be required by a disabled child, by the prospect of unbearable financial burdens, and by the realization that their child is not "perfect."

Self-care is important for the family energy level and the child. There are many techniques available to help the family work with the child with special problems to attain independent activities of daily living — i.e., self-feeding, toilet training, sleeping through the night and dressing.[7]

Behavior modification and biofeedback programs have been found to be very successful in helping children gain control of a variety of behaviors. The nurse, working with the developmental disabilities team, may provide the continuity of care for the patient, work with the family to ensure understanding of and compliance with the regimen or established protocol, and work with others to modify regimens to best fit the needs of the family and the child.

Institutionalization is usually accompanied by a feeling of guilt on the part of the family, a sense that they *should* have managed. They may neglect their other children, which in turn creates another source of guilt. In a very real sense, too, they mourn the loss of a "normal" child. Placing someone in an institution can be confusing and demoralizing, and parents may appear to be resentful, surly, or rejecting. The community health nurse can help by listening, comforting, and encouraging them to express their anxieties even though this might take the form of blaming the doctor, making accusations, or creating a scene. The nurse can do much to turn parental action to more fruitful directions. What is obvious to an outsider is not always so apparent to those blinded by close involvement with a problem. Families need reassurance that the child will be happy if he is doing what he *can* do, that improvement is possible for many, that the family does not stand alone, and that supporting agencies are available. The child, too, may need special attention, lest he be affected by the parents' despair. Putting things in perspective is often the greatest help in enabling the family to cope on its own.

7. A major concern in continuing care is *interpreting the needs of the child with disabilities.* A retarded child has the same needs as other children for attention, cuddling, affection, and such training as can be assimilated. (The problems of parental support are different only in degree.) The feelings of the child with problems may be more openly expressed, and accomplishments may be limited; however, the equal opportunity for learning is essential to healthy growth.

It is important that parents understand the probable limits of development, so that they do not expect the impossible; yet it is equally important that they set their sights on the highest possible goals. Learning will be slow — often one little thing at a time. Routines are important to follow; they chart a reliable, secure course to follow. Praise and approval are crucial.

Training must be initiated early so that as many children as possible may be made ready to take advantage of special classes within the regular school system. This usually means that the child should be toilet-trained and able to follow instructions. As much as possible, life should be run along normal lines — that is, the care provided should be similar to that of other children in the family. Regular school is preferable to special schools when the educational system is equipped and staffed as necessary.

Parents must also be prepared to accept a longer period of dependency with a developmentally disabled child than with other children. The child with developmental lag will nurse longer, demand attention until much older, and take longer to learn simple mechanical skills such as tying shoe laces or feeding himself. As they reach adolescence, children with developmental disabilities need information about changes in their bodies and their feelings, just as other children do. The family will be helped by anticipating these changes, having a plan for teaching, and possibly talking with other families with similar concerns.

Some families overreact to the special child. Parents may reject siblings or isolate themselves from the community. The children may withdraw from their friends, or avoid bringing them home. Parents may hover too closely, never going out together so that one can remain home with the affected child. Such isolation and social avoidance is, of course, a very real threat to the "normal" members of the family group, often creating stress, marital dissension, and mutual blame. All families — but especially those who are coping poorly — should be encouraged to take some remedial action such as joining the local chapter of the National Association for Retarded Citizens, or discussions with like-experience parents, or professional counseling. Sometimes the nurse will have to literally bully the family into taking such steps.

Parents and children will need continuing encouragement to persist in efforts toward integrating the child with developmental disabilities with the larger social group. At school or in the playground, for example, siblings often have to protect their brother or sister with cerebral palsy from the thoughtlessness of others, from the disappointment of not being chosen for games, or from the irritation of others as he displays poor impulse control. Classmates of the deaf child will need coaching to promote understanding and acceptance of his different or diverting behavior. Others must learn to share in the goal of helping the child with special problems to see himself as a worthy, contributing member of his society.

8. Through seeking out and providing support to families suffering from physical or cultural deprivation, abusive behavior, or severe psychiatric disorders, the community health nurse may help to *moderate the impact* of such conditions. Parents in families where the norm of behavior is cool or undemonstrative may need to be taught very basic skills such as how to hold an infant lovingly, how to talk to him, or how to provide toys for the child which will enhance perception and motor responses. The community health nurse should always be on the alert for ways to locate and activate both formal and informal sources for support; warm grandparents, neighbors, a special teacher, or an enrichment class.

9. The nurse should *serve as a liason* between families and available sources of diagnosis and care. Many parents, hoping to disprove the diagnosis of mental retardation, or a developmental disability, shop around for medical advice, seeking someone who will discount the problem. In the process, much time can be lost both in care of the affected member and in adjustment by the rest of the family. Reference to diagnostic and treatment centers, special clinics, or other authoritative sources may help resolve the family's ambiguity and ready them for action. (In such cases, appropriate clearance must *always* be made with the usual medical advisers.) Above all, the fostering of a realistic but hopeful attitude toward the problem will prepare the family to participate in its own care.

The community, too, needs a fuller understanding of its role in the prevention and care of developmental disabilities. The community health nurse can bring to the attention of others some of the practical problems and needs of her clients. Through participation in such organizations as the National Association for Retarded Citizens, on school or community committees, through meetings with law enforcement personnel — in fact, in the course of all her activities — she can encourage positive attitudes toward the developmentally disabled and those who try to care for them.

She can document the impact of "labeling" on mentally retarded individuals, the frustration and misery that comes with repeated failure or public shunning; the dangers inherent in the tendency to lump all mentally retarded people together rather than see them as the separate entities they are. When caring for a particular family or client, the community health nurse might talk with neighbors, school personnel and school mates as well.

The care of the family with a developmentally disabled member will require all the skills inherent in community health nursing practice. Despite the obvious limits, much can be done for these families and much can be accomplished through positive community action to prevent and care for these problems which carry so many heavy burdens with them. It is imperative that children with special problems are treated with dignity, understanding, and love — whether or not they can be rehabilitated.

REFERENCES

1. Section 132, Developmental Disabilities Assistance and Bill of Rights Act (PL 95-602) November 6, 1978.
2. Unofficial estimates from the Bureau of Developmental Disabilities, Office of Human Development Services, Department of Health and Human Services, May 1980.
3. Surgeon General's report: *Healthy People.* Washington, D.C., U.S. Government Printing Office, DHEW, PHS Pub. No. 79-55071, 1979, p. 37.
4. American Public Health Association: *Control of Communicable Diseases in Men,* 12 ed. Washington, D.C., American Public Health Association, 1975, p. 273.
5. Barnard, K. E., and Douglas, H. B. (eds.): *Child Health Assessment.* Washington, D.C., U.S. Government Printing Office, DHEW Pub. No. (HRA 75-30), December 1974, p. 4.
6. Erickson, M. L.: *Assessment and Management of Developmental Changes in Children.* St. Louis, Mo., C. V. Mosby Co., 1976.
7. Ibid., Chapters 14 to 16.

SUGGESTED READINGS

Apgar, V., and Beck, J.: *Is My Baby All Right?* New York, Trident Press, 1972.
Baker, B. L., et al.: *Steps to Independence: A Skills Training Series for Children with Special Needs.* Champaign, Ill., Research Press, 1976.
Barnard, K. E., and Eyers, S. J. (eds.): *Child Health Assessment, Part 2: The First Year of Life.* Washington, D.C., U.S. Government Printing Office, DHEW, HRA 79-25, June 1979.
Bradley, R. H., and Caldwell, B. M.: Early home environment and changes in mental test performance in children from six to thirty-six months. Dev. Psych., *12*:93, 1976.
Buscaglia, L.: *The Disabled and Their Parents: A Counseling Challenge.* Thorofare, N.J., Charles B. Slack, 1975.
Committee for the Study of Inborn Errors of Metabolism, Division of Medical Science, Assembly of Life Science, National Research Council: *Genetic Screening. Programs, Principles, and Research.* Washington, D.C., National Academy of Science, 1975.
Conley, R.: *The Economics of Mental Retardation.* Baltimore, Johns Hopkins Press, 1973.
de la Cruz, F. F., and LaVeck, G. D. (eds.): *Human Sexuality and the Mentally Retarded.* New York, N.Y., Brummer/Mazel, 1973.
Erickson, M. L.: *Assessment and Management of Developmental Changes in Children.* St. Louis, Mo., C. V. Mosby Co., 1976.
Frankenburg, W. K., and North, A. F.: *A Guide to Screening for the Early Periodic Screening, Diagnosis and Treatment Program under Medicaid.* Washington, D.C., U.S. DHEW Social and Rehabilitation Services, 1974.
Fuchs, F.: Genetic Amniocentesis. Sci. Amer., *242*:47, 1980.
Gordon, J. M.: Community nursing care study: Life in a community that cares. Nurs. Times, *73*:1272, 1977.

Johnson, S. N.: *High-Risk Parenting: Nursing Assessment and Strategies for the Family at Risk*. Philadelphia, J. B. Lippincott Co., 1979.

Lis, E. F., and Ruess, A. L.: A perspective on the growth and development of handicapped children. *In* Wallace, H., Gold, E., and Lis, E. (eds.): *Maternal-Child Health Practices*. Springfield, Ill., Charles C Thomas, 1973.

Milunsky, A.: Current concepts in genetics: Prenatal diagnosis of genetic disorders. New Eng. J. Med., *295*:377, 1976.

Moore, C. B., and Morton, K. G.: *A Readers Guide for Parents of Children with Mental, Physical or Emotional Disabilities*. Washington, D.C., U.S. Government Printing Office, U.S. DHEW, PHS Pub No (HSA) 77-5290, 1976.

Murray, A.: Implementing a behavior modification program. Nurs. Times, *73*:171, 1977.

Saintz, M. L.: *The Nurse and the Developmentally Disabled Adolescent*. College Park, Md., University Park Press, 1977.

Saxon, W.: Behavioral contracting: Theory and design. Child Wel., *58*:523, 1979.

Schuelt, V. E., et al.: Diet discontinuation policies and practices of PKN clinics in the United States. Am. J. Pub. Health, *70*:498, 1980.

Smith, S. S.: *No Easy Answers: The Learning Disabled Child*. Washington, D.C., U.S. Government Printing Office, U.S. DHEW PHS, (ADM) 77-526, 1978.

Tudor, M.: Nursing intervention with developmentally disabled children. MCN, *3*:25, 1978.

Wilkin, D.: Community care of the mentally handicapped — Family support. Nurs. Mir., *146*:39, 1978.

Nursing Problem Classification for Children and Youth. Washington, D.C., U.S. Government Printing Office, DHEW Pub. No. (HSA) 77-5201.

RESOURCES

Alexander Graham Bell Association for the Deaf, 3417 Volta Place, N.W., Washington, D.C. 20007.

American Academy for Cerebral Palsy, 1255 New Hampshire Avenue, N.W., Washington, D.C. 20036.

American Academy of Child Psychiatry, 1800 R Street, N.W., Washington, D.C. 20009.

American Association for the Education of the Severely and Profoundly Handicapped, P.O. Box 15287, Seattle, Washington 98115.

American Association of University Affiliated Programs for the Developmentally Disabled, 1100 17th Street, N.W., Washington, D.C. 20036.

American Association on Mental Deficiency, 5201 Connecticut Avenue, N.W., Washington, D.C. 20015.

American Coalition for Citizens with Disabilities, 1346 Connecticut Avenue, N.W., Washington, D.C. 20036.

American Foundation for the Blind, 15 West 16th Street, New York, New York 10011.

American Physical Therapy Association, 1156 15th Street, N.W., Washington, D.C. 20005.

American Speech and Hearing Association, 9030 Old Georgetown Road, Bethesda, Maryland 20014.

Association for Children with Learning Disabilities, 5225 Grace Street, Pittsburgh, Pennsylvania 15236.

Child Welfare League of America, 67 Irving Place, New York, New York 10003.

Children's Defense Fund, 1763 R Street, N.W., Washington, D.C. 20009.

Epilepsy Foundation of America, 1828 L Street, N.W., Washington, D.C. 20036.

International Association of Parents of the Deaf, 814 Thayer Avenue, Silver Spring, Maryland 20910.

National Association for Retarded Citizens, 2709 Avenue E East, Arlington, Texas 76011.

National Easter Seal Society for Crippled Children and Adults, 2023 West Ogden Avenue, Chicago, Illinois 60612.

National Foundation/March of Dimes, Box 2000, White Plains, New York 10602.

National Tay-Sachs and Allied Diseases Association, Room 1617, 200 Park Avenue South, New York, New York 10003.

SIECUS (Sex Information and Education Council of the U.S.), 72 Fifth Avenue, New York, New York 10011.

Spina Bifida Association of America, P.O. Box G-1974, Elmhurst, Illinois 60126.

United Cerebral Palsy Association, 66 East 34th Street, New York, New York 10016.

CHAPTER 23

SUBSTANCE ABUSE:
A SELF-INFLICTED
RISK

Substance or drug abuse is not a new problem. People have used alcoholic beverages, cocaine, and opium for centuries as well as a variety of other mood-inducing or sedative potions. (Tobacco is of more recent date.) A more recent development, however, is the extraordinary prevalence of substance or drug abuse among all segments of society.

The rapid proliferation and adoption into medical practice of new and powerful agents to relieve tension, induce sleep, change mood, and relieve pain has led to indiscriminate and often harmful use of certain drugs, whether legally prescribed or secured from illicit sources. Advertising has glamorized cigarette smoking and the use of alcohol and has encouraged the belief that there is a pill for every kind of pain or discomfort.

Many sociologists believe that this increase of abuse has been caused by the uncertainties and stresses of living in the midst of continual change, by increasing mobility and changing family patterns, and by the resultant loss of personal and community identity. Whatever the reason — and despite a plethora of state and local agencies and programs created to reduce the volume of substance and drug abuse — the "drug problem" still exists and continues to flourish.

The definition of abuse may differ from one agency or resource to another; and, as a consequence, estimates of prevalence vary widely.

Drug abuse, for example, may be defined as addiction to or dependence upon a drug, or it may be interpreted as *any* use of such a substance.[1] Estimates of marijuana "abuse" may or may not include those people who have merely tried marijuana once or those who smoke sparingly. An "alcoholic" may be any heavy drinker, or may refer to a drinker who is unable to accomplish his or her usual work or meet normal responsibilities. "Cure" of alcoholism may be taken to mean total abstinence, or simply restriction of intake to a level compatible with meeting responsibilities. "Substance" may include or exclude tobacco, coffee, or food.

Individuals and/or families are reluctant to admit drug usage, fearing social disapproval, legal action, or loss of the source of drug supply. The result is general under-reporting of usage, especially in the case of hard drugs such as heroin. It is impossible to know how accurate statistics on drug abuse really are, so, in considering reports, it is important to "read the label" carefully.

Drugs also differ greatly in the amount and type of effect created, both psychologic and physiologic. Occasional or social drinking is viewed differently from alcohol dependence, with its stress on families and physical disability. There is a great difference in impact between the use of marijuana and that of heroin. Some planners suggest that efforts to control marijuana should be relaxed or subordinated to more urgent needs, because the risk it presents is minimal. The risks created by heroin, on the other hand, are great and clearly indicate that every possible effort must be made to control availability and to prevent and treat addiction. Unfortunately, the control methods in use today appear to be grossly inadequate. There is a pressing need for development of new treatments and approaches that will combat substance abuse.

Solutions to the problem of substance abuse rest almost entirely on the decisions and motivation of the individual user. Efforts to control access to a drug by increasing the cost or making its sale illegal have never been more than marginally successful. Prohibition of the sale of alcoholic beverages, for example, spawned a wave of organized crime of major consequences and apparently increased rather than decreased the consumption of alcohol.

Obviously, efforts must be made to keep drugs away from the school grounds, and to require prescriptions for dangerous drugs. It makes sense to prohibit smoking in areas where it may be detrimental to the health of non-smokers. But the *main* thrust must be directed toward creating an informed and motivated potential consumer group who can make the necessary decisions regarding smoking, drinking, and drug use.

The immediate rewards of drug use are enticing, making it more difficult to change drug behavior. The self-doubting, anxious, harassed man or woman who resorts to alcohol finds surcease from his or her personal demons, or develops a feeling of being on top of the problems, or feels capable of being liked. A cigarette provides a relaxing pause for the overbusy worker. A shot of heroin brings relief from the intolerable craving for the drug, or escape from a threatening world. The marijuana smoker may achieve a sense of conviviality and of group identity. LSD creates the illusion of sensory expansion and limitless delights — when it works! The joys of abstinence do not compete easily with these rewards. The ultimate costs to be paid seem comfortably distant and are all too easily banished by the drug itself.

SMOKING

The serious consequences of cigarette smoking to health have been well documented. Careful epidemiologic investigations over two decades have made it clear that those who smoke are indeed risking their lives. Two government reports provide the following facts:[2]

1. At every year of age over 35, death rates are higher for smokers than for non-smokers. In 1966 deaths from all causes among men aged 45 to 64 for those who smoked was 1,329 per 100,000 of the population. For non-smokers the rate was 708 per 100,000.

2. Smokers have higher death rates from coronary heart disease than do non-smokers, and tobacco acts independently and conjunctively with hypertension and elevated serum cholesterol to increase the risk. The 1966 study showed that the coronary heart disease death rate for smokers was 615/100,000 compared to 304/100,000 for non-smokers, and the rates from all heart and circulatory disease 802 and 422/100,000 respectively. *Cessation* of smoking is associated with decreased risk of death from coronary heart disease.

3. Cigarette smoking is the most important cause of chronic obstructive bronchopulmonary disease in the United States, and cigarette smokers have a higher death rate from emphysema and chronic bronchitis. The risk of developing chronic obstructive lung disease is three to twenty times greater for smokers, depending on age and the amount smoked.

4. Cigarette smoking is the major cause of lung cancer among men in the United States, and a significant factor in lung cancer in women. The risk of lung cancer decreases with cessation of smoking.

5. Smoking during pregnancy results in more premature births and in lower birth weight of the child, and probably increases the risk of an unsuccessful pregnancy.

6. There are community as well as individual consequences of smoking. Smoking may pollute the air sufficiently to increase its carbon monoxide content. It can cause discomfort to others, especially those with allergies. For smokers on low incomes, the cost of cigarettes may have serious financial consequences, cutting into funds required for fundamental needs.

The smoking of pipes and cigars is generally not implicated in these caveats, provided pipes and cigars are used moderately and smoke is not inhaled. The exception is increased risk of cancer of the lips and the oral region, which does appear more frequently among pipe, cigar, and cigarette smokers.

Who Smokes — And Why?

According to a 1978 survey taken by the U.S. Department of Health, Education and Welfare, 38 per cent of adult males were reported as being cigarette smokers, compared to 53 per cent in 1955.[3] Adults who were divorced or separated were more apt to be smokers than were married couples.

In a 1975 survey, almost one-third of the women employed outside the home were smokers, compared to 27 per cent of housewives; among this group, white collar workers were more likely to smoke (34 per cent) than were those employed in other occupations (32 per cent). Among unemployed men, this situation was reversed — fewer white collar workers were smokers (36 per cent) than in other occupations. Among men, those in relatively affluent families (family income of $20,000 or more) were less likely to smoke (35 per cent) than were those with incomes of $7,500 to $10,000 (46 per cent).[4]

The per cent of teenagers 12 to 18 years of age who smoke has decreased during the past five years, particularly among males. This decline reverses the trend of increased smoking demonstrated during the years 1968 to 1974. Eleven per cent of teenage males were smoking in 1979, compared to 15 per cent in 1968. The proportion of teenage females who smoked in 1979 was 13 per cent, slightly higher than it was in 1968, but a decrease from 15 per cent in 1974.[5]

Why Do They Smoke?

Most adults are aware of the dangers of cigarette smoking. In the 1975 survey referred to previously (see Reference 4), 90 per cent of the respondents agreed that smoking is harmful. The great majority of teenagers are well informed regarding the dangers of smoking. Why do they smoke?

Among adults who are heavy smokers, there are some who have developed a psychologic dependence upon cigarettes. The yearning for a cigarette outweighs the risking of serious health consequences. Although they are aware of the dangers, most smokers tend to believe that "It won't happen to me."

For young people, probably the strongest influence is the example set by the family. Teenagers are much more likely to start smoking if a parent or an older sibling smokes, or if a parent is missing from the home.

Young people are also influenced by a desire to impress others and a tendency to think in the present, rather than in the future. A naiveté concerning the power of addiction leads them to think, "Why not smoke? I'm young and I can stop later." They may hold (or hide behind) such fallacious ideas as "cigarettes are harmless if they have filters," or that "smoking is essential to avoid gaining weight." The example set by popular students, teachers, and peers is also a strong influence.

Whatever the reasons for smoking, they seem to be compelling ones; for despite media campaigns and all-out educational efforts, smoking still retains its hold on a large proportion of the population.

MISUSE OF DRUGS

The Problem

Drug abuse has been described as "a Gordian knot of environmental, intrapsychic, and pathophysiologic issues."[6] It is a problem for health agencies and members of the health professions, for educational institutions, for law enforcement and welfare agencies, for every concerned parent or family member, for all citizens who value safety — and for the community health nurse.

Why People Take Drugs

Drugs are powerful substances. Used properly for specific curative purposes, they are beneficial. Used improperly, they can be fatal. *All* drugs should be taken circumspectly and prescribed with caution.

Drug abuse can, and often does, occur in conjunction with *medically prescribed substances.* Modern advertising has encouraged a belief (shared by many patients and physicians alike) that there should be a pill for every pain, stress, or discomfort. Understandably, people want to avoid pain; but doctors seem reluctant to suggest that some pains and miseries just have to be borne. Often, however, the "nervous" or anxious individual will push for surcease from symptoms of even minor problems, usually rejecting non-drug approaches such as adequate exercise, relaxation techniques, or rest. The result is that patients who actually need no medication are not satisfied unless they "get something" from the doctor; they demand drugs, and this demand can lead to overuse.

Drug overuse may also occur because of *poor control measures* in patient care — especially in the absence of a central health history. In some cases, an individual may go from one doctor to another, acquiring small amounts of drugs from each, without ever revealing these multiple sources to the principal physician involved.

Drug overuse or abuse may result also from *technical lag,* where drug-related pathology may not be clear until the drug has been in use for some time. A good example of this is the association between treatment of post-menopausal symptoms with estrogens and the increased incidence of cancer of the uterus — an association not discovered until years after the drug was well established in medical practice.[7] Many efforts are underway to provide post-marketing monitoring of new drugs by the Federal Food and Drug Administration, as well as by medical and pharmaceutical professional associations and by drug manufacturers, but the task is clearly a monumental one.

There are other routes to drugs than through medical advice and prescriptions. A person may try drugs to satisfy his or her curiosity about all that they have heard, or to gain acceptance among peers, or to feel important, or to "get even" with parents who are perceived as unsympathetic or domineering. Some take drugs to enhance their perceptions and increase creativity, others to seek oblivion, or to savor the encounter with danger.

In many cases, an individual's description of a drug experience may lure another person into experimenting for himself; this is so common that some professionals often describe addiction as being a communicable disease. Some take drugs "because they are there"; others are enticed by pushers; still others turn to drugs in the face of crises such as failure in school work, divorce, or acute illness.

Once on drugs, the support and friendship of fellow users and the characteristic, exceedingly strong sense of community that develops among users provide additional incentive. Physical and psychologic dependency develops rapidly with the use of some drugs such as heroin, more insidiously with drugs that do not usually produce physical dependency, such as marijuana.

The prevalence of drug abuse is high; users exist in all strata of society and extend across a wide age range — from 8 years old to senescence. It is estimated that 2 per cent of the population age 18 and over or 2,500,000 persons have a serious drug problem. Of these, approximately 450,000 to 500,000 are heroin dependent. In 1977, 60 per cent of 18- to 24-year olds had tried marijuana, about 20 per cent had tried stronger substances such as cocaine and hallucinogens, and about 30 per cent had illegally used drugs available only under a doctor's prescription. Barbiturate mortality has declined from over 2,600 in 1970 to under 1,300 in 1976.[8]

In the years between 1975 and 1979 there occurred an appreciable rise in marijuana use by high school seniors. While 47 per cent of the students of the class of 1975 used marijuana at least once during their lifetime, 60 per cent of the students of the class of 1979 had done so. Use of cocaine has increased in this group as well (see Table 23–1).[9]

There are many kinds of drugs used, and cross-over is frequent — i.e., a person taking LSD may also use heroin, or drug users may on occasion turn from hard drugs to alcohol.

There are several categories of addictive drugs. The *sedative-hypnotics* include alcohol, barbiturates, tranquilizers, and other central nervous system depressants. *Stimulants* include amphetamines and cocaine (cocaine acts as a stimulant, although it is designated a narcotic under the U.S. Controlled Substances Act). *Hallucinogens* include LSD and PCP (or angel dust), which is the most widely used hallucinogen among teenagers today. The chief problem substance among the *narcotic* agents is heroin. *Marijuana* and other *cannabis derivatives* differ from the other categories in that they have not been proven to lead to physical dependence, although psychologic dependence (habituation) can occur. Marijuana can act either as a stimulant or a depressant. The results of studies of the long-term effects of marijuana use are inconclusive except

Table 23–1 TRENDS IN LIFETIME PREVALENCE OF THIRTEEN TYPES
OF DRUGS FOR THE NATION'S HIGH SCHOOL STUDENTS

		Per Cent Ever Used				
Drug	Class of 1975	Class of 1976	Class of 1977	Class of 1978	Class of 1979	'78–'79 change
	N = (9400)	(15400)	(17100)	(17800)	(15500)	
Marijuana	47.3	52.8	56.4	59.2	60.4	+1.2
Inhalants	NA	10.3	11.1	12.0	12.7	+0.7
Adjusted[a]	NA	NA	NA	NA	18.7	NA
Hallucinogens	16.3	15.1	13.9	14.3	14.1	−0.2
Adjusted[b]	NA	NA	NA	NA	18.6	NA
Cocaine	9.0	9.7	10.8	12.9	15.4	+2.5 sss
Heroin	2.2	1.8	1.8	1.6	1.1	−0.5 ss
Other opiates[a]	9.0	9.6	10.3	9.9	10.1	+0.2
Stimulants[c]	22.3	22.6	23.0	22.9	24.2	+1.3
Sedatives[c]	18.2	17.7	17.4	16.0	14.6	−1.4
Tranquilizers[c]	17.0	16.8	18.0	17.0	16.3	−0.7
Alcohol	90.4	91.9	92.5	93.1	93.0	−0.1
Cigarettes	73.6	75.4	75.7	75.3	74.0	−1.3
Amyl and butyl nitrites[d]	NA	NA	NA	NA	11.1	NA
PCP[d]	NA	NA	NA	NA	12.8	NA

Notes: Level of significance of difference between the two most recent classes:
s = .05, ss = .01, sss = .001. NA indicates data not available.
  [a]Adjusted for underreporting of amyl and butyl nitrites.
  [b]Adjusted for underreporting of PCP.
  [c]Only drug use that was not under a physician's orders is included here.
  [d]Data based on a single questionnaire form. N is one-fifth of N indicated.
  (From 1979 Highlights. Drugs and the Nation's High School Students, Washington,
D.C., USDHEW, NIOA.)

in very heavy users, who show behavioral changes and a higher
incidence of physical injury.

The *consequences* of drug abuse are severe. For the user, physical
debility, malnutrition, infections (from needles), upper respiratory illness, and hepatitis are among the physical consequences. Behavioral
problems can include moodiness, confusion, unlawful activity, and
bizarre or irrational actions. These physical and behavioral complications can result in decreased productivity, estrangement from the family,
and isolation from the community. The abuser is frequently a danger to
the rest of the population; he or she also acts as a drain on community
resources, since drug-related diseases or mental illness often require
extensive community services. Drug usage also encourages organized
crime, and control measures require a substantial percentage of community funds.

The impact of drug use on the user's family is profound. Parent-
child, sibling, and marital relationships are severely strained by the

social censure attached to drug use and by the erratic and irrational behavior of the user. Families of users are torn by guilt, misery, false hopes, resentment, and tremendous frustrations in the face of a problem of gargantuan proportions.

Drug abuse is not a series of independent or separate problems. "Crossover" — moving from one drug to another is common. This suggests that there may be a drug-susceptible personality, and that dependency is not limited to only one drug.

The Potential for Treatment is Limited

The philosophy underlying current treatment of drug misuse is based on decreasing the availability of illegal drugs, reducing the desire of susceptible individuals to use drugs, and providing treatment and rehabilitation when it is needed. Programs at the national level have increased in recent years in all these areas. The Bureau of Narcotics and Dangerous Drugs, the Customs Bureau, the Internal Revenue Service, and the Office of Law Enforcement are among agencies contributing to this effort. They are supported by less complex, local, often volunteer action groups. Despite stepped-up efforts, control of supplies appears to be partial at best — as soon as one pusher, drug route, or source of supply is thwarted, another appears, more ingenious than the last.

Methadone, a synthetic opiate used to prevent withdrawal symptoms in heroin addicts during the detoxification process, has proven a disappointing though useful drug. It was hoped that methadone might be a safe and acceptable substitute for heroin, which could be adopted by addicts to wean them from the drug. However, detoxification has seldom led to lasting abstinence, although it has some strong short-term benefits.

Attempts to modify drug behavior are generally unsuccessful, probably because of the lack of motivation on the part of the drug users. According to Louria, "There is at present a growing realization that the rehabilitation of the drug user is difficult even if the user is well-motivated, and it almost always fails if the user is not motivated."[10] Many field workers still cling to stereotypes about drugs and drug users — as well as do parents and the general public: for example, "once a heroin user always a heroin user," or, "drug users are criminals" — limiting their effectiveness. Educational programs for teachers may prove of minimal value in changing drug behavior among students, since it is hard for the drug user to relate to non-users — to see them as anything but "outsiders." Training *may* increase the teacher's perceptiveness in dealing with students who have drug problems, but best results appear to come from using "like experience" personnel (former users), provided they do not expect too much of the client ("If I did it, he can too").

Clearly there is need for much more research: epidemiologic to clarify the nature of dependence and dangerous behavior; pharmacological to identify possible treatment aids; and behavioral to tease out the roots and influences in drug related behavior.

MISUSE OF ALCOHOL: A GROWING PROBLEM

The *use* of alcoholic beverages is widespread and socially accepted, and the majority of the estimated 95 million users of alcoholic beverages present no special problem. The use of alcohol constitutes a "drinking problem" when the individual:

1. Must drink to cope with his problems or responsibilities, drinks almost every day.

2. Is frequently intoxicated, a minimum of once a week.

3. Goes to work or drives a car while intoxicated.

4. Sustains an injury, or comes into conflict with the law as a result of drinking.

5. Continues to drink when drinking is clearly prejudicial to health — i.e., in the presence of severe kidney impairment, for instance.

6. Behaves in a manner uncharacteristic of behavior when sober — e.g., abuse of family members, or bizarre social behavior.

It is estimated that almost nine million people in the U.S. satisfy one or more of these criteria — approximately 10 per cent of the total drinking population.

Who Are the Drinkers?

Two out of three adults over the age of 21 use alcohol.[11] Men are more apt to engage in heavy drinking than are women. About four-fifths of all men and three-fifths of all women are drinkers, and about 10 per cent of these are problem drinkers.[12] Recent trends indicate, however, that women are rapidly closing the gap. Some researchers speculate that this is the result of incongruencies in the education of women and the traditional role of the woman as homemaker. Some women feel bored and frustrated when confined to homemaking activities; this creates one kind of stress or tension. On the other hand, women in the labor market experience a different variety of stress and tension. Whatever her occupation, if the woman feels contented in her work, she is not likely to turn to alcohol for solace. If the pressures are not balanced by a sense of reward, alcohol is apparently a handy palliative.

How does someone become an alcoholic? There is no single or simple answer. Some people seem bent on this form of self-destruction from an early age; others fall into it gradually. Some personality types seem to be more susceptible to alcoholism than others. Many refuse to acknowledge that they *are* alcoholics. For most, the process is accomplished by a series of "little" decisions: the decision to take the first drink; the decision to have one more; the decision to buy drink with money which should go for other necessities; the decision to drink despite a known illness. Important decisions are made by the family and associates of the drinker as well — the decision to "help" by not revealing the drinker's true problem; the decision to "let him work it out himself;" the decision to treat drunkenness as a joke — all can have devastating effects.

Alcohol abuse occurs in all social and economic groups. Of the estimated six to nine million alcoholics in the United States, only about 5 per cent are skid-row types.[13]

An estimated 10 per cent of the adult population has a serious drinking problem. Alcoholism mortality (from cirrhosis, alcoholism, or alcoholic psychosis) has remained at about 2 per 100,000 population from 1950 to 1975. In 1975, an additional 51,000 fatalities were indirectly attributed to alcohol use, including 18,000 motor vehicle fatalities. The social costs were estimated to be $43 billion in lost production, health and medical services, accidents, crime and other social consequences.[14]

Of increasing concern is the rising incidence of alcohol abuse among young people and school-age children. Alcoholic beverages are generally easier to secure than drugs, produce a satisfying level of escape, and are harder for adults to decry in view of the adult experience. Drinking is also considered to be a symbol of maturity, a "macho" sign of sophistication. Many young people are introduced to alcohol in their own homes, and often observe family and friends becoming boisterous and merry on alcohol. This is both a strength and a weakness in handling the problem. When drinking is experienced and supervised in the home, young people are more likely to be taught *responsible* drinking than if they indulge secretly with contemporaries. Alternately, parents who have developed irresponsible patterns in their own drinking may communicate this life style to their children. The attitude of "Isn't he a scream?" said of the "funny" drunk may well be transferred.

The *consequences* of alcohol abuse affect both the user and the family, as well as the community. The *hard drinker* may expect to live 10 to 12 years less than those without drinking problems, to be the responsible party in a large proportion of automobile accidents, to require more medical care, and to suffer great limitation of income due to erratic work habits. He is far more likely to be involved with the law than are his non- or limited-drinking contemporaries.[15]

The family with an alcoholic parent is subject to great stress and upheaval; often there is general disintegration of the family social structure as a result of the uncharacteristic behavior of the sick person, and replication of the parental destructive use of alcohol is frequent. When one member relinquishes the responsibilities of homemaking and family support, others must change roles to fill the gap. The economic stability of the family may be disrupted when alcohol keeps the principal wage-earner from working or prohibits his normal advancement on the job. Involvement in arrests or public exhibitions of drunkenness can create tensions between parents or between parent and children, or may produce serious mental health complications. Reduced expectations for family income, social life, future security, and childrens' education play havoc with family relationships.

Costs to the community are also large. Families including a problem drinker are much more likely to need support from social workers and guidance personnel, economic aid, and legal assistance than other families. Medical costs may also be incurred by the community — for preventable illness, for others injured by the alcoholic, for family members reacting to the stress produced by the drinking member. A drop in family income results in less productivity, diminished buying power, and a smaller tax return to the community.

The *potential for prevention* and mitigation is present but currently limited. Dependence on alcohol develops from a multitude of essentially personal decisions, and is nourished by internal, physical, social, and environmental conditions that affect concepts of self, perceptions of problems, and the ability to resist external pressure. Only by affecting this broad frame of interlocking and reinforcing conditions can one influence drinking behavior.

Prevention programs have mainly centered on mass education programs aimed for at-risk populations. Early intervention programs in the workplace, offering treatment and counseling, can be of tremendous help.

Apparently many people manage to cure themselves of serious detrimental drinking habits. The American Drinking Practice survey made in 1969 found that 32 per cent of the adults surveyed did not drink; of these non-drinkers, only one-third said they formerly drank.[16] Self-help groups such as Alcoholics Anonymous are widely available and apparently well patronized. However, there is nothing approaching sure cure or an easy cure for alcoholism at present.

Three out of four alcoholic men and women are married, living at home, holding a job, and are reasonably well-accepted within their communities. For those in this category who want to change, the outlook is good.[17] If rehabilitation is measured in terms of ability to maintain a decent family life, a reasonably good working record, and acceptance in the community, 50 per cent to 75 per cent (depending upon personal characteristics) may expect a successful outcome.[18] Personal attitudes are the most significant factors in establishing a prognosis. If, on the other hand, "cure" is defined as absolute and continuing abstinence, the statistical results drop to very low numbers.

Goals for Control May Be Limited

It is wise to set modest goals for control of alcoholism or excessive drinking. While some alcoholics find it possible to control their drinking or stop drinking altogether, many cannot. They may, however, be able to schedule drinking at other than work times — abstaining or drinking sparingly during the work week, and drinking only at weekends. Or they may be prevailed upon to avoid drinking when children are present. For example, in some industrially based programs, "success" may mean getting an individual to the point where he can hold a job, even if he is unable to stop drinking altogether or to achieve promotion in his work. The overall goal may be to strive for *responsible* drinking rather than abstinence, both in preventive and curative efforts.

THE COMMUNITY HEALTH NURSE AND SUBSTANCE ABUSE

Medical workers must realize that a tremendous effort of will is demanded to change established dependency on tobacco, drugs, or alcohol. This makes a very strong case for avoiding *initial* introduction of dangerous substances — i.e., not starting the use of drugs, tobacco, or alcohol at all — as the most fruitful approach. If the youth who is tempted to "just try" heroin or to smoke cigarettes can be persuaded to say "no", a great deal of later anguish and agony can be avoided.

Much of the community health nurse's impact in control of substance abuse will result from merging this concern with other concurrent activities, rather than from special programs. While the nurse may serve on the staff of an alcohol advisory service or in a drug detoxification center, these programs are not designed to reach those who need attention for *prevention* of the abuse. Preventive efforts should be targeted for those between the ages of 10 to 13 and their parents. This age group is at risk of initiating substance abuse, be it cigarettes, alcohol, marijuana or drugs. Besides information about specific negative effects and problems encountered with specific abusive agents, efforts need to focus on value clarification, decision making and knowing how to say "no" to peer group pressure.

Another important element in prevention for this preadolescent age group is positive role models they can identify with. Older siblings, high school sports "stars," and popular singers or television stars can be very effective in teaching about substance abuse.

Parents of children that "hang out together," neighborhood residents, or parents' associations can openly communicate about the risks and set limits on behaviors that will be tolerated, and seek active participation of all parents in monitoring behavior and enforcing rules.

In every situation the crucial group is the peer group — their morals and values are most contagious. Individuals — especially young individuals living in neighborhoods where rates of crime, delinquency, and drug use are high — are at special risk. The availability and general acceptance of drugs increase the pressure on the uninitiated to conform to the drug pattern.

Once these vulnerable groups are identified, efforts may be concentrated within the supportive network to help individuals to cope with their problems. Parents may be urged to give more than usual support and understanding to one of their children whose coping skills are weak and where resistance to failure and despair are low, and to avoid comparison with others whose protective armor is stronger. Parents and youth leaders should put extra effort into securing community alternatives to congregating at street corners or in the shopping malls where it is easy to drift into drug use.

It is important for the nurse to think about the example her own behavior sets. Whether or not to use tobacco, alcohol, mood-altering prescription drugs, or illegal drugs is an individual decision. Each nurse must decide for herself whether her behavior reflects her professional commitment to health and her responsibility to the community.

Early detection and case finding is important to the control of substance abuse. In her ongoing work with families and groups in the community, the nurse can observe for symptoms of drug abuse or alcohol abuse. Family assessments should include information about smoking, drinking and drug behavior. The nurse may need to seek consultation for herself in recognizing signs and symptoms of certain drugs frequently used that may require prompt treatment.

Knowing the community is vitally important — for example, which blocks or shopping centers have heavy drug traffic, local bars in the neighborhood, or at-risk apartment houses. Working with other community groups, alerting police to particular problem areas, and sharing information with self-help groups such as drug treatment centers can provide a broader attack on the problem.

Early case finding of pregnant women using drugs is important for the mother and the baby. In a study of over three hundred pregnant narcotic addicts in New York City, 90 per cent had had either no prenatal care or inadequate care, and over half of the newborn babies showed congenital neonatal addiction, with recognizable symptoms.[19] Furthermore, this group experienced more prematurity and more complications than other groups.

Nursing *strategies* for working with families in resolving problems related to substance abuse are varied. They may include prompt referral for emergency medical or psychiatric treatment, referral to self-help groups, counseling and support, direct physical care and providing information on health matters. She may also participate in therapeutic group sessions when people with similar problems seek ways of quitting or controlling a particular habit. In these formal, or informal groups, the presence of some knowledgeable person who is aware of the psychologic process of securing behavioral change may be helpful. Someone who can guide the group but not lecture is important.

The community health nurse may engage in *active treatment* in special care units such as methadone maintenance or detoxification centers, or as an adjunct to clinic care. In such instances, additional training is usually provided.

Focal to nursing care for drug-related disorders is observation of the patient's behavior, and securing information about what transpired before care was instituted. Through questioning and observation, significant clues may be uncovered — exaggeration of mood, fluctuating levels of awareness, evidence of illogical thinking or distorted perception, impaired motor coordination, irregular levels of consciousness, tremors, respiratory distress — all are typical indicators. Most life-threatening are the depressants, and symptoms of somnolence, stupor, or coma indicate critical need for care. Such information must often come from someone other than the patient (who may be fuzzy or nonresponsive) who may know what drug was being taken — a member of the drug family, or the client's regular family.

Progress May Be Slow

Habits are difficult to break and backsliding is frequent. The nurse should encourage families, i.e., every day without a drink, or without a cigarette is a good day. Families need to expect some back sliding and not have unreachable expectations; if they falter in resolve, they should simply be encouraged to start again.

Frequently, people using various drugs or other substances have other health care problems or need general information on nutrition or for that matter, how to safely administer drugs. Self-help groups involved in detoxification can use help in obtaining needed medical care, treating wounds, and simply learning how to care for their bodies.

Self-help groups, such as Alcoholics Anonymous and Narcotics Anonymous, have been helpful in rehabilitating members. Often cessation is not total or is not maintained over time, but even decreasing the amounts of alcohol or drugs used is progress.

The nurse can mobilize support for the family so that they can have a better understanding of their own attitudes and behaviors. Support is especially important to members of the family who are not involved in substance abuse behavior. Groups organized by local health agencies, industries, schools, churches, or close neighbors are prime sources of support for problem sharing and decision making.

Families will need help to anticipate backsliding and not react in utter despair. Sources of medical care may need to include psychiatric care or group counseling for the entire family. If treatment, such as

Antabuse, methadone, or antidepressants are used, the family will need to understand the amount prescribed, the importance of regular use, potential side effects and ramifications if not taken.

For individuals unable to stop their habit, the nurse should try to help the person toward more responsible drinking, smoking, or drug taking. For example, it is possible for many people to have an alcoholic beverage without becoming intoxicated by drinking slowly so as to reduce the impact of the alcohol — sipping rather than gulping — and by eating before or while drinking. Another device for the drinker to use is to learn to space out his drinks. The drinker should be sensitized to thinking ahead: it is possible to arrange *in advance* whether to drive home from a party or to rely on assistance from a friend or to call a taxi.

The nurse should contribute to the *improvement of community facilities* for care. She should make known to existing facilities and agencies the ways in which she can support their efforts and develop appropriate communication patterns for referral and a mutual reporting network.

When adequate facilities are not available — or if existing ones are for some reason unacceptable — the community health nurse should transmit this information to appropriate community sources, either directly or through the nurse administrator.

It is impossible to remove all harmful or potentially harmful substances from the environment. The focus of programs to control abuse of substances of all kinds must be on strengthening the capacity of individuals and communities to live with these substances.

REFERENCES

1. Drug dependence is defined by the World Health Organization as the following: A state, psychic and sometimes also physical, resulting from the interaction between a living organism and a drug, characterized by behavioral and other responses that always include a compulsion to take the drug on a continuous or periodic basis in order to experience its psychic effects, and sometimes to avoid the discomfort of its absence. World Health Organization, Expert Committee on Services for the Prevention and Treatment of Dependence on Alcohol and Other Drugs: *Technical Report Series* #407. Geneva, World Health Organization, 1969, p. 6.
2. Source figures from two reports: (1) U.S. Department of Health, Education, and Welfare, Public Health Service: *The Health Consequences of Smoking*, 1972. Washington, D.C., U.S. Government Printing Office, Pub. No. 75-7516, 1972, pp. 1–10. (2) U.S. Department of Health, Education, and Welfare, *Facts About Smoking and Health*. Washington, D. C., U.S. Government Printing Office, Pub. No. 75-8717, 1975, p. 6.
3. U.S. Department of Health, Education, and Welfare, Public Health Service: *Promoting Health/Preventing Disease: Objectives for the Nation*. Atlanta, Ga. August 1979, p. 77.
4. U.S. Department of Health, Education, and Welfare, Public Health Service: *Adult Use of Tobacco*. Atlanta, Ga., Center for Disease Control, 1975.
5. U.S. Department of Health, Education, and Welfare, Public Health Service: *Health in the U.S.: Chart book*. Washington, D.C., U.S. Government Printing Office, Pub. No. (PHS) 80-1233, 1980, p. 25.

6. Greene, M. H., and Dupont, R. L. (eds.): The epidemiology of drug abuse. *A. J. Pub. Health, 64* (Supplement):1, 1974.

7. Mintz, M.: New unit to monitor perils in the use of prescription drugs. *Washington Post.* December 27, 1976, p. C–12.

8. U.S. Department of Health, Education, and Welfare: *Promoting Health . . .*, p. 85.

9. U.S. Department of Health, Education, and Welfare: 1979 Highlights. Drugs and the nation's High School Students. Five Year National Trends. Washington, D.C., U.S. Government Printing Office, Pub. No. (ADM)80–930, 1979, p. 25.

10. Louria, D. B.: A critique of some current approaches to the problem of drug abuse. Am. J. Pub. Health, *65*:581, 1975.

11. U.S. Department of Health, Education, and Welfare: *Thinking About Drinking.* National Institute on Alcohol and Alcoholism, Pub. No. 4561, 1972, p. 4.

12. American Public Health Association: *Mental Health: The Public Health Challenge.* 1975, pp. 148–49.

13. Mueller, J. F.: Treatment of the alcoholic — Cursing or nursing? Am. J. Nurs. *74*:245, 1974.

14. *Promoting Health*, p. 84.

15. Bauer, K.: Averting the self-inflicted nemesis (SINS) from dangerous driving, smoking and drinking. *In* Mushkin, S. J. (ed.): *Consumer Incentives for Health Care.* New York, 1974, p. 7.

16. Ibid, p. 14.

17. U.S. Department of Health, Education, and Welfare: *If Someone Close To You Drinks Too Much.* Washington, D. C., U. S. Government Printing Office, Pub. No. 7523, 1975, p. 14.

18. Ibid.

19. Stone, M. L., Salerno, L. J., Green, M., and Zelson, C., Narcotic addiction in pregnancy. Am. J. Obstet. Gynecol. *109*:716, 1971.

SUGGESTED READINGS

Alexander, M.: The vector in heroin addiction. New Eng. J. Med., *288*:423, 1973.

Allie, B. A.: Marijuana and the adolescent. J. Natl. Med. Assoc. *70*:677, 1978.

Apgar, F. M.: Our children are going to pot: Comments from a health educator. *J. School Health, 50*:40, 1980.

Bauer, K. G.: Averting the self-inflicted nemeses (SINS) from dangerous driving, smoking and drinking. Mushkin, S. J. (ed.): *Consumer Incentives for Health Care.* New York, Prochst, 1974, pp. 3–33.

Brink, P. J., Behaviorial characteristics of heroin addicts on a short-term detoxification program. *Nurs. Res., 21*:38–45, 1972.

Bukolash, D.: Essentials the nurse should know about chemical dependency. J. Psych. Nurs. 16:33, 1978.

Burkhalter, P. K.: *Nursing Care of the Alcoholic and Drug Abuser.* New York, McGraw-Hill Book Co., 1975.

Cameron, D. C., and Ling, G. M.: Fools paradise. World Health Org. Tech. Rep. Ser. No. 551:16, 1974.

Chafetz, M. E.: New federal legislation on alcoholism — Opportunities and problems. A. J. Pub. Health, *63*:206, 1973.

Cuskey, W. R., and Prem Kumar, T.: A differential counselor role model for the treatment of drug addicts. Health Serv. Rep. 88:663, 1973.

Dansky, K. H.: Bridge to the turned on. Am. J. Nurs. 70:778, 1970.

Deschin, C. S.: *The Teenager in a Drugged Society: A Symptom of Crisis.* New York, Richard Rosen Press, 1972.

Dickinson, Sister Corita: The alcoholic: An unperson? Nurs. For., *14*:194, 1975.

Dole, V. P., et al.: Long-term outcome of patients treated with methadone maintenancy. Ann. N.Y. Acad. Sci. *311*:181, 1978.

Edwards, G., Demon drink. WHO Chron. *29*:10, 1975.

Elaine B., Clare M., June S., and Janet A.: Helping the nurse who misuses drugs. Am. J. Pub. Health. *64*:9, 1665, 1974.

Estes, N. J., Counseling the wife of an alcoholic spouse. Am. J. Nurs. *74*:1251, 1974.

Foreman, N. J., and Zerwekh, J. V.: Drug crisis intervention. Am. J. of Nurs. 71:1736, 1971.

Forrest, G.: *The Diagnosis and Treatment of Alcoholism.* Springfield, Ill., Charles C Thomas, Pub., 1975.

Fortin, M. L.: Detoxification, then what? A community nursing course in alcoholism. Am. J. Nurs. 80:113, 1980.

Goshen, C. E.: *Drinks, Drugs, and Do-Gooders.* New York, Free Press, 1973.

Graham, J. D. P. (ed.): *Cannabis and Health.* New York, Academic Press, 1976.

Green, D. E.: Nurses are kicking the habit. Am. J. Nurs. 70:1936, 1979.

Greene, M. H., and Dupont, R. H. (eds.): The epidemiology of drug abuse. Am. J. Pub. Health, 64: Supplement, 1974.

Hanlon, J. J.: *Public Health Administration and Practice,* 6th ed. St. Louis, Mo., C. V. Mosby Co., 1974, pp. 473–496.

Hecht, M.: Children of alcoholics are children at risk. Am. J. Nurs. 73:1764, 1973.

Heineman, M. E., and Estes, N. J.: A program in alcoholism nursing. Nurs. Outlook, 22:575, 1974.

Hoberman, P.: Substance Abuse: Alcohol, drugs, tobacco and food. *In* American Public Health Association: Chapter 6, *Mental Health, the Public Health Challenge. Washington, D.C., 1975, pp. 148–153.*

Hofman, F. G., with Hofmann, A. D. *A Handbook on Drug and Alcohol Abuse: The Biomedical Aspects.* New York, Oxford University Press, 1975.

Horn, D.: Smoking and disease — what must be done. WHO Chron. 31:355, 1977.

Johnson, B. D.: *Marijuana Users and Drug Subculture.* New York, John Wiley, 1973.

Johnston, L. D.: Drug use during and after high school: Results of a national longitudinal study. Am. J. Pub. Health, 64:29 (Supplement), 1974.

Kandel, D., Single, E., and Kessler, R. C.: The epidemiology of drug use among New York State high school students: Distribution, trends, and change in rates of use. Am. J. Pub. Health, 66:43, 1976.

Khan, I., et al.: WHO's programme in drug dependence with special emphasis on developing countries. N. Inst. Drug Abuse Res. Manag. Ser. 19:26, 1978.

Lavenhar, M. A.: The drug numbers game. Am. J. Pub. Health, 63:807, 1973.

Levengood, R., Lowinger, P., and Schoof, K.: Heroin addiction in the suburbs: An epidemiologic study. Am. J. Pub. Health, 63:209, 1973.

Levy, R., and Brown, A. R.: Untoward effects of drug education. Am. J. Pub. Health, 63:1071, 1973.

Lieberman, F., Caroff, P., and Gottesfeld, M.: *Before Addiction: How to Help Youth.* New York, Behavioral Publications, 1973.

Lipp, M. R., Benson, S. G., and Allen, P. S.: Marijuana use by nurses and nursing students. Am. J. Nurs. 71:2339, 1971.

Louria, D. B.: A critique of some current approaches to the problems of drug abuse. Am. J. Pub. Health, 65:581, 1975.

Martin, R. M.: *The Role of the Nurse in Drug Abuse, Treatment, Preparation, and Practice.* Kansas City, Mo., American Nurses' Association, 1972.

Mayo, J. A.: Psychopharmacological roulette: A follow-up study of patients hospitalized for drug overdose. Am. J. Pub. Health, 64:616, 1974.

McKee, M. R.: Drug abuse knowledge and attitudes in middle America. Am. J. Pub. Health, 65:584, 1975.

McLellan, A. T., et al.: Changes in drug abuse clients — 1972–1978: Implications for revised treatment. Am. J. Drug Alcohol Abuse, 6:151, 1979.

Morgan, A. J., and Moreno, J. W.: Attitudes toward addiction. Am. J. Nurs. 73:497, 1973.

Mueller, J. F.: Treatment for the alcoholic: Cursing or nursing? Am. J. Nurs., 74:245, 1974.

National Institute on Alcohol Abuse: *Second Report to the U.S. Congress on Alcohol and Health.* Washington, D.C., U.S. Government Printing Office, July 1974.

National Institute on Drug Abuse: *Marijuana and Health.* Eighth Annual Report to the U.S. Congress, Washington, D.C., U.S. Government Printing Office, 1980.

Pillari, G., and Narus, J.: Physical effects of heroin addiction. Am. J. Nurs. 73:2105, 1973.

Ray, R., et al.: The association between chronic cannabis use and cognitive functions. Drug Alcohol Depend. 3:365, 1978.

Redfield, J. T.: Drugs in the workplace—Substituting sense for sensationalism. Am. J. Pub. Health, 63:1064, 1973.

Seiden, R. H., Tomlinson, K. E., and O'Carroll, M.: Patterns of marijuana use among public health students. Am. J. Pub. Health, 65:613, 1975.

Seltzer, C. C., Friedman, G. D., and Siegelaub, A. B.: Smoking and drug consumption in white, black and oriental men and women. Am. J. Pub. Health, 64:466, 1974.

Sigell, L. T., et al.: Popping and snorting volatile nitrites: A current fad for getting high. Am. J. Psych. 135:1216, 1978.

Sparer, G.: OEO drug treatment programs. Pub. Health Rep. 90:455, 1975.

Stanton, M. D.: The family and drug misuse: A bibliography. Am. J. Drug Alcohol Abuse, 5:151, 1978.

Stitzer, M. L., et al.: Reinforcement of drug abstinence: A behavioral approach to drug abuse treatment. Natl. Inst. Drug Abuse Res. Manag. Ser., 25:68, 1979.

Tennant, F. S., Jr., et al.: Children at high risk for addiction and alcoholism identification and intervention. Ped. Nurs., 6:26, 1980.

Tennant, F. S., Jr., Mohler, P. J., Drachler, D. H., and Silsby, H. D.: Effectiveness of drug education classes. Am. J. Pub. Health, 64:422, 1974.

U.S. Department of Health, Education, and Welfare: *If You Must Smoke.* Center for Disease Control, Atlanta, Ga., Pub. No. CDC 75–8706, 6:26, 1980.

U.S. Office of the Assistant Secretary for Health, Office on Smoking and Health: *Smoking and Health: A Report of the Surgeon General.* Washington, D.C. 1979.

Vourakis, C., and Bennett, G.: Angel dust: Not heaven sent. Am. J. Nurs. 79:649, 1979.

World Health Organization: Controlling the smoking epidemic. Report of the WHO Expert Committee of Smoking Control. WHO Tech. Rep. Ser. 636:7, 1979.

Wynder, E. L., et al.: Tobacco and health: A societal challenge. New Eng. J. Med., 300:894, 1979.

CHAPTER 24

LONG-TERM ILLNESS

Long-term illness is a major public health problem in virtually every industrialized country of the world. Long-term illnesses range from mental retardation to the disabling and traumatic effects of accident; from heart disease, cancer, stroke, and arthritis to loss of hearing or sight, and from emphysema to psychiatric illness. These disorders are linked together by chronicity and by similarities in the social and medical problems they present. Kurlander defines chronic disease as meeting one or more of the following criteria:

1. It is permanent.
2. It leaves a residual disability.
3. It is caused by nonreversible pathologic conditions.
4. It requires special rehabilitative training of the patient.
5. It requires long supervision or care.[1]

Chronic diseases are a major cause of death. In 1977 heart disease, cancer, and stroke, the most prevalent chronic diseases, accounted for 595.1 of the total 878.1 deaths for each 100,000 of the population.[2] While the mortality from heart disease has decreased since 1968 (between 1968 and 1977 the age-adjusted rate decreased 21.6 per cent), heart disease remains the most common cause of death (210.4 per 100,000 population), followed by cancer (133 per 100,000 population) and stroke (48.2 per 100,000).[3]

The prevalence of chronic disease — (i.e., the number affected at a given point in time — is also impressive. It has been estimated that 47 million Americans suffer from some sort of chronic obstructive lung condition, 4 million from epilepsy, and 250,000 from multiple sclerosis.[4, 5] One-half to one per cent of the population is estimated to be mentally retarded, and about 15 to 20 per cent are estimated to have some form of mental illness.[6, 7] These examples demonstrate the magnitude of the problem of chronic illness.

The proportion of people with health problems increases with age, and as a group the elderly are more likely to suffer from multiple, chronic and other disabling conditions. Eighty per cent of people over

65 have one or more chronic conditions, and their medical treatment accounts for about 30 per cent of the nation's health care expenditures. Over the past decade, 42 to 47 per cent of people over 65 have limitations due primarily to chronic conditions. The average number of days of limitation ranges from 31 to 38 days per person per year.[8]

THE IMPACT OF CHRONIC ILLNESS GOES BEYOND MERE NUMBERS

Chronic illness produces stress in the individual, the family, and the community. It may threaten one person's sense of identity or the community's confidence in its power to intervene in human catastrophes. It may negate the family's most cherished goals, and create heavy financial drains upon both family and community. While many of those with chronic illness will be able to manage independently, the large number who are disabled and of limited means can find chronic illness a crushing burden.

The chronically ill person may feel socially isolated, unable to fill his usual family roles, and devoid of the energy required for social interchange. He may have to give up a job. Disagreeable manifestations of the illness, such as odors or unsightly expectoration, may lower his self-image. Feelings of helplessness, loss of bodily control, or intractable pain can cause deep depression or decrease his will to live. The best of medical care may be defeated by such responses.

For the family, too, chronic illness poses a considerable threat. Family members often feel overwhelmed by the demands for care, plagued by feelings of guilt or inadequacy, and sometimes cheated out of a life of their own. Children may feel neglected, in the way, or unduly restricted. Family members involved in intensive at-home care can themselves experience social isolation. Sheer fatigue and neglect of other home and community responsibilities may produce high levels of stress.

The economic burdens of chronic illness are also great, both to the family and to the community. Technologic advances make more sophisticated (and more expensive) care possible. For some elderly people on fixed low incomes, purchase of medications, equipment, and dietary prescriptions may mean real deprivation. The use of dialysis in the treatment of chronic renal failure can bankrupt a family, or make care available only to those able to afford it, or may compel the community to make difficult moral decisions when the available machines are fewer than are needed. An enormous demand for care has been created by the large numbers of sick people involved, the constantly growing potential for treatment, and aggressive public demand for more care for the elderly. The community, even as the family, must weigh these needs against competing needs for health and welfare and the limits of available resources.

Patient care represents only the tip of the iceberg of the family and community responses required for solution to the problems of chronic illness.

THE CARE OF CHRONIC ILLNESS IS A MAJOR COMPONENT IN COMMUNITY HEALTH NURSING SERVICES

The nature of chronic illness, and particularly of disabling chronic illness, is such that community health agencies must assume a large share of the responsibility for care. This is true because:

1. The great majority of those with disabling chronic illness receive most of the care they need outside the hospital or other institution, usually in their own homes (the natural arena of community health services).

2. The health of the family and that of the affected person are so interdependent that treating them separately is virtually impossible. (The traditional unit of community health nursing is the family.)

3. Experience has shown that it is possible, although not always simple, to adapt treatment to home care, with greater reliance on family or other informal resources for the actual care. Professional services may be needed for some aspects of treatment, but this is apt to be incidental to the broad health care plan. What is required is mobilization, training, and support of indigenous care agents (fundamental community health nursing concerns).

4. The most pressing needs of the chronically ill are oriented to health rather than to illness. Specific treatment is necessary, but often subordinate to such general measures as strengthening family functioning, encouraging prudent health behavior, managing stress, or dealing with fatigue.

For all of these reasons, a large share of care for chronic illnesses will continue to rest with community services. This may raise troublesome problems: needs may create demands that exceed the resources for care. Equally important health care programs may be crowded out by the insistent and sometimes seemingly insatiable demands for long-term care. Staff within the agency may have to be changed to meet the needs of this special group. More aggressive care and complex home-based treatment will require additional preparation and consultation on the part of the staff. In the light of the responsibilities created by long-term illness, a new balance may have to be struck between hospital and community health nursing staff and new considerations given to the ratio between populations served and community health personnel available.

Primary Preventive Measures Are Limited

Opportunities for primary prevention of chronic conditions (preventing initial occurrence of the condition) are often limited because either the etiology of the disease is obscure or preventive measures have not yet been developed.

The association between smoking and chronic respiratory disease or lung cancer offers an opportunity for primary preventive action through changing smoking behavior. Protecting the expectant mother from exposure to infectious disease, radiation, or inadequate obstetrical care may help prevent injury to the fetus. Genetic counseling that leads to voluntary restriction of conception may help reduce the transmission of certain genetic faults. However, specific primary prevention of many diseases such as epilepsy, muscular dystrophy, multiple sclerosis, and some mental retardation must wait for further research.

Efforts continue in many fields to discover causes, to detect associated behaviors or symptoms, or to identify people or populations who seem susceptible to particular conditions. Correlations between breast cancer and child-bearing patterns or familial history of breast cancer, smoking and heart disease, stress and mental breakdown are examples.

To date, the most helpful measures to prevent chronic illness seem to be non-specific ones, based on probable, presumed, or demonstrated relationships to one or more diseases. In promoting these measures, one should:

1. Discourage smoking, especially cigarette smoking.

2. Avoid unnecessary exposure to environmental pollution such as burning leaves, careless use of insecticide sprays, or industrial pollution which occurs when preventive equipment is not used in factories or in disposing of chemical wastes.

3. Insist upon immunization against communicable diseases for individuals and contacts — polio, rubella, influenza.

4. Help identify genetic risks through careful study of family history, and provide or secure genetic counseling as indicated when there is a risk of heritable or family-linked conditions such as diabetes, sickle cell anemia, or mental disorder.

5. Promote adequate prenatal and delivery care and provide advice on family planning.

6. Secure prompt and adequate care of respiratory conditions, high blood pressure, or other acute illnesses that may become chronic.

7. Endorse a prudent life style, including a diet sufficiently low in calories and animal fats to prevent obesity, regular exercise, adequate sleep, healthy sexuality.

8. Provide prompt care and surveillance as necessary for conditions which are known to predispose individuals to later problems: hypertension, anemia, obesity, stress.

9. Sponsor vigorous accident prevention measures in home, school, industry, and on community streets and highways.

Research in causation and associated factors related to chronic disease is being widely and aggressively pursued; it is important to be alert for new information in professional literature.

Much of what the community health nurse does in the prevention of chronic illness will be included as part of other on-going activities. Immunization may be part of preschool, school, or prenatal services. Accident prevention will enter into all activities as a major concern in school or industrial environments and in planning community health efforts. Family histories including a genetic pedigree may be part of a health maintenance program, prenatal care, or community health education endeavor. The community health nurse may participate in, or use the findings of, screening programs for hypertension or other danger signals. Services directed to elderly populations can offer educational and counseling and opportunities for action to prevent chronic illness.

Secondary Prevention Offers Promise

Secondary prevention is concerned with the early recognition and treatment of conditions in order to make them less destructive. In this area, it is possible to move more surely and effectively. Among measures recommended for secondary prevention are the following:

1. Maintaining regular comprehensive medical surveillance — including emotional and developmental assessment — throughout life, and with increased frequency at points of greater vulnerability (such as early childhood, adolescence, pregnancy, late middle and advanced age).

2. Introducing formal and informal screening measures in the home, in school, in industry, and in the community. Although screening measures do not diagnose illness, they serve to identify those who need more definitive study. Self-examination of the breast and evaluation of changes incident to arthritis are screening measures adapted to the family level. General screening, multiphasic screening, or screening for special conditions such as tuberculosis, cancer, heart disease, or behavioral disorders may be conducted at the community level. (The nurse's role in family and community screening processes is discussed more fully in Chapter 18.)

3. Setting of specific testing programs to identify asymptomatic disease such as cervical cancer, glaucoma, or hypertension.

4. Using current services as a means of uncovering conditions requiring further investigation. For instance, in the course of prenatal visits to an expectant mother, the nurse may find a family member who has symptoms suggestive of cancer; or she may discover a child who is developing unusually slowly or who is exhibiting bizarre or unexpected

behavior. Such "case finding" is admittedly opportunistic, but a sensitive eye can discern many conditions needing further study.

5. Alerting vulnerable groups to the need for early recognition of symptoms of particular chronic conditions. For example, older age groups might be especially susceptible to glaucoma; certain ethnic groups seem more vulnerable to hypertension; families of the chronically ill may be unusually liable to stress. These groups could be apprised of available diagnostic facilities and of the importance of observing symptoms of the disease or disorder. Reaching such populations may require a variety of channels: incidental contacts made during home visits, using individuals as emissaries to spread the word to others in the community; and the utilization of ready-made groups such as parent-teacher organizations, farm cooperatives, church groups or 4-H clubs. Although every member of the health team will be engaged in these alerting procedures, the nurse's share will be considerable, especially in less populated areas.

6. Strengthening existing preventive services. Prenatal care, school examinations, and the prompt use of the family medical adviser for preventive as well as curative care are examples of programs that could be fortified to encourage early identification of disease and subsequent treatment of illness.

Early detection and preventive services are frequently inefficiently or unproductively used because the public is unaware of available resources. The community health nurse should encourage use of all available sources of assistance, and should vigorously follow up any and all cases she has detected requiring definitive diagnosis or care.

Tertiary Prevention Can Help

Unfortunately, for many chronic illnesses there is at present no way to either prevent or contain the disease. The early discovery of lung cancer does not necessarily lead to an improved prognosis. Arthritis and emphysema run their course relentlessly. For many with chronic illness, "health" means a truce with pain, disability, or indignity rather than freedom from disease or its symptoms. Tertiary preventive care (minimizing as far as possible the deleterious effect of the illness) can help make the situation more tolerable and avoid unnecessary discomfort or restriction. The major opportunity, as Strauss points out, is to improve the quality of life.[9] This preventive thrust extends not only to the patient, but also to the exhausted family, to the anxious fearful child, and to the uneasy, sometimes awkward relative or friend. All are faced with the problem of adjusting to the same stressful situation. By providing or supervising care through interpretation and support, and by mobilizing resources for care, the community health nurse may help maintain individual and family functioning at the highest possible level.

Nursing Needs Will Vary Widely

The nature and the direction of nursing provided to the family with a chronically ill member will be determined by the impact of the condition on individual function and also by the degree to which the family is able to cope with the problem. It will also vary at different points in the course of the illness.

Not All Chronic Illness Is Disabling

Many people who are chronically ill are able to carry on their usual activities despite the existence of a chronic condition. They may be able to manage quite well without assistance from community service, or, if under community care, they may not require the services of the community nurse. For example, people with epilepsy, if under medical supervision, may be expected to lead essentially normal lives as can many people with early stages of arthritis. Most diabetics are also able to carry on their usual activities with little or no assistance. If families have adequate support from their medical or clinic advisers, no community health care may be needed. Others may need short term care to bolster treatment provided in the home, or they may need help and advice to aid them in finding available community resources.

Most Chronic Illness Has a Predictable Course

Five phases of chronic illness may be identified.

1. *The prediagnosis phase* of chronic illness may be fraught with uncertainty and stress. The threat of disability or disfigurement, a concern about the costs of care, and worry about interruption of work or school may result in extreme tension. If the family has not built strong supportive relationships, the patient (or the parent or other responsible person) may try to "protect" others in the family from knowing the facts, even though he may feel alone and unsupported as a consequence.

2. *The phase of acceptance* of the condition can be deeply disturbing. The patient's first reaction may be denial, shock, rage, or despair. "Why me?" is the inevitable and unanswerable question of each. However, sometimes the reaction is one of simple relief at having a hidden worry transformed into a reality that can be confronted. As the illness progresses, a few patients will continue to deny the existence of the disease; however, for most, acceptance is usually achieved, although with varying degrees and types of accommodation.

3. *The phase of action* — when treatment and care are initiated — may also create some anxiety in the patient or in the individual administering care. Until the skills of observation and of therapeutic

methods are well established, the anxiety may be alleviated by action itself: "doing something" provides a sense of some control over the situation.

4. *The phase of the long hard pull* is often characterized by periodic discouragement or, in the case of a family care giver, just plain fatigue. The time demand for care may be overwhelming. The home nurse or the patient may become irritable, impatient, and careless in carrying out necessary routines. At this point, support becomes very important. When the disease is characterized by remissions, new stresses will be created by periods of false hope alternating with continued curtailment of activities and increased dependence.

5. *The phase of separation* may be reached when care becomes too complex for the family to manage and nursing home or hospital care is required, or when death is imminent. For the family, separation will mean grief and, frequently, feelings of guilt. For the patient, hospitalization can symbolize rejection and, as it is often proof of a downhill course, it can precipitate despair.

THE GOALS OF COMMUNITY HEALTH NURSING ARE DIRECTED TOWARD PATIENT, FAMILY, AND COMMUNITY

The goal of community health nursing in chronic disease care is to support the family and other care agents in improving the quality of life of the chronically ill while protecting the family and contributing to community understanding and action in the care and control of chronic illness.

Specifically, the community health nursing effort is designed to

1. Maintain the ability to function in both patient and family.
2. Support the patient's care regimen.
3. Maximize the comfort and safety of the patient.
4. Mobilize and coordinate community and family care efforts.
5. Reduce patient and family stress occasioned by illness and by eventual separation.
6. Observe and report new patterns or unexpected occurrences that might advance the knowledge of disease processes or the effects of treatment.

Maintenance of Function on the Part of Patient and Family

For the person with chronic illness, a well-known slogan applies: "It's not how long you make it; it's how you make it long." The quality of life of the patient with a long-term illness is very much affected by the degree to which he can do those things he considers important and maintain his independent and contributing role within the family.

Physical Function. Maintaining physical function means independence to the patient. Nurses are familiar with the need to maintain an adequate range of motion in postsurgical care of the mastectomy patient. The struggle for any patient to control those activities necessary for daily living — feeding himself, washing himself, combing his own hair, moving about — is a vital one.

Outside the hospital, direct nursing care must be predominantly a family responsibility. Success may be limited, and the cost in both time and energy can be high. It may take long tedious hours of patient practice to enable the stroke victim to talk or to feed himself again, or to teach the colostomy patient to manage the techniques of elimination.

Professional personnel are usually available only intermittently. Special personnel, such as a physical therapist, may not be available at all, either to help directly or to give advice. In many instances, it will fall to the community health nurse to provide the major portion of care. She can help in the following ways:

1. Determine, through conference with others involved in care, reasonable goals for the patient that can be set for the restoration of function. It is important that these be honestly presented to the sick person.

2. Increase her own skill by working with agency personnel, such as physical therapists; or by self-initiated training, wherein she arranges to participate in rehabilitative care in a hospital or to undertake formal class work. The nurse would also be wise to establish rapport with someone skilled in the treatment of long-term illness whom she can turn to for consultation and advice — for instance, a clinic nurse or a private physician or a regular consultant in her own or another agency.

3. Evaluate and increase the competence of the family or of auxiliary workers to carry out required care.

4. Supervise and encourage the patient, the family, and auxiliary workers as they carry out necessary procedures.

Social Function. Ability to function at the social level is as important to the quality of life as the ability to function physically. The ability to contribute — to help with preparation of a meal or to do handwork for others — may do much to improve depleted self-image. Providing social stimulation can help make the days of the chronically ill person more pleasant, less tedious, and often less lonely. The nurse's visit, during which she talks to the patient about events, plans, local news, may assume great importance; visits from neighbors, relatives, and friends help bring the outside world into the sickroom. Ex-patients, patients with similar experiences, or volunteers (such as members of the Ostomy Society or of "Reach for Recovery") may share the listening and supporting functions of care.

It is imperative to prevent stagnation or immobilization that may contribute to a decline in the capacity to function. In encouraging activity, the nurse must enlist the entire family. Valuable support can be provided by volunteers: teenagers are especially good at reading to patients, for example. Voluntary agencies can provide not only direct service to the patient through their own workers, but can also be a source of consultation, teaching materials, and educational opportunities for the nurse and family.

Support of the Patient's Care Regimen

An important aspect of nursing the chronically ill is to assess and maintain adherence to the prescribed treatment regimen. Maintaining the regimen may be a difficult task. Estimates reported of adherence to a medication regimen for tuberculosis ranged from 29 per cent to 86 per cent.[10] Even allowing for differences in the criteria for adherence used by the various investigators, it is likely that there are wide variations in performance.

There are many reasons for non-compliance.[11, 12, 13] What seems most common is that the patient and/or the care-giver feel that "the juice is not worth the squeeze." The pills may give too little relief and cost too much; the treatment may be tedious and painful so that it is better to suffer from the disease than from the treatment; it may be easier to wash the sheets than to diaper the patient. An overprotective spouse may decide it is not worth struggling with the tears, complaints, pain, fatigue, and the entreaties of the patient in order to persevere with the treatment or the exercise. To some extent, the patient has the right to choose — he may elect to discontinue dialysis in favor of a peaceful death, or to refuse painful treatments even though so doing will shorten his life. But in general the nurse will encourage both patient and family to conform. The following steps may help achieve a high proportion of compliance.

1. Be sure the patient and the person giving care understand the purpose and the importance of the treatment. There is no need for the diabetic child to understand just how diabetes develops, but he and any responsible attendant must know the effects of insulin, and the relationship between insulin intake, food intake, and exercise. The person with tuberculosis must understand the importance of taking prescribed medication regularly, and the relationship between the medication and communicability of the disease.

It is particularly important that the family understand the potential danger of self-prescribed medications. Often, people with chronic diseases are under the care of several medical advisers, and will be taking several medications simultaneously. In such cases, both the nurse and the family should be alert for any symptoms of possible drug reaction. Also, the drugs prescribed may be numerous and difficult to distinguish from one another. In many instances, several drugs may have to be tried before finding one that is effective. In the interim, the patient may become discouraged at the lack of progress.

2. Be sure the patient and/or the person providing care know exactly *how* to do what is required and *why* it is done that way. The insulin syringe is held a certain way to avoid infection; the unsteady patient is supported in such a manner to prevent a fall. The process of show and tell should be continued until the home attendant feels reasonably comfortable in performing the treatment or measuring the medication or handling the equipment.

Written check lists or reminder sheets may lend confidence. If the care is to be given by a non-professional, the family and the patient, as well as the care-taker, should feel confident of her skills.

3. When treatment extends over a long time, provide *frequent reinforcement* and encouragement. Especially in the "long hard pull" phase of the illness when there may be a tendency to be less careful in carrying out the regimen, or a temptation to experiment with unorthodox or unauthorized techniques, or well-advertised non-prescription drugs. Inasmuch as drugs are administered by the nurse or family in the absence of a medical or nursing supervisor, considerable responsibility is placed upon the community health nurse to familiarize herself with the possible complications and contraindications for any drug pre-scribed. The necessary information may be supplied by the family's physician, or the hospital nurse; in some instances a medical committee of the agency or a special nursing consultant may be a helpful source. However it is accomplished, the nurse must be sufficiently informed to carry out the procedures required, and must take whatever time necessary to *become* fully informed.

Maximize the Comfort and Safety of the Patient

In many instances, providing comfort is the most imperative need of both patient and family. The skill with which the patient is bathed, fed, and put into or removed from bed has much to do with his ability to tolerate unavoidable discomforts. Skin care, positioning, and careful control of exercise to avoid fatigue all help prevent more serious discomfort. "Keeping mother comfortable" is reassuring to the family as well as to the patient. To achieve this end, the community health nurse may help by:

1. Providing personal care for a short part of the day or at intervals when the need is greatest.

2. Teaching and supervising the family, the home health aide, or any other provider of care.

3. Referring the family to other sources of care such as the Visiting Nurse Association, or the American Red Cross for adult education classes in home nursing.

4. Assisting the family in finding sources for equipment or supplies. For example, a Visiting Nurse Association or a community loan chest may be able to supply a hospital bed; the local chapter of the American Cancer Society may help provide dressings.

5. Teaching the family to notice and report immediately any change in the patient's condition. It would be wise to leave a list of things which it is especially important to observe, and a telephone number to be called should there be a need to report any change.

6. Maintaining a safe environment. It is important to protect the chronically ill patient from the possibility of infection. Contact with family or friends who have "just a little cold" or with children who have been exposed to an infectious disease should be emphatically discouraged. Even a minor cold can be serious for the victim of emphysema.

Other safety measures should also be followed, such as placing potent drugs out of the patient's reach, or keeping a small light burning so he will not stumble if he must get up at night. Taking extra care with heating pads, lamps, or other electrical equipment is a vital precaution, especially if the patient is disoriented or confused.

The Health and Safety of the Care-Giver Is Also Vitally Important

The family member turned nurse is apt to undertake an impossible load, concentrating all attention on the sick person and ignoring her own needs. The community health nurse's responsibility includes measures to protect the home care giver, to help her resolve her divided loyalties. The nurse may be able to develop ways of cutting the time required for care without danger to the sick person. The family member responsible for care needs time for rest, for exercise, for other essential household tasks, time to lead her own life. Fatigue is very dangerous. The patient's room should be made convenient for the home nurse, with the bed at a suitable height, supplies properly arranged or stored, and a comfortable chair for those times when "care" is conversation.

Relief time should be provided daily, weekly, and monthly. Sometimes it is possible for a demanding patient to spend some part of the year in the home of another child or relative. Nurse's aides or volunteer neighbors or relatives may provide occasional care. Some countries have developed infirmary style facilities where sick people may stay while the family goes on a holiday: here, one must improvise!

MOBILIZATION AND COORDINATION OF RESOURCES

The chronically ill person is probably using multiple sources of care in a constantly changing configuration. He may be in and out of the hospital, then under the care of a diagnostic and treatment center, then under the supervision of the family physician. The physical therapist, occupational therapist, speech therapist, neurologist, cardiologist, and psychiatrist may be in constant or intermittent attendance. Any change in the treatment pattern can involve several new agents of care.

In addition to all this institutional support, help may also be coming from informal sources — neighbors, relatives, former work-mates, friendly aid church groups. The family may need help initially in locating these various sources; once the resources have been mobilized, both family and care contributors will need some means of coordinating their efforts.

The community health nurse may serve as coordinator or case manager. On the other hand, coordination may be provided by another agency, a comprehensive care clinic perhaps, or Health Maintenance Organization. Whether as organizer-manager or as a contributor to care, the community health nurse must be involved in coordinating activities. The essentials of coordination include:

1. A coordinated plan of care developed by or known to the family and other major providers of care. Some multi-disciplinary agencies have evolved a problem oriented record system which is used by all workers who provide care and which is obviously a great advantage in coordination of effort. However, few agencies have responsibility for the entire spectrum of care, and many are built around a single patient rather than a family unit system. In most cases, additional coordinating efforts will be required.

The achievement of a coordinated plan is by no means simple, since agencies will vary in concepts of the care required. The psychiatric hospital may feel care should be directed solely at the patient, with the goal being to provide support and reassurance in a tranquil environment. The community health nurse would probably feel that care of the patient should be conducted on a level that is compatible with the health of the entire family. The resulting proposals could be very different in structure and content.

The nurse may want a written outline for care, as a guide for her own actions. The overall plan, however, may have to be stated much less formally. Through occasional conferences, exchanges of information by mail or by telephone, and periodic reviews of the care plan, it is possible to achieve a reasonable level of coordination.

2. Prompt exchange of essential information is a critical factor in care. Periodic reports, open lines of communication, informal relationships with other agencies and sources of care will all keep the information flowing. Written communication is often too slow to be useful, and when reduced to the stylized format of a standard report may not convey the message clearly.

3. Periodic review of all the components of care in order to detect duplications, inadequacies, unproductive elements, or missed opportunities is essential in long-term care, where the nature of the need is

constantly changing. It is particularly important in such a review to note the degree to which the overall plan incorporates the decisions and protects the integrity of the family as a whole.

MANAGEMENT OF STRESS IS CRUCIAL

Control of stress adds to the family's ability to cope with the illness and with eventual separation. Families will vary in the strength they can muster to deal with stress and in the amount of external support they will require. The degree and type of support needed will also vary at different points in the disease.

The point of initial diagnosis may be exceedingly traumatic. Some families will meet this with complete despair: most will suffer from great anxiety and discouragment. For some, however, it may be a welcome relief from the uncertainty and ever present worry of the prediagnostic phase. They are relieved to have met the true enemy at last and to confront the problem in specific terms.

A question frequently raised is "Should the patient be told the truth?" As Brauer points out, this is far from a simple question.[14] The answer must be carefully considered by the physician and the family as well as by the nurse. Indeed, the question must be "Which patient, what truth?"

The apparent stoic who demands "the truth" may actually be hoping for reassurance rather than facts. The family, too, may react to the truth in different ways. If the diagnosis is catastrophic and the outlook dim, they may in some instances act as though the patient were already dead; or they may become so frightened that they are unable to provide the support needed by the sick member. Furthermore, so much of chronic illness remains a mystery that "the truth" may turn out to be wrong — as when the patient survives far beyond the time expected. Failure to tell the patient may increase his feelings of helplessness, deprive him of the opportunity to share his fears and anxieties. The nurse may help the family to decide what is best for this particular person at this particular time.

The *how* as well as the *why* of helping the family at this point assumes critical importance. In general, it seems useful to encourage open expression of feelings: the patient should know that his rage or depression is acceptable behavior in the nurse's eyes; and the family must know that they can discuss their own disappointments and frustrations freely, without fear of being judged, as they struggle to adapt their life to the new demands and limits imposed by the chronic illness.

The community health nurse can help reduce stress by reassuring the family members that they are able to deal with the situation and that help is available. They may derive great strength from her stance of confident expectation: it is important to provide an anchor, someone to whom the family can turn when they need help. This may be the nurse or some other professional worker. When a home health aide provides the major part of care the family will probably turn first to her, and the professional nurse will serve in an auxiliary position. Properly briefed, the aide may prove a close and welcome support.

Action is also a useful antidote to stress. Finding out about a prosthesis if mastectomy is likely, restructuring the household routine or rearranging equipment so the disabled stroke patient can do more for herself and for others, finding tasks that are within the patient's physical abilities — all are therapeutic actions.

Another difficult point comes a few months after diagnosis when the reality of the long hard pull becomes clear. Care of the chronically ill person, especially one who is greatly incapacitated, can be grueling. It is not surprising that families become tense and upset when the illness seems likely to drag on forever. The optimism of the sick person may lag, demands for family attention become more insistent, the principal care giver may begin to feel trapped. The need for relief measures becomes urgent. The nurse can help by urging another relative to take over for a few weeks, or arranging short-term nursing home placement. The nurse herself can support the family by listening, by encouraging the family to see their problems in realistic terms, by helping them to accept assistance, and by referring them to case work or to other counseling services when necessary.

Nonmedical problems may be a source of stress. One great concern of families is the fear that they cannot meet the financial obligations imposed by prolonged illness. They may be justifiably worried about medical and hospital bills, and about the inability of the patient to continue to contribute to the family's income, or about future expenses such as the need for nursing home care. The nurse can help by referring the family to sources of information about insurance benefits or about community facilities for care, including the special provisions under the Social Security Act for illness and for total or partial disability. The nurse should familiarize herself with the general provisions of legislation affecting the chronically ill so that she can judge whether or not the family should investigate these possibilities for further help. Provisions for the care of veterans and for industrial compensation are other possible sources of financial aid. When the nurse's information is inadequate, or the financial problem is complex, the help of the social welfare staff should be sought.

Stress is inevitable at the separation phase. When separation is due to the need for special care not possible in the home, there may be a strong feeling of guilt on the part of the family, a feeling that they should have made greater efforts to cope. The patient may feel rejected and hurt at being "sent away," and fearful of the new experience. He may openly and bitterly blame the family for taking this step, and plead for a change of plans. Perhaps even harder for the family is the situation in which the patient — a very retarded child, perhaps, or a disturbed adult — may not understand what is happening.

The nurse can help the family and the patient to verbalize their concerns; she can reassure the family that they have indeed considered all possible choices, and she can explain the contributions and conditions of the facility to which the patient will go.

When death occurs or is imminent, the family may need additional nursing support. It is well to remember that the period of bereavement and adjustment stretches beyond the death of the patient. Many families will continue to need nursing attention for some time.

The community health nurse can help the family to *appreciate and support the efforts of the hospital or nursing home personnel* to make this an "affirmative" time for the dying patient — to help the patient *live* until he dies.[15] To the family, the hospital or institution staff may seem callous and insensitive. The family may fear the effects of the liberal use of narcotics; they may not understand the basic rationale that dictates maximum control of pain for the patient at this time. They may feel that the staff is cruel in answering the dying patient's queries honestly, that they thus remove any hope the patient may have had for recovery. Talking to the personnel responsible for institutional care can reassure the family and help them to support and feel comfortable about the steps that are being taken. They may also be helped by knowing how difficult it is for the staff, as well as for the patient and for the family, to face the fact of death.

The patient's style in facing crises, including this one, may be to put up a brave front and appear cheerful and self-contained, reserving for himself the process of confrontation with dying. Other patients need to talk about death, and find relief in discussing their feelings and concerns. All patients may need reassurance that steps will be taken to control the pain and that they will not be allowed to die unattended.

For the family with a member who has a disabling chronic disease, whose care is provided primarily in the home or other non-institutional setting, the contribution of community health nursing can be very great indeed. The number of chronically ill cases is already enormous, and likely to grow. The needs for present and anticipated care will strain the community health nursing system to the utmost, even if funds and personnel are sharply increased. The job can be done only if each nurse exercises ingenuity in practice, in the use of other resources, and in planning and evaluation of her own services to the chronically ill and their families.

REFERENCES

1. Kurlander, A. R.: Chronic and degenerative disease. *In* Porterfield, J. H. (ed.): *Community Health Services.* New York, Basic Books, Inc., Publishers, 1966, p. 67.

2. Monthly Vital Statistics Report. *Advance Report, Final Mortality Statistics*, DHEW Pub. No. (PHS) 79-1120, *28*:3, 1979.
3. Ibid., p. 4.
4. American Lung Association: *Facts in Brief*. New York, American Lung Association, 1975.
5. Metropolitan Life Insurance Co.: *Statistical Bulletin*. *56*:3, 1975.
6. Lieberman, E. J. (ed.): *Mental Health. The Public Health Challenge*. Washington, D.C., American Public Health Association, 1975, p. 139. Note: Previously reported incidence of mental retardation has been higher; the lower rate is the result of redefinition of mental retardation.
7. Regier, D. A., Goldberg, I. D., and Taube, C. A.: The defacto U.S. mental health services system. Arch. Gen. Psych., *35*:690, 1978.
8. Surgeon General's report: *Healthy People*. Washington, D.C., U.S. Government Printing Office, U.S. DHEW, PHS, Pub. 79-55071, 1979, p. 74.
9. Strauss, A.: *Chronic Illness and the Quality of Life*. St. Louis, Mo., C. V. Mosby Co., 1975.
10. Kuemmerer, J.: *Adherence to Medical Recommendations for Oral Antituberculosis Drugs*. Doctoral Thesis, Baltimore, Johns Hopkins School of Hygiene and Public Health, 1968, p. 10.
11. Becker, M. H., et al.: Selected psychosocial models and correlates of individual health-related behaviors. Med. Care, *15*:27 (Supplement), 1977.
12. Marston, M. V.: Compliance with medical regimens—A review of the literature. Nurs. Res., *9*:312, 1970.
13. Vincent, P.: Factors influencing patient non-compliance: A theoretical approach. Nurs. Res., *20*:509, 1971.
14. Brauer, P. H.: Should the patient be told the truth? *In* Skipper, J. K., and Leonard, R. C. (eds.): *Social Interaction and Patient Care*. Philadelphia, J. B. Lippincott Co., 1965, p. 167.
15. Martinson, I. M.: Quality care for dying patients dependent on nurses. Am. Nurse, *11*:5, 1979.

SUGGESTED READINGS

Abt Associates, Inc.: *A National Profile of Catastrophic Illness – Final Report*. Cambridge, Mass., National Center for Health Services Research, U.S. DHEW July, 1977.
Anderson, C. A.: Making the right moves in discharge planning: Home or nursing home? Let the elderly patient decide. Am. J. Nurs., 79:1448, 1979.
Around the Clock Aids for the Child with Muscular Dystrophy. New York, Muscular Dystrophy Association of America.
Arthritis Foundation: *Primer on the Rheumatic Diseases*, 7th ed., New York, The Arthritis Foundation, 1973.
Bachscheider, J. E.: Self-care requirements, self care capabilities and nursing systems in the nurse management clinic. Am. J. Pub. Health, *64*:1138, 1974.
Barsch, R. H.: *The Parent of the Handicapped Child: The Study of Child Rearing Practices*. Springfield, Ill., Charles C Thomas Publishers, 1968.
Benoliel, J. Q.: Childhood diabetes: The commonplace in living becomes uncommon. *In* Strauss, A. L. (ed.): *Chronic Illness and the Quality of Life*. St. Louis, Mo., C. V. Mosby Co., 1975, pp. 89–98.
Benoliel, J. Q., Overview: care, cure, and the challenge of choice. *In* Earle, A. et al. (eds.): *The Nurse as Caregiver for the Dying Patient*. New York, Columbia University Press, 1976.
Bergner, M., et al.: The sickness impact profile: Validation of a health care measure. Med. Care, *14*:57, 1976.
Blau, S. and Schultz, D.: *Arthritis — Past, Present, and Future*. New York, Doubleday and Co., 1973.
Breslow, L.: Early case-finding, treatment and mortality from cervix and breast cancer. Prev. Med., *1*:141, 1972.
Brickner, P. W., Boyle, M. T., Dyque, T., Holland, P., and Madden, P. M.: Outreach to welfare hotels, the homebound, the frail. Am. J. Nurs., 76:762, 1976.

Chang, B. L.: Generalized expectancy, situational perception, and morale of the institutionalized age. Nurs. Res., 27:316, 1978.

Cherniak, R. M.: Handord, R. G., and Swanhill, E.: Home care of chronic respiratory disease. J.A.M.A., 208:821, 1969.

Cospers, B.: The yo-yo factor in chronic illness. Nurs. For., 13:207, 1974.

Daniels, L. M., et al.: What influences adherence to hypertension therapy? Nurs. For., 18:231, 1979.

Danowski, T. S.: Diabetes As a Way of Life, 3rd ed. New York, Coward, McCann and Goeghegan, Inc., 1974.

Debuskey, M. (ed.): The Chronically Ill Child and His Family. Springfield, Ill., Charles C Thomas Publishers, 1970.

Dehn, M.: Rehabilitation of the cardiac patient. The effects of exercise. Am. J. Nurs., 80:435, 1980.

Drake, R. E.: Guidelines for helping patients and families cope with traumatic illness. In Reinhardt, A. M., and Quinn, M. D.: Family Centered Community Nursing. St. Louis, Mo., C. V. Mosby Co., 1973, pp. 228–236.

Dunlop, B. D.: Expanded home-based care for the impaired elderly: Solution or pipe dream? Am. J. Pub. Health, 70:514, 1980.

Eagerhaugh, S.: Getting around with emphysema. In Strauss, A.: Chronic Illness and the Quality of Life. St. Louis, Mo., C. V. Mosby Co., 1975, pp. 99–107.

Esberger, K.: Dying and the aged. J. Gerontol. Nurs., 6:11, 1980.

Franck, P.: A survey of health needs of older adults in northwest Johnson County, Iowa. Nurs. Res., 28:360, 1979.

Frazier, C. A.: Parent's Guide to Allergy in Children. Garden City, N. Y. Doubleday and Co., 1973.

Futrell, M., et al.: Primary Health Care of the Older Adult. N. Scituate, Mass., Duxbury Press, 1980.

Hackler, E. N., and Howell, A. T.: Re-socializing the stroke patient. Nurs. Outlook, 21:776, 1973.

Hammond, E. A., and Begley, P. K.: Screening for glaucoma: A comparison of ophthalmoscopy and tonometry. Nurs. Res., 28:371, 1979.

Hancheft, E., and Torrens, P.: A public health nursing project for adult patients with heart disease. Pub. Health Rep., 82:683, 1967.

Hanlon, J.: Public Health Administration and Practice, 6th ed. St. Louis, Mo., C. V. Mosby Co., 1974, Chapter 24.

Hauver, V. H., and Goodman, J. A.: The evaluation of performance and cost in a hypertension control program. Medical Care, 18:485, 1980.

Hawken, M., et al.: Practical aspects of anticonvulsant therapy. Am. J. Nurs., 79:1062, 1979.

Heart Facts, 1974. New York, American Heart Association, 1974.

Jones, E. W., McNitt, B. J., and McKnight, E.: Patient Classification for Long-Term Care: User's Manual. Washington, D.C., U.S. Government Printing Office, DHEW, PHS, Pub. No. (HRA) 74-3107, 1973.

Kane, R. L., and Kane, R. A.: Long-Term Care in Six Countries — Implications for the U. S., Fogarty International Center, Bethesda, Md., Superintendent of Documents. Washington, D.C., U.S. Government Printing Office, (Stock No. 017-053-00058-2) 1976.

Katz, S., Ford, A., Downs, T. D., Adams, M., and Rusby, D.: Effects of Continued Care: A Study of Chronic Illness in the Home. U.S. DHEW Pub. No. 73-3010, Washington, D.C., U.S. Government Printing Office, 1973.

Kaufert, J. M., et al.: Assessing functional status among elderly patients: A comparison of questionnaire and service provider ratings. Med. Care, 17:807, 1979.

Kelly, J.: Epilepsy symposium nursing management. Nurs. Mir., 147:17, 1978.

Knef, H.: The Verdict. New York, Farrar Strauss and Giroux, 1975.

Kübler-Ross, E.: Death: The Final Stage of Growth. Englewood Cliffs, N. J., Prentice-Hall, Inc., 1975.

Lenneberg, E., and Rowbotham, J.: The Colostomy Patient. Springfield, Ill., Charles C Thomas Publishers, 1970.

Levine, E. S.: Lisa and Her Soundless World (A children's book). New York, Behavioral Publications Inc., 1974.

Martinson, I. N., Armstrong, G. D., and Geis, D. P. et al.: Facilitating home care for children dying of cancer. Cancer Nurs., *1*:41, 1978.

McFarlane, J.: Children with diabetes, special needs during growth years. Am. J. Nurs., 73:1360, 1973.

Morse, J.: Aspiration and achievement — A study of 100 patients with juvenile rheumatoid arthritis. Rehab. Lit., *33*:290, 1972.

Neill, K.: Behavioral aspects of chronic physical disease. Nurs. Clin. North Am., *14*:443, 1979.

Neugebauer, R., et al.: Epilepsy: Some epidemiological aspects. Psychol. Med., 9:207, 1979.

Powers, M. M.: Factors influencing attitude, knowledge, and compliance of hypertensive patients., ANA Pub., 1979 (D-67), 11.

Requarth, C. H.: Medication usage and interaction in the long-term care of the elderly. J. Gerontol. Nurs., 5:33, 1979.

Roberts, I., The elderly: A challenge to nursing-planning care at home. Nurs. Times, 74:154, 1978.

Shamansky, S. L., and Hamilton, W. M.: The health behavior awareness test: Self-care education for the elderly. J. Gerontol. Nurs., 5:29, 1979.

Shomaker, D. M.: Use and abuse of OTC medications by the elderly. J. Gerontol Nurs., 6:21, 1980.

Strauss, A.: *Chronic Illness and the Quality of Life*. St. Louis, Mo., C. V. Mosby Co., 1975.

Suezsk, B.: Chronic renal failure and the problem of funding. *In* Strauss, A.: *Chronic Illness and the Quality of Life*. St. Louis, Mo., C. V. Mosby Co., 1975, pp. 108–118.

Wang, M. K.: A health maintenance service for chronically ill patients. Am. J. Pub. Health, 60:713, 1970.

Weissert, W., Wan, T., and Livieratos, B.: *Effects and Costs of Day Care and Homemaker Services for the Chronically Ill: A Randomized Experiment*. Hyattsville, Md., National Center for Health Services Research, DHEW, Jan. 1979.

Wieczorek, R. R., and Horner-Rosner, B.: The Asthmatic Child: Preventing and Controlling Attacks. Am. J. Nurs., 79:258, 1979.

Multiple sclerosis. Am. J. Nurs. (continuing educ.), *80*:274, 1980.

The patient with scoliosis. Am. J. Nurs. (continuing educ.), 79:1587, 1979.

U.S. Department of Health, Education, and Welfare, Social Security Administration: *Demographic and Economic Characteristics of the Aged*. Washington, D.C., U.S. Government Printing Office (HEW 3. 49:45), 1975.

CHAPTER 25

POPULATION CONTROL AND FAMILY PLANNING

The uncontrolled growth of population has been recognized as an important and worldwide problem with serious social, health, and economic implications. In poor or industrially underdeveloped nations, population control may be required for survival. The growing numbers of people to be fed and provided with other basic necessities may outrun the country's production capabilities, or exceed the amount that could conceivably be met with substantial international aid. Poverty, a short life span, lack of employment, substandard health, and low levels of energy are the usual accompaniments of serious overpopulation. Furthermore, the effect of increased fertility is felt quite rapidly. For example, if families in the United States were to have an average of *two* children, one hundred years from now there would be 350 million people in the country. If the number of births was increased by just one to an average of three children, in that same period the population would grow to almost one billion.[1]

All countries must share in the concern of population control. The Commission on Population and the American Future states:

This country, or any country, always has a "population problem" in the sense of achieving a proper balance between size, growth, and distribution on one hand, and on the other the quality of life to which every person in the country aspires.[2]

In industrially advanced countries, the threat inherent in overpopulation is not the danger of famine, abysmal poverty, debility, and early death but that of a debasing of the quality of life that has been achieved as a result of technical, medical, and social advances. Simply stated, the fact is that when there are fewer people, there is more of everything to go around — more food, more jobs, more educational opportunity, more space for homes and recreational areas. Planned (selective) reproduction allows for a better reproductive product and better conditions within which the child can live and grow.

Obviously, limiting population growth will not in itself ensure a better quality of life for all. Unless public policy and collective action are directed toward assuring equitable distribution of benefits, problems of poverty, deprivation, hunger, and exploitation will exist along with new abundance for the elite.

Before the advent of modern medicine and widespread birth control, populations were kept in check by terrible natural restraints — war, pestilence, famine, and high infant mortality. We have eliminated some of the old problems, and created a whole set of new ones. Modern benefits — without the support of a moral stance and clearly stated socially oriented, positive values — may lead only to inactivity, boredom, and decadence. Even the most enlightened public policy and personal concern cannot assure the opportunity for a good life for all people.

In addition to the impact of controlled fertility on population size, there is a strong feeling among many groups that the means of controlling family size should be available, as a human right, to those who want it. Children, too, have a right to be wanted, protected, and loved; and proper spacing and control of family size can help ensure this right. While speaking at an International Women's Year session Helvie Sipila, Assistant Secretary General of the United Nations, stated it this way:

> The state should enable its citizens to control their reproductive behavior as safely, effectively and efficiently as possible. New laws should be introduced and enforced, guaranteeing access to all relevant information, education and services — including, as appropriate, contraception, abortion and voluntary sterilization.[3]

This philosophy was reiterated in the Report of the National Commission on the observance of International Women's Year 1976 when they endorsed a statement declaring the "fundamental rights of all women to information and means necessary to control voluntarily and freely the number and spacing of their children."[4]

Population control is the combination of public policy and public and private action designed to produce a level of population growth compatible with the resources that are likely to be available, and assuring the achievement of a good life as defined by the specific group concerned. It involves plan rather than chance and consideration for the future as well as for the present.

Public population policy should reflect considerations of the social, economic, and human consequences of uncontrolled growth. Planning should be based not only upon desirable levels of population but also upon the constraints that operate in the very sensitive area of reproduction. For example, people in some areas may fear that they will be left without progeny to care for them in their old age; they must be convinced that even if fewer children are born, an adequate number will reach maturity. The freedom of the individual to choose is a precious thing to most people, and efforts to control reproduction may seem a very real threat. For this reason, the right of the individual to choose must be jealously guarded.

Family planning is the process by which families, couples, or sometimes individuals decide how they will regulate their reproduction, and take necessary action to do so. It is much more than limiting the size of families. It involves deciding how many children are desired and at what intervals, selecting a method of fertility control or in the case of infertility, means of inducing fertility compatible with beliefs, values, and preferences; and dealing with any failures that may occur in fertility control. It is a voluntary decision. Any attempt to preempt the family's right to decide by tying welfare or other benefits to limiting family size must be considered as unethical and ultimately harmful to the family and to the community. Family planning is the family's way of determining one important aspect of its future, and sometimes a way of permitting full development of its members. It is a means of regulating reproduction processes so as to maintain the physical, social, and economic well-being of the family and to assure each child a reasonable chance for an adequate life.

Studies have repeatedly shown that most couples (regardless of ethnic group or income status) desire a relatively small family. Edmands' study of a group of low-income families found that most desired a limited number of pregnancies, but that there was a wide disparity between the desire to limit family size and the knowledge to do so.[5] The most recent cohort of women at the end of their childbearing years averaged 3.2 children per woman.[6] The future average family size is expected to decline.[7]

While documentation of the impact of uncontrolled reproduction upon family life is still presumptive, there are obvious problems. Frequent or mistimed pregnancies may place a great strain upon the mother's health and vitality, especially for those on marginal incomes or with already uncertain health. An unwanted pregnancy can place a substantial drain on an already stringent budget, and result in a downward revision of the family's expectations. The mistimed baby may arrive just as the mother was planning to re-enter the labor market. The teenage pregnancy may lead to a hasty marriage with little chance of success, and force both young parents to abandon plans for higher education.

The number of unwanted births is calculated in many ways, and estimates vary widely as to the proportion of babies that are unwanted or pregnancies that are mistimed. According to results from the 1976 National Survey of Family Growth, an estimated 8.1 million, or 12.0 per cent, of a total of 67.8 million live births occurring to mothers aged 15 to 44 years were unwanted. This represents a slight decrease in the proportion of unwanted births since a similar survey in 1973. A larger proportion of black mothers reported not wanting another child at conception than did white mothers, even when parity was accounted for. Education and income level were also factors — i.e., the highest proportion of wanted births was among women whose education or income was highest.[8]

Fortunately, most parents, when faced with an unwanted or mistimed child, find their protective instincts prevail, and they are able to welcome and love the newcomer despite an inopportune arrival. For some, however, there is no reconciliation, and in those cases there is a strong risk that the child may be rejected, neglected, or even physically or psychologically abused. Some studies suggest that unwanted children have more problems than other children, both at home and at school.

THE MEANS FOR FERTILITY CONTROL ARE AVAILABLE

There is at present no single perfect method of fertility control. The search goes on for a contraceptive that is effective, safe, and free from undesirable side effects as well as coitus independent, readily accessible, and reversible. Each method currently available has characteristics that can make it troublesome or ineffectual for some people. Some women suffer uncomfortable side effects from birth control pills; some cannot retain an IUD; for many people, there are methods which are unacceptable because they conflict with religious beliefs or are distasteful to the individual. Therefore, decisions about the particular method to be used must be made by the user; the advising professional must take into consideration the clients personal likes and capabilities.

There is, however, a wide range of extremely low risk, highly effective methods of contraception, as well as some less effective but more acceptable methods that may be preferred for personal reasons. The three most effective methods of contraception are oral contraceptives ("the pill"), the intrauterine device (IUD), and sterilization of one or both partners. The first two are reversible, that is, they can be discontinued to allow for pregnancy when desired. The third, sterilization, must at this time be considered permanent, although studies of the possibility of reestablishing fertility are underway.

In the 1976 National Survey of Family Growth, 22.3 per cent of the sample of currently married women, 15 to 44 years of age, used oral contraceptives; 6.1 per cent used an intrauterine device; and 7.2 per cent used a condom as their birth control method. In this group, 28.3 per cent were surgically sterilized.[9] In the same survey, post-married women reported higher rates of oral contraceptives (28 per cent) use as well as a slightly higher rate of surgical sterilization (30.1 per cent).[10]

Oral Contraceptives and the IUD: Highly Effective, Reversible Measures

Oral contraceptives use a combination of estrogens and progestogens to produce systemic changes that prevent ovulation. The pills are taken in accordance with a prescribed schedule once a day for 20 or 21 days during the menstrual cycle. "Sequential" pills are designed to mimic the natural hormone change by varying the amounts of estrogens and progestogens during the menstrual cycle. They are decreasing in popularity because they tend to be less reliable and because they appear to be associated with increased incidence of mammary tumor.

The risk in oral contraceptives was brought to public attention in 1969 and 1970 when it was noted that users appeared to have an increased susceptibility to embolism and cancer. However, the risk is slight and in most instances the benefits outweigh the dangers, since childbearing itself can be hazardous. Oral contraceptives combined with smoking have also been implicated in thrombophlebitis. As a result, there has been a trend toward reducing the amount of estrogens prescribed, which may reduce the risk even more and yet still afford a high level of protection. Side effects that influence the acceptability of oral contraception include nausea, tenderness of the breast, bloating, and (less frequently), vaginal infections. These effects usually disappear with time. However, women will vary in reaction to one or another specific pill: a pill that produces strong side effects in one woman may be totally acceptable to another. Regulation of oral contraceptives is the responsibility of the Food and Drug Administration, since they are considered to be drugs.

The intrauterine device, commonly referred to as the IUD, is also a highly reliable method of fertility control and the second most popular method in the United States. The IUD is a small device, usually made of plastic, that is introduced into the uterus (by a physician or other specially trained person) where it remains in place and prevents conception. The exact mechanism by which the IUD acts is not known, but it is extremely effective and has very few side effects. The IUD can be removed by the physician whenever the client so desires. The devices are made in a variety of shapes and designs so that, in most cases, a woman can be fitted with one that is both secure and comfortable. No one type of IUD is most successful with all women, and some women cannot tolerate any: problems can include occasional bleeding, or discomfort, and susceptibility to infection. There is a heightened possibility of ectopic pregnancy or spontaneous abortion, although these complications do not occur frequently.

Less Effective Reversible Measures May Be Used in Special Situations

These measures include sexual procedures that prevent pregnancy and various "barrier" devices that prevent the union of sperm and ovum. The major procedural approaches are abstinence, either total or at presumably fertile periods, and coitus interruptus. The rhythm method, designed to avoid sexual contact at fertile periods in the menstrual cycle, is based on careful physical study of the individual woman. The fertile period is charted by close observation and recording of symptoms, and intercourse is avoided during that period in the menstrual cycle. The self-discipline demanded of the participants makes it difficult for some to follow this regimen. Some couples report that sexual feelings are intensified during fertile periods, making temporary abstinence very frustrating. Some find that such planning and conscious control of sexual expression are a threat to conjugal adjustment. At best, the rhythm system is much less effective than other methods available; however, some couples may choose it because it conforms to their religious or ethical values.

Coitus interruptus, withdrawal of the penis before ejection of semen during intercourse, has long been practiced as a means of avoiding unwanted pregnancy. Its disadvantages lie in the tensions it can cause in both partners, and the danger that personal control will not be adequate to the situation. On the whole, it is rated relatively low in effectiveness; however, as one adherent said, "It's handy and it's cheap."

Barrier methods, primarily the condom and the diaphragm, are also selected by many couples, although they are less reliable in the control of conception. Barrier methods utilize cheap and readily available supplies, are simple to use and allow for control by either partner. Before the introduction of the pill, these methods — especially the use of the diaphragm by the female partner — were major control methods; however, because they are less effective, they are now used only by a small proportion as the primary procedure (7.2 per cent reported using condoms and 2.9 per cent reported using diaphragms in the United States).[11]

In some countries, and in the United States to a far lesser degree, the use of the condom is being promoted because it is useful in unplanned sexual encounters and is so readily accessible. It is consistent, too, with the trend toward having the man assume greater responsibility.

Permanent Contraceptive Measures

Voluntary sterilization of either or both partners is being used more widely. For many couples who already have a family of the desired size, there may remain ten or fifteen years during which the woman continues to be fecund. It is wise, too, to avoid conception at this stage because the later years of potential childbearing are much more hazardous to mother and baby than are the earlier years. There is greater danger, too, to women over the age of 40 in the use of oral contraceptives. Voluntary sterilization is a preferred strategy for such older couples because it offers virtually complete protection without any side effects or inconvenience. People who are carriers of genetic defects may also want to consider this permanent block to conception.

Surgical methods of sterilization have been simplified and are becoming much more available. Tubal ligation for women and vasectomy for men may be performed without hospitalization and at very little risk. The development of the "mini-lap" surgical maneuver for tubal ligation allows for a very small incision, local anaesthetic, and minimal (if any) hospitalization. Costs are low if compared to the purchase of other fertility control supplies over a period of years. Sterilization does not affect sexual desire — indeed, sexual relationships may be greatly improved when there is no longer any fear of unwanted pregnancy. Voluntary sterilization is now legal in all states.

Interruption of Pregnancy by Abortion is Increasingly Common

While there is no disagreement that abortion is a far less desirable method of limiting family size than is contraception, there are occasions when it appears to be preferable to continuing a hazardous or strongly unwanted pregnancy. For example, a fetus that is badly damaged due to accident or genetically transmitted disorders, a subteen pregnancy, and a woman who has proven to be a grossly inadequate mother may all be considered cases for abortion.

For some individuals and groups, abortion may be unacceptable because of ethical or religious beliefs. However, abortion is entirely a voluntary procedure, and there is no need for any individual or group to be either urged or compelled to accept or even consider it.

It is hoped that when programs for fertility control can reach all groups or populations who need them, and as contraceptive methods become more available and attractive, resorting to abortion will be unnecessary for all but a very few cases.

The Supreme Court's landmark decision of January 22, 1973, overruled restrictive statutes concerning abortion, and determined that states may not prohibit a woman's right to an abortion during the first three months of pregnancy. Thereafter, the state may regulate abortion according to its own statutes so long as the means apply reasonably to the mother's health. States may mandate other regulations such as a requirement for the approval of a husband or parents as appropriate.

This decision has led to much greater availability of legal abortion and has resulted in a drastic reduction of unsafe and often demeaning illegal abortions that in the past caused so many maternal deaths. From 1973 to 1977, reported legal abortions in the United States increased by an annual average of 15 per cent. In 1977, over 1,079,000 were reported with 15- to 19-year-olds accounting for one-third of these.[12] Illegal abortion was most frequently found among married women in low income groups, at the mid-childbearing period.

Experience has shown the safety of early termination of pregnancy, with risk increasing as the pregnancy progresses: the risk is three to four times higher in the second trimester than in the first.[13] Early abortion may be accomplished safely in ambulatory care facilities. Of increasing interest is very early abortion, sometimes called menstrual regulation since it is not possible to establish pregnancy at that point. This is performed within 14 days after expected menstruation, which involves very little danger and allows procedures that can be tolerated by very young women. It may also be more acceptable to those whose attitudes toward abortion are ambiguous.

Abortion involves complex legal issues, balancing the rights of the woman and of the unborn child, often vacillating between medical and moral considerations. As abortion becomes a recognized and respectable medical intervention within a wider range of services, its procedures have been refined and regulated. However, abortion services have not kept pace with the demand for such care.

INFERTILITY AS WELL AS OVERFERTILITY CAN BE A PROBLEM

In 1976 about 6.9 million couples, or 25 per cent of all married couples with the wife of childbearing age, had fecundity impairments.[14] The causes of infertility are numerous, and to arrive at an evaluation and possible corrective measure usually requires extensive study of both husband and wife. Problems include physical anomalies, obstruction of the fallopian tube, hormonal deficiencies, chronic alcoholism, exposure to excessive radiation, or inadequate number or vitality of sperm in the semen. The likelihood of conception varies with the age of the couple, the frequency of intercourse and the length of exposure. Emotional disorders or menstrual stress may also be factors.

Couples should understand that infertility is correctable in many instances, although 5 to 10 per cent of all married couples probably cannot conceive. They must realize the complexity of identifying the cause, and the importance of their own observations and participation in arriving at a diagnosis. New knowledge of hormonal effects and the potentials of artificial insemination may bring hope to childless families. Also, for some infertile couples, adoption may be an acceptable alternative.

RESOURCES FOR FAMILY PLANNING ASSISTANCE HAVE INCREASED DRAMATICALLY

Despite the rapid growth of facilities, services are not yet reaching all those who need them, or are not available early enough to provide for optimum use of contraceptive measures, or for very early pregnancy care.

As stated in the Surgeon General's Report of 1979, in the United States there are an estimated 6,000 clinics providing family planning services. Although 80 per cent of married women aged 15 to 44 are contraceptive users, 25 per cent of sexually active unmarried women aged 15 to 19 never use contraceptives and about 45 per cent of them only occasionally.[15]

Family physicians have traditionally supplied some fertility control or birth control services to their patients. In the past, such information tended to flow to the middle and upper income level families, whereas the *need* was highest among low income groups, who had neither the money nor the sophistication to secure such services. Today, care is being extended to a much larger population: national emphasis has moved family planning into standard medical practice and created organized resources specially designed to serve those desiring care but not previously reached.

In the future, efforts will probably incorporate family planning and population control measures into general health services such as maternity care and mental health and health advisory services rather than relying on separate facilities and agencies. This should ensure broader and more efficient coverage.

THE ROLE OF THE COMMUNITY HEALTH NURSE IN FAMILY PLANNING

There are many ways in which the community health nurse may participate in family planning and population control activities — whether as a direct participant in a family planning center or as a catalyst, linking people to appropriate services of help and supplying specialized agencies with needed information about families and communities. The school nurse has access to the students, many of whom are beginning sexual activity, and their parents, who may be finding it difficult to accept the "new morality" — an important group to reach.

Opportunities for uncovering needs, for counseling, and for referral are plentiful in the course of providing care in maternal health facilities or industrial or school services. In general, community health nursing efforts may be directed toward the following:

1. Identifying, counseling, and, when appropriate, making referrals for people who desire and are not now receiving information or services in family planning.

2. Providing and interpreting family planning instruction or community resources to those families needing, contemplating, initiating, or maintaining fertility control measures.

3. Contributing to the development of new services or methods, and evaluating these services and methods in the light of the specific population groups being served.

Some Trends and Indicators in Family Planning

The unmet need may be computed in many ways — e.g., by atypical birth rates in given populations, by surveys of those regulating abortion or sample surveys of specific populations, and by counting unwanted births. These calculations may be more useful in groups than with individual families, since it is the desires and the values of a particular family that function as the criteria.

The expected family size in the United States is close to the replacement level of 2.1 children per family. Trends in the birth rate from 1910 to 1976 are shown in Figure 25–1. The graph shows a steeply declining course from 1910 to the 1930's. There was a brief upswing in the period after World War II (the so-called "baby boom"), but the curve rapidly resumed its downward path. This consistent decline, combined with the current pattern of smaller families, suggests that control of fertility has already been accepted as general practice.

Despite this drop, the size of the population in the United States will *increase* in the immediate future, as the post-war boom babies reach childbearing age. Until they move beyond this stage and the smaller cohorts of childbearing age take over, the lowered fertility rate is not likely to be reflected in population figures.

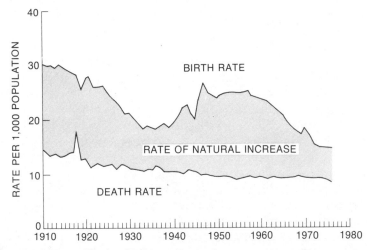

Figure 25–1   Rates of births, deaths, and natural increases: United States, 1910–1976.

Reaching Out to Those Who Need Help

For some members of the population, offering or making services available is not enough; many need to be sought out. Typical groups with special needs include those with a history of unwanted children; debilitated women or those with serious chronic illness or adverse genetic histories; couples who have their desired number of children; families with grossly inadequate general health care (often also the lowest income families); members of ethnic groups where parental attitudes toward childbearing and family size differ from those of adolescents or young adults in the family.

People may be reluctant or distrustful about using available facilities, shy about discussing their problems, or avoiding contraceptives in the erroneous belief that they represent a threat to their sexuality. Edmands found that many mothers in low income groups felt it was difficult to raise questions and appreciated having the nurse or other worker initiate the discussion.[16] Sometimes clients hesitate to talk with a nurse whose name suggests she may be a Catholic, or a client of that faith may not wish to make overt inquiries (although a substantial number of those using contraceptive facilities are Catholics).

Alternatively, some clients are afraid that the nurse will try to put pressure on them to take some action they do not want to take: one woman living on welfare said to the author, "Having babies is one thing *nobody* can stop me from doing!" Reassurance that decisions are the prerogative of the family and that the professional is a source of information rather than of harassment may in itself be helpful. "Outreach" strategies — taking the initiative without preempting the families' right to decide — are important.

Setting up various lines of communication is a good tactic. The teachers of adolescent-aged students, family physicians, and personnel officers in industry all may pass the word to people who have never before been contacted. The nurse can let it be known that information and advice are available about fertility control in the course of other services; the word will spread. Special programs for groups in low-income neighborhoods can also help. For instance, one health department, working directly with prostitutes, combined surveillance for sexually transmitted diseases with instruction or referral for control of conception. Sometimes surveys taken within groups under general care may be useful to help determine the unmet need for care — high school or grammar school students, for example, or maternity patients, or clients in a neighborhood clinic. The nurse should be alert, too, for couples who may want help with problems of infertility.

Above all, it is important to remember that *placing and keeping clients under care is essential:* strategic assistance can help reinforce the skills of family problem solving, help avoid unwanted births, and help prevent needless sterility.

Helping Families Evaluate the Options

Helping families ascertain all the possible avenues of fertility control — from no controls at all to sterilization — may help them in making their decisions. Before making any determinations, families have the right to all relevant information. They should know that there is no such thing as a perfect or foolproof method for control of fertility, and they should be advised of the relative effectiveness of all methods. They should be told about side effects, possible interference with sexual activity, and the range of dangers involved. They need to consider the acceptability of one or another method to *them.* For example, some couples or individuals may not be concerned that a particular method is coitus related, while others may feel that use of the condom or diaphragm destroys the spontaneity and enjoyment of sex. Others may fear the risks involved in using the pill, despite the relatively small percentage of that risk. Some couples or individuals may eagerly opt for sterilization despite the fact that it is at this time considered irreversible, while others will be haunted by doubts and pessimistic worries: "What would we do if we lost one of the children?" Some may consider themselves "less" of a man or a woman if they choose sterilization.

The worker must guard against unconscious bias that leads her to advocate a particular method or prevents discussion of the option of no controls. For example, some groups feel that excessive persuasion is used with welfare patients or with mentally retarded individuals. Some specific ethnic groups may even fear that fertility control represents an attempt at genocide. Implicit in all policy and program statements for family planning is that the choice to use or not to use, or the selection of one method over another, must rest with the client. The professional's only obligation is to make sure that any decision is an informed one. Aggressive procedures are useless in this deeply personal aspect of family life. Calmness and patience must be observed in all deliberations.

In the case of abortion, the situation can be particularly tense. Careful and unhurried pre-abortion counseling is imperative. Even under the best of circumstances, anxiety is inevitable, and there are usually unexpected feelings of guilt or bereavement after the abortion. It is important that there be ample opportunity for the client to express her feelings and to talk them out thoroughly. Gedan points out that adolescents may resist doing all the revealing, and that the most effective counseling can be accomplished by "a conversation between equals."[17] Sometimes clients will respond as they think they are *expected* to respond, agreeing verbally but never intending to follow the plans or program they are working out with the nurse or social worker.

The client considering abortion may truly fear the wrath of parents or husband; or the condemnation of a family physician or religious adviser; she may confuse legal authorities with the agency which the worker represents. The pregnant woman may be reluctant to involve her partner in the decision to seek abortion, when in fact he may feel deep concern and be anxious to share in the decision. Abortion is an issue which invariably involves more than just one individual: when treated as a problem to be solved by the couple or by the whole family, the decision may strengthen rather than weaken affectional bonds.

The individual must be prepared, too, for less than excellent care. Facilities may be overcrowded, personnel poorly equipped to handle the emotional aspects of the problem, the process of qualifying for care and arranging payment may be tedious. The nurse should prepare the client for such a situation by building support *outside* the hospital or clinic. The patient should know that all possible options for action and for care have been examined and that the best available facilities have been secured.

Infertile couples also need support. The couple may find infertility an embarrassing topic to discuss: inability to conceive often presents a powerful threat to the individual's sense of identity. There may be great reluctance to bring these concerns into the open, or one partner, in an effort to reassure the other, will deny feelings of unhappiness or loss. Skill in eliciting feelings as well as facts is important. Infertile couples who do not respond to treatment may rush into adoption proceedings without first studying or resolving their own feelings of inadequacy or frustration. They should be encouraged to make this decision with great caution and deliberation.

Continuing surveillance may be maintained by the clinic or other facility or may be primarily assumed by the community health nurse for some or all of those using organized family planning services. The community nurse may also work with private physicians in following up cases.

The first year after institution of some program of fertility control is the most critical. Most "drop-outs" occur during that period. A 1970 national study indicated that, in the case of oral contraceptives, 16 per cent discontinued taking the pills during the first three months, and 41 per cent had discontinued at one year.[18]

Discontinuance may be associated with bleeding or spotting, difficulty in establishing a regular menstrual cycle, fear of cancer or other serious disease because of publicized reports. Some clients feel they have been pressured into going to the clinic and reassert their independence by resisting the prescribed regimen. In some instances, control measures were discontinued because pregnancy occurred despite the pill or device. In view of this, it is a good idea to be sure contraceptive users know just how to call for help if anything goes wrong.

Some who continue and then stop the control procedures may have decided to have a child, in which case the family should be prepared to seek prenatal care early in the pregnancy.

Another critical point in general surveillance is the time families have achieved the desired number of children. This is a point at which couples may wish to consider a change in the method of fertility control they have been using. It may take time for the couple to talk through their feelings about permanent control via sterilization or other recommended changes in treatment. Acceptance of permanent infertility may at first seem like a threat to manhood or to femininity. However, the relative risks of childbirth for older women should be explained to help them make an informed decision. Information about the costs of different methods, the effects on sexuality, and so forth may be important.

THE COMMUNITY HEALTH NURSE MAY ADD TO KNOWLEDGE IN THE FIELD OF FERTILITY REGULATION

Through observation and analysis made in the course of providing care, the community health nurse may discover interesting clues to reproductive behavior. Studying the incidence and nature of side effects of different oral contraceptives used by her clients may reveal new evidence. Do certain types of women tend to have more side effects than others using the same drug? Why are some more able than others to follow the prescribed regimen? Why do some women continue with the prescribed treatment even though uncomfortable side effects persist? What motivates people to seek help with fertility regulation? Why does the woman who has steadily resisted advice on fertility control through eleven births suddenly say "enough!" and request the help she has so stoutly refused before? Why do some young and vigorous people seek sterilization?

The community health nurse must use a variety of strategies — initiating action; providing data on needs, or knowledge of the needy to specialized groups; using group approaches or individual family methods; talking, listening, doing, and referring. As noted earlier, nursing efforts in fertility control will for the most part be an integral part of other services to families — maternal and child health care, school health services, health education efforts, and disease control projects.

The enlistment of clients to help disseminate information is especially valuable in this field. The man who has had a vasectomy or the woman who has had a tubal ligation may be willing to explain it to others; a sexually active teenager who has recognized her own responsibility to protect herself against unwanted pregnancy may be willing to lead a discussion of her peers.

Family planning control is an excellent vehicle for other health care service. Post-abortion care provides a good opportunity to discuss not only contraception but also general family communication problems, the importance of early maternity care, the need for objective consideration of health problems, the value and characteristics of à healthy sexuality, parent-child relationships. Screening for cervical cancer and for sexually transmitted disease, checking on blood pressure, and general nutrition level may also be included. Sometimes, however, nurses become overenthusiastic in the course of collecting information. It is important to set reasonable limits on demands for clients' time. The object of the nursing effort is to help, not impose.

Widespread and intelligent control of fertility can contribute to the realization of national goals and policies. There are many advantages, both physical and emotional: within the family, it may contribute to happier and richer family life; for the individual, it may lead to a sense of being in control of one's life, to a healthier sexuality, and to a sense of meeting one's responsibilities to the community. Family planning support is an essential part of community health nursing practice.

REFERENCES

1. *Population and the American Future: Report of the Commission on Population Growth and the American Future.* Washington, D.C., U.S. Government Printing Office, 1972, p. 22.
2. Ibid., p. 13.
3. Quoted in *Association for Voluntary Sterilization News*, March 1975, p. 4.
4. *To Form a More Perfect Union: Report of the National Commission of the Observance of International Women's Year, 1976.* Washington, D.C. Script Doc., 1976, pp. 267–268.
5. Edmands, E.: A study of contraceptive practices in a selected group of urban Negro mothers in Baltimore. Am. J. Pub. Health, 58:263, 1968.
6. U.S. Bureau of the Census: Population estimates and projections, *Current Population Reports*, Series P-25, No. 704, Washington, D.C., U.S. Government Printing Office, July 1977.
7. Ibid.
8. Advance data from *Vital and Health Statistics*, National Center for Health Statistics, U.S. DHEW, No. 56, January, 1980.
9. Advance data from *Vital and Health Statistics*, National Center for Health Statistics, U.S. DHEW, PHS, No. 36, August 18, 1978, p. 2.
10. Advance data from *Vital and Health Statistics*, National Center for Health Statistics, U.S. DHEW, PHS, No. 40, September 22, 1978, p. 2.
11. Ibid., No. 36 (August 18, 1978), p. 2.
12. *Healthy People, Surgeon General's Report*, DHEW, Pub. No. 79–55071, p. 84, 1979.
13. American Public Health Association: *Recommended Program Guide for Abortion Services*, Washington, D.C., 1972.
14. *Advance data, National Center for Health Statistics*, U.S. DHEW, No. 55, January 24, 1980.
15. *Healthy People, Surgeon General's Report.* U.S. DHEW, PHS, Pub. No. 79–55071, p. 85, 1979.
16. Edmands, p. 58.
17. Gedan, S.: Abortion counseling with adolescents. Am. J. Nurs., 74:1856, 1974.
18. Sear, A. M., and Turner, M. N.: Factors associated with short term oral contraceptive discontinuation. Fam. Plan. Persp., 6:230, 1974.

SUGGESTED READINGS

American Public Health Association, Program Area Committee on Population and Public Health: *Family Planning: A Guide for State and Local Agencies.* New York, American Public Health Association, 1968.

American Public Health Association: *Recommended Program Guide for Voluntary Sterilization.* Am. J. Pub. Health, *62*:1265, 1972.

Anonymous: Does Anyone Care? Am. J. Nurs., *73*:1562, 1973.

Association for Voluntary Sterilization: *The Case for Voluntary Sterilization.* New York, 1971.

Cohn, H. D., and Lieberman, E.: Family planning and health: Congruent objectives of Malthus and Spock. Am. J. Pub. Health, *64*:225, 1974.

Corey, M.: United States organized family planning programs in fiscal year 1974. Fam. Plan. Persp., *7*:98, 1975.

Davis, J. E.: Vasectomy. Am. J. Nurs., *72*:509, 1972.

Doran, C.: Attitude of thirty American Indian women toward birth control. Health Ser. Rep., *87*:658, 1972.

Edmands, E. M.: A study of contraceptive practices in a selected group of urban Negro mothers in Baltimore. Am. J. Pub. Health, *58*:263, 1968.

Ennis, B., and Siegel, L.: *The Rights of Mental Patients.* New York, Avon Books, 1973, pp. 1 and 25.

Finkel, M. L., and Finkel, D. J.: Sexual contraceptive knowledge, attitudes and behavior of male adolescents. Fam. Plan. Persp., *7*:256, 1975.

Fischman, S. H., et al.: Nurse-midwifery and family planning in the United States: Data from the 1976–1977 American College of Nurse-Midwive's study. Adv. Plan. Parent, *13*:78, 1978.

Freeman, E. W.: Abortion: Subjective attitudes and feelings. Fam. Plan. Persp., *10*:150, 1978.

Furstenberg, F. F., and Crawford, A. G.: Family support: Helping teenage mothers to cope. Fam. Plan. Persp., *10*:322, 1978.

Gedan, S.: Abortion counseling with adolescents. Am. J. Nurs., *74*:1856, 1974.

Gilbert, S.: Artificial insemination. Am. J. Nurs., *76*:259, 1976.

Goldstein, P. J., and Zalar, M. K.: The family planning nurse specialist. Am. J. Obstet. Gynecol., *114*:646, 1972.

Gonzales, B.: Voluntary sterilization. Am. J. Nurs., *70*:2581, 1970.

Hanlon, J. J.: *Public Health Administration and Practice,* 6th ed. St. Louis, Mo., C. V. Mosby Co., 1974, Chapter 4.

Howard, J., and Roule, K.: A survey of public health nurses' knowledge and attitudes about family planning. Am. J. Pub. Health, *62*:962, 1972.

Huvall, L. K.: Issues in contraception: Today's pill and the individual women. MCN, *2*:359, 1977.

Kaufman, S. A.: *New Help for Childless Couples.* New York, Simon and Schuster, 1965.

Kelly, M.: Birthright—an alternative to abortion. Am. J. Nurs., *75*:76, 1975.

Kistner, R. W.: The infertile woman. Am. J. Nurs., *73*:1937, 1973.

Manisoff, M.: *Family Planning: A Teaching Guide for Nurses,* 3rd ed. Planned Parenthood Federation of America, Inc., 1972.

Manning, B. E.: RESOLVE — A support group for infertile couples. Am. J. Nurs., *76*:258, 1976.

McCallister, D., Thiessen, V., and McDermott, M.: *Readings in Family Planning: A Challenge to the Health Professions.* St. Louis, Mo., C. V. Mosby Co., 1973.

Ogg, E.: *Voluntary Sterilization* (Public Affairs Pamphlet #507). New York, Public Affairs Pamphlets, 1974.

Omran, A. R., et al.: *Family Formation Patterns and Health, An International Collaborative Study in India, Iran, Lebanon, Philippines, and Turkey.* Geneva, World Health Organization, 1976, Ch. 8.

Park, C. B., Han, S. H., and Choe, M. K.: The effect of infant death on subsequent fertility in Korea and the role of family planning. Am. J. Pub. Health, *69*:557, 1979.

Selle, H. F., Holmes, D. W., and Ingbar, M. L.: The growing demand for midtrimester amniocentesis: A systems approach to forecasting the need for facilities. Am. J. Pub. Health, *69*:576, 1979.

Stolley, P. D., et al.: Thrombosis with low-estrogen oral contraceptives. Am. J. Epidemiol., *102*:197, 1975.

Taylor, D.: Contraceptive counseling and care. *In* Mercer, R. T.: *Perspectives on Adolescent Health Care.* Philadelphia, J. B. Lippincott, 1979.

Turner, C., and Darity, W. A.: Fears of genocide among black Americans as related to age, sex, region. Am. J. Pub. Health, *63*:1029, 1973.

Van Ginneken, J.: Prolonged breastfeeding as a birth spacing method. Studies Fam. Plan., *5*:201, 1974.

Wallace, H. M., Gold, E. M., and Dooley, S.: Relationships between family planning and maternal and child health. Am. J. Pub. Health, 59:1355, 1969.
World Health Organization: *Family Planning in the Education of Nurses and Midwives.* Geneva, Public Health Papers #53, World Health Organization, 1973.
World Health Organization, Expert Committee: *Family Planning in Health Services.* Technical Report Series, 476, 1971.

RESOURCES

Planned Parenthood Foundation of America
810 7th Avenue
New York, NY 10019
> Local groups — check the telephone directory: information, publications, community action groups, national and local programs, research.

Association for Voluntary Sterilization
708 3rd Avenue
New York, NY 10017
> Publications, information, research, political action.

Birthright: offices in most large cities. Help to unwed pregnant girls to secure nursing care so that they can have their babies (as alternative to abortion). Individual units vary widely in services offered.

State and local Health Department family planning services.

CHAPTER **26**

SPECIAL
COMMUNITIES

For the most part the communities (or populations) with which the community health nurse works are defined by geographic, political, or social boundaries and are inclusive of all individuals within that area. However, there are some "special" populations — communities within communities, with which community members identify — that are capable of generating as well as moderating problems in health maintenance care. These special populations may include the following:

1. Ethnic groups — American Indians, Spanish-speaking populations, black populations, and groups with strong second country affiliation such as descendants of Indochinese, Chinese, or Central European immigrants— who want to preserve their cultural "roots."

Such identification is generally considered a helpful way to promote group pride and identity. It is no longer imperative to "talk American" as soon as possible after immigration, nor is it necessary to feel ashamed of acting in "old country" ways. The old goal of the melting pot has been replaced by an appreciation of the values of preserving the differences among the diverse cultural segments of the population.

2. Groups sharing economic or social deprivation — e.g., deteriorated or poverty-stricken neighborhoods, homeless or drifting populations (such as those in skid row) who congregate for mutual support, and impoverished marginal farmers or other rural dwellers who lack adequate support — and groups trying new patterns of development and distribution of "wealth".

3. Work groups: employees in industrial plants or large mechanized farms, migrant workers, or school populations.

4. Groups in total care facilities, such as a nursing home population, prison populations, and some military units.

In general community health practice, work with one or more of these special communities is to be expected. For example, on a daily basis, the community health nurse may be in contact with families of an ethnic origin different from her own.

These special population segments may represent one facet of the work of the community health nurse, or they may constitute her full-time work load. In either case, it is necessary to study and understand these communities, to clarify their impact on the overall health care effort, to develop adaptations of services to accommodate their needs, and to relate them to the population as a whole.

In working with such special populations, the primary consideration is: How do the factors that establish group identity affect the health and health care needs of individuals and their families?" The family living in poverty may gain strength from others, or may cooperate with one another for improvement of the situation. Learning how to "make it" with too little of everything is a skill that can be shared with other groups and with health professionals. Other families in similar circumstances may feel defeated, helpless, inert, and despairing. Membership in a particular cultural group, such as an American Indian or black community, may build pride and self-confidence in the individual; on the other hand, such membership may have a negative effect. The prison experience affects individuals very differently, but its importance as a community force cannot be questioned.

A second consideration is what resources exist in these special populations for improvement of the general health conditions? Can this experience offer education and support leading to better health practices that will carry over to life "outside"? Can the industrial plant "host" a cancer detection clinic for the spouses of employees, support public health programs, participate in epidemiological studies of working populations? Can the schools help with community programs to deal with adolescent pregnancy or sexually-transmitted disease?

It is important to ask, "Does this particular group have problems that differ from those of the general population?" For example, it has been clearly shown that those living in poverty are subject to greater incidence of illness and malnutrition, and are less likely to seek out available care than are some other population groups. Coal miners have a special society milieu, as well as a shared danger and pride in their work, that affects the kinds of help they are willing to use, the nature of family life, and the satisfactions for which they strive. Prisoners, deprived of the presence of family and friends, and unable to control their activities, may feel hostile, frustrated, and helpless.

Most special groups have strengths as well as problems to impart to their members. The ability to *survive* among the very poor — the ingenuity, the closeness to one another that sometimes exists, has a real potential for mutual help. The hardihood of the very old is a constant surprise. Unexpected strengths may appear when the population is seen in the light of its own goals and values.

Another important consideration for the community health nurse is her obligation to recognize the similarities and differences between her values and those of the special group with which she is working. Working with culturally diverse groups challenges the nurse's own cultural convictions and enables her to re-evaluate values in light of human needs. The nurse should not feel it is necessary to take on the attitudes, habits, or beliefs of the special populations she is working with in order to be accepted by them. In fact, knowing and accepting one's own values is an important first step in working effectively with special communities.

In dealing with special communities, the community health nurse will be concerned with the following:

1. Analyzing the population, based on statistical information as well as on comments from members and group leaders.
2. Defining special health problems or hazards arising from or associated with the environment and/or living habits, as well as identifying resources.
3. Setting goals and priorities with leaders of the group and other concerned citizens, based on needs of the community.
4. Providing services in ways sensitive to the different cultural values and attitudes of the special community and appreciating the value differences between herself and these special groups.
5. Evaluating the impact of nursing services on the special community.

The discussion of special communities that follows serves as a sampling of frequently encountered groups.

Ethnic Communities [1]

If community health nurses are indeed population-oriented, the identification of population characteristics of a particular ethnic group is important for developing nursing programs. The community health nurse should view these biological and cultural variations as they relate to health care, avoiding stereotyped images of ethnic groups and appreciating the rich variations among peoples.

Biologic Variations. Frequently occurring differences among ethnic groups are skin color and hair texture, facial features, bone and body structure and size, rate of growth for children, and susceptibility or resistance to certain diseases.

Pigment in the skin and texture of the hair require different kinds of care and observational skills. Redness cannot be observed easily on dark skin, thus the nurse must rely on such indicators as pain, or warmth or tenderness for detection of inflammatory process. Anemia may be assessed by observing the conjuctive and buccal mucosa as well as ashen skin color.[2]

Physical growth and development are different among cultural groups. Oriental children might appear unusually small if norms for this group were not known in contrast to Caucasian norms. Studies have shown black children to be taller, heavier, and to have greater motor achievement than white children of the same age.[3]   Susceptibility to certain diseases is also a known cultural event. Sickle cell disease and hypertension in blacks, Tay-Sachs disease, Buerger's disease in Jews, myopia in Chinese, increased susceptibility to tuberculosis in blacks and American Indians, and diabetes mellitus in American Indians and Jews are well documented. Different rates of specific types of cancer have also been found to be associated with different ethnic origin. Inherited resistance to selected diseases is also important. Black Americans have a low incidence of multiple sclerosis and skin cancer. American Indians have a low incidence of duodenal ulcers. The low incidence of heart disease in Orientals is being investigated as well.[4]

Cultural Variations.   Food preferences, beliefs about birth and death, responses to pain, health practices and body care, role of the family, and words and concepts used to identify problems are related to the subculture we belong to.

Mexican Americans who follow cultural beliefs use "hot" and "cold" food as healing methods for specific illness.[5] A similar theory is followed by Chinese Americans in meal preparation — i.e., Yin (cold) and Yang (hot). A hot diet is offered postpartum, since a woman is in a "cold" condition due to blood loss. Fruits, vegetables, and cold drinks — Yin foods — would be avoided. Adherence to specified treatments depends on how these treatments fit into the hot/cold theory of these cultures.

Encouraging families to use more milk in their diet may have deleterious effects among blacks and American Indians. The incidence of lactose enzyme deficiency is high in these groups, and ingestion of milk may cause increased production of gas. Depending on the environment and culture, certain foods that are usually considered to be essential may not be readily available. It is important to assess the total intake before judging a particular diet as inadequate.

Birth and death have important implications along with diverse rituals, according to a group's cultural norms. The nurse must be sensitive to the various cultural implications if she is to give the necessary supportive care. The Jewish briss (ceremony of male circumcision performed eight days after birth) and the different meaning of death for certain Indian tribes are examples of these.[6] For oriental families, pregnancy and birth are considered a dangerous period during which the mother and child must be guarded by specific rituals.[7]

The health care practices and folk care beliefs of certain communities may differ from the "germ" theory of western Anglo-Saxon medicine. Frequently, health care is mixed with religious significance, disease may be punishment for being out of harmony with nature or for bad behavior.[8]

Many "counter-culture" communities have developed their own

healing methods. For these groups, aspects of Chinese, native American, chiropractic and homeopathic medicine have been incorporated into beliefs about health care. For example, diet therapy must be consistent with "low" or "high" vibrations for that cultural group or the therapy will be disregarded.

Women of many cultures find it impossible to use birth control devices and methods or to seek care for themselves and their children, unless their husband or other significant family member gives them permission to do so. Patterns of family interaction are different in all cultures and must be respected and worked with. In Latino-Chicano families, family and kinship extends beyond the immediate family to encompass in-laws, grandparents, and the "compadre system" — i.e., godparents and good friends. Family roles are clearly defined in terms of male dominance and respect for elders. The community health nurse must recognize these roles and take care not to expect individuals to act contrary to traditional norms. She needs to ascertain who has the decision-making role, and then work with this person.

DEVELOPING A PROGRAM

In developing a nursing program, the community health nurse will work *with* community groups in defining their needs and goals. Part of this process will involve identification of group leaders (such as other health workers, religious persons, or school teachers) who are interested and involved in determining needs, goals, and resources and who are willing to work to see these goals accomplished. Giving recognition to those who have traditionally provided health care (such as "granny" midwives and medicine men) will strengthen the program and facilitate case-finding efforts. The community health nurse will need to identify demographic characteristics; special health problems; usual economic, educational, and work patterns; folk beliefs and practices; and attitudes toward existing health care resources.

The literature is replete with information for many special groups, especially black and Hispanic groups. The American Indians are presented as an example of the nursing process.

American Indians: A Case in Point[10]

There are nearly 700,000 Indians and native Alaskans in this country — many of whom are living on federal Indian reservations and in remote rural communities, maintaining much of their traditional culture. In recent years, younger families have been moving to the cities in search of employment.

Analysis of Population. The characteristics of the native American population are quite different from those of the general population.

Almost half of the native Americans are below the age of 18, the median age being 18.6. Only 11 per cent of native Americans are 55 years or older, a figure much lower than that of the general population.[11] The total birth rate for Indian women 15 to 44 years of age (as of 1976) is 30.7 per 1,000 population, which is greater than the overall United States rate of 14.7 per 1,000 population.[12] The post-neonatal death rate is also high — 10.1 per 1,000 live births in 1976 — primarily as a result of pneumonia, diarrhea, and other infectious diseases.[13]

Special Health Problems.   Certain health problems are of special concern. These are accidents, alcoholism, depression, and other mental health problems, maternal and child health deficiencies, poor nutrition, and problems of aging. Trachoma and tuberculosis are much more prevalent in the American Indian population than in the general population, as is diabetes mellitus. The generally low level of education, high level of unemployment, poor housing and sanitation, and unsafe water supply are all linked to these special health problems.[14]

Deaths due to accidents, cirrhosis of the liver, homicide, and suicide accounted for 34 per cent of the crude death rate in 1975. These four causes of death are frequently related to alcoholism and have a large degree of human participation, an important aspect in planning nursing care.[15]

Resources.   There are many positive cultural resources in this special population as well. The strength of the family, tribal solidarity, the religious philosophy of living in harmony with nature, and much of traditional Indian medicine have value for health efforts with this community.

Recognition of the medicine man and the belief in the supernatural cause of illness can be blended with the needed immunizations, mental health programs, and maternal and child health programs, making these activities more acceptable to the Indian population. Special ceremonies — such as holy day feasts, healing ceremonies, the menstrual ceremony for protecting the woman and family from danger, the blessing way, and the first anniversary after the death of a villager — must be observed. Certain tribes believe that the expectant woman should not discuss or make plans for the unborn child because a tragedy may befall the fetus. The community health nurse will need to find ways of working with this cultural fact to provide needed health care.

The American Indians' use of folk medicine does not mean a rejection of Western medicine as effective, but simply a desire to utilize all measures available to them. Cultural taboos and traditions may at times be in conflict with recognized Western medicine. When family members react to this, there is a tendency to label them as uncooperative. It is up to the community health nurse to use every method to enhance communication and understanding at this time.

The nurse needs to determine the usual activities of the patient and family. Is the family dependent on rug weaving or do they herd sheep? Do they live in a hogan, cabin, mobile trailer, or government housing? Is there running water, heat and refrigeration? Who makes the decisions about health care in the family—the husband, grandmother, or medicine man? The answers to these questions determine how the family and the nurse will plan and work toward health.

Access to health and social services is often limited for the American Indian population. Many of the reservations and communities are located in isolated, rugged areas. For native Alaskans, transportation is made more difficult due to lack of roads. The Indian Health Service (IHS), a branch of the U. S. Public Health Service Administration, is the main provider of health services. The IHS offers a variety of services including preventive programs, environmental services, dental health, mental health, public health nursing, health education, and hospital and clinic services.

Although many services are provided on the reservations and innovative efforts have been made to provide services where they are needed, access and acceptability of health care services remain a problem. The health needs of this population continue to outweigh the number and types of services provided as well as the numbers of qualified persons to provide the services, despite the efforts of both government and private organizations.

Many initiatives have been taken to recruit native Americans for careers in health. Included among these are nursing programs within associate and baccalaureate degree programs, and allied health programs in a variety of disciplines such as dentistry, social work, and medicine.[16] The Indian Health Service also takes advantage of other federal legislation, such as the Area Health Education Centers (AHEC), in providing trained medical personnel to work in underserved areas.

Tribal organizations and local community leaders are becoming more actively involved in determining health needs, resources, and planning of health affairs. In the past decade, tribally established community health boards have helped develop local program policy, determine needs and priorities, and allocate resources. There is also a National Indian Health Board, the National Tribal Chairmen's Association, and the National Congress of American Indians having impact on health issues at the national level. There are also native corporations for regional areas, such as the United Southeastern Tribes, that manage and provide a variety of health services. These and other groups, especially at the local level, will need to be consulted and worked with if the community health nurse is going to effect a useful strategy for delivering her services.

PROVIDING SERVICES SENSITIVE TO THE BELIEFS OF OTHERS

All people share an interest in health and illness, but individuals from different cultures tend to perceive situations in terms of their own complex cultural traditions. When clients' expectations differ from those who are providing services, failure to accept available health services is likely to occur. If practitioners have an understanding of the values of their clients and a positive attitude and respect for them, the potential for identifying ways of providing services acceptable to others is greater. If practitioners disregard established health customs, clients may avoid them.

Encouraging folk medical healers to participate in helping families with health problems and accepting the need for certain ancient rituals are ways of being supportive to the family and encouraging positive health practices.

Cultural variation in regard to health beliefs and health seeking behavior are great. Some subgroups are more "middle class" in their attitudes and practices, while other groups will follow strict tradition. There can be as much variation among peoples of a designated culture as between peoples of different cultures.

EVALUATING THE IMPACT OF SERVICES

The community health nurse must always be critical of the services she provides. Good intentions and "missionary zeal" can lead to negative outcomes if they are not accompanied with sound planning, consideration, and acceptance of others' cultural values. Large differences in mortality rates from specific diseases will take time to remedy, especially if there are no significant changes in economic or living conditions. The nurse will need to set realistic goals with clients, families, and local groups, and measure success in relation to them.

In working with different cultures and communities, the nurse is concerned with cultural components in etiology and incidence of disease as well as with the behavior of people in the face of illness and their coping abilities with everyday problems. The emphasis should be on determining what people want and aiding them in the process of obtaining their goals rather than on working for predetermined goals. The nurse must consider the position of women, along with that of nurses, in different subcultures and the political structure influencing decision making.

The individual nurse needs to discover what the value similarities and differences are between her cultural orientation and the subculture she is working with. She must learn to respect each value system and look for ways of creating a dynamic interaction of both. Such a transaction enables the nurse to develop as a person as well as to better determine the work expectations of the special community under her care.

REFERENCES: ETHNIC COMMUNITIES

1. The authors wish to thank Patricia Deiman, Nurse Consultant, Division of Nursing, Bureau of Health Professions, HRA, DHHS, for her assistance in the preparation of the section on ethnic communities.
2. Roach, L.: Assessment: Color changes in dark skin. Nursing, 72:2, 1972.
3. Pediatric Multiphasic Program—Height and weight of 7,500 children of three skin colors. Am. J. Dis. Child., *124*:866, 1972.
4. Branch, M. F., and Paxton, P. P.: *Providing Safe Nursing Care for Ethnic People of Color.* New York, Appleton-Century-Crofts, 1976, p. 11.
5. Abril, I.: Mexican American folk beliefs—How they affect health care. MCN, 2:168, 1977.
6. Primeaux, M.: Caring for the American Indian patient. Am. J. Nurs., 77:91, 1977.
7. Chung, H. J.: Understanding the Oriental maternity patient. Nurs. Clin. North Am., *12*:72, 1977.
8. Snow, L.: Folk medical beliefs and their implications for care of patients. Ann. Int. Med., *81*:82, 1974.
9. Byerly, E., Molgaard, C., and Snow, C.: Dissonance in the Desear: What to do with the Goldenseal? Presented to the Fourth National Transcultural Nursing Conference, Snowbird, Utah, September 1978.
10. The authors wish to acknowledge the assistance of Rosemary Wood, Chief Nurse, Indian Health Service, Public Health Service, Department of Health and Human Services.
11. Public Health Service, Department of Health, Education, and Welfare: *Indian Health Program.* Washington, D.C., U.S. Government Printing Office, p. 20.
12. Ibid.
13. Primeaux, p. 58.
14. *Indian Health Program*, p. 9.
15. Wood, R.: Newsletter from the Chief Nurse. Indian Health Service, Feb. 23, 1977, pp. 4–5.
16. *Indian Health Program*, pp. 12–16.

SUGGESTED READINGS

Abrahams, R.: *Positively Black*, Englewood Cliffs, N.J. Prentice-Hall, Inc. 1950.
Bass, M. A., and Wakefield, L. M.: Nutrient intake and food patterns of Indians on Standing Rock reservation. J. Am. Diet Assoc., *64*:36, 1974.
Bauwens, E. E. (ed.): *The Anthropology of Health*, St. Louis, Mo., C. V. Mosby, 1978.
Bazell, R.: Health care: What the poor people didn't get from the Kentucky Project. Science, *172*:458, 1971.
Bello, T. A.: The third dimension: Cultural sensitivity in nursing practice. Imprint, *23*:36, 1976.
Blackfeather, J.: Community health nursing—Indian health. Imprint, 27:34, 1980.
Boxof, R. P.: The Navajo attitudes toward available medical care. Am. J. Pub. Health, *62*:1620, 1972.
Bramley, D. G., and Longino, C. F. (eds.): *White Racism and Black Americans.* Cambridge, Mass., Schenkman Publishing Co., Inc., 1972.
Branch, M. F., and Paxton, P. P.: *Providing Safe Nursing Care for Ethnic People of Color.* New York, Appleton-Century-Crofts, 1976.
Brink, P.: *Transcultural Nursing—A Book of Readings.* Englewood Cliffs, N.J., Prentice-Hall, Inc., 1976.
Brown, M. S.: A cross-cultural look at pregnancy, labor, and delivery. *JGN Nurs* 5(5):35–8, September, October, 1976.
Bruhn, C. M., and Pangborn, R. M.: Food habits of migrant farm workers in California. *J. Am. Diet Assoc.*, *59*:347, 1971.
Chamberlin, R. W., and Radebaugh, J. F.: Delivery of Primary Health Care: Union Style. N. Engl. J. Med., *294*:611, 1976.

Chang, B.: Some dietary beliefs in Chinese folk culture. J. Am. Diet Assoc., 65:436, 1974.

Clark, M.: Health in the Mexican-American Culture, 2nd ed. University of California Press, Los Angeles, Calif., Berkeley, 1970.

Comer, J. P., and Poussant, A. F.: *Black Child Care*. New York, Simon & Schuster, 1975.

David, H. P.: Healthy family functioning: A cross-cultural appraisal. Bull. World Health Organ., 56:327, 1978.

Dubos, R. Determinants of health and disease. In *Man, Medicine, and Environment*. New York, Mentor Books, pp. 87–113.

Dunbar, T., and Kravitz, L.: *Hard Traveling: Migrant Farm Workers in America*. Cambridge, Mass., Ballinger Publishing Co., 1976.

Erhard, D.: Nutrition education for the "Now" generation. J. Nutr. Educ., 2:135, 1971.

Farris, L. S.: Approaches to caring for the American Indian maternity patient. *Am. J. MCH*, 1:82, 1976.

Ford, V.: Cultural Criteria and Determinants for Acceptance of Modern Medicine Among the Teton Dakota, Rosebud Indian Reservation, South Dakota, *Commun. Nursing Research* 6:41–62, Sec. 73.

Frankenburg, W. K., Dick, N. A., and Carland, J.: Development of preschool-aged children of different social and ethnic groups: Implications for developmental screening. J. Pediatr. 87:125, 1975.

Fuchs, M., and Bashshur, R.: Use of traditional Indian medicine among urban native Americans. Med. Care, 13:915, 1975.

Grivett, L. E., and Pangborn, R. M.: Origin of selected Old Testament dietary prohibitions: An evaluation review. J. Am. Diet Assoc., 65:634, 1974.

Harrison-Ross, P., and Wyden, B.: *The Black Child: A Parent's Guide to Raising Happy and Healthy Children*. Berkeley Publishing Co., New York, 1974.

Herrera, T., and Wagner, N.: Behavioral approaches to delivering health services in a Chicano community. *In* Reinhardt, A. M., and Quinn, M. D. (eds.): *Current Practice in Family-Centered Community Nursing*. St. Louis, Mo., C. V. Mosby Co., 1977.

Hill, R.: *The Strengths of Black Families*. New York, National Urban League, Inc., 1971.

Home Health Service in Chinatown. Washington, D.C., U.S. Government Printing Office, U.S. Dept. of HEW, Bureau of Community Health Services, 1973.

Hongladarom, G. C., and Russell, M.: An ethnic difference — lactose intolerance. Nurs. Outlook, 24:764, 1976.

Jenkins, S.: Tuberculosis: The native Indian viewpoint on its prevention, diagnosis, and treatment. Prev. Med., 6:545, 1977.

Lerninger, M.: Transcultural nursing: A promising subfield of study for nurses. *In* Reinhardt, A. M., and Quinn, M. D. (eds.): *Current Practice in Family-Centered Community Nursing*. St. Louis, Mo., C. V. Mosby Co., 1977.

Lundell, S.: Folk medical beliefs and their implications for care of patients: Ann. Int. Med., 81:82, 1974.

Lynch, H. T., et al.: Cancer of the colon: Socioeconomic variables in a community. Am. J. Epidemiol., 102:119, 1975.

Mandell, F.: Gypsies: Culture and child care. Pediatrics, 54:603, 1974.

McKenzie, J. L., and Chrisman, N. J.: Healing herbs, gods, and magic: Folk health beliefs among Filipino-Americans. Nurs. Outlook, 25:326, 1977.

McQueen, D. V.: Social aspects of genetic screening for Tay-Sachs disease. Soc. Biol., 22:125, 1975.

Nartsney, R. A. (ed.): *Hispanic Culture and Health Care*. St. Louis, Mo., C. V. Mosby Co., 1978.

National League for Nursing: *Ethnicity and Health Care*. New York, NLN, Inc., 1976.

Orgne, M.: Health care and minority clients. Nurs. Outlook, 24:313, 1976.

Paul, B. D.: *Anthropological Perspectives on Medicine and Public Health, Social Interaction and Patient Care*. Philadelphia, J. B. Lippincott Co., 1975.

Rudolf, G., et al.: *The Social Reality of Ethnic America*. Lexington, Mass., D.C. Health, 1974.

Segall, A.: Sociocultural variation in sick role behavioral expectations. Soc. Sci. Med., 10:47, 1976.

Snow, L. F.: Sorcerers, saints and charlatans: Black folk healers in urban America. *Cul. Med. Psych.*, 2:69, 1978.

Spector, R.: *Cultural Diversity in Health and Illness.* New York, Appleton-Century-Crofts, 1979.

Stokes, L.: Delivering health services in a black community. *In* Reinhardt, A. M., and Quinn, M. D. (eds.): *Current Practice in Family Centered Community Nursing.* St. Louis, Mo., C. V. Mosby Co., 1977.

Symposium on cultural and biological diversity and health care. Nurs. Clin. North Am., *12*:1, 1977.

Trends Affecting U.S. Health Care Systems. Washington, D.C., U.S. Government Printing Office, DHEW No. (HRA) 76–14503, prepared by Aspen System Corp., 1976.

Weisenberg, M., et al.: Pain: anxiety and attitudes in black, white, and Puerto Rican patients. *Psychosom. Med.,* 37:123, 1975.

Weslager, C. A. *Magic Medicines of the Indians.* Somerset, N. J., Middle Atlantic Press, 1973.

White, E. H.: Health and the black person: An annotated bibliography. Am. J. Nurs., 74:1839, 1974.

The School

The first school nursing service was established in New York City in 1902, at the instigation of Lillian Wald of the Henry Street Settlement. Troubled because children with skin diseases, left untreated, were being excluded from school for long periods of time, she offered a one-month demonstration of nursing by a Henry Street nurse. This was so successful that within a few weeks twelve nurses were appointed to work in schools.[1]

Since its inception, school nursing services have grown in size and scope both as part of health-related nursing programs in communities, and as specialized nursing programs within the structure of the school. In 1976, there were 19,798 nurses employed by Boards of Education.[2]

Nurses employed in health-care community agencies provide substantial amounts of school nursing care as part of their regular service to families and communities. A 1972 study of allocation of nursing services found that 39.1 per cent of the total available time for public health nursing was allocated to school health, compared to 29.9 per cent for home visiting and 16.1 per cent for clinic services.[3]

Although there is much discussion as to whether school nursing should be provided as a part of a general community nursing service or as a separate and school-based service, there is little evidence that one administrative pattern is more desirable than the other. Incorporating school nursing into the general community health programs — that is, a single nurse serving the school and the community at large — has some advantages: it unifies in-school and out-of-school care; it is economical of nursing time; and it allocates nursing time in the school according to a community-wide nursing priority system. In contrast, the school-based program has the following advantages: more specialized nursing care; readier financing (school funding may be more flexible or more assured than health agency funding); a closer integration of the health and educational efforts on behalf of the protection and development of the school-age population.

The trend in recent years has been toward specialized staffing, and the rapid development of programs for school nurse practitioners may be expected to accelerate this movement.[4] Whatever the sponsorship or organization, both school and community health agencies are bound to share the total responsibility.

The school offers a unique channel for community nursing; it reaches virtually all children at some point. The Bureau of the Census reported school enrollment of over 60 million persons in 1977 — 1,618,000 in nursery school, 3,191,000 in kindergarten, 29,234,000 in elementary school; 15,753,000 in high school, and 10,217,000 in post-secondary institutions.[5]

The school may become an arm of community action, including health action, either by serving as a center for adult education and after-school activities or through the utilization of school children as emissaries in health educational efforts. Recent emphasis on the "community school" — one that is committed to involvement in the community it serves as well as to the education of its pupils — has extended the traditional concerns of the school. Some proponents envision a school open 12 months a year, 12 or more hours a day. Programs would be designed for all age groups, including the aged and the very young. The school would thus become a kind of community center. Other agencies could participate in the programs, use the facilities of the school, and take advantage of the closeness generated by the comprehensive community approach.

ORGANIZATION OF SERVICES

The organization of nursing in school health programs varies widely. Nurses may be employed on a full- or part-time basis by local educational units, with the nurse coming under the direction of an educational administrative officer such as the principal or director of health and physical education programs.

The nurse may be employed locally, but be required to meet certain state-mandated requirements as to education or experience. Nurses may be employed by educational agencies, but required to meet standards of, or to accept supervisory assistance from, other agencies; for example, school nurses may be appointed by the local Board of Education, but be required to meet qualifications set by a health authority. School nurses may be employed by health authorities, and be allocated as necessary for nursing in the schools. Whatever the patterns of employment, it is important that school and community health efforts on behalf of the school population be coordinated. In one county, the public health agency offered three different levels of nursing care in the schools, to meet the needs and preferences of the school.[6]

Briefly, the function of the school nurse is threefold: (1) to extend and enhance the personal care and educational services afforded the total school population; (2) to contribute to the maintenance and improvement of the physical and social environment of the school; and (3) to relate the school health program to other community health care efforts.

As might be expected, there are wide variations in the specific programs and activities of nurses in the school setting, depending on the preparation of the nurse and the availability of other health or health-related personnel such as counselors, health educators, or physicians. The school health nurse practitioner, for example, can provide a much more intensive program than would be expected of a community health nurse who may provide a few hours of care weekly. The outreach activities of school nursing personnel will vary widely. Also, in some communities, school personnel maintain close and continuing contact with parents and conduct a number of pre-school programs. In other communities the school health activities are more narrowly focused on children enrolled in the school.

Common health problems in the school setting include not only the ills and ailments of school children, but also those of the teaching and service staff.

Among school children, some problems of the past have become less critical. Whooping cough, measles, poliomyelitis, and chickenpox have been brought under control and need less intensive containment measures. Persistent attention is needed to deal with accidents, misuse of drugs, and pregnancy among the school-age population. Violence in the school setting also presents health care needs.

Another area of increasing interest is the emphasis on provision of the full range of educational experiences for handicapped children, keeping them in the mainstream of education rather than on the fringes.[7]

The concept behind this is that separate but equal education is no substitute for the challenge of integrated education. Many children with severe developmental disabilities such as lack of bowel and bladder control or frequent seizures are moving into the general school resource, with a consequent demand for more intensive nursing support. Teachers, school nurses, and others in the school system need preparation in special treatments, medications, and procedures for handling braces, crutches, and wheelchairs. There have been a variety of problems in securing acceptance of these children by their peers, teachers, and the general community. School nurses have had to work hard to find and provide resources for children with developmental disabilities. Frequently the families, especially mothers, of these children have been valuable resources in sharing knowledge and techniques in coping with normal daily activities. Money for such care comes from many sources, including federal programs under the Social Security Act, e.g., MCH — Title V; EPSDT—Title XIX; Health and Nutrition—Title IV, Education and Training of the Handicapped — Title X.

Problems of health maintenance — oral hygiene and care of dental cavities, nutrition problems including overweight, sleep and eating habits — are often encountered in the school population. These conditions may provide teaching material for general courses, and be incorporated in classes on science or family living.

Health Assessment of the School Community

Health assessment of the school population is more than the sum of illness, injury, or negative health behavior of the total group. Variations in health conditions among subgroups, the hazards created by the school itself, and the patterns of interchange between school and community as well as among different subgroups of the population must be ascertained and analyzed.

Cohesiveness within school groups is a big factor in defining and implementing health programs. For example, the success of busing in achieving better racial balance in the school is dependent on the ability of the school and children and staff to exploit this opportunity to produce a cohesive, accepting group able to learn from one another. If the prevailing attitude is one of resentment, fear, or distaste, serious mental health threats may develop.[8]

Communication of the school with community health agencies and with various levels of staff strengthens the teaching opportunity as a social learning experience. Ease of access to management and informal patterns of working together are indications of healthy communication.

Environmental factors may also present hazards. School crossings without traffic lights, unsafe equipment, undesirable loiterers, high absence rates throughout the total school population or for a designated group, or the unsupervised play for young children in the period between dismissal from school and return of parents from work, are examples of school community problems.

Characteristics of the School Community

1. The *purpose* of the school is to prepare its students to live effectively in their society as children and later as adults — to be comfortable in a highly sophisticated technical environment and, at the same time, remain sensitive and responsive to human needs. This broad mandate is second only to that of the family itself.

2. The school is *deeply rooted* in most communities. While the state has central authority for ensuring adequate education for all of the children, local boards or committees provide the administrative decisions required to implement the statewide commitment. The level of concern of local school boards is almost universally high.

3. The *school population* includes diverse groups — students, teachers, administrators, consultants, counselors, maintenance personnel, and health personnel. All of these must be considered in establishing the health program.

4. The *school nurse is often the link* between the school and community health resources. Through referral and the exchange of information between school and community, the nurse is in a position to identify needs that require community or school action.

5. The *school environment* itself may be a hazard to health. Buildings in disrepair, inadequate crossing signals, and poor provisions for bicycle traffic are some examples of environmental concerns. The social environment may also produce health threats — lack of social integration in student groups, and isolation of subgroups, (such as Spanish-speaking families or children from very low income areas) — may cause stress.

School experience is *mandatory* for specified age groups — children must attend until the age of 16 and communities must provide the facilities required. Because attendance at school is required, the schools must provide a milieu for growth and not one that will endanger the health of students. Students should not have to plow through a group of drug purveyors to get into school, or sit in classrooms with flaking asbestos ceilings, or be exposed to communicable disease unnecesarily.

6. The school system often has *built-in stress hazards:* competition for grades, for recognition in sports (a frequent road upward for disadvantaged youth), or for the recognition inherent in being elected to a school office or committee. Cross-cultural activities designed to reduce intergroup tension may also produce stress in the early phases of these programs.

Developing a Nursing Program in the School

Developing the school-based nursing program involves assessment of problems, establishment of feasible goals specific to this population, carrying out needed activities, and evaluating process and results of the program. However, there are some areas of special concern in this setting.

The establishment and efficacy of the program concern several groups in the school setting and in the community. For example, the school nurse is concerned with control of communicable diseases — an area of equal importance to other nursing groups in the community (such as the public health nurse, or the State Health Department). Health goals must be related to the overall educational goals of the schools. Safety programs are of concern to physical education personnel and to groups such as parent-teacher organizations. Immunization programs are a major concern of health agencies. Developing sensible health habits is a concern of educators and service personnel in many agencies.

The nursing program must be planned to account for all of these shared concerns and to relate programs in nursing to the public's concerns for a healthy and informed citizenry.

Health Assessment of the School Population

Health assessment measures in the school are almost always a multiprofessional undertaking that involves the child himself, his family, the teacher, school counselors, psychologists, attendance officers, school social workers, physical education instructors, and volunteer or paid assistants and technicians as well as nurses and physicians. The school nurse, because of her awareness of the need to use all measures — from the simple and incidental observation of the teacher to the multidiscipline comprehensive health examination — for the detection of health aberrations, will encourage everyone in contact with the school child to be alert to any developmental or health deviation. Those in contact with children should have available to them informational materials that will allow them to observe intelligently and direct them to the person to whom they should report any observed or suspected deviation from expected health behavior.

Pre-school Measures

Ensuring a healthy school population depends on activities that are undertaken before the child is actually enrolled in school as well as on those performed at the time of the child's initial entry into the school community. Even though it is undeniably better to think of health care of children as a continuous program beginning at the point of conception, the fact is that it often takes the stimulus of impending school enrollment to get some things done. It is hoped that the child entering school will have had a complete medical and dental appraisal; that he will have completed his immunization series (including recommended booster shots); and that any reparable defect, especially impairments of vision and hearing, will have been corrected.

The school nurse may confer with parents prior to the child's entry into school and help to establish special examination or immunization clinics when the services of a family physician or of other medical facilities are not available. Head start activities, designed to enrich the preschool years as a preparation for school, require nursing support, since health care is an integral aspect of the program.

Observation by the Child and the Family

However effective and efficient school measures for detection of health problems may be, they cannot take the place of intelligent observation and action on the part of the pupil and his family. Even the kindergarten child can learn to recognize when he has a cold and to report this to the teacher. The nurse may reach children by integrating this information into class content, such as personal hygiene or home-making, or by providing opportunities for students to help with health observations or screening measures. A valuable route that may be available in the secondary school is the Future Nurses' club, the Future Homemakers' club, or the Health Careers' club. These social activity groups usually include students who have an interest in health careers and who are especially ready for health instruction. These students may also exert considerable influence on their peers in health matters.

Several methods of communication may be used to involve family members. Parents who are present at the time of school medical examinations may be advised on health symptoms or may be invited to participate more extensively in health instruction (such as classes in home nursing), or to volunteer assistance in the health program. The parent-teacher association may offer meeting-time for the nurse to discuss school health problems; or the nurse may talk informally with individual parents at the time of the meetings. However, neither of these methods are likely to reach those who most need such instruction, such as those in the low-income group or those living in isolated locations. Since these parents seldom attend such school activities, the nurse may have to plan to reach them in the home. If the nurse is carrying general as well as school nursing responsibilities, she may plan to see these parents either individually or in clusters in a neighborhood; or she may enlist the services of a nurse in the general program, of a school health aid, or of a volunteer to make teaching visits to selected families.

"Notes to take home" is another measure for reaching parents with health information. This approach has the obvious advantage of reaching large numbers of parents, especially mothers; however, it is perhaps the least effective measure, since the notes may be lost or disregarded.

Provisions for Observation by the Teacher

The teacher as the individual having the most contact with the child during the school day is a key person in health observation. The community health nurse in the school may improve the quality of the teacher's observations by:

1. Arranging for the inclusion of health content in teachers' meetings. These meetings, usually held just before the start of the school year, offer an excellent opportunity for reaching teachers, especially those new to the school system. At this time, it is possible to orient new teachers to the role and the services of the school health nurse and other

health personnel, to arrange for briefing in observation techniques, and to inform teachers of the availability of nursing and other health services. This is also an opportunity for returning teachers to catch up with changes in the program or in the health personnel and to find out about the plans of the health-care group for the year ahead. Arrangements for such contacts are made through the school principal, school superintendent, or the student personnel office.

2. Scheduling teacher-nurse conferences. These conferences are usually planned by the nurse and teacher with the approval of the responsible school administrator. The teacher-nurse conference is the backbone of the teacher education program. It is here that the nurse and the teacher have an opportunity to discuss the problems of individual children, especially those whose health appears to be threatened. It is the occasion for a more general interchange in which each becomes informed of the problems of the other with respect to the health and education program; there is also an opportunity to agree on courses of action that have to do with an individual child or with the class as a group.

Sometimes the problem is not so much with an individual child as it is with the group as a whole. The teacher may find a group of inattentive or irritable students or a class in which a few students appear to dominate over the others to an undesirable degree. Sometimes culture-based group attitudes — such as attitudes toward premarital intercourse — may have health implications. Recently there have been efforts to reorganize school populations to make them more representative of the community as a whole rather than of their immediate neighborhood. In this effort, the school population becomes more diversified with respect to sociocultural backgrounds and, often, in learning interests. This may, however, create interpersonal, mental, and emotional health problems for both students and teachers.

The teacher-nurse conference should be carefully planned. The time should be set when the teacher has no scheduled class or when the children can be engaged in some activity that does not require the teacher's concentrated attention. Sometimes a teacher aide or parent volunteer can take over the class during the conference. The teacher should have had a prior opportunity to look at each child individually (usually with the guidance of a teacher observation form) for any possible health problem and to evaluate changes in those children under special observation.

Sometimes the teacher will want the nurse to meet the children as a group and may suggest that the nurse give a short talk to the class. This may serve a useful purpose, but the nurse must be careful not to divert her time to formal instruction when the real need is to explore general health matters with the teacher or to confer with individual students who have health problems.

The nurse should review her records of this particular class prior to the conference in order to bring to the conference a report on the progress made with children who are under nursing care.

The overall scheme for teacher-nurse conferences should be cleared with and understood by the school administration officer, since he is responsible for the total school effort. Anything that interrupts the usual teaching schedule or that incorporates into the school program content not under his supervision is of concern to him. His support is essential in gaining the cooperation and interest of the teaching group.

3. Alerting teachers when special observations are needed, for example, when there is an increased incidence of influenza or when teenage pregnancies are prevalent and frequently unreported. This provides an opportunity for "spot" briefing, or outlining and describing the symptoms that may be observed if, for instance, emotional problems are paramount; discussions of typical behaviors of children who are anxious, withdrawn, and depressed may help sharpen the teacher's observations.

Screening Measures

In some states, there are laws requiring that specific screening measurements be made at stated intervals. In virtually every school there are policies requiring such screening. Screening in the school setting may take many forms:

1. Informal screening of each child each day may be performed by the classroom teacher for evidence of deviance from usual health behavior.

2. Screening examinations for vision and hearing may be conducted by technicians, teachers, parents or other volunteers, and nurses.

3. Special screening measures may be instituted for a particular problem (such as tuberculosis infection) for selected children at unusual risk, for children referred by the teacher, or for specific individuals with known problems.

4. Dental screening may be conducted by the dentist, dental hygienist, or dental assistant.

5. Periodic physical examinations may be performed by the school or family physician and nurse practitioner at specified intervals.

6. Self-completed or family-completed health inventories or health histories may be required. When the family physician takes the responsibility of completing the provided form, he submits it to the school where it is then reviewed by the school nurse or school physician.

The nurse may have a major part in planning and implementing the screening program. The scheduling must be such that it interferes as little as possible with the formal educational process. Volunteers or technicians may need orientation to the programs or to the school, or they may need specific and comprehensive training by the school health personnel. The nurse must arrange to have time available not only to be present at the examination, to train or orient other workers, and to make the necessary physical arrangements but also to complete the required follow-up care for problems that are uncovered. In arranging her schedule, the nurse will want to be sure there is additional time available for this latter activity; it is of little use to discover health problems if nothing is done about them.

In general it is felt that it is beneficial for a parent to be present when the child is receiving a physical examination. This allows the health staff to clarify the health situation immediately. This parental participation is also felt to have a strong motivating effect that makes correction of the problem more likely.

In carrying out screening procedures, the nurse should avoid spending time in routine procedures. By delegating this kind of work to aides, volunteers, or technicians, she can be free to circulate; to talk with teachers, parents, and children; and to take the first steps in assuring follow-up care for problems.

HEALTH CARE OF THE SCHOOL POPULATION

Planning nursing care for the school population is a multifaceted task. The case load of the community health nurse in the school is the total school population, which includes both the students and the employees of the school. The extent of the responsibility of the nurse will be spelled out in policy statements; in some situations the nurse may participate in school sponsored medical examinations for teachers, whereas in other instances this is not a part of the school health program. The nurse in the school may or may not participate in preschool examination and surveillance, adult health education, or home visiting. Within these understandings, the nurse in the school will define the need for different categories of care for specified groups in the school population.

Using the measures that are available and effective in identifying health problems, it will be possible for the nurse to focus on those individuals or groups who appear to have a substantive health problem or who are at unusual risk. This will include those children with multiple handicaps or health deviations, those from disorganized families who exhibit signs of social alienation, or those with chronic diseases requiring therapeutic maintenance. From this information she will develop a case load of children who are in need of intensive nursing supervision. For the remainder of the children, general surveillance will be adequate, and nursing efforts may be directed toward keeping the alertness level of teachers and parents high. Some nurses like to categorize students into three levels, thereby allowing for an intermediate service load that requires less than intensive care but more than simple surveillance.

A valuable index of need for nursing care is the absence record of individuals, groups, or specific schools. The frequency of absence in the school as a whole is, of course, important. Even more important, however, is the pattern of absence and the reasons for absence from school. The child whose absences are frequent, of short duration, and not accompanied by the need for medical care merits study with respect to general vitality level and, perhaps, attitude toward school; whereas illnesses of long duration suggest a more definite medical problem. If the absences appear to coincide with school examinations or special programs (such as physical education), the search for causes may take a different tack. When a whole school is characterized by frequent absence — especially of girls — at points of family crisis, the need may rest in sociocultural value orientations or in the community's failure to provide adequate home help. Absence patterns that consistently affect a specific group of children might alert the nurse to the possibility of group experimentation with drugs or other unapproved activities.

Establish a Nursing-care Philosophy. It is important to establish a philosophy that will serve as a basis for and as a general guide to the nurse and to those who assist her in the provision of nursing care. This philosophy will depend somewhat upon the prevailing educational philosophy. The nursing-care philosophy might include concepts such as these:

1. The goal of nursing care is to keep the child in school and maximize his participation in school activities. This might lead to the decision to have handicapped children receive treatments in school rather than at home, to refer children to special classes only when these classes are necessary for the progress of the student (not to relieve the anxiety of the school staff), to deal with group attitudes toward handicapping conditions in a way that will provide sensible peer support for the handicapped child, or to make arrangements with the school cafeteria to provide special foods for children requiring them so that they need not eat apart from their classmates.

2. Preventive and anticipatory services represent the major thrust of the school nursing program. This suggests that emergency care of children and staff be delegated where possible and that volunteer or technical assistance be maximized to reach students who are in need of more substantive health counseling. It further supposes that the nurse will have the required background of information on the conditions expected and on the preventive measures available in this group as a basis both for her own work and for the delegation of nursing work.

3. The participation of parents and children in health decisions will be maximized. Thus, parents may serve as volunteers, older students may teach health to younger groups, and health-care proposals will, as far as possible, be posed in terms of possible alternatives in action.

4. The family is the unit of service in the personal care aspects of nursing. This requires that the school nurse not only involve the family in the care of the child but also concern herself with the effect of the

child's condition or behavior in the family and help secure required care for other members of the family.

Developing a Health Care Network

The school nurse frequently is the organizing link between the children and their families and the community health resources. The nurse must involve diverse talents and groups in meeting the needs of the school-age population. This means working with school principals, Boards of Education, the PTA, the local medical society and a variety of other concerned groups in establishing program policy and developing interest in health-related programs. The nurse may need to develop volunteer groups to work in screening programs or to help meet basic needs to assist high risk families in the community. The nurse will need to develop linkages with providers of services, be they physicians, social workers, truant officers, teachers, or, as frequently happens, a combination of all of the above.

Nursing Activities

The school health nurse contributes to the health care and health education of the school population in five ways:

1. By participating in health assessment measures, including observation, screening, physical examination, and epidemiologic investigation.

2. By providing or arranging for care of injuries and of emergency or continuing illness.

3. By counseling or arranging for counseling with students or other personnel who have health problems (including, of course, emotional health problems).

4. By involving parents, teachers, and pupils in planning and conducting health-care activities and in decision making relative to their own health.

5. By contributing to the development of health-related learning experiences for students through curriculum development; by special activities such as clubs or study groups; or through consultation with teachers or other personnel.

Physical Assessment

A growing trend is for schools or health departments to hire nurse practitioners to provide primary-care services to school children. These nurses, who usually have special training for these responsibilities, provide physical examinations to children and manage the health problems or concerns of most students based on standard protocols, referring more complex problems to physicians or other specialists.[9]

First-Aid Care of Emergencies and Illness. Prompt and effective first-aid care of emergencies is essential to the safety program. Even though the nurse herself may provide emergency treatment, in most instances she must rely on others who are on the scene to give immediate care. Every school should designate personnel who have had preparation in first-aid care and who are available to assist in emergency situations. The school may have its own policies or procedures relative to emergency care, or it may adopt the American Red Cross Textbook or other standard text as the manual for care. The American Red Cross or another organized community training facility may provide instruction, or there may be qualified first-aid instructors on the school faculty. Emergency care supplies should be available where needed and should be maintained at all times.

It is also important that procedures be established for notifying the family of illness or injury, for transporting children who must go home, for placing the child when there is no one at his home during the day, and for securing necessary medical care. Sometimes a readily available physician is assigned to school health work; more often, there are designated physicians or institutions near the school from whom emergency care may be secured. Directions for obtaining emergency care, along with the phone number (and, when relevant, the name of the person to be called) should be posted in a prominent place.

School facilities should provide a place where it is possible to isolate a child suspected of having communicable disease and a cot where children may rest if they are ill or injured. If volunteers are used for transportation, the drivers should be adequately insured.

Counseling and Psychosocial Evaluation. Many of the problems and concerns of the school-age population are not solved by medical treatment. They are social, emotional problems, frequently with a developmental basis, that the child and family must learn to solve for themselves. Social and mental health counseling may be available in the community, provided in part by Big Brother/Big Sister programs, or the nurse may need to develop such a resource, using herself and others.

Health Education of the School Population

It is important that the individual student and his family have sufficient knowledge to permit them to recognize health problems, to foresee health problems, and to take appropriate action when the need arises.

Much of the content of health education will be provided in courses in family health or family living, in biology classes, in physical education classes, and in courses in the humanities and government. The nurse's function is to reinforce and supplement this general information by assisting with materials or suggested content.

The nurse's greatest contribution to health education will lie in efforts with individuals or small groups that have expressed specific health concerns. Thus, a child coming for a bandage for a cut finger may be taught about prevention of accidents or of infection, or the young girl with frequent menstrual discomfort may be helped to a better understanding of her own development.

The nurse may be asked to serve as a member of a school health committee. Such committees are usually made up of representatives from those departments in the school that have a major concern with health and health teaching, of parents, of students, and of appropriate community agencies. The committee usually reports to the administrative officer, to the school principal (if the committee is school-wide). The nurse who spends a portion of her time in such a generalized program should take this responsibility as seriously as does the nurse who spends full time in the school.

The Health Record

Good records contribute greatly to the effectiveness and continuity of care in the school setting. As with other services, the problem-oriented record has many advantages. (See Chapter 5.) In general, a cumulative health record is combined with the general cumulative school record; and, when there are special health problems that require more intensive care, there may be a special and separate health service record. The health record is shared with discrimination. For example, the child's general cumulative record might include developmental data or information on conditions that require special seating, lighting, or particular continuing observation or support by the teaching staff. This information will be immediately available to all authorized school personnel. For those students with intensive nursing needs and a separate nursing record, a notation on the cumulative record indicates that the child is in this special case load. Thus, others will be alerted to talk to the nurse if they observe any special difficulty with the child, and the nurse may still maintain this special record to ensure the confidentiality of its contents.

Evaluation of Nursing Process

The evaluation of nursing processes and outcomes is complicated in the health setting by the wide dispersion of responsibility. However, health progress often *can* be measured, even though one could not say the progress was due specifically to the nursing effort. A properly constructed record should make it easy to see at a glance whether or not the problems identified have in fact been referred to care, whether or not the care was received, and the results of care.

With nursing programs that involve a large number of students (as in follow-up care after a school medical examination), it is sometimes helpful, as an aid to measuring progress, to keep a separate "check off" index file or posting sheet in order to identify quickly the group still needing interpretation of correctional procedures.

Bryan, discussing the special problems of school nursing in culturally deprived areas, lists several indicators of parental action that were pertinent to her program.[10] Similar specific identification of desired and measurable outcomes would be most helpful in other school settings.

The nurse in the school should assure herself that care has been received when it is provided by agencies other than the school, and she should institute the requisite planning and follow-up procedures. Case conferences with nurses in the health department or the visiting nurse association or with the parents and the family medical adviser are essential. Though such procedures are time-consuming, the lack of precision in care that occurs without such careful clearance is even more costly.

Special studies may be needed to identify children with high risks for health problems. A study of children who were frequently absent was completed in the Delaware School System. They found that absence was associated with family attitudes toward school, illness of other family members, and fear or dislike of school on the part of the child.[11] The effectiveness of care can be improved if it is possible to identify the associated factors for illness or noncompletion of recommendations for health care. Such knowledge helps the nurse to plan more carefully in order to accommodate these impediments to care. When final outcomes are unsatisfactory because of failure of community support, the careful documentation of these conditions by the school nurse may play an important part in securing corrections.

The Improvement of the School Environment

The school environment is second only to the home environment in its effect upon the health and development of children and youth. A healthful school environment should be free from hazards or barriers to health in order to be conducive to the proper physical and social development of the child and to the child's education, which is a joint commitment of the school and the family. These characteristics might describe the desirable environment in any setting, but the problems of the maintenance of a healthful environment in the school are somewhat specialized.

Physical Hazards

Safety in the school takes a prominent place in establishing a suitable environment for the child. The responsibility for maintaining a safe environment is shared by many people: the administrative staff, who plan for new equipment and buildings; the teachers of health education, who maintain activity areas and control the behavior of children on the playground, in sports, and in practices; the maintenance superintendent, who sees to it that good housekeeping practices reduce accident hazards; the classroom teacher, who observes and reports unsafe conditions; and the sanitarian, who inspects the premises for compliance with regulations. Often there will be a safety committee or council in the school, and the nurse's contribution may be mainly through her observation and her reporting to, or her participation on, this committee. In smaller schools, the nurse may be required to take more initiative in studying the safety of the environment and in securing correction of undesirable or unsafe conditions.

Communicable Diseases

Freedom from undue exposure to communicable disease is assured by maintaining the recommended immunization level in the school; by prompt recognition (by alerted teachers and parents) of any deviation from usual health when communicable disease is prevalent; and by the exclusion from school (or temporary isolation if already at school) of those with symptoms of communicable disease.

The school nurse must be knowledgeable about the symptoms and treatment of communicable diseases, she must know the immunization level of the school population, and she must be aware of the level of expertise of those responsible for the continuing screening of children. She needs also to be familiar with local regulations governing exclusion and readmission to school when communicable disease is suspected or diagnosed.

Psychosocial Environment

The psychosocial environment may have a significant impact on the health of the school child. A curriculum that is too difficult or too crowded may produce stress. A curriculum that is not sufficiently challenging — or, to use the modern student phrase, "not relevant" — may be equally stressful for the bright or more committed student. Schedules that do not permit interspersing of constricting and free activity or that include long class periods may also create stress. Excessive homework may also be a problem, especially when family support for such study is low.

Situations that lead to discouragement, fatigue, or loss of self-confidence or self-respect are also health deterrents. Interpersonal stress among student groups arising from interracial or intercultural conflict, too much emphasis on formal testing, and track systems in which one group becomes known as "the dummies" or that lead to the development of sharply defined subgroups are examples of stress-producing situations that may result in emotional or social health problems. The school nurse may initiate outreach measures designed to merge some efforts of those with differing background. The student living in poverty and in constant contact with crime may show ability in dancing, this talent could be made apparent in a school play, but the student might need support or encouragement to get to a tryout. The opportunity to help the librarian as a paid or volunteer worker might open a new world to another student. The "not yet but likely" criminal may be urged to help protect elderly people in a deteriorated neighborhood as they shop or go to clinics. Sometimes socially approved activities prove as attractive as delinquency, but the opportunities must be made available.

The nurse may serve as ombudsman for children who are at odds with the school or neighborhood agencies with which they must deal. She may also encourage disadvantaged students to talk of some of the positive aspects of dealing with poverty; using low-cost foods, learning about handcrafts and shopping in the thrift store may lead to a new, more positive kind of recognition.

Dress may also be a stress factor. Inability to secure proper clothing may cause a youngster to feel inferior; lack of cleanliness or careless dress may reflect and reemphasize a sense of defeat and lack of personal worth. Some teachers have found that "dress up days" have a very real influence on the manners and sense of self-esteem of the students, provided, of course, that the dressing up is within the capability of the children's family.

Inducements to Good Health Practice

The environment should offer inducements to good health practice. Adequate lighting in the school setting is crucial. Although there has been considerable disagreement as to exactly how much illumination is needed, Byrd reports American Medical Association support for the level of 10 foot candles of light in hallways and similar areas, 30 foot candles for reading, and 50 foot candles for fine work.[12] The Illuminating Engineering Society recommends 50 foot candles for reading and 100 to 150 foot candles for very fine work.[13]

The nurse should help children develop good habits in the use of available lighting; she should urge that fixtures be kept clean, that bulbs be replaced promptly, and that there be "brightness balance," that is, a balance in brightness between the seeing task area and the area immediately adjoining it (the recommended balance in reading areas is 3 to 1). Glare should be avoided.

The seating of school children and opportunities to move about during the classroom session are also important prerequisites to maintenance of good posture and the reduction of fatigue. Adequate facilities for handwashing, with plentiful and suitable soap and towels, are also necessary.

Provisions for in-school feeding are important. In large school systems, cafeterias may be under expert management, and the nurse's only concern may be the ways in which the facility is used: the availability of good food choices, scheduling to avoid dangerous overcrowding, and student behavior in the cafeteria as it relates to health. The sanitarian will be concerned with the preservation of good maintenance practices. The nurse, however, should be alert to the opportunity provided in the cafeteria for good food choices, the educational opportunities the food service may provide, and the quality of the socialization that occurs.

The presence of inducements to poor health practice may be a concern. The availability of soda, candy, and cigarette vending machines may contribute negatively to the health environment.

The existence of good role models in the teaching, administrative, and student personnel staff is also a powerful factor in health behavior. The example set by the teaching and the administrative staff and the degree to which they are able to incorporate sound health teaching into the total curriculum have a profound impact on children's perceptions of health and of health care. The teacher's lesson that school children should stay at home to avoid infecting others when they have evidence of a communicable disease makes little impression if she herself comes to school coughing and sneezing with a cold.

The nurse should seek out all possible measures for establishing and reinforcing a joint nurse-teacher approach to health problems. Circulating the annual report of the nurse to the teaching staff or using teacher's meetings or teacher-nurse conferences to discuss the plans for the nursing service in the school are examples of approaches that might be used. When any unusual circumstances arise, the nurse, acting in coordination with the school medical adviser, may send a reminder to teachers. For example, if a polio immunization program is being started in the community, the teachers might be informed of the importance of this preventive measure, the method that is being used, and the children or adults who should be encouraged to secure immunization. If nutritional conditions among students appear to be below par, suggestions about observation of children for symptoms of malnutrition or about the use of hot lunch supplementary feeding programs may help. The nurse might work with a nutritionist in the school or in the local or state health department to be sure the materials she is using are pertinent and up-to-date.

Students are also a valuable health resource. A valuable channel for the school nurse is the membership of the future nurses club or the health careers club. These clubs attract students who have a special interest in health and who may later enter one of the health occupations. The school nurse is often the sponsor for these groups. Help with materials and further information may be secured from the National Health Council.

Students may serve as volunteers in various health activities in or out of the school. When students are expected to observe or work in community agencies as part of the education program, the nurse may help the instructional staff in arranging such observations and, for some students, experience in health agencies.

The nurse may also be called upon to help teachers and students with special projects in other subject matter areas in which the content involves health. For example, a history student might be interested in health conditions at a given era, or a science student may be interested in some of the health problems of space explorations.

THE RELATIONSHIP OF SCHOOL NURSING
TO THE HEALTH OF THE FAMILY AND
THE COMMUNITY

A supportive and participating community is an essential environmental condition. The ability of the school to contribute to the health of the child will depend upon community support in providing funds and in setting general policy regarding conditions for school health care.

A community that is interested in what the school is doing for its children, in understanding the basis for the school health program, and in participating in its development and evaluation can profoundly influence service outcomes.

The nurse may contribute to securing a supportive and participating community by using her work with children as a channel to "reach out" to the parents and to the neighborhood. Mothers and fathers may be invited to conferences where decisions are being made about school examinations and the ways in which parents will be notified and asked to participate. A group of parents may volunteer to interpret the upcoming program to other mothers in their neighborhood and may encourage them to participate by attending the examination session.

The nurse can also do much to interpret the school health program and the needs and plans of the school community to official and volunteer agencies in the community, to parents or to those whose children are not in school, and to the family physician, who may need to follow up on the problems uncovered in a school examination or who, in some instances, may be resentful of the school's interference with the care of his patients.

The nurse may also attend and become involved in the general community activities of the school apart from their health aspects, or she may engage in community teaching such as home-nursing classes. Thus, she may come to know and to appreciate the parents and neighbors and help them to recognize the very real interest of the school in their welfare.

Through the health program in the school, the nurse contributes to the general health care of the school-age child. Through service planning sessions, case discussion, epidemiologic studies, and referral, the nurse in the school keeps other health agencies informed as to the needs and the problems of school-age children and plans the school nursing program in such a way as to support the general community efforts on behalf of the school-age child. Data regarding nursing needs or health conditions found in the school are helpful to the generalized community health nurse in program planning, just as the activities of the school health nurse with respect to such community activities as vaccination for poliomyelitis contribute substantially to the total community effort.

In summary, the school must be seen as a powerful channel for reaching the public with important health information and guidance. It offers not only a way to assure each child of the opportunity to maximize his learning experience free from unnecessary disease and accident, but also a chance to increase his ability to cope with health conditions that cannot be remedied and to prepare him for the important health decisions he must make immediately and later, when he reaches adulthood.

REFERENCES: THE SCHOOL

1. Roberts, M.: *American Nursing, History and Interpretation*. New York, Macmillan Co., 1954, p. 84.
2. *Facts About Nursing, 1976–1977*. Kansas City, Mo., American Nurses Association, 1978, p. 39.
3. Division of Nursing, U.S. Department of Health, Education, and Welfare: *Surveys of Public Health Nursing, 1968–1972*. (HRA 76.8), Washington, D.C., U.S. Government Printing Office, 1975, pp. 105–106.
4. See for example: American Nurses Association and American School Health Association: *Recommendations on Educational Preparation and Definition of the Expanded Role and Functions of the School Nurse Practitioner*. Kansas City, Mo., American Nurses Association. See also Igoe, J.: The school nurse practitioner program. *In* Hall, J. E., and Weaver, B.: *Distributive Nursing Practice, A Systems Approach to Community Health*. Philadelphia, J. B. Lippincott Co., 1977.
5. U.S. Bureau of the Census: *Current Population Report*, No. 321, Washington, D.C., U.S. Government Printing Office, 1977, p. 20.
6. Edwards, L., and Kelly, E.: A three-level school program. Nurs. Outlook, 25:388, 1977.
7. Education for the Handicapped Act (PL 94–142), 1975.
8. Coles, R.: *Children of Crisis*. Boston, Little Brown & Co., 1967.
9. For example see: *Analysis and Planning for Improved Distribution of Nursing Personnel and Services. Inventory of Innovations in Nursing*. HEW, PHS, NRA, Bureau of Health Manpower, Division of Nursing, November 1976, pp. 33–36. Also see American Nurses Association and American School Health Association: *Recommendations on Educational Preparation and the Definition of the Expanded Role and Functions of the School Nurse Practitioner*. Kansas City, Mo., ANA, 1973.
10. Bryan, D.: Redirection of school nursing services in culturally deprived neighborhoods. Am. J. Pub. Health, 57:1164, 1967.
11. Basco, D., et al.: Epidemiologic analysis in school populations as a basis for change in school-nursing practice. Report of the second phase of a longitudinal study. Am. J. Pub. Health, 62:491, 1972.
12. Byrd, O. E.: *School Health Administration*, 4th ed. Philadelphia, W. B. Saunders Co., 1966, p. 388.
13. American Institute of Architects: *Standards of School Lighting*. Illuminating Engineering Society, 1962.

SUGGESTED READINGS: THE SCHOOL

American Academy of Pediatrics: *School Health: A Guide for Health Professionals.* Evanston, Ill., 1977.

American Nurses Association and The American School Health Association: *A Joint Statement of the American Nurses Association and the American School Health Association. Recommendations on Educational Preparation and the Definition of the Expanded Role and Functions of the School Nurse Practitioner.* Kansas City, Mo., American Nurses Association, September 1973.

Basco, D., et al.: Epidemiologic analysis in school population as a basis for changing school nursing practices. Report of 2nd phase of a longitudinal study. Am. J. Pub. Health, 62: 491, 1976.

Benell, F. B.: *Drug Abuse and Venereal Disease: Misconceptions of a Selected Group of College Students.* New York, Simon & Shuster, 1973, pp. 584–587.

Blaser, L. E., and Scharf, R. H.: School teachers as case finders. Nurs. Outlook, 19:460, 1971.

Bryant, N. H.: School nurse utilization at International School, Bangkok, Thailand. Nurs. Res., 22:164, 1973.

Downs, F. S.: The omsbudsman is a nurse. Nurs. Outlook, 19:473, 1971.

Edwards, L., and Kelly, E.: A Three-level school health program. Nurs. Outlook, 25:388, 1977.

Epstein, E. and Orkui, M.: Could that maddening itch be lice or mites? Patient Care, 7:94, 1973.

Hamessley, M. L.: *Handbook for Camp Nurses and Other Camp Health Workers.* New York, Tiresias Press, 1973, p. 159.

Hanlon, J. J., and McHose, E.: *Design for Health, School and Community,* 2nd ed. Philadelphia, Lea & Febiger, 1971, p. 406.

Heit, P.: The Berkeley model. Health Educ. 8:2, 1977.

Igoe, J.: *The school nurse practitioner program. In* Hall, J. E., and Weaver, R.: *Distributive Nursing Practice: A Systems Approach to Community Health.* Philadelphia, J. B. Lippincott, 1977.

Jenny, J.: Preventing dental disease in children. Am. J. Pub. Health, 64: 1147, 1974.

Lawrence, M. M.: *The Mental Health Team in the Schools.* New York, Behavioral Publications, 1971, p. 169.

Lore, A.: Adolescents: People, not problems. Am. J. Nurs., 73:1232, 1973.

McNeil, J., and Bergner, L.: Use of mobile unit to provide health care for preschoolers in rural King County, Washington. Public Health Report, 90:344, 1975.

Nader, P.: *Options for School Health: Meeting Community Needs.* Germantown, Md., Aspen Publishers, 1978.

Natapoff, J.: Children's views of health: A developmental study. Am. J. Pub. Health, 8:995, 1978.

Nemir, A.: *The School Health Program.* Philadelphia, W. B. Saunders Co., 1970.

Nichols, D. D.: Some recent data on community college health services progress. J. Am. Col. Health Assoc., 22:61, 1973.

Oda, D. S.: The role of the community nurse in school systems. *In* Archer, S. E., and Fleshman, R.: *Community Health Nursing Patterns and Practice.* N. Scituate, Mass., Duxbury Press, pp. 346–360, 1979.

Oda, D. S.: Increasing role effectiveness of school nurse. Am. J. Pub. Health, 64: 591, 1974.

Pelton, W. J., et al.: *The Epidemiology of Oral Health.* Howard Press, 1969.

Quinn, D.: No room at the inn. Gaps in services for troubled youth and the role of the CHN. *In* Reinhardt, A. M. and Quinn, M. D. (eds.): *Current Practice in Family-Centered Community Nursing.* St. Louis, Mo., C. V. Mosby Co., 1977, p. 248.

Rice, A. K.: Common skin infections in school children. Am. J. Nurs., 73:1905, 1973.

Smiley, O. R.: Public health nurses and teachers in school health programmes: A problem in communication. Int. Nurs. Rev., 23:141, 1976.

Smith, V.: A study of injuries. J. School Health, 41:108, 1971.

Starfield, B., and Sharp, E.: Medical problems, medical care and school performance. J. School Health, 41:184, 1971.

Tuthill, R. W., Williams, C., Long, G., and Whitman, C.: Evaluating a school health program focused on high absence pupils: A research design. Am. J. Publ. Health, 62:40, 1972.

RESOURCES: THE SCHOOL

American Nurse's Association, 2420 Pershing Road, Kansas City, Mo. 64108. Membership, publications, programs, standard setting.

American Public Health Association, Washington, D.C. School Health Section.

American Red Cross — Local Chapter. Programs in care of infants, first aid, safety, home care of the sick, water safety, publications, volunteer services.

American School Health Association, Kent, Ohio 44240. Publications, standards.

National League for Nursing, 10 Columbus Circle, New York, N.Y. 10019. Membership, educational materials, educational opportunities.

School personnel with special health interest. Committees (accident prevention, studying and recommending action for specific problems — such as unmarried adolescent mothers).

The Occupational Health Setting

The health of those who work is a vital public concern. The total labor force — those at work or seeking work — has been increasing. In 1975 there were 94,793,000 people in the labor force, compared to 77,178,000 people in 1965. It is estimated that by 1985, 110,690,000 people will be a part of the labor force. These figures include all segments of the adult population — men and women, persons of low or high income and of urban or rural residence. Almost a third of their life is spent at work. Workers need — and they expect — a safe work environment that is conducive to good physical and mental health. Health insurance and health care are important fringe benefits. Furthermore, work itself and the ability to stay employed are of deep importance to most adults. For the head of the family, it is a symbol of his or her role as provider; for the professional worker, it is an outlet for creative skills;

and for the mother, it may be a chance to provide more things for the children or to get away from the isolation of the home setting. For employers, the health of the worker is inextricably linked with production; absence or inefficiency due to poor health may lead to expensive lags in production and may affect many workers other than the one who is ill or injured. For the country, the achievement of full production is a necessary condition for improving the standard of living; therefore, the health of the working population is a serious government concern as well.

Nursing has been an accepted component of industrial health services for a long time. The first industrial nurse in the United States, Ada Stewart, was employed by the Vermont Marble Company in 1895. The work she did was largely as a visiting nurse and would probably be described today as "generalized public health nursing."

SOME CURRENT TRENDS AND PROBLEMS

According to Ashford (from a study commissioned by The Ford Foundation), "Health, work, and environment rank among the most important areas of social concern today, and the point where these concerns converge — the work place — has become a microcosm of national conflict."[1] Labor, management, and environmentalists have voiced concern over the growing evidence of occupational origin of such diseases as pneumoconiosis among coal miners, cancer caused by asbestos, and beryllium disease and liver cancer caused by vinyl chloride. An increase in the reported injury rate (29 per cent from 1961 to 1970) has also been the cause for some labor-management disputes. This has been, in part, responsible for passage of federal legislation — i.e., The Coal Mine Health and Safety Act of 1969, Occupational Safety and Health Act of 1970 (OSHA), and The Toxic Substance Control Act of 1976.[2]

Defining "safe levels" for a growing variety of toxic substances — particularly as they relate to chronic diseases — causes lawmakers, labor, and management a great deal of difficulty. "Do we prohibit use or consumption of a material until it is proven safe, or do we allow it to be used until it is proven harmful?" — this is a pivotal question in the enforcement of the new laws.

A second trend affecting occupational health is the broadening of the perceived mission of this service. Lavenne describes the trend in this way:

Industrial medicine . . . began with accidents in works and factories, went on to occupational diseases and their prevention, and now must concern itself more and more with questions of adaptation of work to man, and man's adaptation to his work.[3]

A new term has been coined to describe the process of achieving this mutual adaptation: *ergonomics* — the application of biologic and engineering sciences to achieve the best adjustment of man to his work, and to improve efficiency and well-being.[4]

A third trend affecting occupational health programs is the rapid extension of production technology. The picking of tomatoes is moving toward automated, rather than hand, processes. The capacity to produce tomatoes of uniform size, a necessary precursor to automated picking, is within sight. This changes the whole nature of the occupational health problem of the tomato harvester. Workers will need training in the handling and maintenance of equipment and in work habits that will decrease accidents. The increased speed of harvesting will make even more difficult the problem of adequate housing and sanitation for workers who are present only a fraction of the year; it may even make the migrant crew obsolete.

There are rapid changes in synthetic and natural materials used for industry and agriculture, with an estimated 300 to 500 new chemicals put on the market each year. Some chemicals have known toxic effects while others have not been tested. Monitoring levels of exposure and developing an information base for defining "safe" levels is part of the mandate for occupational health nurses. The nurse in occupational health must develop special knowledge of the science areas that are related to the work processes, and she must constantly relearn the conditions of the work situation as they affect health.

A fourth significant trend affecting occupational health is the great extension of insurance coverage for the working population. Although compensation insurance, which provides benefits for work-related accident or illness, has long been common, more extensive general health insurance is now prevalent. This provides greater coverage for nonindustrial health problems and may extend insurance coverage to the family of the worker. The prepaid multispecialty group practice is an option in many health benefit plans and is required by law (Health Maintenance Organization Act of 1973) for certain employers. Some workers, such as the United Mine Workers of America in the Appalachian mining towns, developed their own hospitals and HMO's to serve the medical needs of workers and their families.

Large industries are tending toward reasonably comprehensive inplant care of employees, but the problem of providing care to the small plant is still largely unresolved. It is in this sphere that the greatest potential for imaginative use of nursing personnel may lie.

OBJECTIVES OF THE OCCUPATIONAL HEALTH PROGRAM

As a member of the occupational health-care group, the nurse shares in the implementation of the objectives of the occupational health program. These are:

1. To protect employees against health and safety hazards in their work situation.
2. Insofar as practical and feasible, to protect the general environment of the community.
3. To facilitate the physical, mental, and emotional placement of workers in work that they can perform with an acceptable degree of efficiency and without endangering their own health and safety or that of others.
4. To assure adequate care and rehabilitation for occupational injury and illness and for the nonoccupational conditions that are specified in the organization's policies.
5. To encourage and assist in measures for personal health maintenance, and to contribute to each worker's ability to cope with his own health needs and those of his family.[5]

The American Association of Occupational Health Nurses (AAOHN) has established the following definition:

"Occupational Health Nursing is the application of nursing principles in conserving the health of workers in all occupations. It involves prevention, recognition, and treatment of illness and injury and requires special skills and knowledge in the fields of health education and counseling, environmental health, rehabilitation, and human relations."[6]

The primary difference between occupational health nursing and non–work-related health care of the presumably well-adult population lies in the work setting and the demands it places on the worker. Accessibility to a large segment of the population, which is provided by the work setting, makes occupational health care an exceedingly attractive channel for public health effort.

THE HEALTH PROBLEMS OF PEOPLE AT WORK

The health problems of people at work are of two types: (1) those that are characteristic of all adults of working age and (2) those that are generated by the work environment or work processes.

Problems Brought to the Job

The mortality for the working population is similar to that for the general population; heart disease, cancer, stroke, and accidents are the leading causes of death. Upper respiratory infections play a major role in illness and cause interruption of work or decreased work efficiency. Other common problems of this age group include alcohol or drug abuse, venereal disease, poor nutrition, and lack of rest and weight control that lead to stress, fatigue, or lowered resistance to disease.

These problems are of concern to the occupational health-care group because they result not only in hardship to the individual and his family but also in absenteeism, an inability to maintain satisfactory work performance, and a need for changes in work assignment.

From a public health point of view, this age group represents a major channel for early recognition and control of long term illness, since it is during these years that the symptomless evidence of disease may first appear and that deleterious health practices have such a profound effect.

Within each work group, there will be subgroups that bring particular problems to the job. The worker recruited from a very low-income neighborhood may bring with him the problems characteristic of the poverty syndrome; women of childbearing age will bring the problems associated with pregnancy and child rearing; the executive may bring a stressful attitude derived from a keen drive for success.

Problems Generated by the Job

Job-induced health problems may arise from the use of toxic or irritating materials or from exposure to extremes of heat, cold, light, or noise. Miners, construction and transportation workers, and blue-collar and lower supervisory personnel in manufacturing industries are at greater risk for occupational disease and injury of this type. Agricultural workers also have a high job illness/injury rate. The work processes involved often make such exposure unavoidable, and the counteractive measures of wearing protective clothing or adopting an attitude of constant vigilance may in turn create a degree of stress.

Exposure to carcinogens and other toxic substances such as asbestos, DDT, and vinyl chloride in the work place is thought to be a major contribution to chronic disease in this country. Studies report that 80 to 90 per cent of cancer could be environmentally caused.[7] (See Table 26–1.)

Accident risk — ranging from the possibility of mine collapse to that of paper cuts — may also be associated with work conditions. Machines may be dangerous in themselves, and require constant care on the part of the worker.

Stress may also arise from highly competitive or monotonous work, or work that does not permit the individual to make choices. Processes that make a man feel like a machine instead of a person, and poor interpersonal relationships among workers also appear to have negative effects on worker morale and health.

Thus, in analyzing the work to be done, the nurse in occupational health must look at the conditions affecting people in the age and sex group that is characteristic of a specific working population and at the culture and the social environment of the community as a whole. She must then look at the health implications of the work environment: the physical characteristics of the plant, the processes and the materials involved, and the interpersonal environment that prevails.

Table 26–1   COMMON OCCUPATIONAL CARCINOGENS

Agent	Organ Affected	Occupation
Wood	Nasal cavity and sinuses	Woodworkers
Leather	Nasal cavity and sinuses; urinary bladder	Leather and shoe workers
Iron oxide	Lung; larynx	Iron ore miners; metal grinders and polishers, silver finishers, iron foundry workers
Nickel	Nasal sinuses; lung	Nickel smelters, mixers, and roasters; electrolysis workers
Arsenic	Skin; lung; liver	Miners; smelters; insecticide makers and sprayers; tanners; chemical workers; oil refiners; vintners
Chromium	Nasal cavity and sinuses; lung; larynx	Chromium producers, processors, and users; acetylene and aniline workers; bleachers; glass, pottery, and linoleum workers; battery makers
Asbestos	Lung (pleural and peritoneal mesothelioma)	Miners; millers; textile, insulation, and shipyard workers
Petroleum, petroleum coke, wax, creosote, shale, and mineral oils	Nasal cavity; larynx; lung; skin; scrotum	Contact with lubricating, cooling, paraffin or wax fuel oils or coke; rubber fillers; retort workers; textile weavers; diesel jet testers
Mustard gas	Larynx; lung; trachea; bronchi	Mustard gas workers
Vinyl chloride	Liver; brain	Plastic workers
Bis-chloromethyl ether, chloromethyl methyl ether	Lung	Chemical workers
Isopropyl oil	Nasal cavity	Isopropyl oil producers
Coal soot, coal tar, other products of coal combustion	Lung; larynx; skin; scrotum; urinary bladder	Gashouse workers, stokers, and producers; asphalt, coal tar, and pitch workers; coke oven workers; miners; still cleaners
Benzene	Bone marrow	Explosives, benzene, or rubber cement workers; distillers; dye users; painters; shoemakers
Auramine, benzidine, alpha-Naphthylamine, magenta, 4-Aminodiphenyl, 4-Nitrodiphenyl	Urinary bladder	Dyestuffs manufacturers and users; rubber workers (pressmen, filtermen, laborers); textile dyers; paint manufacturers

Based on data from the National Cancer Institute. As published in American Public Health Association: *Health and Work in America—A Chart Book*. Washington, D.C. November 1975, p. 15.

DEVELOPING THE NURSING PROGRAM IN AN OCCUPATIONAL HEALTH SETTING

Identification of Nursing Needs

As in any other setting, the nursing needs of the work population will represent the relationship between the health problems of the group; the degree to which they are able to cope with these problems;

the services provided by other health workers; and the capacity of the occupational nursing staff in terms of time, skills, and authorization. The pattern developed will vary from plant to plant. A thorough assessment of the industry along with a knowledge of the daily problems and needs of both management and workers is essential.[8]

Emergency Care

Needs for emergency care will be present in some degree in all settings. However, there will be great differences in the nature of the accident risk. In a steel plant, for example, major accidents may be a primary concern; whereas in a bank, the accidents will be for the most part minor in nature. The need for emergency care of illness will also vary greatly. When the work force contains a significant complement of older workers, care for coronary attack or stroke may be required often enough to necessitate special preparation to deal with these problems expeditiously, such as CPR programs for all employees. When the work force is largely female and young, minor illnesses will more likely be the pattern. It is important to know the nature, as well as the extent, of the possible emergency care load in order to determine the degree to which the nurse or other professional health worker must plan to provide care and the extent to which reliance may be placed on first-aid personnel equipped with short training. It is important to know the kinds of accidents that are most common: for instance, whether most accidents are falls from high equipment, foreign objects in the eye due to failure to wear safety goggles, or dermatitis arising from the use of irritating substances. A careful review of accident and emergency records for the past year will tell the nurse much about what to expect in the way of emergency care.

Occupational Illness and Disease

Needs for other than emergency nursing care of occupational or nonoccupational illness or injury include case finding, prevention, and care. Exposure to physical, chemical, or biological agents may cause dermatologic irritation, allergic sensitivity, toxicity, narcosis, carcinogenicity, and asphyxia and may produce pathophysiologic as well as psychologic disorders. Case-finding needs are based on expected or possible incidence of specific conditions, which, in turn, are estimated on the basis of the incidence of these conditions in the general public in the age, sex, and racial groups represented in the industry and also on the basis of the conditions that might be anticipated as a result of the particular industrial processes used. Again, a review of a sampling of records of those receiving service during the previous year and an analysis of medical examination results will provide much information. Review of the complete work history is also important since many occupational diseases have a long latency period. The nurse must use an epidemiologic approach to case finding — recording information so that the relationship between complex situations or a single stress agent, environment, and disease can be determined. An important part of the epidemiologic approach is frequent observation of workers in the work place. A record of the frequency and patterning of absences will also be a clue to illness patterns of the group.

It is harder to establish an estimate of emotional or health behavioral problems. The nurse must be able to recognize unusual behavior, such as dizziness or drowsiness, fatigue, increased tardiness or absenteeism, vague ailments, domestic problems, or overt bizarre behavior. The causes for these symptoms can be stress on the job or at home, alcoholism, drug use, or exposure to toxic substances such as carbon disulfide, acetates, lead, mercury or other heavy metals, and pesticides. The nurse is in a key position to find cases early, determine etiology, and assure appropriate treatment through review of records, knowledge of working conditions, and familiarity with the worker's family.

Rehabilitation

The employee, his family, and the employer all have an interest in rehabilitation after illness or injury. Nursing activities may include organizing a rehabilitation program involving community resources as well as those within the organization, counseling the worker and his family, providing direct care during working hours, and helping in the selection of and adjustment to a new job.[9]

Health Education

Health counseling or health education needs are identified by the problems uncovered in screening or medical examination programs and by the expected health problems of analogous age and socioeconomic groups in the general population. Records of the previous year will indicate the rate of positive findings in medical examinations or screening procedures and the counseling or educational services that were previously provided. However, in most instances, records will indicate a less than optimum level of recognition of such need. Direct observation of factors such as food choices in the cafeteria, weight trends, or on-the-job behavior may provide further clues.

The need for referral to care agents other than the nurse, either in or out of the plant, may be estimated by reviewing a sample of records to determine whether or not referral would have been useful. Even readily available sources in the plant, such as a nutritionist or psychologist, may be inadequately used, and referral to community agencies or family physicians may be minimal. Again, past practice may or may not be a good index of the level of the need, since nurses vary widely in their sensitivity to referral needs.

Preventive Care

The need for specific preventive measures may be estimated by comparing the actual recorded experience of the group against a list of desirable preventive measures for a typical group of similar age. Desirable measures might include:

1. Medical examination: annual or biennial.

2. Immunization: recommended schedules may be secured from the medical director, from the local or state health department, or from a medical advisory panel.

3. Periodic screening: depending on medical advice, the age of the group, and the nature of the industry might include screening for specific occupational hazards such as toxic effects of materials used or contact dermatitis, vision and hearing tests, weight checks, cervical smears for detection of cancer, tuberculin testing or x-ray examination, tonometry for detection of glaucoma, tests for diabetes, blood pressure and hemoglobin determination.

Needs of the Organization

Support of general personnel and production policies of the firm may also require special nursing measures. If the industry is making a special effort to employ socially disadvantaged groups, for example, the nurse might be expected to develop a special intensive health counseling plan and to arrange her own program to reach these workers early and frequently. She might make home visits in order to understand the problems this group faces in adapting to regular work or to identify and deal with family health or health-related problems that may be impeding an individual's work progress. A program of weight control and dietary reform for executives might be backed up by nursing action to secure the cooperation of their families. She might encourage their spouses to use the service of an agricultural extension staff or of a gas or electric company in planning family fare consistent with the prescribed dietary plan. New recruits in a military setting might receive a little extra nursing attention or referral to volunteer sources of support until they become accustomed to being away from their homes and families, since some will never have had that experience before.

The nurse in occupational health must keep abreast of new legislation as it affects the work setting. This involves knowing the required record-keeping systems and required monitoring system of equipment and hazardous materials. She should be able to inform the employer of new criteria developed at the state and federal levels and interpret the effect of proposed regulations on the health and safety program in terms of costs and benefits.

Interpretation of the firm's policies and of the legal rights and obligations of employers and employees may sometimes be indicated in order for the nurse to explain why certain procedures are necessary.

In the process of seeking out nursing needs, the nurse will be able to identify individuals and groups that are at special risk or that need more than the usual amount of nursing care or support. Based on this information, she will build the register of cases requiring intensive or continuing supervision.

Nursing Goals

Nursing goals should be explicit and time-related. Once nursing needs are determined, the nurse can take a realistic look at what may be accomplished through nursing in a given time period. She will then want to establish, for her own guidance, a set of specific goals (or desired nursing outputs). These goals will, of course, be influenced by the company's philosophy of care. Examples of goals she may want to set are as follows: that 80 or 90 per cent of pregnant workers will be under medical care within the first trimester; that the rate of eye accidents associated with failure to wear goggles will be reduced by x per cent; that recommended immunization procedures will be offered to the entire working staff, and that 75 per cent will accept these immunization procedures. Specific goals add direction to nursing activities and provide a basis for evaluation and interpretation of the service to nonhealth personnel.[10]

Establishment of the Health-Care Relationship Network

Establishing the health-care relationship network in the industrial setting takes time and thought. Within the plant, the nurse is working with new partners. The physician director upon whom she relies for many decisions may often be there only on a part-time or an on-call basis. The safety engineer, the systems analyst, the personnel director, the shop steward (union representative), the foreman and various management officers, the industrial psychologist or vocational counselor, the rehabilitation worker, and the insurance company health consultant staff offer new kinds of support and, in turn, expect different things from the nurse from those expected of her by the usual community health working group. The nurse needs to know and be known by each of these people; she must understand their relative contributions to employee health and must establish ways of reporting to and planning with them that are both effective and efficient in the use of time.

The health of the worker represents only one facet of the health care of the family, and the health care of the industrial community represents only one part of the total community health care. Relationships with hospitals, clinics, voluntary and official health and welfare agencies, educational facilities, and private family physicians must be established and maintained at an easy and productive level. Person-to-person contact, careful information exchange, and case conferences will work here, as they do in the general community health program, to provide a good base for a congenial and effective working relationship.

Identifying Priorities in Nursing Activities

It is axiomatic that nursing time is never adequate to do all that could be done. The occupational health nurse, like all others, will have to select among alternative actions in order to get the greatest results for the nursing time invested. A list of those individuals or groups with unusual need for nursing care will serve as a starting point in arranging activities.

Another basic objective is to achieve visibility and coverage. Much of what the occupational health nurse is able to do results from a good understanding of her function by those who use nursing care or who are responsible for referring others for such care. Referral for nursing care is more likely to be pertinent if the nurse is known to workers and management groups. Getting around the plant should be a high-priority activity, since it provides the nurse with an opportunity to observe conditions that affect health and also makes her a familiar figure to the work force. When there is more than one work shift or when the work force is scattered throughout several locations, the nurse will want to be sure that she is available to all of the various groups that are entitled to use her services. This may affect the scheduling of conference time in order to reach those who change shifts in the early morning or the late afternoon. The arrangement and planning of nursing activities must also take account of the need to respect the integrity of the work flow. For example, removing one worker from a production line for a conference on prenatal care may disarrange the work of several others in her unit. Arranging these activities in conjunction with the work supervisor will avoid such conflict.

Policies and Standing Orders

Policies and standing orders should be in writing and complete. Sometimes, especially in small plants, the nurse must work without the help of an on-the-spot physician. It is important that she safeguard the patient and protect her own professional integrity by having clearly written policies and standing orders. Such statements, however, cannot be substituted, either professionally or legally, for the nurse's own professional judgment. There may be occasions when standing orders should not be followed: for example, if there is some indication of sensitivity to a common drug. However, well-written and frequently reviewed policies are an essential basis for action. Written and signed standing orders are essential for the safety of the patient, and they also serve to interpret to others the limits of the nurse's authority with respect to dispensing drugs or to taking other action in the absence of an immediate medical diagnosis.

The Nurse's Role in Safety

Safety is everybody's business in the occupational setting. In many instances, first-aid care is given by short-trained workers in the work unit. Much safety teaching is done on the spot by the foreman or the training officer as he introduces the new workers to the job or as he engages in a continuing reinforcement of the safety education program. According to one training officer, "The habit of safety is caught as well as taught" — pointing out the importance of having every one set a good example to others in safety practice.

The nurse may be responsible for the coordination of first-aid efforts and for maintaining first-aid supplies. Whether or not it is written into her job description, the nurse in occupation health must be constantly alert to gaps in the safety system and must assure as far as possible that accidents are prevented and that victims are treated promptly and properly when they do occur.

The provisions of workman's compensation laws vary from state to state, but in general they provide for liability of the employer and for certain medical and disability benefits to employees suffering industrial injuries. For the worker to be compensated, the injury must arise out of, or in the course of, employment. In general, the same benefits apply whether or not the injured person was negligent.

Some nursing time should be allowed to add to the knowledge of occupational health. Although few nurses in occupational health have had the opportunity to engage in rigorous research, virtually every one has a chance to add to knowledge of the health problems and health care of the working population. This may take the form of participating in epidemiologic investigations, such as tracing the factors associated with an outbreak of dermatitis; of evaluating different methods of providing care, such as involving the worker himself in health decisions as compared to keeping the majority of decisions in the hands of the health professionals; or of describing and analyzing patterns of absence from work.

Health Records

Records play an especially significant role in occupational health services. They provide an official record that may protect the rights of the employee and of the employer, and they may serve as legal evidence regarding the circumstances surrounding a particular injury or illness.

Since the nurse is often the first observer at the time of injury or illness, her record is particularly valuable.

The cumulative health record of the employee is important in understanding his health progress and in relating changes in his health to changes in the work situation. Since many adults do not visit a personal physician on a regular basis, a well-kept occupational health record may provide the only reasonably comprehensive picture of an individual's health progress. As such, it could be an invaluable aid to the physician or to the hospital medical staff should the employee require intensive care.

The analysis of health records has already been mentioned as an excellent basis for establishing health needs, for planning health programs, for documenting the need for extra plant care facilities, and for evaluating the nursing and health services provided. Health records should be considered confidential documents. When a health condition requires work adjustment, the condition and the limits it imposes may be interpreted by the physician in a written statement to management, but the record itself should be available only to qualified health personnel. Policies relating to the divulgence of health information should be clearly stated and rigorously followed. Sometimes this confidential health information takes the form of a record analysis of the reasons for the patterns of absence, the characteristics of an "absence-prone" group, or of a record audit in which an outside consultant is requested to analyze the service provided as it relates to personnel needs.

Whatever the form, the nurse is in a good position to add to the knowledge about the needs for and processes of occupational health care. The nurse trained in community health is especially helpful in dealing with areas of health care as distinguished from care of disease or injury.

THE NURSE IN OCCUPATIONAL HEALTH
MAY NEED SPECIAL PREPARATION

The nurse in the occupational setting faces practical problems somewhat different from those she would expect to find in other settings. She is much more "on her own." One study conducted in 1964 involving over 10,000 occupational health nurse respondents indicated that most nurses work without supervision: 40 per cent of the respondents reported that they worked alone, and another 16 per cent stated that they worked with other nurses but without a supervisor. Furthermore, only one-fourth worked with a full-time physician, and nearly a third reported that they had no physician available on a regular basis; however, 95 per cent had access to a physician on an on-call basis.[11] A 1972 Conference Board survey of 858 companies found that 24 per cent of companies with 500 or more employees have occupational nurses only. If the company is in a rural area, nurses are working alone 50 per cent of the time (see Fig. 26–1).[12] Thus, many nurses in the occupational setting will need more than the basic nursing preparation.

New and constantly changing methods of production and of manpower utilization create health and nursing needs of considerable complexity. The nurse in the occupational setting needs to be unusually aware of physiologic responses to the conditions of work, such as the effects of heat, cold, stress, and noise; she needs a sufficient grasp of biochemistry to recognize the potential or actual toxic effects of materials used in particular occupational settings; she must be familiar with emergency nursing; and she must understand the dynamics of produc-

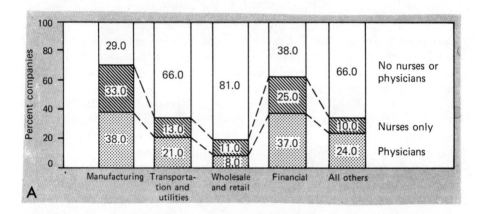

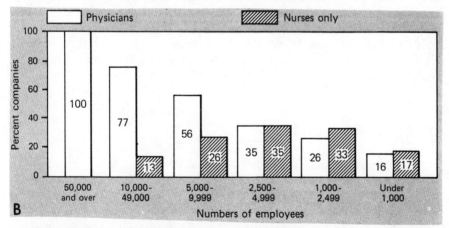

Figure 26–1 A study of 858 companies with 500 or more employees showed that wholesale and retail firms employed the lowest percentage of physicians and nurses. *A*, Companies employing medical personnel by company type and kind of personnel (full-time), 1972; *B*, companies employing medical personnel by company size and kind of personnel (full-time), 1972. From The Conference Board: *Industry Roles in Health Care.* New York, Conference Board Report No. 610, 1974, p. 23. As published in American Public Health Association: *Health and Work in America — A Chart Book.* Washington, D.C., November 1975, p. 95.

tion and of management in order to fit her program into the whole fabric of the productive effort.

The need for the nurse to make preliminary diagnostic decisions has already been noted. This, too, suggests the need for special preparation in relevant clinical fields. The administrative responsibilities of the occupational health nurse who works alone or without the structure of an organized occupational health program are also great; they may range from program development and budgeting to setting up first-aid stations or clinics. An analysis of the areas of knowledge or skills required in this field has been developed by a special subcommittee of the Permanent Commission and International Association on Occupational Health.[13] This report should be read by anyone contemplating employment in occupational nursing. Federal grants for education are available to nurses under the NIOSH Educational Resource Center Program, and some university nursing programs have developed occupational health nurse practitioner curriculums. There is no doubt that formal post-baccalaureate education could make a significant contribution to the development of requisite competencies.

In her on-the-job development, as in so many other things, the occupational nurse must be on her own. Most large city and state health departments and some insurance carriers have nurse consultants who may be called upon for help. When community nursing agencies supply part-time nursing to industry, they are likely to secure a nurse who is knowledgeable in the occupational health field to direct the work and to provide leadership to others engaged in the occupational health program. Professional associations in nursing and in public health, including the American Association of Occupational Health Nurses, can provide assistance through publications and programs. Experts in other fields within the industry may make willing and valuable consultants. Each nurse must seek out and use these sources for professional support.

SPECIAL WORK GROUPS

Every work group has its own special problems; however, agricultural workers, including migrant workers and workers in small industries (500 or less), face unique risks.

Agricultural Workers

As of 1975, 3.5 per cent of the total work force were farm workers.[14] The farm workers of this country suffer a disproportionate number of occupational illnesses and injuries. In 1973, the incidence rate for illness and injury was 11.6 per 100 full-time workers, the fourth highest in the country.[15] As of 1972, 81 per cent of farm workers were not covered by any form of group health insurance.[16]

Statistics on the health of farm workers are not readily available. Many states do not cover agricultural workers under Workmen's Compensation laws; few records are kept; and no single group is responsible for agricultural health. Inaccessibility to health facilities, seasonal variations, and the transient quality of the work further confounds the problem.

One special hazard faced by farm workers is that of accidents, usually from heavy farm equipment. Because of the distance of the farm from centers of population and the shortage of skilled workers, the farmer is forced to do many things that in urban centers would be undertaken by specialists. He is, at once, electrician, carpenter, mechanic, operator of large equipment, animal keeper, and manager.

Although a small number of farmers have had specific training, for the most part training has been a family or self-initiated process. Because farming is a family occupation, women and children may be temporary members of the work force. They may, for example, drive tractors or handle other large equipment at peak periods of the farm cycle. Thus the danger of accident is higher on farms than in other settings.

The farm worker is also exposed to dusts, pollens, and a variety of chemicals that may have harmful health effects, some of which are cumulative. Insecticides, rodenticides, and pesticides are examples of such materials. Organophosphates — one class of frequently used pesticides — are virtually nerve gases, affecting the level of red cells and the nervous system.

Another hazard faced by the farm worker is exposure to diseases of animals that may be transmissible to man: for instance, anthrax, rabies, or tularemia.

Perhaps just as serious as exposure to pollutants or to disease is the problem of inaccessibility of health care. Federal support for construction has increased the number of hospitals available to farm residents and, to a limited degree, has improved the operation of rural hospitals; however, the distances involved often lead to sparingly used facilities.[17]

The number of physicians available is less than that found in urban centers, and the age of the physicians who are available tends to be higher. As a result, care may be delayed or home remedies may be used, especially during busy seasons. The fatalism that seems to characterize the farm worker group may also contribute to the failure to deal with disease until it is well advanced or severely incapacitating.

Migrant Workers

The health problems of migrant agricultural workers are sufficiently different to require special programs. More than 700 of the nation's 3,100 counties depend on farm workers from outside the local area during the peak harvest season. This work is provided largely by migrant laborers who travel in defined "streams" or routes as they move from one harvest area to the next. (See Figure 26–2). It is estimated that approximately 400,000 to 450,000 people move in the migrant stream each year.[18]

The migrant laborer travels with his family. He is recruited and supervised by a "crew leader" who deals with the farm owners and serves as a leader of the work group. It is the crew leader who owns much of the equipment, such as the buses and trucks in which the group travels. He is the camp manager, he provides food and the transportation from the campsite to the fields, he allocates the work, and he serves as a banker and as an intermediary with the employer and with the communities to which the migrants travel.

The agricultural migrant population is poor and, for the most part, unskilled. Many are separated from the mainstream of the communities they serve by language barriers or by cultural patterns. Most have little formal education.

The migrant's record for health is poor. Although comparative statistics on a national level are difficult to obtain, it is generally believed that infant mortality and mortality from accidents, and from a variety of infectious diseases are greater for this group.

The problems that the migrants bring with them are aggravated by the conditions of the work itself. For the most part, work is piecework and pay is determined by the amount each one harvests. This tends to encourage long hours; the traditional farmer's day of "can't see to can't see" often prevails. It also encourages children's participation in the

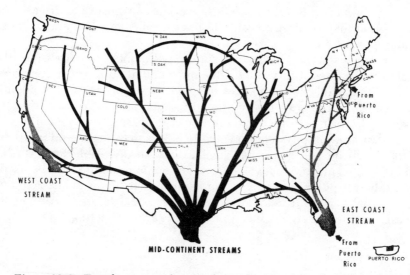

Figure 26–2 Travel patterns of seasonal migratory agricultural workers. (From *Migrant Health Program Current Operations and Additional Needs.* U.S. Department of Health, Education and Welfare, U.S. Government Printing Office, Washington, D.C., December, 1967.)

labor force; children over 9 years of age are generally included in the work in the fields.

Because the work requires a large number of workers for a very short period of time, housing is apt to be isolated from the general community and minimal in construction and facilities. Crowded conditions prevail, and facilities for cooking are often primitive. Local and state regulations do require specific provisions for sanitation, but these laws vary greatly.

Often migrant workers find they are not socially welcome in the communities they serve; they may be considered "wild" or "different." Residence requirements may bar them from health or welfare services. Their frequent moves make it extremely difficult to maintain continuity of care.

The federal government has long been concerned about the plight of the migrant worker, and the Migrant Health Act of 1962 and its amendments greatly expanded federal activity in this area. The goal of this legislation is to raise the level of health services provided to migrants to the level of those provided to the general population. Direct services may be sponsored by federal funds; more commonly, however, state programs are partially subsidized by federal contributions. The Comprehensive Health Care Act and many legislative actions designed to improve the conditions of the very low income group have also contributed to intensified government efforts on behalf of agricultural migrant families. A potent factor in this legislation is the support afforded for family health clinics. In many areas, these clinics are held after the working day in order to reach all who need help.

Nursing adaptations required for this population are designed to deal with the poverty syndrome and with problems arising from the mobility of the group and the inadequacies of the environment.

The approaches that work with other groups living in poverty are equally pertinent to the migrant population. Intensified care, "reaching out," taking special care to assure that true communication exists, and strengthening the family's sense of worth and competence are essential.

Because the needs of this group are so great, most agencies find that a combination of volunteer and paid workers is required. In one area in Ohio, for example, the regular health staff was supplemented by volunteer groups who recorded stories and songs in Spanish for a Spanish-American group of children left in camp while their parents were in the field; besides providing entertainment, this activity helped to strengthen the migrant workers' sense of identity with a specific culture. Sometimes lawyers serve as volunteers, since migrants often need help in understanding their legal rights and obligations. Literacy and homemaking classes may be organized to supplement the health services.

The problems of sanitation and nutrition are unusually great for this group. Even such simple things as handwashing may be hard to arrange. Parents will need considerable help in adapting the family diet to foods that can be prepared with the limited equipment and time available.

Such changes of habit are not easily accomplished. Powdered milk, for example, is inexpensive, is usable when refrigeration is limited, and can be easily transported. However, for families who are unaccustomed to its use, the taste may be unacceptable. Also, the need for milk may not even be recognized.

Child care represents another grave concern. Children are often inadequately protected against communicable disease, are fed under unsanitary conditions, and are inadequately supervised when the parents are at work in the fields. Day care centers are badly needed, but they are difficult to organize. In some communities, volunteers acting under the aegis of local social agencies or the VISTA program have provided day care services for children of migrant workers.

Family planning is another service that frequently misses the migrant group. Their isolation and transitory stay in the community make it difficult to locate sources for family planning and to secure the necessary follow-up care.

Although the diseases from which the agricultural migrant population suffers will probably parallel those of others who are poor and in farm work, communication problems may increase the difficulty of identifying problems and providing care. The short stay and, often, the cultural and language barriers of the migrant workers preclude the slow development of trust and the easy interchange that grows with familiarity and extended contact over a long period of time. Thus the nurse has to seek more diligently for possible problems. There are, for example, great differences among camps in the number of venereal disease cases reported. There is little reason to suppose that there is an actual difference in the occurrence of these diseases; rather, the difference in rate is more likely the result of failure to report symptoms that require care.

The need for emotional support and motivation toward health care is also extremely high in this group. The migrant life is so rigorous that the need for other than frankly curative health care may have a low priority. The social isolation in, and sometimes frank rejection by, the communities in which they work can only be emotionally damaging. With such pressures, health care requires an exceptional effort on the part of all of the health professional group.

With the migrant population, the need to provide for continuity of care is paramount. Since the migrant stream transcends state lines and covers many communities in the course of the year, continuity is difficult to achieve. The nurse should familiarize herself with the stations along the migrant stream and establish communication with the health organizations and personnel who will care for the family later. Referral forms and procedures may need to be developed. The United States Public Health Service encourages the use of a wallet-sized personal health history to be carried by each person as he moves along the migrant stream. This is a valuable adjunct to agency records. If, in addition, each nurse assumes the responsibility for informing the health organization at the next station on the stream about those who require special care and, as far as possible, refers the family needing care to a particular person, continuity of care is more likely to be achieved.

It would be an error, however, to assume that the failure of families to seek or to secure care in the new community is due entirely to mechanical failure of the referral system. All too often the worker and his family do not truly understand the nature of their problem or are not persuaded of the importance or of the need for care. Careful teaching, demonstrated concern on the part of health personnel, and the use of interpreters to assure that the message is understood are essential to secure the motivation required for the family to seek follow-up care.

The Small Industry

Approximately 50 million people in the United States work in industries employing less than 500 workers. Therefore, they are not covered by the Occupational Safety and Health Act and may not employ safety and health professionals.[19]

Part-time nursing service may be provided through voluntary and public health agencies in the community, thus providing health benefits comparable to larger establishments. Hours and conditions of the service are agreed upon by the agency and the industry, and contracts are drawn up. Frequently an advisory committee is formed, made up of representatives of management, the community health nurse, local or state occupational health units, insurance company, and labor unions that can be an asset in establishing policy and interpreting programs to workers.

The nurse is usually the only immediately available representative of health services and the first source of health care. She will work with a designated physician, physician panel, or clinic from whom she will secure standing orders and policies relative to referral for medical care. For many of the health education aspects of the work, she will be on her own.

When such service is provided through an agency, there is usually one person with special preparation in occupational health nursing who serves in a supervisory and coordinating role and who either provides the service or works with the nurse who is actually visiting the plant and providing service. The nurse in this setting carries the same responsibilities that would characterize work in any other occupational health setting. She has the same responsibility for assuring that emergency care is available and appropriate, for promoting the general health of the workers, for protecting them against hazards in the environment, and for providing intensive care to those with special problems. Because she is the only regular health worker in the setting, and because she may be only a part-time employee, it is especially important for the nurse in this type of industrial establishment to be visible and to take the time to familiarize herself thoroughly with the work force and with the work processes. Because of the absence of specialists in personnel, in safety, and in management, she will have more than the usual responsibility for initiating certain facets of the program or for proposing changes that will improve care. For example, a system for employee counseling and health education may need to be established from scratch, or a totally inadequate record system may have to be revised and updated in order to support the day-to-day responsibilities of the nurse's job.

The community health nurse will come with the strengths of knowing how to use community resources and work with families. She will need to learn about the Occupational Safety and Health Act, prevention of occupational accidents, and the etiology of occupational diseases. The agency and the nurse will need to align themselves with experts in the areas of occupational safety engineering, industrial hygienists, and occupational medicine.

REFERENCES: THE OCCUPATIONAL HEALTH SETTING

1. Ashford, N. A.: *Crisis in the Work Place: Occupational Disease and Injury.* A Report to the Ford Foundation. Cambridge, Mass., MIT Press, 1976.
2. Lee, J.: *The New Nurse in Industry — A Guide to the Newly Employed Occupational Health Nurse.* Center for Disease Control, U.S. Department of Health, Education, and Welfare (NIOSH Pub. No. 78–143), Washington, D.C., U.S. Government Printing Office, 1978, pp. 77–85.
3. Lavenne, F.: Down the mines: Heat, dust, and danger. World Health, p. 28, March, 1969.
4. Carpenter, D.: Machines made to measure. World Health, March, 1969, p. 6.
5. These objectives have been adapted from the statment of objectives in The American Medical Association's publication, *Scope, Objectives, and Functions of Occupational Health Programs.* (Revised, 1971) p. 26.
6. Lee, J.: *The New Nurse in Industry,* p. 3.
7. Ashford, N. A.: *Crisis in the Work Place. . . ,* p. 11.
8. Serafini, P.: Nursing assessment in industry. Am. J. Pub. Health, 66:757, 1976.
9. Bernhardt, J. H.: The role of the occupational health nurse in employee rehabilitation. Occup Health, Nurs., 23:9, 1975.
10. Webb, S.: Objective criteria for evaluating occupational health programs. Am. J. Pub. Health, 65:31, 1975.
11. Gray, J.: Why define occupational health nursing? Nurs. Outlook, 15:52, 1967.
12. American Public Health Association: Health and Work in America—A Chart Book. Washington, D.C., 1975, p. 95.
13. Report of the Nursing Subcommittee in the Nurse's Contribution to the Health of the Worker, 1973. ISBN No. 0:9500840.
14. Manpower Report of the President. U.S. Department of Labor and Department of Health, Education, and Welfare. April 1975, p. 35.
15. American Public Health Association: *Health and Work in America.* Washington, D.C., 1975, p. 52.
16. Ibid., p. 36.
17. Hospital Survey and Construction Act, (PL 725).
18. Senate Subcommittee on Migratory Labor. Committee on Labor and Public Welfare, 91st Congress, p. 34.
19. Brown, M. L.: The quality of the work environment. Am. J. Nurs., 75:1755, 1975.

SUGGESTED READINGS: THE OCCUPATIONAL HEALTH SETTING

Baughn, S.: A nursing theory and model for occupational health nursing. Occup. Health Nurs., 25:7, 1977.

Browning, R. H., and Schulman, S.: An analysis of contract-service in the migrant health service referral system. Am. J. Pub. Health, 65:1177, 1971.

Caplan, R., et al.: *Job Demand and Worker Health.* Washington, D.C., U.S. Dept. H.E.W., PHS, Center for Disease Control, NIOSH, April 1975.

Cassel, J.: The use of medical records: Opportunity for epidemiological studies. Occup. Med., 5:185, 1963.

Cline, S.: *Alcohol and Drugs at Work.* Washington, D.C., Drug Abuse Council, Inc., 1975.

Community Health Nursing for Working People. U.S. Dept. of H.E.W., PHS, Environmental Health Service (No. 1296) 1971.

Coles, R.: Migrants, Sharecroppers, and Mountaineers. Boston, Little, Brown and Co., 1971.

Daniel, M.C.: Special programs on health and safety. Occup. Health Nurs., 22:14, 1974.

Fuenjes, J.: The need for effective and comprehensive planning for migrant workers. Am. J. Pub. Health, 2, 1974.

Geary, J. A., and Crane, J.: Following the migrant stream. *In* Hall, J. E., and Weaver, B. (eds.): *Distributive Nursing Practice, A Systems Approach to Community Health.* Philadelphia, J. B. Lippincott Co., 1977, pp. 519–528.

Hanlon, J. J.: *Public Health Administration and Practice.* St. Louis, Mo., C. V. Mosby Co., 1974, pp. 576–85.

Health and Work in America: A Chart Book. Washington, D.C., Am. Pub. Health Association, 1975.

Howe, H. F.: Preventing occupational health and safety hazards in small employee groups. Am. J. Pub. Health, 65:1581, 1971.

Karvonen, M.: Fitting the job to the worker. World Health, July, 1974, p. 30.

Last, J. M. (Ed.): Maxcy–Rosenau Public Health and Preventive Medicine. Regulation and Control of Occupational Health Problems, 11th ed., New York, Appleton-Century-Crofts, 1980.

Lee, J. A.: *The New Nurse in Industry: A Guide for the Newly Employed Occupational Health Nurse.* U.S. Dept. H.E.W. Center for Disease Control, Washington, D.C., U.S. Government Printing Office, Jan. 1978.

McMichael, A. J.: An epidemiologic perspective on the identification of workers at risk. Occup. Health Nurs., 23:7, 1975.

Macúch, P.: Dangers of a long day. World Health, July, 1974, p. 10.

Occupational Safety and Health Act of 1970. P. L. 91, 596.

Peterson, J.: *Industrial Health.* Prentice-Hall, Inc., Englewood Cliffs, N.J., 1977.

Rieke, F. E.: Industrial clinic services to small industries. Am. J. Pub. Health, 65:69, 1972.

Ross, D. S., and Bamber, L.: Costs of accidents. Occup. Health, 27:49, 1975.

Sauereisen, P. F.: OSHA's special problems in smaller plants. J. Occup. Med., 15:432, 1973.

Spickard, J. H.: Nuclear reactors—the employee monitoring and safety program. J. Occup. Med., 15:343, 1973.

Stellman, J., and Daum, S.: *Work is Dangerous to Your Health.* New York, Pantheon Books, 1973.

Sterns, W.: The expanded roles of the occupational health nurse. Occup. Health Nurs., 23:18, 1975.

Webb, S.: Objective criteria for evaluating occupational health programs. Am. J. Pub. Health, 65:31, 1975.

World Health Organization: *Early Detection of Impairment in Occupational Exposure to Health Hazards.* Technical Report Series #571, Geneva, 1975.

World Health Organization: Environmental and Health Monitoring in Occupational Health. Technical Report Series #535, Geneva, 1973.

RESOURCES: THE OCCUPATIONAL HEALTH SETTING

American Associaton of Occupational
  Health Nurses (AAOHN)
575 Lexington Avenue
New York, New York, 10022

Occupational Health Nursing (Journal)
Chas. B. Slack, Inc.
6900 Grove Road
Thorofare, New Jersey 08086

American Board for Occupational Health Nurses,
  Inc. (ABOHN)
P.O. Box 638
Thousand Palms, California 92276
A. H. Mayrose, Snyder, Executive Secretary

American Industrial Hygiene Association (AIHA)
25711 Southfield Road
Southfield, Michigan 48075

American Medical Association (AMA)
Department of Environmental, Public,
  and Occupational Health
535 N. Dearborn Street
Chicago, Illinois 60610

Journal of the American Medical Association
Archives of Environmental Health
535 N. Dearborn Street
Chicago, Illinois 60610

American Occupational Medical Association (AOMA)
150 North Wacker Drive
Chicago, Illinois 60606

Journal of Occupational Medicine
P.O. Box 247
Downers Grove, Illinois 60515

Society for Occupational and
  Environmental Health (SOEH)
1714 Massachusetts Avenue
Washington, D.C., 20036

U.S. Department of Health and Human Services
National Institute for Occupational Safety and Health (NIOSH)
Parklawn Building
5600 Fishers Lane
Rockville, Maryland 20852

U.S. Department of Labor
Occupational Safety and Health Administration (OSHA)
200 Constitution Avenue, N.W.
Washington, D.C. 20210

Correctional Institutions: A Captive Population

There has been a resurgence of public concern about protection of the health of individuals held in corrective institutions. These institutions vary in the services afforded, but three general types may be identified: (1) the short detention unit; (2) the minimum security institution used for individuals presenting minimum risk; and (3) the standard or maximum security facility, which provides close surveillance.

Health care for inmates of correctional institutions is a major issue for correctional officers, the courts, legislatures, and health care professionals. Approximately 500,000 inmates in 4,500 institutions, ranging in size from large prisons housing thousands of inmates to small jails housing a few, are in need of adequate health care.[1] Health care delivery systems of most prisons and jails are inadequate, and correctional institutions in general are having difficulties meeting minimal standards of care.

Health care for prisoners has usually been at the "prerogative of the correctional institution," isolated from community practice and scrutiny. For most, incarceration has meant diminished access to quality medical care, although there is a recognized need for general health programs as well as attention to specific health problems for this population.

Correctional institutions are constantly under attack because of conflicting views about local, state, and federal correctional systems. Society generally has not come to grips with the purpose of incarceration — i.e., prevention, deterrence, reform, containment, control, punishment, therapy, and rehabilitation. These objectives are difficult to achieve because of overcrowding and limited financial resources. Some critics would abolish the whole system, while others would strengthen it. An important fact in considering health services for correctional facilities is that custody and security of the population are foremost. Cooperation with the larger correctional system is vital to the everyday activities of providing nursing care to prisoners.

Recent studies suggest that incarceration is not a very productive deterrent to future delinquency. There are numerous experimental programs being developed to reverse negative behavior patterns. Many of these programs depend on the creation of a "family" or community support system for the incarcerated individual to reinforce positive behavior.

THE POPULATION IN THE PRISON COMMUNITY

The population that is served by the prison nurse includes the incarcerate, the service staff, the guard and, to some degree, the family of the incarcerated individual. For example, a young wife may be helped to sort out her feelings about her husband's predicament by talking out her frustrations and anger and by vocalizing her attitudes toward the situation. The nurse may help visiting friends and family to understand the prisoner's needs for support and understanding and for frequent contact with them.

Institutional staff members may need help with their own health problems and guidance with their role in strengthening the rehabilitation efforts for the inmates under their jurisdiction. The guard may bring with him fear, racial prejudice, and harsh patterns of discipline from his own background that must be dealt with.

Statistics for children in custody include juveniles held for court action and those held in detention centers, shelters or half-way houses, correctional facilities, and diagnostic centers. As of June, 1974, there were 76,471 juveniles held in public or private correctional facilities. The largest percentage, approximately 70 per cent, were male. Usual offenses were for felonies, misdemeanors, drug offenses, or status offenses.[2]

The largest offense groups for adults in state operated facilities are burglary and robbery. The highest proportions of prisoners serving time for crimes of violence come from large cities. Most individuals incarcerated are male, between the ages of 20 and 30 years, and black. Members of races other than white or black made up a small proportion of inmates — less than 5 per cent, in most jurisdictions.[3]

The typical inmate was a high school dropout, with the median number of years of schooling completed being approximately 10.5 years.[4]

Length of sentence varied by state, the highest median sentence being 25.6 years in Ohio and the lowest being 4.3 years in South Dakota.[5]

In jails, the sex, race, and age statistics are very similar to those in prisons. What is important to note is the disparity between the number of persons in "temporary" detention and those actually sentenced. According to a Boston study, only 17 per cent of the total Boston jail population were given prison terms each year.[6]

"Temporary detention" can range from a day or two to as long as a year. Structural facilities for vocational and recreational programs are frequently nonexistent in these settings because the prisoner's stay is thought of as temporary. Health care services usually consist of a cursory screening program and "sick call." Yet being detained in jail before a trial and experiencing the fears of an uncertain future can be more stressful than actual imprisonment. At this point in the correctional system, the prisoner is at greater risk of suicide or of other abusive behavior to himself and others.

SPECIAL HEALTH PROBLEMS

Health problems of prisoners are closely related to violence (trauma), drug and alcohol abuse, and psychiatric problems. They are also at risk for the usual health problems of the larger community — whether these are communicable disease or chronic conditions such as epilepsy or hypertension.

A study of the Tennessee State Penitentiary found higher injury rates and higher infections and parasitic disease rates for prisoners than those reported for the adult-male U. S. population of comparable age groups. The higher injury rate for prisoners may be explained by an increase in violence during imprisonment and closeness of confinement with persons prone to violence. Poor hygiene and poor sanitary conditions would be suspect in explaining the higher rates of infections and parasitic diseases.[7] Increased aggravation of chronic conditions, such as ulcers, was also found at much higher rates in the prison population.

1. Hazards of the Incarceration Process:

Incarceration is a time of crisis for the inmate and his family. Major stressors specific to the condition of detention have been identified as:

a. Losses, such as loss of job, freedom, family contacts, dignity, food choices, privacy, and sexual activity;
b. Threats, such as violence or the threat of homosexual advances;
c. Physical discomfort related to sleeping, eating, and other personal functions;
d. Drug and/or alcohol withdrawal;
e. Fears, such as fear of impending trial, or of infidelity of spouse or other companion.[8]

Depending on an individual's coping level, these stresses cause people to react in different ways. Some become sullen, depressed and not infrequently suicidal, while others may react in overt hostility. Whatever reaction, it is upsetting to himself, the other inmates, and the guards, for the prevailing goal is to "keep things quiet," and belligerence is a threat to the correctional officer's self-esteem.

The fears of the family, both for the well-being of the inmate as well as their own, are intense. Incarceration not infrequently results in the breakup of marriage and puts wife and children on the welfare rolls. Rumors about prison life and cruel treatment make the family apprehensive about their loved one. Quick access to outside help for support of emotional response to this new situation as well as economic support for the family may be needed.

2. Hazards of the Environment:

Public health approaches to environmental problems in correctional facilities are similar to those necessary for any institution. These include a structure that meets codes for fire and safety, ventilation and heat control, safe water supply with proper plumbing and sewage disposal, lighting, noise control, vermin control, and general housekeeping and food service. In large facilities a sanitary supervisor may be employed to monitor proper environmental practices. In smaller institutions, the nurse may need to help train a correction officer interested in sanitation.[9]

The greatest environmental contributers to unhealthy living conditions in correctional facilities are overcrowding and lack of space for recreational activities, both indoors and outside the prison building. Overcrowding results in tension and unrest as well as lack of privacy. It also contributes to the rapid spread of infectious diseases. The lack of recreational activities and space results in the universal problem for prisoners — boredom. Larger facilities have developed a variety of programs for education and vocational training and prison industries, as well as diverse sports activities. The ability to exercise, to relate in positive ways to other residents, and to engage in productive endeavors helps to alleviate stress and anxiety. These programs are not always available, especially in jails and smaller facilities or in prisons where these activities are seen as contrary to security measures.

Although the American Medical Association, the American Correctional Association, and the American Public Health Association all have standards related to the above problems, funds and strategies for implementation of these standards across the country have been slow to materialize. Many states, triggered by inmate riots, have set up advisory health commissions to oversee and recommend improvements in prisons.[10]

3. Special Problems of Probation and Parole:

Indeterminate sentences of uncertain duration are a cause of much frustration and anxiety for inmates and their families. While in detention centers, the prisoner faces uncertainty about type of sentence. Once sentenced, he still faces uncertainty concerning the amount of time committed, which can vacillate with subjective decisions based on "good" behavior or rehabilitative progress. Fears at the time of parole due to questions of what will be expected, obtaining and keeping a job, and changing relationships with family make this a time of crisis as well.

The total context of family, friends and neighbors, and all the positive and negative forces that may exist in this system for the prisoner must be utilized in a new way if he is to function successfully "on the outside." There may be problems with housing, overdue bills, illness in other family members, and family conflicts that need to be worked on lest they seem overwhelming. The community health nurse can be a catalytic force in helping the family mobilize to work on these problems and build on their strengths before the time of probation. The family may need assistance in anticipating problems and in determining ways in which these problems can be solved to avoid another crisis. Ongoing support to the family, such as family therapy through a neighborhood mental health center, may be useful to individual members in the family. Questions such as "Will husband and wife be compatible?" or "Will the prisoner be safe in society?" must be discussed openly, and with sensitivity.

The issues of probation and parole are also difficult for correction officers. These individuals are being asked to predict human behavior, something at which none of us is very good. Attempts have been made at identifying predictions of "success," using factors such as age, race, years of schooling, family support systems, and record of prior convictions.[11] Although potentially helpful, none of these methods are fail-safe. Techniques and standards are still only guides, and personal decisions must be made.

4. Special Health Concerns for Women and Juvenile Prisoners:

Most of the literature on inmates describes the majority population — i.e., adult males — and little is said about the special needs of incarcerated women and children. The environment itself may be more stressful to women, who are not segregated by severity of crime but placed together because they are female — again, in overcrowded conditions. Because the facilities for women are smaller, they frequently do not provide recreational, medical, or rehabilitation services.

Other special needs are related to reproduction and child care. Approximately three-quarters of the female prison population are mothers — usually black, unmarried, and between the ages of 21 and 30 years.[12] The incarcerated mother needs help in coping with the concerns of the separation of mother and child, the need for finding suitable alternative care for children with relations or foster homes, and all the other health issues involved in child care. She must turn to the prison staff, the social workers, and the community health nurse for such assistance.

It is not unusual for incarcerated women to be pregnant, necessitating the full range of prenatal, nutritional, and health educational services. Screening programs for drug abuse, alcoholism, and venereal disease are usually part of the intake procedure; however, recognition and treatment of these problems are particularly important for the pregnant woman.

Some penal institutions have special programs to assist the female prisoners to cope with these issues. They include day care centers at prisons, half-way houses, unrestricted visitation for children, and work release programs. The community health nurse, with her knowledge of resources and people in the community, may be able to assist families in using these resources, thereby reducing the stress of imprisonment.

Special needs of children and adolescents held in custody fall into three categories: (1) health problems common to all children and adolescents during the period of rapid growth and body change; (2) health problems related to complications resulting from their life style, including poor nutrition, venereal disease, hepatitis, unwed pregnancy, emotional illness, and drug abuse; and (3) health problems resulting from undiagnosed congenital abnormalities and other untreated diseases. These problems require special expertise and follow-up care for adequate treatment, often difficult to obtain in the correctional setting.

The community health nurse will need to work with the parents and other family members of these children as well, involving and coordinating other care-givers. Children with antisocial behavior may come from a variety of home environments, and the community health nurse will need to use her best skills in working with these families-in-stress.

Rather than use conventional prisons and jails, many departments of correction use community facilities such as farms, camps and half-way houses for minors. These facilities need to plan for ongoing health care of residents, and the community health nurse may be helpful in assisting them to establish ties with prepaid group practices, private physicians, or clinics and hospitals in the area so that the special health needs of these children can be met.

DEVELOPING A HEALTH CARE NETWORK

In developing a health care network, the nurse must design and effect a plan that ensures the collaboration of security and medical personnel, of the inmate subculture, of community resources, and of the prisoner and his or her family.

Security personnel or correctional staff form a hierarchy of command — from a commissioner, to wardens, to assistant wardens, and then to correctional officers. The goal is security, with no disruptions. The custodian, the lowest man in the hierarchy, is a pivotal person — powerful in that he controls access to health care, yet vulnerable because of the stress of potential disturbances of a violent nature. The nurse does not need to declare herself either for or against inmates or custodians, but can assist both sides in averting crisis behavior. According to Cohen, when an inmate becomes severely depressed, he may attempt suicide or become overly aggressive and a threat to himself, other inmates, and the security officers. A screening mechanism, developed for use by the guards in a detention center, helped to teach guards about alternative interpretations to abusive behavior, symptoms of distress, and new ways of working with these problems. The guards could then alert others in the correctional system to prisoners who needed immediate medical attention or who needed further assessment.[14]

By sharing information about the inmates' fears and difficulties as well as respecting the needs of the custodial staff, the nurse can gain cooperation that will make life easier for everyone.

The inmate subculture, though informally organized, has its own rules and ethics. This code involves being loyal to other inmates, keeping information from guards, and maintaining a calm exterior. There is also a hierarchy based on the crime committed, age, strength, and leadership skills. Older and weaker inmates are often taken advantage of by stronger, tougher prisoners unless they are protected by other prisoners or by physical separation. Peer approval and protection are important aspects of daily living.

Other people important to the prisoner are his lawyer, the correction officers regularly assigned to him, and his family. The nurse is also important, since she provides medication and access to the doctor. If the health program is to work, the nurse must find ways of exploiting existing reciprocal relationships among these groups. This may mean working with families of prisoners and helping them meet their needs so they are in a better position to offer support to the prisoner. Or it may mean working with corrections officers to help them cope with the stress of their job so they can see the needs of prisoners in a more positive light. Whatever the health effort, it must fit in with the overall goal of security and "keeping things quiet."

Possible Services and Activities

The health program for the incarcerated population will depend on the size and resources of the institution, the community and its resources, the available staffing, and the specific needs of prisoners, their families, and the correctional staff.

The American Public Health Association, the American Medical Association, and the U. S. Department of Justice have each established minimal standards for health care in correctional institutions.[15, 16, 17] Still, the health care delivery systems of most correctional facilities are inadequate and, to varying degrees, do not meet the above standards for physical examinations, dental care, medical records, staffing, facilities, and equipment. All facilities are under pressure from the courts to upgrade the health care they provide so as not to violate the constitutional ban against cruel and unusual punishment. There are serious constraints, and deficiencies — i.e., a lack of resources, a dearth of staff willing to work in this setting, and little knowledge about how to effect change in a complex system.

The community health nurse can assist correctional staff in determining both the health needs of the inmates and the proper mix of resources to meet those needs. The community health nurse can encourage the formation of an inmate health committee to meet with staff to discuss health needs and services. She can assist in implementing health standards that are within existing capabilities and can work with existing community resources (such as the state or local health department, local hospitals, prepaid groups, and community mental health programs) to begin addressing those programs not met by the facility. Generations ago, the jailhouse, like the poorhouse, was a part of the community. Now, most correctional institutions are wholly cut off from the community around them, forgotten by the public.

The correctional health care system can gain enormous benefits from re-establishing ties with other community agencies. For example, inmates may visit homes for the aged to provide entertainment, or talk to schoolage groups about how one can get involved in crime without intent. They may be encouraged to cultivate a capacity for self expression such as art or writing. Of necessity, small jails in remote rural areas are part of the total community. Larger institutions in urban areas need to become a part of the community as well. Establishing training relationships with schools of nursing, medicine, and other helping professions, is one way of getting the outside community more involved in these institutions. One university videotaped and shared discussions about crime and punishment between students and inmates. With this interaction, students were more informed about the complex issues within the criminal justice system and the inmates were able to test and determine what "normal society" felt about crime and punishment.

With institutions so overcrowded and frequently nonproductive, some officials are seeking alternatives to incarceration for non-violent offenders. Crimes in the area of immigration, postal theft, forgery, and white collar crimes are usually considered non-violent. Alternative sentencing — a constructive sentence somewhere between probation and imprisonment — is being tried by many judges and is gaining public acceptance as a reasonable approach to dealing with the crime problem. It offers retribution to the victim, rehabilitation to the offender, and savings to society. Offenders are sentenced to community service work related to their crime — for example, a woman convicted of shoplifting was sentenced to service in a nursing home, and a man convicted of burglary, who was also a barber, was ordered to give free haircuts at the local Salvation Army Men's Social Service Center.

Another successful approach to greater community involvement has been to develop advisory councils with representatives of the local medical and dental associations, the bar association, the legislature, and other key groups in the community.

The strength of the community health nurse's advocacy position comes from the direct services she can provide to the prisoner and his family. As a clinician, she will assess the personal strengths of her inmate-patient, his coping abilities, nutritional state, sleeping patterns, and physical health and endurance. Her interventions may include facilitating transfer to a pleasanter cell, appearing with a glass of water or juice, and encouraging visits and letters from family and friends. She can assist the inmate to anticipate certain discomforts, give him opportunity for ventilating his feelings in an acceptable way, help him anchor his expectations in reality, and help him see his own responsibilities for overcoming anger and despair. Visits from the clergy may help build morale, making it easier for him to think about adapting and coping with the problems at hand. The nurse may be able to discern early signs of distress in her inmate-patients and with proper care prevent abusive and violent behavior. By sharing information, teaching early signs of stress, and respecting their experience, she can enlist the support of correctional officers.

As stated earlier, working with families of prisoners is critical to their coping with their present situation as well as to the inmate's successful re-entering into the community. The community health nurse needs to find out what the incarceration process has meant to a particular family, determine what resources are available to them, and evaluate what can be done to restore or strengthen the family's capacity to accommodate.

By truly caring about people in difficult situations — by leaving no stone unturned in helping the inmate and his family to cope with their problems — the nurse builds trust and hope, which are essential to reform.

REFERENCES: CORRECTIONAL INSTITUTIONS

1. Report to the Congress by the Comptroller General of the U.S.: A Federal Strategy is Needed to Help Improve Medical and Dental Care in Prisons and Jails. Dec. 22, 1978, GGO-78-96, p. 1.
2. U.S. Department of Justice, Law Enforcement Assistance Administration, National Criminal Justice Information and Statistics Service: Children in Custody, (Fed.) 1977, pp. 1–4.
3. Census of Prisoners in State Correctional Facilities, 1973. National Prisoner Statistics, December 1976. U.S. Department of Justice, pp. 5–7.
4. Ibid., p. 7.
5. Ibid., p. 8.
6. Metropolitan Boston Detention Study. Brighton, Mass., Massachusetts Joint Correctional Planning Commission, 1972.
7. Jones, D.: *The Health Risks of Imprisonment.* Lexington Books, D.C. Heath & Co., 1976, pp. 170 and 171.

8. Cohen, E. G.: Crisis Intervention in a detention center. *In* Miller, M. H., and Flynn, B. (eds.): *Current Perspectives in Nursing: Social Issues and Trends.* St. Louis, Mo., C. V. Mosby Co., 1980, p. 47.
9. Novick, L., and Al-Ibrahim, M.: *Health Problems in the Prison Setting: Clinical and Administrative Approach.* Springfield, Ill., Charles C Thomas, 1977, Chapter 16.
10. GAO Report to Congress: *A Federal Strategy is Needed to Help Improve Medical and Dental Care in Prisons and Jails.* December 1978, pp. 30–33.
11. Gottfredson, S. M., Wilkins, L. T., and Hoffman, P. B.: *Guidelines for Parole and Sentencing.* Lexington, Lexington Books, 1978.
12. Al-Ibrahim, M.: *Health Problems in the Prison Setting.* Springfield, Ill., Charles C Thomas, 1977, p. 78.
13. Brecher, E., and Penna, R.: *Health Care in Correctional Institutions.* Washington, D.C., National Institute of Law Enforcement and Criminal Justice, Law Enforcement Assistance Administration. U.S. Department of Justice, 1975, p. 36.
14. Cohen, E. G.: Crisis intervention in a detention center. *In* Miller, M. H., and Flynn, B. (eds.): *Current Perspectives in Nursing: Social Issues and Trends.* St. Louis, Mo., C. V. Mosby Co., 1980, p. 49.
15. American Public Health Association: *Standards for Health Care in Correctional Institutions.* Washington, D.C., 1976, 62 pp.
16. American Medical Association: *Standards for the Accreditation of Medical Care and Health Services in Jails.* Chicago, Ill., 1978, 21 pp.
17. Brecher, E., and Penna, R.: *Health Care in Correctional Institutions,* p. 36.
18. Crime Talk: Human Behavior, Feb. 1979, p. 36.

SUGGESTED READINGS: CORRECTIONAL INSTITUTIONS

American Academy of Pediatrics. Health standards for juvenile court residential facilities. Pediatrics, 52:452, 1973.
Brecher, E., and Penna, R.: *Health Care in Correctional Institutions.* Washington, D.C. National Institute of Law Enforcement and Criminal Justice, Law Enforcement Assistance Administration, U. S. Department of Justice, 1975.
Clendenen, R. J., et al.: Project newgate: The first five years. Crime & Delinquency, 25:55, 1979.
Cohen, E.: Crisis intervention in a detention center. *In* Miller, M. H., and Flynn, B. (eds.): *Perspectives in Nursing: Social Issues and Trends.* Vol. II. St. Louis, Mo., C. V. Mosby Co., 1980.
Cooper-Smith, F.: Caring for women in prison. Nurs. Times, 75:907, 1979.
Curran, W. J.: Due process, jury trials and juvenile justice. Am. J. Pub. Health, 61:1901, 1971.
Goldsmith, S.: The status of prison health care. Pub. Health Rep., 89:569, 1974.
Gottfredson, S. M., Wilkins, L. T., and Hoffman, P. B.: *Guidelines for Parole & Sentencing.* Lexington, Lexington Books, 1978.
Hastings, G. E., et al.: Nurse practitioners in a jailhouse clinic. Med. Care, 18:731, 1980.
Hawkins, G.: *The Prison Policy and Procedure.* Chicago, Chicago Press, 1976.
Holly, H.: Jail matron, R. N. Am. J. Nurs., 72:1621, 1972.
Jones, D.: *The Health Risks of Imprisonment.* Lexington, Mass., Lexington Books, 1976.
Ketterling, M. E.: Rehabilitating women in jail. J. Rehab., 36:36, 1970.
Litt, I. F., and Cohen, M. I.: Prisons, adolescents and the right to quality medical care. Am. J. Pub. Health, 64:894, 1974.
McDowell, H.: Leadership at the cell-block level. Am. J. Nurs., 75:423, 1975.
Menninger, K.: *The Crimes of Punishment.* New York, Viking Press, 1968.
Murtha, R.: Change in one city's system. Am. J. Nurs., 75:421, 1975.
New York State Nurses Association, Council on Nursing Practice: Standards for Nursing Service in the Prison Health System. N.Y.S.N.A., Guilderland, New York, 1980.
Novick, L.: The contractual model for prison care. Med. Care, 14:694, 1976.
Novick, L., and Al-Ibrahim, M. S.: *Health Problems in the Prison Setting.* Springfield, Ill., Charles C Thomas, 1977.

Robinson, D.: Prisoners as patients. New Engl. J. Med., 287:101, 1972.

Rosenheim, M. K.: Kids on ice — Children in confinement. Am. J. Pub. Health, 63:390, 1973.

Steidl, S.: Prisoner-Patient. Nursing 78, 8:120, 1978.

Symposium Proceedings — Health Care in Correctional Institutions: Problems and Issues by Southern Health Foundation, Inc., 1977.

Torok, L.: Straight Talk from Prison. New York, Human Sciences Press, 1974.

Twin, E., et al.: Hospital operates health program at jail. Hospitals, 49:51, 1975.

U.S. General Accounting Office: Report to the Congress of the U.S.: A Federal Strategy is Needed to Help Improve Medical and Dental Care in Prisons and Jails (GGD-78-96) Dec. 22, 1978.

Windstead-Fry, P.: Health care in prisons: Change in one city's system— Mental health nursing of inmates. Am. J. Nurs., 75:425, 1975.

RESOURCES: CORRECTIONAL INSTITUTIONS

American Correctional Association
4321 Hartwick Rd.
College Park, Maryland 20740

American Medical Association (and State and local units)—Standards for the Accreditation of Medical Care & Health Services in Jails
535 N. Dearborn St.
Chicago, Ill. 60610

American Public Health Association, Task Force on Jails and Prisons
1015 Fifteenth St. N.W.
Washington, D.C. 20005

Law Enforcement Assistant Administration, U.S. Dept. of Justice
730 Peachtree St. N.E.
Atlanta, Ga. 30303

American Academy of Pediatrics, Committee on Youth
1801 Hinman Ave.
Evanston, Ill. 60204

American Bar Association
1155 E. 60th St.
Chicago, Ill. 60637

CHAPTER 27

PROSPECTS AND EXPECTATIONS

The prospects for community health nursing within the complex world of the future seem bright. The characteristics exhibited by community health nursing now and in the past (adaptiveness; wide acceptance; meshing with the community and other health structures; and the capability for open, close, and continuing service relationships) should have great relevance for problems and services that are likely to arise in the future. There will be continuing and substantive changes in practice, in service programs, in organization, and in professional education to adapt to the anticipated — and, even more, to the unanticipated — developments ahead. It is on these assumptions that the following expectations are based.

Community Health Nursing Personnel Seems Likely to Increase Both in Absolute Numbers and as a Proportion of the Total Nursing Pool

There are a number of indicators that suggest the need for expansion of community health nursing service. Most obvious, the still-growing population of the immediate future will generate an increased demand for care. The "graying" population will require nursing support in and outside the home. A growing commitment to *healthiness* (as differentiated from freedom from disease) will lead to much more preventive care and counseling. The management of stress, the initiation of changes in health behavior, and the enlistment of groups in their own health care require all the educating, coordinating, and supporting care that are traditionally the concerns of community health nursing.

Worry about costs and speculation concerning the imminence of a national health insurance program will intensify the present trend of transferring care from hospitals to the home. This trend is economical and serves as a means of improving the quality of care through greater involvement of the family as well as informal resources in the community. Whether this increase is likely to primarily affect professional personnel or those with shorter training is hard to determine. The present outlook suggests a need for more workers at both ends of the scale — home health aides as well as nurse practitioners and clinical specialists.

The Role of the Community Health Nurse Will Remain Fluid

The roles of all health workers change as new categories of personnel continue to surface and as individual fields of practice enlarge their areas of concern. Each locality or agency will have its own special parameters and staff configuration. Community nursing must be sufficiently flexible to permit services to flow wherever they are needed, provided the services fall within the general purview of community health. Thus, community health nurses may engage in primary care, serve as nurse/family practitioners, work directly with local physicians' groups in support of their patients, or engage in school nursing — depending upon the local situation.

Community Health Nursing Practice Will Become More Sophisticated

The general trend in nursing is toward a more theoretical, independent practice, and this move will be reflected in community health nursing. The development of nurse practitioners and clinical nursing specialists will also have an impact on community health as well as on all other fields of nursing.

The expectation is that more and more complex illnesses will be cared for in the home; this, in turn, will set new requirements for community health practice in the area of therapeutic intervention. Furthermore, the mounting collaborative effort toward improving the physical or social environment will demand more sophisticated management.

Since there are inevitably a multiplicity of factors underlying every problem, assessment often involves evaluation of several interacting and reinforcing conditions, with the necessary data being secured by subtle and probing investigation. Often there is no correct answer to a problem; one can only choose the best possible solution within the available constraints and opportunities. The line between parental support and parental overprotection, for example, is not easily drawn. Assessment will be improved but also complicated by expanded and automated systems for retrieving health data. The demand for the community health nurse's accurate and specific assessment of family interacting and coping will increase.

The Nurse-Family Community Relationship

In the future, conditions which threaten health will require long-term, constantly available, and uncomplicated sources of advice and assistance. Those involved with family care should be prepared to deal with small problems and remedial measures as well as with more substantive ones, to develop independent action within the family, and to mobilize the big guns of our medical, social, and political system when they are needed.

Although in principle community nursing has been accepted for a long time, in practice it has rarely received the same thoughtful planning and action as that given to the care of individuals and families. As health care becomes a right rather than a privilege, the entire community population — instead of the "case load" — must become the equal concern of the nurse. Community assessment must be as much a part of practice as is family assessment. Intervention must include measures to serve and promote change in the community as well as in families. Politics, economics, and theories of social change will be as basic (indeed, already are!) as the more traditional tenets of biomedical and nursing science. This concern for the community in no way negates the fundamental place of personal care within the total effort of community health nursing practice.

The Managerial Aspects of Practice Will Increase

If any health care program is to be truly comprehensive, there must be constant monitoring of the relationship between needs and services, resources and actions, and goals and results. Within this health care system, the community health nurse would be a logical candidate for management of the family care component. This includes implementation of alerting systems, liaison with different providers of health care, and development of measures to evaluate responses to action. The computer will play an important part in such monitoring, but human expertise will be crucial to the relevance and effectiveness of the system. Such planning and supervision are not something apart from nursing, rather, they are essential elements of the nursing process. Indeed, monitoring, alerting, planning, referral, and evaluative feedback (traditional aspects of community health nursing) are the basic ingredients of such managerial efforts.

The "Cluster"

The increasing complexity and extent of extra-hospital nursing require personnel trained at various levels of skill and responsibility. Nursing "clusters," combining multilevel specialists and a general staff, are likely to become common service units. When assigned to a defined population, these units provide a mechanism for unified planning and action.

QUESTIONS AND CHANGES

What is known about community health practice is a mere "speck" in a "sea" of questions and uncertainties. Is the hallowed home visit worth its high cost, or would less expensive interviews be as effective? Does team nursing save money, or does it cost more because of administrative and supervisory costs? Is there any indication that fully prepared or specialty-level nurses obtain different results from those of short-trained aides? Are there some situations in which the short-trained worker can do *more* than the nurse with higher-level achievement? What are the ethical considerations in using reinforcement techniques to secure specified behaviors? What principles are relevant in deciding whether the doctor, social worker, or nurse should undertake specified functions or activities?

Added to these questions is the fact that community health nursing is affected by changes in many other areas; thus, alteration in hospital discharge policies, the inclusion of home visiting in a health maintenance organization, or the hiring of a new social worker can all modify the practice and procedures of a nurse or of an entire agency. For this reason, every community health nurse as well as every other nursing professional must regard patterns of practice as subject to continual change, trial, and evaluation.

One cannot read or think about the future without some trepidation. The prospective changes seem enormous. The ecologic balance is threatened, and mankind seems unable or unwilling to take the necessary steps for survival. New and more tenacious threats to health surge in as old ones are conquered. Yet the potential for biomedical-technological "breakthroughs" of the future are unprecedented; gonorrhea vaccine and nuclear-powered hearts in the 1980's, chemical control of behavior and cloning (parthenogenics) in the 1990's and a variety of biological-computer combinations are all possible realities for the future.[1]

The scope of community health nursing, the techniques, and the demands for new knowledge, will also change; however, the demands for excellence and for continued adaptation to the needs of the family and the community will remain constant.

The Meaning of Excellence

For the nurse who is a true professional, the urge to excel is compelling, unremitting, and lifelong. For society, the pursuit of excellence in its helping professions is a necessary protection against the misuse of a powerful social force. For the recipient of community nursing service, professional excellence in the nurse is that intangible quality that makes the nurse "special" and the service "great."

Excellence in community health nursing is neither an "extra," nor is it a matter of choice. It is becoming more and more clear that without excellence in practice, the process of helping can degrade the human spirit even while it is catering to the physical needs of patients. Care may stifle independence and sap vigor through the very act of loving, but unknowing, ministration.

Community health nursing touches the lives of people over long periods of time. This sustained relationship, coupled with the human values attached to nursing skills, means that the social impact of nursing is great. For this reason, the search for excellence must be seen as a mandate rather than an opportunity. How will we — and others — judge our practice?

The Criterion of Relevance

If one were forced to choose a single criterion for excellence, it is likely that *relevance* would serve such a purpose. *Relevance* implies a goodness of fit between worker and work that should maximize both efficiency and effectiveness. In community health nursing practice, the concept of relevance might be discussed in terms of purpose, people and program.

Relevance to Purpose

Relevance to purpose implies congruence in the services provided, the method by which these services are provided in relation to the purposes of nursing, of the health movement, and of the specific action unit in which the nurse is functioning.

Thus, if the purpose of nursing is to help families cope with their problems, practice must give evidence of extending family capability through teaching and guidance and of sharply identifying and dealing with the real problems of real people.

If the purpose of the health system is to provide care for the whole community, the nurse's program must be developed within this same context of concern. Nursing service that provides exquisite care to a small segment of the population but no service at all to the rest of the population is not relevant in terms of the health system's purpose; less exquisite, but better distributed, care may be closer to the ideal of excellence.

If the purpose of a particular agency is to reach out aggressively to unserved groups, a traditional service not particularly geared to the needs of the low-income group would fail to meet the criterion of relevance; whereas unconventional activities that may not even appear to fall within the realm of nursing may be very relevant indeed.

Relevance to People

Relevance to people implies congruence between nursing action and the needs, expectations, and desires of the people served. A concept of needs that is directed toward disease-related care or to standard preventive procedures is unlikely to meet this measure of relevance unless it also allows for the basic human needs of security, recognition, or achievement.

Relevance to people must also take into account the degree to which nursing is supporting and meeting the needs of other workers in the health effort. For example, a community health nurse might use a home health aide in such a way as to provide for the continuing growth in responsibility and competence in the aide; on the other hand, the nurse may allow the aide to provide excellent care to patients while stifling any of her attempts in taking initiative or in experimenting with new ways. Such failure to support coworkers may also detract from the value of the nursing effort.

Another facet of "people-relevant" practice is congruence with the ways in which people are accustomed to act. Nursing referral patterns that do not take into account the local dependence upon the aid of the family physician or the interagency communication by memo in a highly informal interagency setting are examples of irrelevant nursing behavior.

Relevance to Program

Program relevance concerns the degree to which nursing is integrated with other ongoing health and welfare programs. For example, one nurse might hear that a new community mental health center is developing and respond by immediately seeking a conference to know how to modify nursing to support this new venture. Another, and less relevant, nursing action would be for the nurse to do nothing until asked.

The Criterion of Maximum Actualization

Excellence in community health nursing is characterized not only by relevance but also by a high level of actualization — that is, by the achievement of the greatest possible effect for the amount of nursing time and competence expended.

One great enemy of productivity is nonservice time — time spent in travel, in visits made to families that are not at home, and in routine preparations or reports not directly involved with service itself. Case and service reports or telephone or mail contacts with physicians are essential to the service provided; and even though all possible economies should be effected in completing these activities, the time so spent should not be called nonservice time. Time spent in the routine checking of supplies or in visits made simply to secure information may be considered nonservice time. Such nonservice time should be constantly analyzed to see if it can be reduced — if telephoning in advance might reduce unsatisfactory home calls or if the use of aides might release nursing time spent in accounting for the laundry in the clinic.

Actualization is greater if the services provided are of sufficiently high *impact* to produce the changes or the action that is desired. A large number of brief contacts with parents may do little to influence the parents' concept of good child-rearing practices; whereas a much smaller number of well-planned and leisurely conferences might be effective in exploring and changing ideas. A visit made to a discharged psychiatric patient who has been home from the hospital for six months will almost certainly have little impact, but a nursing visit may be welcomed and highly effective if made shortly after his discharge from the hospital. Timing, method, and content all affect the degree of impact.

Maximum actualization is also related to the *wise choice among alternative courses of action.* Unfortunately, far too much nursing care is provided to families in a follow-the-book manner — visits are made at specified times to families in which tuberculosis is present; group work is provided for expectant mothers or parents but not to other groups with similar problems; nursing contacts are equated with home visits, so that telephone contacts are not counted as service accomplishments but as "office time." The result may be that nursing service is organized with too little attention paid to possible alternatives. Thus, selection among several courses of action must include discovering new alternatives as well as selecting among those already in use.

Maximum actualization implies that nursing time is not used to do those things that can be done as well or better by some other available or potentially available resource. Much has already been said about the unused potential of those served by community health agencies: the capacity of individuals and groups to make health decisions, to plan action for health care, to seek out and refer those needing community health services, and to teach and support one another. There is no doubt that nursing effort could be much more effective if these resources were fully used.

Volunteer or paid nurse assistants may also represent an underused resource. This kind of help is presently limited to jobs far below the level of decision making and independent action of which these workers are capable. For example, the volunteer or clinic aide may be useful in planning and evaluating the program, as well as in handling routine tasks; moreover, such participation may enhance the nurse's efforts in this area.

In the preceeding italicized sentence, it is important to note the phrase "available or potentially available resource." Even though the school teacher may be able to do many things ordinarily undertaken by the community health nurse, the teacher may in fact not be an "available" resource for weighing and measuring children (unless such activity has been incorporated as a teaching measure) because of the demands of her work. The mental health clinic might be better able to help parents deal with a rebellious, handicapped adolescent than is the community health nurse; however, if the clinic has a waiting time of several months, the nurse might feel that this clinic is not in fact an "available" resource.

The Criterion of Growth

Excellence is characterized by a continuing increment in the skills of professional practice and in the scope of professional influence. Such growth is as important to the seasoned nurse as it is to the novice.

Growth in professional skills may be indicated by an increase in technical and professional knowledge and process and also by the development of specific personal skills that are basic to professional practice. Thus, the nurse in community health may need to improve her knowledge of modern care of the cancer patient or of the legal implications of emergency care in industry, or she may need to develop her ability to work with people of a cultural background that is different from her own.

The "growing nurse" is constantly increasing the impact of her interchange with recipients of nursing service, broadening the range and the complexity of the decisions she is making, and increasing the degree to which she assumes a leadership stance.

The Criterion of Creativity

Of all traits considered desirable in today's world, the capacity for creativity or innovation is perhaps the most valued. Creativity is not something that exists apart from the daily work routine. It is only while one wrestles with daily problems and works with available facilities and people that the problems can be identified; and it is with these real dilemmas that an innovative and creative approach is demanded. The nurse who never toys with a "way-out" idea or who never takes time to speculate on what would happen if the system could be changed is unlikely to go far in original thinking and action. On the other hand, innovative thinking must also be geared to the "can do" answer; there must be at least some chance that the idea is feasible. Challenging the establishment appears to be common among the young (and some people who are not so young) today, and it is a valuable habit for one who wants to live creatively; however, the true test of creativity is to apply the same degree of energy and persistence toward resolving today's problems.

THE ACHIEVEMENT OF EXCELLENCE TAKES TIME AND PLANNING

The achievement of excellence within the nursing service as a whole is a primary concern of the supervisory and the consultant staff. In the long run, however, it is the nurse herself who must set both the goals for her own development and the course of action for meeting these goals.

Goals Give Direction

If excellence is to be achieved, it is important to know just what kind of change is desired. This will be related to career goals and life commitments. For some nurses, work will be an interlude between school and marriage, while for others it will be an absorbing career. For many, nursing will fall somewhere between these two objectives. For some the quiet pleasure of doing a good job in a small sphere at the direct service level — to do tangible good — is the exciting challenge. For others, the challenge lies in exerting a different kind of influence — to develop something new, to lead others to greater achievement, or to influence public policy or social action on a broad front. Goals will be different, and the courses of action to achieve excellence will be different; nevertheless, in every case the contribution of excellent nursing has the potential for bettering the situation in which nurses work.

As with service goals, goals for self-improvement will be systems-oriented. There will be long-range goals to fit one's self for leadership or to continue to deepen the quality of practice in a direct care situation. Within these long-range goals there will be other goals, such as to improve one's capacity to deal with groups, to strengthen one's content knowledge in tuberculosis or in psychiatric nursing, to gain greater assurance in working with members of other disciplines, or to start some small field studies that are both compatible with full-time employment and sound in concept and technique.

Assessment Shapes the Plan

It is important to know by what route these goals for self-improvement are likely to be realized and by what means achievement can be measured. An accurate reading of the present status is a necessary basis for estimating the needs for change and for measuring progress. Part of this evaluation of needs and progress may come from the supervisor's periodic evaluation of performance. Most of the evaluation, however, must come from an honest and thoughtful comparison of present performance with the nurse's own concept of ideal professional behavior.

Improvement must rest on a clear understanding of the barriers to progress, whether they be a lack of knowledge, a lack of personal or interpersonal skills, or administrative restrictions that impede change. Often nurses feel that their jobs do not allow sufficient freedom to try out new ideas. This may be true in some instances. However, this perception may be an excuse rather than an actual reason for a lack of action; it is sometimes surprising how far a regulation can be stretched if one just asks! For example, one nurse who wanted to try evening visits to families was told that regulations did not allow for overtime and that the agency could not take responsibility for workers being out during the evening. When it was explained that the nurse wanted an opportunity to talk to the fathers of the household, it was found that visits on Saturdays would accomplish this purpose and be quite compatible with the regulations.

The study of one's performance should not stop with estimating how well things are working under the present system for providing care; it should also include speculation as to whether or not a result would have been better if the problem had been approached differently. For example, the nurse who is achieving good response from expectant mothers in a one-to-one relationship using home visits might ask if perhaps results would be even greater if a group approach were used.

Excellence is a Way of Life

Many suggestions can be made about ways in which the quality of professional performance can be brought to the excellence level, but the achievement of excellence really requires the adoption of a consistent way of life based on analysis, challenge, and innovation.

The habit of analyzing failures alone, with others who are more experienced or with those who hold an objective viewpoint, is perhaps the most valuable habit of all. Analyses of failure make possible the identification of factors that require different approaches, personal skills that need strengthening, and the things that appeared *not* to influence the outcome. For example, in caring for a coronary patient at home, the family may appear unwilling or unable to change its style of living to the degree necessary to support the patient. Without careful analysis, the nurse may try to meet the situation by providing more of the same — more intensive instruction, more home visits, and more exhortation. Analysis will help determine what information is entirely adequate and that the family is fully aware of the nurse's availability and willingness to provide support; in this case the difficulty may lie instead in the efforts of the family to deal with a demanding adolescent. In order to keep her at home, they have, in effect, set up a noisy junior canteen in the home.

Cultivating exposure to new ideas is also an important way to move toward excellence. The habit of professional reading, of attending professional meetings, and of sitting in on meetings of other groups provides stimulation for new ideas and new approaches.

The habit of making experience work for development is also valuable. For some people, working for five years is the same as repeating one year of experience five times. For others, it is a continuing opportunity for growth. To achieve excellence in practice is a professional obligation, and the quest for excellence can be an exciting and rewarding personal adventure.

REFERENCE

1. Selim, R.: Health in the future: In the pink or in the red? Futurist, *13*:340, 1979.

SUGGESTED READINGS

Bandman, E. L., and Bandman, B. (eds.): *Bioethics and Human Rights: A Reader for Health Professions.* Boston, Little Brown & Co., 1978.
Blum, H. L.: Social perspective on risk reduction. Family & Comm. Health, 3:41, 1980.
Mahler, H.: People. Sci. Am., *243*:78, 1980.

APPENDIX A: FAMILY COPING INDEX*

INTRODUCTION

Purpose

The purpose of the Family Coping Index is to provide a basis for estimating the nursing needs of a particular family.

Nursing Need

A family nursing need is present when:
1. The family has a health problem with which they are unable to cope. Health problems include threats to health and need for intelligent action for health promotion as well as disease or disability.
2. There is reasonable likelihood that nursing will make a difference in the family's ability to cope.

Public health nursing visits may be required for purposes other than nursing needs of the family — for instance, to secure epidemiologic or research data, or to establish the reason for absence from work or school. This form is not concerned with establishing such institutional needs.

Generic Nature of Nursing Needs

Basic to the use of this form is the concept that nursing needs can be defined in nursing terms, that is, in relation to the nursing intervention that is required. For example, "diabetes" or "illegitimacy" do not represent definitions of nursing need, although such medical and social conditions make demands on the family which may or may not give rise to nursing needs.

---

*Developed by Marie Lowe, Richmond IVNA City Nursing Service and Ruth B. Freeman, Johns Hopkins School of Hygiene and Public Health, 1964

The definition of a family nursing need must be based on nursing itself. The health problem, the attitudes and knowledge of the family, the availability of medical and hospital resources will determine in some measure the "mix" of nursing skills required by a particular family at a particular time, but regardless of the type of problem, the area and extent of nursing practice required can be analyzed using a single rubric. The diabetic, the unmarried mother, and the school child may require quite different patterns of nursing care, although all patterns will be made up of the same elements of nursing practice — including physical care, therapeutic measures, education, and family counseling. Differences in the pattern of nursing required may differ as widely within a particular medical diagnostic category as among medical categories. One family in which diabetes is a problem will need extended direct service and education, modification of the family attitudes and behavior, referral to organized or informal community resources. Another family may need virtually no nursing — the family may be knowledgeable about the disease, able to use community resources well, and accustomed to providing support to its members.

Diagnosis of nursing needs in terms of the nursing intervention required should help the nurse to organize and plan nursing care with precision so that the care given is tailored to fit the particular family situation.

It should inhibit ritualistic response — that is, giving "routine" and undiscriminating care to prenatal patients or diabetic patients or well babies.

Relation of Coping to Nursing Need

Coping may be defined as dealing with problems associated with health care with reasonable success.

To maintain health the individual or family must be able to deal with the problems of participating in preventive, curative or rehabilitative measures to make social adjustments that are required by the health situation; to make wise decisions in relation to seeking and using health services, and to contribute in whatever ways they can toward maintaining the health of others. This capacity to deal with the situation — to cope — is central to health competence of the family.

Coping has been selected as an index of nursing need because the particular contribution of nursing to health care is to strengthen or supplement the capacity of the individual or family as it encounters the stress of illness, or the opportunity to prevent disease and promote health.

When the family is unable to cope with one or another aspect of health care, they may be said to have a "coping deficit." However, a coping deficit in a family cannot be equated as a nursing need according to the definition. The likelihood that nursing will make a difference in coping must also enter into the equation. If a family is coping poorly with family health maintenance — if diet is poor and use of preventive measures resisted—one must ask whether the causes are such that the educational and supportive efforts of nursing are likely to result in change. Not even nurses can do everything. In some instances review of previous efforts, taking a careful family history, periodic appraisal of family progress, may make it clear that nursing cannot be expected to change the situation. It may then be decided that nursing needs are limited to helping in periods of crisis or acute illness. The Index provides a means for indicating the anticipated change in the family's capacity to cope with its problems, as well as their present coping capacity.

Sometimes the difference that nursing is expected to make is in the direction of minimizing regression or preventing a decrease in coping capacity. For example, old-fashioned comforting of patient and family may minimize despair and help channel affection toward useful ends; continuing occasional nursing care for bed-bound patients may provide needed relief for the family and enable them to continue care without hospitalization. While no *positive* change can be expected with nursing, *negative* change might be anticipated if nursing were not provided. Nursing would still be expected to make a difference.

The Family Unit

The form is designed to record *family* rather than individual coping capacity. In public health nursing the family cannot be seen only as a factor to be taken into account in caring for the individual patient — the family *is* the patient. The health of the home helper is influenced by the presence of a hemiplegic patient just as the patient's care is influence by the helper; the health of siblings of the handicapped child is threatened by the family demands arising from the patient's condition just as the patient's health is affected by the level of understanding and support the siblings can provide. The functioning of the family as a whole, as well as of each of its members, is affected by the presence of a health problem.

DIRECTIONS FOR SCALING

The Family Coping Estimate (See Fig. A) consists of two parts—a point on the scale and a justification statement. The scale enables you to "place" the family in relation to their ability to cope with nine areas of family nursing at the time observed, and as you would expect it to be in 3 months or at time of discharge if nursing care were provided. Coping capacity is rated from 1 (totally unable to manage this aspect of family care) to 5 (able to handle this aspect of care without help from community sources). Check *not applicable* if the particular category is not relevant to the situation. When each of the nine categories has been

FAMILY COPING ESTIMATE

Family_____   Nurse_____   Date_____

Initial_____   Periodic_____   Discharge_____

Coping Area	Rating x-status 0-est. change Poor....................Exc.	Justification
Physical Independence	1 2 3 4 5 Not Applicable ☐	
Therapeutic Independence	1 2 3 4 5 Not Applicable ☐	
Knowledge of Condition	1 2 3 4 5 Not Applicable ☐	
Application of Principles of Personal Hygiene	1 2 3 4 5 Not Applicable ☐	
Attitude Toward Health Care	1 2 3 4 5 Not Applicable ☐	
Emotional Competence	1 2 3 4 5 Not Applicable ☐	
Family Living Patterns	1 2 3 4 5 Not Applicable ☐	
Physical Environment	1 2 3 4 5 Not Applicable ☐	
Use of Community Resources	1 2 3 4 5 Not Applicable ☐	
Comments		

Figure A Reverse side is used for nursing care plan. (Developed jointly by the Richmond IVNA City Nursing Service and the Johns Hopkins School of Hygiene and Public Health, 1964.)

rated, the result will be a profile of family coping capacity in relation to the family nursing required, and by the changes you expect to occur in the course of nursing service.

The justification consists of brief statements or phrases that explain why you have rated the family as you have. These statements should, as far as possible, be expressed in terms of behavior or observable facts rather than in adjectives (for instance, not "good" diet—but, "family food includes basic five" or "watch TV together, share housework willingly"). It may take some time to develop these statements at first — to be sure, the words say what you want them to say. The pertinency of these statements is crucial as you try later to judge how the family has changed.

The index should be completed for each new family admitted for more than incidental service — that is, families in which you expect to make more than three visits. You may be able to do this on the first visit, but if you feel you do not have enough information to make the required judgment, you may want to delay it until the second or even third visit. However, if it is to help you define and plan to meet nursing needs, it must be completed early in the course of care.

The evaluation should be repeated (1) at three-month intervals if the family is carried for a long period of time; (2) whenever there is a drastic change in the situation (for example if the sick member goes to the hospital, or a chronically ill patient develops an acute episode); and (3) at discharge.

General Considerations

1. It is *coping capacity* and not the underlying problem that is being rated. The family may have a member with a serious and incapacitating cardiac condition under constant threat of recurrence. There is no doubt that his condition is critical. However, if the family understands the disease, has mobilized to adapt to it, knows how to recognize changes in condition and to use available resources and feel confident of their ability to handle a crisis, their *coping capacity* is excellent. If, on the other hand, the family is anxious, unfamiliar with community resources, or fails to realize the importance and the nature of prescribed treatment their coping capacity would be *low*.
2. It is the *family* and not the individual that is being rated. If a man is unable to care for himself due to severe disability, but the necessary care is being provided by members of the family, family coping is adequate even though the individual himself is not able to manage. If the patient is receiving excellent care by the family, but the family is resentful, under a dangerous level of stress or other members of the family are being deprived of needed care, the *family* is not coping, even though the *patient's* condition is good.

Scaling Cues

The following descriptive statements are "cues" to help you as you rate family coping. They are limited to three points: *1*, or no competence; *3*, moderate competence; and *5*, complete competence. You will find, however, that most families will fall somewhere in between these points. Mark the point you feel most nearly describes the level of competence they have. The descriptions are not complete but suggestive. In the long run it is your own professional judgment that will be needed to make a decision. When there is no problem or the area is not relevant, check the "no problem" column.

1. Physical Independence

This category is concerned with ability to move about, to get in and out of bed, to take care of daily grooming, walking, etc. Note that it is the *family* competence that is measured — even though an individual is dependent, if the family is able to compensate for this the family may be independent. However, the quality as well as quantity of ability is important; hence, if the *focus* of care is poor — if a mother is giving care to a handicapped child that he could give himself, or if one person is giving care that should be shared with other members — the independence might be considered incomplete. The *causes* of dependence may vary — lack of physical independence in the family may be due to actual physical incapacity, to lack of "know how," to unwillingness or fear of doing the necessary tasks.

1 = Family failing entirely to provide required personal care to one or more of its members. *Example:* arthritic patient unable to get out of bed alone, no one available to help; patient "cannot" give his hypodermic medication because of fear.

3 = Family providing partially for needs of its members, or providing care for some members but not for others. *Example:* mother may be doing well with own and husband's care, but failing to give daily care efficiently to newborn baby; daughter may be giving excellent physical care to aged mother but at cost of neglecting children somewhat, or with poor body mechanics that place undue strain upon herself.

5 = All family members whether or not there is infirmity or disability in one or more members, are receiving the necessary care to maintain cleanliness, including skin care, are able to get about as far as possible within their physical abilities; are receiving assistance when needed without interruption or undue delay.

2. Therapeutic Competence

This category includes all of the procedures or treatment prescribed for the care of illness such as giving medications, using appliances (including crutches), dressings, exercises and relaxation, special diets, etc.

1 = Family either not carrying out procedures prescribed or doing it unsafely. For example, giving several medications without being able to distinguish one from the other, or taking them inappropriately, applying braces so they throw the limb out of line, measuring insulin incorrectly. Family resents, rejects, or refuses to give necessary care.

3 = Family carrying out some but not all of the treatments — for example, giving insulin but not adhering strictly to diet; carrying out procedures awkwardly, ineffectively, or with resentment or unnecessary anxiety. For example, crutch walking may be done, but with

the helper using poor body mechanics, or not giving the patient enough security and confidence; patient may give own hypodermic, but say "I dread it every time." May be giving medications correctly, but not understanding purposes of the drug, or symptoms to be observed.

5 = Family able to demonstrate that they can carry out the prescribed procedures safely and efficiently, with the understanding of the principles involved and with a confident and willing attitude.

3. *Knowledge of Health Condition*

This category is concerned with the particular health condition that is the occasion for care. For example, knowledge of the disease or disability, understanding of communicability of disease and modes of transmission, understanding of general pattern of development of a newborn baby and the basic needs of infants for physical care and TLC.

1 = Totally uninformed or misinformed about the condition. For example, believes tuberculosis is caused by sin, or syphilis cured when symptoms subside; believes stroke patient must be bedridden, and that it is cruel to make them do for themselves; that overweight in the school-age child is "healthy."

3 = Has some general knowledge of the disease or condition, but has not grasped the underlying principles, or is only partially informed. For instance, may recognize need for TLC but not relate this to placing the baby's crib near people when he is awake; or holding him when feeding; may accept fact that patient is dying but not see need to prepare family for this event; may understand dietary and insulin control of diabetes, but not need for special care of feet, etc.

5 = Knows the salient facts about the disease well enough to take necessary action at the proper time, understands the rationale of care, able to observe and report significant symptoms.

4. *Application of Principles of Personal and General Hygiene*

This is concerned with family action in relation to maintaining family nutrition, securing adequate rest and relaxation for family members, carrying out accepted preventive measures such as immunizations, medical appraisal; safe homemaking habits in relation to storing and preparing food.

1 = Family diet grossly inadequate or unbalanced, necessary immunizations not secured for children; house dirty, food handled in unsanitary way; members of family working beyond reasonable limits; children and adults getting too little sleep; family members unkempt, dirty, inadequately clothed in relation to weather.

3 = Failing to apply some general principles of hygiene — for instance, keeping house in excellent condition but expending too much energy and becoming over fatigued as a result; secured initial immunizations but not boosters, or some but not all available immunizations; general diet and homemaking skills good, but father carrying two full-time jobs.

5 = Household runs smoothly, family meals well selected; habits of sleep and rest adequate to needs.

5. Health Care Attitudes

This category is concerned with the way the family feels about health care in general, including preventive services, care of illness and public health measures.

1 = Family resents and resists all health care; has no confidence in doctors, uses patent medicines and quack nostrums, feels illness is unavoidable and to be borne rather than treated; feels community health agencies shouldn't interfere or bother them; practices folk medicine or superstitious rites in illness.

3 = Accepts health care in some degree, but with reservations. For example, may accept need for medical care for illness, but not general preventive measures; may have confidence in doctors generally, but not in the clinic or "free" doctors; may feel certain illnesses are hopeless (such as cancer), or care unnecessary — for instance, dental care for the young child.

5 = Understands and recognizes need for medical care in illness and for the usual preventive services, arranges for periodic physical appraisals and follows through with recommendations, accepts illness calmly and recognizes the limits it imposes while doing all possible to effect recovery and rehabilitation.

6. Emotional Competence

This category has to do with the maturity and integrity with which the members of the family are able to meet the usual stresses and problems of life, and to plan for happy and fruitful living. The degree to which individuals accept the necessary disciplines imposed by one's family and culture; the development and maintenance of individual responsibility and decision; willingness to meet reasonable obligations, to accept adversity with fortitude, to consider the needs of others as well as one's own.

1 = Family does not face realities — assumes moribund patient will get well, that they can eventually pay a hospital bill far beyond their means, that an unwanted pregnancy isn't so; one or more members lacking in any emotional control — uncontrollable rages, irresponsible sexual activities; one or more members alcoholic, family torn, suspicious of one another; evidences of great insecurity, guilt or anxiety.

3 = Family members usually do fairly well, but one or more member evidences lack of security or maturity. For example, thumb sucking in late childhood; unusual concern with what the neighbors will think; failure to plan ahead for foreseeable emergencies; leaving children unattended, "fighting" in the family on occasion.

5 = All members of the family are able to maintain a reasonable degree of emotional calm, face up to illness realistically and hopefully; able to discuss problems and differences with objectivity and reasonable emotional control; do not worry unduly about trivial matters, consid-

er the needs and wishes of other family members, of neighbors and those with whom they work and live in making decisions or deciding upon action.

7. Family Living Patterns

This category is concerned largely with the interpersonal or group aspects of family life — how well the members of the family get along with one another, the ways in which they make decisions affecting the family as a whole, the degree to which they support one another and do things as a family, the degree of respect and affection they show for one another, the ways in which they manage the family budget, the kind of discipline that prevails.

1 = Family consists of a group of individuals indifferent or hostile to one another, or strongly dominated and controlled by a single family member; no control of children, or family so totally dependent on one another that they are being stifled — for example, mother developing habits of dependence in sons so as to threaten future capacity for independence in own family life, no rational plan for managing available money; "battered" child.

3 = Family gets along but has habits or customs that interfere with their effectiveness or coherence as a family. For example, a family fond of one another, have many home activities, but dominated by a father in a kindly way; recreational habits separate family much of the time; children somewhat overprotected; expectations of the children unrealistic — parents expecting children with low academic competence to enter professions, etc.

5 = Family cohesive, does things together, each member acts with regard for the good of the family as a whole; children respect parents and vice versa; family tasks shared; evidence of planning.

8. Physical Environment

This category is concerned with the home and community or work environment as it affects family health. The condition for housing, presence of accident hazards, screening, plumbing, facilities for cooking and for privacy; level of community — (deteriorated or modern, presence of social hazards such as bars, street gangs, delinquency, pests such as rats), availability and condition of schools, transportation.

1 = House in poor condition, unsafe, unscreened, poorly heated, neighborhood deteriorated, juvenile and adult delinquency among neighbors, no play space except streets.

3 = House needs some repair or painting but fundamentally sound; neighborhood poor but possible to protect children from social influence through school or other community activities; house crowded but adjustments to this fairly adequate.

5 = House in good repair, provides for privacy for members and is free of accidents and pest hazards; neighborhood respectable and provided with play space for children; free from undesirable social elements; opportunities for community activity.

9. Use of Community Facilities

This category has to do with the degree to which the family knows about and the wisdom with which they use available community resources for health, education and welfare. This would include the ways in which they use services of private physicians, clinics, emergency rooms, hospitals, schools, welfare organizations, churches and so forth. The *coping ability* does not indicate the level of the *need* for services, but rather the degree to which they can cope when they must seek such aid. Even though a family has a severe housing problem, if they have used all appropriate facilities for enforcing landlord's compliance with sanitary regulations to secure public housing, their coping capacity in relation to *use* of community facilities is high, even though the underlying condition is not corrected.

1 = Family has obvious and serious social needs, but has not sought or found any help for them. For example, a family may be borrowing unreasonable sums of money for medical care, while not using available free hospitals or clinics; or leaving children without any supervision while the mother works; or fail to take steps to register for public housing when it is indicated. Using resources inappropriately, for example, calling ambulance or using emergency services for minor ills.

3 = Family knows about or uses some, but not all of the available community resources that they need. For example, the family may be under welfare care, and know how to use the social worker responsible for their care, but not have recognized that the counselor in the school could help with educational planning, or that the church might provide recreational activities for the children as well as spiritual guidance.

5 = Family using the facilities they need appropriately and promptly. Know when to call for help and whom to call. Feel secure in their relationship with community workers such as social workers, teachers, doctors, etc.

Discussion

The Family Coping Index was developed in 1964 as a tool for practice, as an approach to identifying the family's need for nursing care and assessing the potential for behavioral changes, and as a method of determining in a more systematic way how the nurse can help the family to manage. This tool has been used by a variety of community health nurses in their work with families and by nursing educations in helping students focus efforts on building upon family strengths. Although the

Family Coping Index was not developed as a research tool, the potential for refinement and standardization is present.

There have been related research efforts. Mickey, in a study of extra-hospital nursing needs, used an approach somewhat similar to the Family Coping Index in defining a community's need for nursing services.[1] Methods were included to estimate intensity of health need as well as coping ability. With trained interviewers, rater reliability was high.

In the last several years, there has been much interest in developing nursing problem classifications or nursing diagnoses. An example of one such list is the Nursing Problem Classification for Children and Youth.[2] This system classifies problems into six major groupings: (1) physical problems or long-term illness; (2) behavioral/emotional/learning problems; (3) the child's environment; (4) growth and development; (5) stress and transient situations; and (6) child rearing and home management. These potential problems and needs of children may or may not be defined as a nursing need, depending on how the family is able to cope. Another study of interest is that completed by Simmons in developing a client problem list in the area of community health nursing.[3] Specific physical, social, emotional, and environmental problems of families and individuals are delineated. Family strengths, weaknesses, and approaches to management can be assessed in light of these problems.

The family and the family cycle with predictable development and times of crisis are of interest to many caring professions.[4] Frequently, the focus of discussion is on the individual within the family as opposed to the family unit and its effect on health behaviors of the individual.

Moos and Moos studied 100 families in an effort to distinguish family characteristics that influence personal growth and behavior.[5] Six distinctive clusters of families were identified: (1) expression-oriented; (2) structure-oriented; (3) independence-oriented; (4) achievement-oriented; (5) moral and religious-oriented, and (6) conflict-oriented. Such taxonomies may help in understanding how different family environments are linked to different family outcomes.

The diagnosis of specific problems, such as the existence of pregnancy, the inadequacy of physical surroundings, the child known to be unruly, or the specific medical diagnosis, involves data that are essentially objective or previously defined. However, determining how well the family is coping may involve data that are more subjective, more subtle and hazy. There is no statistical measure of how deeply the family feels about a particular problem, how far they are willing to go in self-help, or whether the "health establishment" recommendation is really relevant to them when all factors in the situation are considered. Thus, professional judgment is essential in the estimation of (1) the meaning and importance of problems to the family and community, (2) the possible avenues of nursing service, and (3) the degree of change which nursing intervention can be expected to effect.

REFERENCES

1. Mickey, J. E.: Findings of a study of extra-hospital nursing needs. Am. J. Publ. Health, 53:1047, 1963.
2. *Nursing Problem Classification for Children and Youth.* DHEW, PHS, Pub. No. (HSA) 77-5201, Washington, D.C., U.S. Government Printing Office, 1977.
3. Simmons, D. A.: *A Classification Scheme for Client Problems in Community Health Nursing.* U.S. DHHS, Pub. No. HRA 80-16, June 1980.
4. Aguilera, D. C. (ed.): Coping with life stressors: A life-cycle approach. Fam. Com. Health, 2:1, 1980.
5. Moos, R. H., and Moos, B. S.: A typology of family social environments. Fam. Proc., 15 357, 1976.

SUGGESTED READING

Gordon, M.: The concept of nursing diagnosis. Nursing Clin. North Am., 13:487, 1979.
Holt, R. H.: Mobilizing family strengths in health maintenance and coping with illness. *In* Reinhart, A. M., and Quinn, M. D. (eds.): *Current Practice in Family-Centered Community Nursing.* St. Louis, Mo., C. V. Mosby Co., 1977, pp. 101–112.

APPENDIX B: THE NLN PROBLEM-ORIENTED RECORD FORM*

*Reproduced by permission of the National League for Nursing, New York, N.Y.

FAMILY NAME _____

FAMILY I.D. No. _____

**FAMILY DATA
AND PROBLEM INDEX**

DATE	ADDRESS	DIRECTIONS—C/O—NEAR	APT/FLOOR	TELEPHONE	HEALTH AREA

FAMILY ROSTER

NAME	RACE	BIRTH DATE	MARITAL STATUS
Man			☐ S ☐ M ☐ W ☐ D ☐ Sep.
Woman: Maiden name:			☐ S ☐ M ☐ W ☐ D ☐ Sep.

Emergency contact: _____   Address: _____   Phone: _____

	FAMILY/HOUSEHOLD MEMBER	SEX	BIRTH DATE	RACE	COMMENTS relationship—occupation—education—etc.
1					
2					
3					
4					
5					
6					
7					
8					
9					
10					
11					
12					

RECORD OF SERVICE

NAME	DATE Adm.	DATE Disch.	PRIMARY DIAGNOSIS	NAME	DATE Adm.	DATE Disch.	PRIMARY DIAGNOSIS

FORM 21-FDPI   DHHA/CHS   © 1974 National League for Nursing

		OTHER AGENCIES ACTIVE			
DATE	FAMILY MEMBER	AGENCY	NAME OF WORKER	TELEPHONE NUMBER	DATE INACTIVE

FAMILY DATA BASE

HISTORY

physical,
functional,
nutritional,
etc.

Sign and date
all entries.

FAMILY PROBLEM INDEX

List all potential, current, or significant past problems that affect the family as a group. Identify family member when appropriate.
Include date of onset or identification and the date of resolution for each problem.

PROB. NO.	FAMILY MEMBER	FAMILY PROBLEMS POTENTIAL/CURRENT–ACTIVE	DATE OF ONSET	DATE RESOLVED	FAMILY PROBLEMS SIGNIFICANT PAST–INACTIVE

CONTINUE ON A NEW FORM

ENVIRONMENT

housing,
sanitation,
transportation,
safety,
etc.

Sign and date
all entries.

ADJUSTMENTS

social,
emotional,
cultural,
vocational,
religious,
etc.

Sign and date
all entries

_____   _____
(Date)   (Signature and title)

PATIENT NAME _____

PATIENT I.D. No. _____

PATIENT PROBLEM INDEX

List all potential, current, or significant past problems that affect the patient. Include date of onset or identification and the date of resolution for each problem.

Page_____

DATE	PROB. NO.	PROBLEMS POTENTIAL/CURRENT—ACTIVE	DATE OF ONSET	DATE RESOLVED	PROBLEMS SIGNIFICANT PAST—INACTIVE

PATIENT NAME _____

PATIENT I.D. No. _____

NARRATIVE/ PROGRESS NOTES

Begin entries pertaining to subjective findings (S), objective findings (O), assessment (A), and plans (P) in the column appropriately headed and write through remaining columns to the right margin. The signature and title of the recorder must appear after each entry.

Page _____

DATE	PROBLEM NO.	S	O	A	P	NARRATIVE/PROGRESS

PATIENT BASELINE DATA

Focus: Health Status and Self-Care System

GUIDE FOR SYSTEMATIC OBSERVATION

(PATIENT DATA BASE)

TO ACCOMPANY FORM 21-PBD

AIR

Source—Quality of environmental air, level of O_2 in a tent, etc.
Inspiration-Expiration—Patency of airway (nasal, tracheal); breath sounds (wheeze, cough, bubbly), manner of tracheostomy care
O_2-CO_2 Exchange—Pale conjunctiva, blue nail beds, Hgb level
O_2-CO_2 Transport—BP, heart sounds, pulse rate and regularity
Cell Utilization—Healing rate, energy level, metabolic rate

COMMUNICATION

Language—Foreign, articulation, grammar
Speech Patterns—Stutter, emissive aphasia
Organs of Speech—Tongue, palate
Non-Verbal—Vocalizations, gestures, writing
Comprehension—Reading, hearing
Educational Level—Eighth grade, Ph.D. in _____

ELIMINATION

Bowel—Patterns, characteristics, management, medication, equipment, etc.
Bladder—Patterns, characteristics, management, medication, equipment, etc.
Other—Wound drainage, perspiration, etc.

EXERCISE

Pattern—Amount, type, timing, etc.
Strength—Hand grasp, extremity vs. resistance, etc.
Voluntary Movement—Gross, fine, joint range of motion
Involuntary—Tremors, seizures, etc.
Productivity—work, recreation, other
Independence—Of movement or assistance required
Equipment—Cane, crutches, etc.

FOOD AND WATER

Physical Appearance—Height, weight, skin dryness and turgor, etc.
Eating Patterns—Usual type and amount of food and fluid intake, factors affecting appetite, etc.
Ability to Ingest—Dental status, ability to swallow, etc.
Ability to Digest and Absorb—Abdominal discomfort, history of G.I. related illness, e.g., ulcers, pancreatitis, etc.
Ability to Metabolize—Healing rate, metabolic rate, energy level
Aids—Special utensils, gastrostomy, etc.
Securing—Financing, transporting, etc.
Storing—Refrigeration, infestation, etc.
Preparing—Cooking facilities, etc.

PSYCHO-SOCIAL

Life Style and Relationships—Marital, social, etc.
Religion—Type, relative importance, etc.
Coping Mechanisms—Problem-solving methods, risk-taking, impulse control, etc.
Basic Needs—Manner of meeting: love, security, control, esteem, etc.
Developmental Stage—Adolescence, productivity—degree of task fulfillment, independence vs. dependence, job or life's work, reproductory phase, etc.

REST AND SLEEP

Patterns—Amount, quality, etc.
Meaning of Rest—What would individual consider restful
Interfering Factors—Pain, noise
Circadian Rhythm—Best hours for sleep, time least and most rest required, etc.
Adequacy—Patient's subjective evaluation: fatigued, rested, etc.
Aids—Pre-sleep rituals, medication

SAFETY AND PROTECTION

Care of Body—Skin, mucous membrane, etc.
Clothing—Adequacy for environment
Housing—Adequacy for environment
Environment—Sanitation, noise, infestation, etc.
Health Maintenance Measures—Dental exams, medical exams, immunization, etc.
Known Untoward Reactions—Allergies, hypersensitivities

SENSORY PERCEPTION

Vision—Acuity, glasses, etc.
Hearing—Acuity, aids, etc.
Touch—Numbness, hypersensitivity
Taste and Smell—Preferences, responses
Pain—Presence, absence, where, when, etc.
Affect—Appropriate, flattened
Memory—Recent, remote
Balance—Sitting, standing, turning
Consciousness—Attention span, seizures
Kinesthetic Awareness—Position, body parts

OTHER

Sources of Health Care—Physician, dentist, clinic or difficulties in obtaining health care
Health History—Disease, injury, operations
Diagnostic Results—Medical, psychological, vocational, etc.
Patterns of Seeking Care—Regularly planned, emergency only, etc.

FACTORS: Physical, Functional, Emotional, Social and Safety

PATIENT NAME_____

PATIENT I.D. No._____

PATIENT BASELINE DATA

Page_____

CODE: √ = Problem present   O = No problem present

PARAMETERS	DATE		SUBJECTIVE AND OBJECTIVE OBSERVATIONS PHYSICAL, FUNCTIONAL, EMOTIONAL, SOCIAL, AND SAFETY
A I R			
Source			
Inspiration-expiration			
O_2-CO_2 exchange			
O_2-CO_2 transport			
Cell utilization			
Other (describe)			
C O M M U N I C A T I O N			
Language			
Speech patterns			
Organs of speech			
Non-verbal			
Comprehension			
Educational level			
Other (describe)			
E L I M I N A T I O N			
Bowel			
Bladder			
Other (describe)			
E X E R C I S E			
Pattern			
Strength			
Voluntary movement			
Involuntary movement			
Productivity			
Independence			
Equipment			
Other (describe)			
F O O D A N D W A T E R			
Physical appearance			
Eating patterns			
Ability to ingest			
Ability to digest and absorb			
Ability to metabolize			
Aids			
Securing			
Storing			
Preparing			
Other (describe)			

©1974 National League for Nursing

FORM 21-PBD   DHHA/CHS   CONTINUE ON OTHER SIDE

PARAMETERS	DATE		SUBJECTIVE AND OBJECTIVE OBSERVATIONS PHYSICAL, FUNCTIONAL, EMOTIONAL, SOCIAL, AND SAFETY
PSYCHOSOCIAL			
Life style and relationships			
Religion			
Coping mechanisms			
Basic needs			
Development stage			
Other (describe)			
REST AND SLEEP			
Patterns			
Meaning of rest			
Interfering factors			
Circadian rhythm			
Adequacy			
Aids			
Other (describe)			
SAFETY AND PROTECTION			
Care of body			
Clothing			
Housing			
Environment			
Health maintenance measures			
Allergic reactions			
Other (describe)			
SENSORY PERCEPTION			
Vision			
Hearing			
Touch			
Taste and smell			
Pain			
Affect			
Memory			
Balance			
Consciousness			
Kinesthetic awareness			
Other (describe)			
OTHER			

Signature and title_____ Date _____

Signature and title_____ Date _____

PATIENT NAME_____

PATIENT I.D. No._____

POSTPARTUM CARE FLOW SHEET

CODE:
C—Care   N—Narrative
S—Supervision   I—Instruction
D—Discussion   E—Evaluation

Grav _____
Para _____
Delivery Date _____

Problem No. _____

Page_____

	PARAMETERS	Baseline	Date of Visit — Year 19____			
SUBJECTIVE	Elimination					
	a. bowels					
	b. urine					
	Emotional Response					
	a. toward husband					
	b. toward baby					
	Fatigue					
OBJECTIVE	General Appearance					
	Lochia					
	Breasts					
	Blood Pressure					
	Pulse					
	Episiotomy					
	Temperature					
	Fundus					
INSTRUCTION	Rest					
	Exercises					
	Care of Breasts					
	Resumption of Intercourse					
	Contraception					
	INITIALS					

FORM 21-PPC/fs   CHHA/CHS   CONTINUE ON OTHER SIDE

PARAMETERS	Baseline	Date of Visit — Year 19___				
Hand Washing						
Hygiene						
Perineal Care						
Diet						
MD Appointment Postpartum Check						
Medications						
INITIALS						

INSTRUCTION

Signature _____

CHILD HEALTH RECORD

CHILD'S NAME _____ PATIENT I.D. No. _____
(Surname)   (First Name)   (M.I.)

Address: _____ Telephone: _____

Sex: _____ Race: _____ Birth Date: _____ Conference Code: _____

Father's Name: _____ Mother's Name: _____
(Include Surname if Different)

Fee Status: ☐ No Fee ☐ Token ☐ Title 19   S.W. I.D. No.: _____

CHILD'S HEALTH HISTORY

PROBLEM	DATES/COMMENTS
Allergies	
Anemia	
Diabetes	
ENT	
Heart	
Hernia	
Intestinal Parasites	
Kidney	
Meningitis	
Obesity	
Pneumonia	
Rheumatic Fever	
Seizure	
Skin	
Speech Defect	
Operations	
Other	
Dates reviewed	_____ _____
	_____ _____

COMMUNICABLE DISEASES: DATES

Chickenpox	Pertussis
German Measles	Polio
Measles	Scarlet Fever
Mumps	Other

DEVELOPMENTAL ASSESSMENT

		AGE OF ATTAINMENT
First 3 mo.	Eyes follow moving objects	_____
	Responds by smiling	_____
	Makes cooing sounds	_____
	Recognizes mother	_____
	Holds head erect	_____
3-6 mo.	Rolls over	_____
	Reaches and Grasps	_____
	Laughs	_____
6-9 mo.	Sits without support	_____
	Creeps	_____
	Distinguishes strangers	_____
	Transfers objects	_____
9-12 mo.	Says mama and dada specifically	_____
	Plays pat-a-cake	_____
	Pulls self to standing position	_____
	Tries to feed self with fingers	_____
12-18 mo.	Waves goodbye	_____
	Walks without support	_____
	Walks up and down stairs	_____
	Combines objects	_____
	Understands words of command	_____
	Speaks a few words	_____
	Tries to feed self with cup and spoon	_____
18-24 mo.	Develops bowel control	_____
	Language — uses 3-word sentences with verbs	_____
	Mimics domestic activities	_____
2 & 3 yrs. till 4th b.d.	Full sentences	
	Develops bladder control day and night	_____
	Asks "Why?"	_____
	Knows own sex	_____
	Counts to 3	_____
4 & 5 yrs. till 6th b.d.	Drops infantile speech patterns	_____
	Plays cooperatively	_____
	Knows numbers and colors	_____

FORM 21-CHR   DHHA/CHS   CONTINUE ON OTHER SIDE

MEASUREMENTS

DATE	HT.	WT.	H.C.

IMMUNIZATION ASSESSMENT RECORD

TYPE	DUE	DATE GIVEN	PRIMARY COMPLETE	REACTIONS
DPT 1				
2				
3				
4				
Booster				
D&T 1				
2				
3				
Booster 1				
2				
Polio T. 1				
2				
3				
4				
Booster				
Measles				
Rubella				
Mumps				

Immunization Record
sent to Health Department

SCREENING TESTS

TYPE	DATE	RESULTS
TBC 1		
2		
3		
PKU		
Gluc/P. 1		
2		
3		
Hemoglobin 1		
2		
3		
Sickle Cell		
Ova/Parasites 1		
2		
Lead 1		
2		
3		
Other		

VISION/HEARING

SNELLEN	DATE	DATE
Right Eye		
Left Eye		
Both Eyes		
R. w/Glasses		
L. w./Glasses		
Both w./Glasses		

AUDIOMETRIC	DATE	DATE
Right Ear		
Left Ear		

Vision/Hearing:_____

_____

SERVICE RECORD

	0-11 Mos.	12-23 Mos.	24-35 Mos.	36-59 Mos.
Initial Comprehensive				
Follow-up 1				
2				
3				
4				
Prolonged Follow-up				
Immunization Only 1				
2				
3	Re-evaluation:			

Next Appt. (Pencil)_____

White Copy—Patient Record
Blue Copy—Billing
Yellow Copy—Physician
Pink Copy—Initiator

DHHA/CHS FORM 21 - ICTP/AS
© 1974 National League for Nursing

INTERAGENCY CARE AND TREATMENT PLAN

TO _____ FROM _____

All entries must be signed with name, title, and date.

Agency Provider No. _____

Patient Name _____

Address _____

Birth Date _____ Soc. Sec. No. _____

Medicare No. _____ Medicaid No. _____

Other Insurance _____ No. _____

☐ REFERRAL—Date: _____ ☐ REPORT—Date: _____

INDEX

Note: In this index, "nurse" refers to "community health nurse" and "nursing" refers to "community health nursing" unless otherwise specified. Page numbers in *italics* refer to illustrations or tables.